Physiology: Theoretical and Clinical Aspects

Physiology: Theoretical and Clinical Aspects

Edited by Johnny Carrey

hayle
medical

New York

Hayle Medical,
750 Third Avenue, 9th Floor,
New York, NY 10017, USA

Visit us on the World Wide Web at:
www.haylemedical.com

ISBN: 978-1-63241-736-7

Cataloging-in-Publication Data

Physiology : theoretical and clinical aspects / edited by Johnny Carrey.
    p. cm.
Includes bibliographical references and index.
ISBN 978-1-63241-736-7
1. Human physiology. 2. Physiology. 3. Medical sciences. 4. Human body. I. Carrey, Johnny.
QP34.5 .P49 2019
612--dc23

Contents

Chapter 19

Preface

Human physiology refers to the study of the bodily functions. The understanding of the human physiology is applied to diagnose the underlying cause of a clinical condition. This field encompasses the development of physiological tests for medical diagnostics. It also involves tests from related medical specialties such as clinical neurophysiology, nuclear medicine and radiology. An understanding of the physiological and pathophysiological pathways is essential in this domain. This book elucidates new techniques and applications of human physiology in a healthcare setting. It strives to provide a fair idea about clinical physiology and to help develop a better understanding of the latest advances within this field. It is a vital tool for all researching or studying physiology as it gives incredible insights into emerging trends and concepts.

The information contained in this book is the result of intensive hard work done by researchers in this field. All due efforts have been made to make this book serve as a complete guiding source for students and researchers. The topics in this book have been comprehensively explained to help readers understand the growing trends in the field.

I would like to thank the entire group of writers who made sincere efforts in this book and my family who supported me in my efforts of working on this book. I take this opportunity to thank all those who have been a guiding force throughout my life.

Editor

Postnatal liver growth and regeneration are independent of *c-myc* in a mouse model of conditional hepatic *c-myc* deletion

Jennifer A Sanders[1]*, Christoph Schorl[2,3], Ajay Patel[4], John M Sedivy[2,3] and Philip A Gruppuso[1,2]

Abstract

Background: The transcription factor *c-myc* regulates genes involved in hepatocyte growth, proliferation, metabolism, and differentiation. It has also been assigned roles in liver development and regeneration. In previous studies, we made the unexpected observation that c-Myc protein levels were similar in proliferating fetal liver and quiescent adult liver with c-Myc displaying nucleolar localization in the latter. In order to investigate the functional role of c-Myc in adult liver, we have developed a hepatocyte-specific *c-myc* knockout mouse, *c-myc*^fl/fl^;*Alb-Cre*.

Results: Liver weight to body weight ratios were similar in control and *c-myc* deficient mice. Liver architecture was unaffected. Conditional *c-myc* deletion did not result in compensatory induction of other *myc* family members or in c-Myc's binding partner Max. Floxed *c-myc* did have a negative effect on *Alb-Cre* expression at 4 weeks of age. To explore this relationship further, we used the Rosa26 reporter line to assay Cre activity in the *c-myc* floxed mice. No significant difference in Alb-Cre activity was found between control and *c-myc*^fl/fl^ mice. *c-myc* deficient mice were studied in a nonproliferative model of liver growth, fasting for 48 hr followed by a 24 hr refeeding period. Fasting resulted in a decrease in liver mass and liver protein, both of which recovered upon 24 h of refeeding in the *c-myc*^fl/fl^;*Alb-Cre* animals. There was also no effect of reducing *c-myc* on recovery of liver mass following 2/3 partial hepatectomy.

Conclusions: c-Myc appears to be dispensable for normal liver growth during the postnatal period, restoration of liver mass following partial hepatectomy and recovery from fasting.

Background

The Myc family includes three closely related genes, *c-myc*, *L-myc*, and *N-myc*, which have been shown to have similar biological activities. The three Myc proteins are basic helix-loop-helix leucine zipper transcription factors that heterodimerize with a binding partner, Max, to bind DNA and either activate or repress the transcription of a large set of target genes [1-3]. An additional member of the family, *B-myc*, encodes a protein that is homologous to the N-terminal domain of c-Myc, but its function remains largely unknown [4]. c-Myc has been shown to regulate genes involved in ribosomal biogenesis, protein translation and the transition from the G0/G1 to S-phase of the cell cycle suggesting that c-Myc

has a functional role in the coordination of cellular growth and proliferation. The expression of *c-myc* is, in general, tightly regulated. Proliferating cells contain high levels of this protein, while the level of c-Myc is significantly decreased as cells growth arrest and differentiate [3]. Dysregulated expression of *c-myc* is associated with the development of many tumors in rodents and humans, including hepatocellular carcinoma [5-7].

c-Myc has been implicated as a regulator of hepatocyte proliferation, growth and metabolism [8,9]. During the process of liver regeneration, quiescent hepatocytes synchronously enter the cell cycle and undergo one, two or more rounds of replication to restore liver mass [10]. Considered an immediate early gene, *c-myc* expression is induced within 30 minutes following partial hepatectomy and has been suggested to be a key factor in the transcriptional response leading to the progression of hepatocytes from G0/G1 to S phase [11]. Transient

---

* Correspondence: Jennifer_Sanders@brown.edu
[1]Department of Pediatrics, Rhode Island Hospital and Brown University, Providence, RI 02903, USA
Full list of author information is available at the end of the article

overexpression of c-Myc in mouse liver results in hepatocyte enlargement and induction of ribosomal and nucleolar genes [12]. Other studies involving *c-myc* transgenic mice have shown that overexpression of c-Myc in the liver induces hepatic glucose uptake and utilization and can inhibit gluconeogenesis [13,14]. While these studies support a role for c-Myc in hepatocyte growth, ribosomal biogenesis and metabolism, they do not address whether c-Myc is required or whether the effects on these processes were due to superphysiological levels of c-Myc.

Previous studies from our laboratory on the regulation of c-Myc during rat liver development revealed several novel findings. First, in contrast to many other organ systems and cell types, rapidly proliferating fetal and quiescent adult liver contained similar levels of c-Myc protein. In adult hepatocytes, c-Myc was localized to the nucleolus, while fetal hepatocytes displayed diffuse nuclear localization. In addition, c-Myc translocated out of the nucleolus in response to a partial hepatectomy [15,16]. These data led us to hypothesize that hepatic c-Myc may play a functional role in liver other than its well established role in hepatocyte proliferation. In order to examine the function of c-Myc in adult liver, we mated mice in which the *c-myc* locus was floxed to mice expressing Cre recombinase under the control of the albumin promoter. The present paper describes the characterization of these mice.

Methods
Animals
c-myc$^{fl/fl}$ mice were gifts of I. Moreno de Alboran [17]. *Alb*-Cre and ROSA26 mice were obtained from Jackson Laboratories (Bar Harbor, ME [18,19]). All mice were C57BL/6 strain housed in a pathogen-free facility and maintained on a 12 hr light/dark cycle. *c-myc$^{fl/fl}$* mice were mated to *Alb*-Cre mice to achieve mice that carried a floxed *c-myc* allele and *Alb*-Cre. Littermates were bred to obtain *c-myc$^{fl/fl}$;Alb*-Cre$^+$ mice and the control mice (*c-myc$^{fl/fl}$;Alb*-Cre$^{-/-}$, *c-myc$^{+/+}$;Alb*-Cre$^+$). Progeny were mated to obtain *c-myc$^{fl/fl}$;Alb*-Cre$^{+/+}$ mice and the control *c-myc$^{+/+}$;Alb*-Cre$^{+/+}$ mice. Breeding pairs that produced litters consisting exclusively of Cre$^+$ pups for at least 5 successive matings were considered Cre$^{+/+}$. *c-myc$^{fl/fl}$;Alb*-Cre$^{+/+}$ and the control *c-myc$^{+/+}$;Alb*-Cre$^{+/+}$ lines were established from these pairs. Pups from both sexes were used for all analyses except 2/3 partial hepatectomy. Blood glucose concentrations were determined using a YSI 2300 STAT plus glucose and lactate analyzer (YSI Life Sciences; Yellow Springs, OH).

For fasting and refeeding experiments, eight week old male and female *c-myc$^{fl/fl}$* and *c-myc$^{+/+}$;Alb*-Cre expressing mice were fed standard rodent chow *ad libitum* (control) or fasted for 48 hr. Where noted, standard

rodent chow was replaced in the cage covers and animals were allowed to feed *ad libitum* for 24 hr (refed). Water was freely available to all mice. Eight to ten week old male *c-myc$^{fl/fl}$* and *c-myc$^{+/+}$ Alb*-Cre expressing mice were anesthetized using isoflurane and subjected to 2/3 partial hepatectomy as described by Higgins and Anderson [20]. All mice were killed by exsanguination under isoflurane anesthesia. Carcass and liver weights were recorded. The liver was divided and fixed in 10% neutral buffered formalin or flash frozen in liquid nitrogen before being stored at -70°C.

To assess Cre activity, female *c-myc$^{fl/fl}$;Alb*-Cre$^{+/+}$ and *c-myc$^{+/+}$;Alb*-Cre$^{+/+}$ were crossed with male ROSA26 mice. Mice were further mated to obtain the following genotypes used for study, *c-myc$^{fl/fl}$;Alb*-Cre$^+$;ROSA26$^+$ and *c-myc$^{+/+}$;Alb*-Cre$^+$;ROSA26$^+$. Mice were genotyped using PCR analysis of tail genomic DNA according to published protocols for *c-myc* [21], *Alb*-Cre transgene [22] and the ROSA26 alleles http://jaxmice.jax.org/protocolsdb/f?p=116:1:3259541732707236::NO:::.

All experiments on mice were performed in accordance with the guidelines of the National Institutes of Health and the Rhode Island Hospital Institutional Animal Care and Use Committee.

DNA Isolation and qPCR
DNA was isolated from triplicate frozen livers obtained from *c-myc$^{fl/fl}$;Alb*-Cre$^{-/-}$, *c-myc$^{fl/fl}$;Alb*-Cre$^±$ and *c-myc$^{fl/fl}$;Alb*-Cre$^{+/+}$ mice at 4, 8, and 10 weeks of age using the DNeasy kit (Qiagen; Valencia, CA). qPCR reactions were performed in triplicate using 25 ng of DNA, 23 µl SYBR green reaction mix, and the 7500 Real-Time PCR system (Applied Biosystems; Foster City, CA). In order to detect the deletion of the *c-myc^{fl}* allele, primers were designed upstream of the 5' lox P site (primers X and Y) and on either side of the 3' lox P site (NB). The primer sequences are as follows: primer X, 5'-CCTC GCGCCCCTGAA-3'; primer Y, 5'-AACCGCTCAGAT CACGACTCA-3'; primer N, 5'-TCCAAACCAGA AACTGAAACATGT-3'; primer B, 5'-ACAATGGGGTC ATTTAGGAC-3'. The relative abundance of the *c-myc^{fl}* allele was calculated by the comparative C_T method using the product generated by primers X and Y as the reference. *c-myc* deletion during liver regeneration was assessed by calculating the ddCt (dCt in liver removed at the time of hepatectomy– minus the dCt in regenerating liver from the same animal) for triplicate mice.

RNase protection assay
Total RNA was isolated from triplicate frozen livers obtained from 8 and 10 week old *c-myc$^{+/+}$* and *c-myc$^{fl/fl}$ Alb*-Cre expressing mice as previously described [15]. RNase protection assays were performed using the mMyc multiprobe template with yeast tRNA as a

negative control (BD Biosciences; San Diego, CA). L32 was used as an internal control to normalize expression data. Quantification of bands was performed by digital analysis using LabWorks software (UVP; Upland, CA).

RT-qPCR

Total RNA was isolated from frozen livers obtained from 4, 8, and 10 week old control (c-$myc^{fl/fl}$;Alb-Cre$^{-/-}$ and c-$myc^{+/+}$;Alb-Cre) and c-$myc^{fl/fl}$;Alb-Cre mice using the RiboPure Kit (Ambion; Foster City, CA). RNA was cleaned using the RNeasy kit (Qiagen) and cDNA synthesized using random hexamers and the TaqMan Reverse Transcription kit (Applied Biosystems). Primer sequences used for amplification of cre were 5'-CGATG CAACGAGTGATGAGG-3' for the sense primer and 5'-GGCAAACGGACAGAAGCATT-3' for the antisense primer. Mouse c-myc primers were obtained from SABiosciences (Frederick, MD). The internal standard $GAPDH$ was amplified using the following primer sequences, 5'-TCCAGTATGACTCCACTCACGG-3' and 5'-TCGCTCCTGGAAGATGGTG-3'. The relative abundance of cre and c-myc was calculated by the comparative CT method using $GAPDH$ as the reference.

Histology and image analysis

Liver was fixed in 10% neutral buffered formalin, paraffin embedded, and stained with hemotoxylin and eosin. Immunohistochemistry was performed for Ki-67 using the indirect immuneperoxidase technique. Briefly, sections were deparaffinized and microwaved in 100 mM sodium citrate buffer, pH 6.0 for 20 minutes, followed by incubation in anti-Ki-67 antibody (Abcam, Cambridge, MA) overnight at 4°C. Slides were scanned with an Aperio Scanscope CS (Aperio Technologies, Inc., Vista, CA). Ki-67 positive cells in ten 20× fields were counted. For Lac-Z staining, liver cryosections (10 µm) were fixed in phosphate buffered saline, pH 7.3 (140 mM NaCl; 2.7 mM KCl; 8.1 mM Na2HPO4; 1.5 mM KH2PO4) containing 0.2% gluteraldehyde, 10 mM EGTA, and 2 mM MgCl2. Sections were washed three times with phosphate buffered saline containing 0.05 mM EGTA, 2 mM MgCl2, 0.12 mM Na deoxycolate, and 0.02% Nonidet P-40 and incubated overnight in the same solution containing 10 mM K3Fe(CN)6, 10 mM K4Fe(CN)6, and 0.5% X-gal. Sections were washed and counterstained with Nuclear Fast Red (Vector Labs; Burlingame, CA). Sections from c-$myc^{+/+}$;Alb-Cre$^{-/-}$; ROSA26$^+$ and c-$myc^{+/+}$;Alb-Cre$^+$;ROSA26$^{-/-}$ mice served as negative controls.

β-galactosidase analyses

β-gal ELISA assays were performed using a kit obtained from Roche (Indianapolis, IN). Briefly, livers were obtained from 6-8 week old c-$myc^{fl/fl}$; Alb-Cre;ROSA26 mice and homogenized by hand using a ground glass homogenizer with 2 ml 1× Lysis buffer (Roche) per 40 mg tissue. Samples were incubated for 30 min at room temperature and centrifuged at 13,000 rpm for 15 min at 4°C. Samples were split into aliquots and frozen in dry ice/ethanol before transferring to -80°C. An aliquot was used to determine the protein concentration using the bicinchoninic acid method (Pierce; Rockford, IL). β-gal ELISA assays were performed according to the manufacturer's directions using 5 µg of liver homogenate.

Statistical analyses

Statistical analyses were performed using GraphPad Prism (San Diego, CA). One-way ANOVA with a post hoc Bonferroni Multiple Comparison test was performed for comparing the relative abundance of the c-myc^{fl} allele by qPCR. Comparisons of the relative abundances of c-myc and cre expression in mice of various genotypes were performed using a Mann-Whitney test. A Spearman rank correlation test was performed to assess the association between c-myc and cre abundance. For results where differences were not significant, no p value is reported.

Results

Deletion of hepatic c-myc

Deletion of murine c-myc by gene targeting results in embryonic lethality at embryonic day 9-10 [23]. In order to assess the functional role of c-Myc in adult mouse liver, we utilized a transgenic mouse line where Cre recombinase is under the control of the $Albumin$ promoter [18]. Conditional deletion of c-myc was achieved by crossing these mice with c-$myc^{fl/fl}$ mice. The F1 generation was intercrossed to obtain c-$myc^{fl/fl}$;Alb-Cre$^+$ and littermate control mice (c-$myc^{fl/fl}$;Alb-Cre$^{-/-}$, c-$myc^{+/+}$;Alb-Cre$^+$). The c-$myc^{fl/fl}$;Alb-Cre$^+$ and c-$myc^{+/+}$;Alb-Cre$^+$ lines were also bred to be homozygous for the Cre transgene. Litters contained the expected frequency of control and experimental animals.

Cre-mediated recombination of the c-myc locus was assessed using a qPCR strategy. Primers (XY) were designed to amplify a region of the c-myc locus upstream of the 5' loxP site. A second primer pair (NB) was designed surrounding the 3' loxP site such that Cre-mediated recombination of the locus would result in a decrease of the NB qPCR product (Figure 1A). Results revealed a significant decrease in the relative abundance of the NB product compared to the XY product in conditional knockout animals, indicating recombination of the c-myc locus.

By one month of age, recombination approached 70% in both male and female c-$myc^{fl/fl}$;Alb-Cre$^+$ expressing mice, while recombination in c-$myc^{fl/fl}$;Alb-Cre$^{+/+}$ mice was significantly higher (Figure 1A).

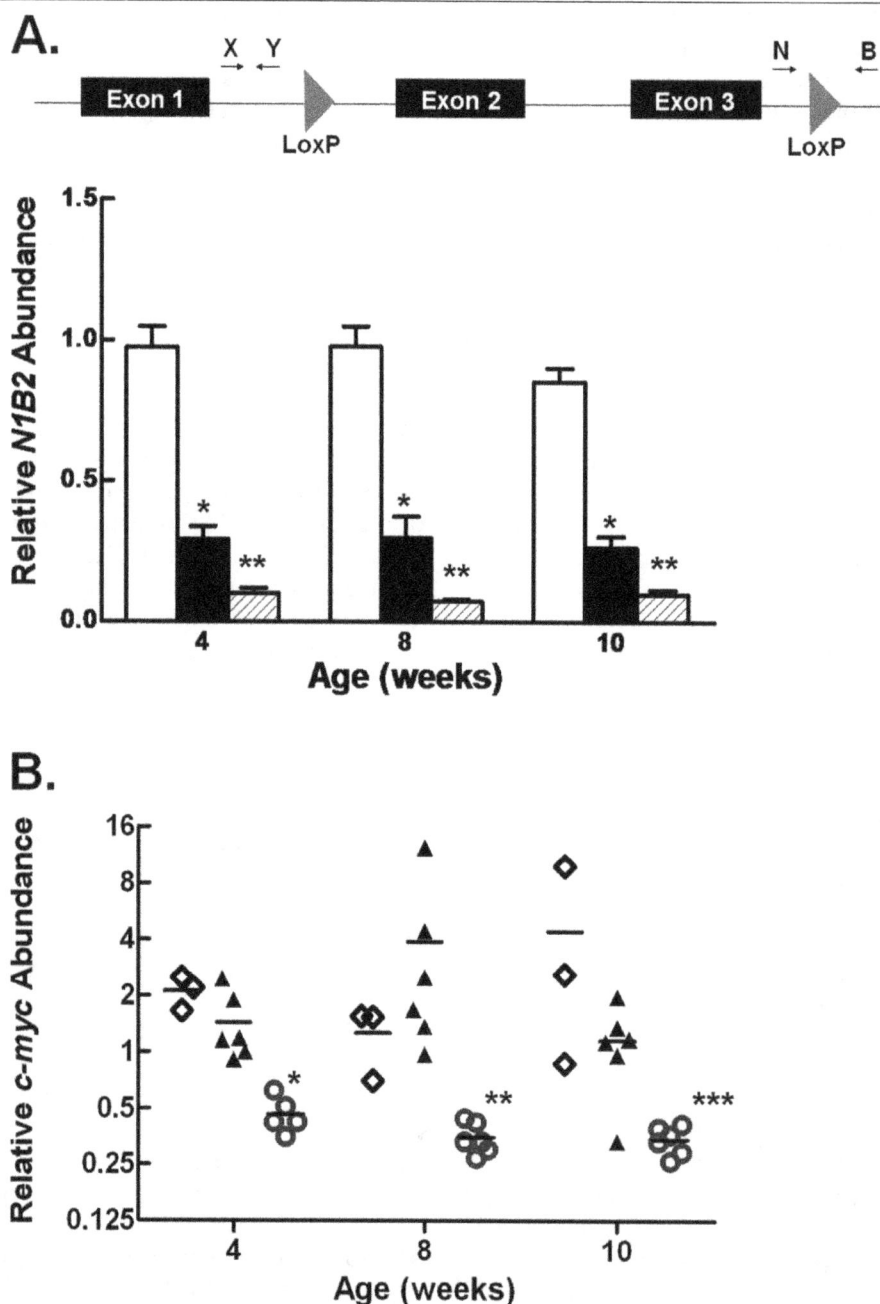

Figure 1 Hepatic *c-myc* deletion in *c-myc^{fl/fl};Alb-Cre* expressing mice. *A. Schematic representation of the c-myc^{fl} allele showing location of primer pairs used in qPCR analyses to determine the relative abundance of the c-myc^{fl} allele. The graph shows the quantification of the c-myc^{fl} allele in liver from male and female c-myc^{fl/fl};Alb-Cre^{-/-} (open bars), c-myc^{fl/fl};Alb-Cre^{+} (closed bars) and c-myc^{fl/fl};Alb-Cre^{+/+} (hatched bars) mice as described in the Methods. Data are shown as the mean + 1 SD. *, P < 0.01 c-myc^{fl/fl};Alb-Cre^{+} versus c-myc^{fl/fl};Alb-Cre^{-/-} . **, P < 0.001 c-myc^{fl/fl};Alb-Cre^{+} compared to c-myc^{fl/fl};Alb-Cre^{+/+}. B. Hepatic c-myc expression in male and female control and c-myc^{fl/fl};Alb-Cre expressing mice as analyzed by RT-qPCR. Data are shown as individual points with the mean. ◊, c-myc^{fl/fl};Alb-Cre^{-/-}; ▲, c-myc^{+/+};Alb-Cre; ○, c-myc^{fl/fl};Alb-Cre. *, P = 0.001 4 wk c-myc^{fl/fl};Alb-Cre vs. controls; **P = 0.0004 8 wk c-myc^{fl/fl};Alb-Cre vs. controls; ***P = 0.0028 10 wk c-myc^{fl/fl};Alb-Cre vs. controls.*

Consistent with previous findings on the temporal expression of the *Albumin*-Cre transgene [24], a similar deletion efficiency was observed in 8 and 10 week old conditional knockout animals, indicating that maximal recombination had been reached by one month of age. Since hepatocytes make up approximately 85% of the total cell population in liver, we estimated that recombination of the *c-myc* locus was near 80% in *c-myc^{fl/fl};Alb*-Cre^{+} and over 90% in *myc^{fl/fl};Alb*-Cre^{+/+} mice.

To examine the influence of Cre-mediated recombination on *c-myc* mRNA, RT-qPCR was performed on total RNA isolated from livers obtained from control (*c-myc*$^{+/+}$;*Alb*-Cre$^{+/+}$, *c-myc*$^{fl/fl}$;*Alb*-Cre$^{-/-}$) and *c-myc*$^{fl/fl}$;*Alb*-Cre$^{+/+}$ mice at 4, 8, and 10 weeks of age (Figure 1B). A 75% reduction in *c-myc* expression in livers from *c-myc*$^{fl/fl}$; *Alb*-Cre$^{+/+}$ male and female mice was observed at one month of age and this reduction in c-*myc* expression remained stable in the liver through 10 weeks of age.

We assessed the effect of the model on c-Myc protein levels by immunoprecipitating c-Myc from total liver homogenates prepared from 4 week old *c-myc*$^{fl/fl}$;*Alb*-Cre$^{+/+}$ and *c-myc*$^{+/+}$;*Alb*-Cre$^{+/+}$ mice (data not shown). c-Myc protein content was low in four week old *c-myc*$^{+/+}$;*Alb*-Cre$^{+/+}$ control mice and below the level of detection in *c-myc*$^{fl/fl}$;*Alb*-Cre$^{+/+}$ mice.

Characterization of hepatic c-myc knockout mice

Our prior studies in the rat showed that c-Myc protein was expressed in quiescent adult hepatocytes, suggesting a functional role for the protein in adult liver other than its role in proliferation [16]. Given the established role of *c-myc* in hepatic proliferation and growth, we measured liver weight to carcass weight ratios in male and female *c-myc*$^{fl/fl}$;*Alb-Cre*$^+$, *c-myc*$^{fl/fl}$;*Alb-Cre*$^{+/+}$ and control mice from one month of age through the first year of life. Liver weight to carcass weight ratios were similar in *c-myc*$^{fl/fl}$ *Alb*-Cre expressing and control mice at all ages analyzed (Figure 2). Despite the increased recombination of the *c-myc* locus in *c-myc*$^{fl/fl}$;*Alb-Cre* homozygous mice, no difference in liver weight was observed in these animals compared to c- *myc*$^{fl/fl}$;*Alb-Cre* hemizygous mice.

c-Myc has been shown to regulate genes involved in glucose metabolism and to be involved in the regulation of cell and nucleolar size [12,25]. In order to determine if loss of c-Myc would result in alterations in glucose homeostasis we analyzed serum glucose levels in fed *c-myc*$^{fl/fl}$ and *c-myc*$^{+/+}$ *Alb-Cre* expressing mice at 4 and 8 weeks of age. Serum glucose was unaffected in the *c-myc*$^{fl/fl}$;*Alb-Cre* expressing mice at both ages (277 ± 19 vs. 271 ± 73.6 and 305 ± 27 vs. 295 ± 20; 4 and 8 weeks respectively).

To investigate whether the organization of the liver parenchyma or hepatocyte morphology was affected in *c-myc* conditional knockout mice, hematoxylin and

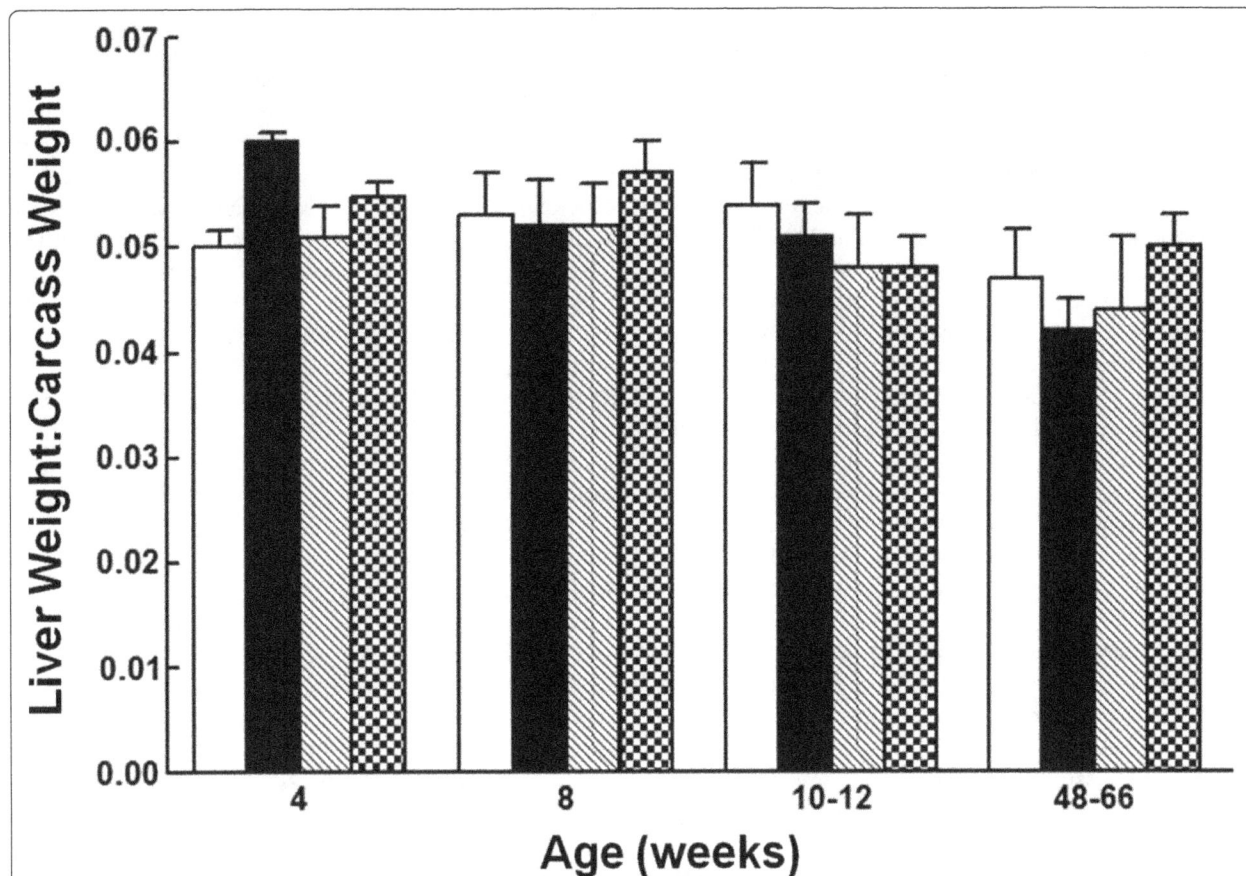

Figure 2 Liver weight to carcass weight ratio in *c-myc*$^{fl/fl}$;*Alb-Cre* expressing mice. Liver:carcass weight ratio was determined for control and *c-myc*$^{fl/fl}$;*Alb-cre* male and female mice at various ages. Data are expressed as mean + 1 SD. n ≥ 3 mice/group. Open bars, *c-myc*$^{fl/fl}$;*Alb-Cre*$^{-/-}$; Black bars, *c-myc*$^{+/+}$;*Alb-Cre*$^+$; Hatched bars, *c-myc*$^{fl/fl}$;*Alb-Cre*$^+$; Stippled bars, *c-myc*$^{fl/fl}$;*Alb-Cre*$^{+/+}$.

eosin stained liver sections were prepared from *c-myc^{fl/fl}*; *Alb-Cre* expressing and control mice at 4, 8, and 10 weeks of age (data not shown). The gross and histological appearance of the liver were similar in *c-myc^{fl/fl}*;*Alb-Cre* expressing and control animals as well as *c-myc^{fl/fl}*; *Alb-cre* hemizygous compared to homozygous animals.

c-myc^{fl/fl};*Alb-Cre* expressing hepatocyte response to nonproliferative and proliferative stimuli

We extended our studies to determine the effect of reducing c-Myc in a nonproliferative model of liver growth, refeeding after a 48 hr fast. Previous studies in our laboratory have shown that rat liver growth during refeeding requires rapid and marked induction of ribosomal biogenesis and translation initiation, two processes where c-Myc has been proposed to have a functional role [26]. Eight week old *c-myc^{fl/fl}* and *c-myc^{+/+} Alb*-Cre expressing mice of both sexes were divided into three groups. Mice were either fed *ad libitum* (control), fasted for 48 hr, or refed *ad libitum* for 24 hr following a 48 hr fast (refed). As no difference in liver weight to carcass weight ratio or total liver protein was observed in *c-myc^{fl/fl}* animals carrying one or two alleles of the *Alb-Cre* transgene, the data from these animals were combined. In agreement with our previous data in the rat [26], fasting for 48 hr resulted in a slight reduction in liver to carcass weight ratio in both control and *c-myc^{fl/fl} Alb*-Cre expressing animals. Refeeding for 24 hr resulted in restoration of liver weight to carcass weight ratio to the level of the control fed mice in both *c-myc^{fl/fl}* and *c-myc^{+/+}* animals (Figure 3A). Total liver protein decreased by approximately 40% in both genotypes with fasting. Recovery of total protein was attained after 24 hr of refeeding in both genotypes, suggesting that full expression of *c-myc* is not required for protein synthesis in this model of liver growth (Figure 3B).

Quiescent adult hepatocytes rapidly enter the cell cycle in response to a reduction in liver mass. Upregulation of c-Myc protein content is an early event in this process, suggesting the hypothesis that liver regeneration following partial hepatectomy requires c-Myc [11,15]. To test this hypothesis, eight to ten-week old male *c-myc^{+/+}* and *c-myc^{fl/fl} Alb-Cre* expressing animals underwent 2/3 partial hepatectomy. Mice were sacrificed 24, 48, or 96 hr post-hepatectomy. Liver weight to carcass weight ratios were determined (Figure 4A). No difference in liver to carcass weight ratio between *c-myc^{fl/fl}*; *Alb-Cre* expressing and control mice was observed at any of the timepoints analyzed. However, a slight decrease in the number of Ki-67 positive hepatocytes was observed in the *c-myc^{fl/fl}* mice compared to wild-type mice 48 hr post-hepatectomy (Figure 4B). To determine if cells lacking in *c-myc* were responsible for liver regeneration, we quantified *c-myc* deletion in each

mouse in the regenerated liver and liver excised at the time of partial hepatectomy. We found that the regenerating liver was as deficient in the *c-myc* allele as was the liver excised at the time of surgery [average fold change (0.84 ± 0.82; 0.80 ± 0.93; 0.78 ± 0.86) 24, 48, 96 hr, respectively]. The persistent loss of the *c-myc* allele was consistent with the conclusion that the recovered liver mass was arising from *c-myc*-deficient cells. Despite any modest decrease in the number of hepatocytes in the cell cycle, the absence of an effect on the recovery of liver weight indicates that the liver is capable of regeneration despite a significant reduction in *c-myc*. As in the non-proliferative model, there was no difference in mice containing one versus two alleles of the *Alb-Cre* transgene. Liver sections obtained from mice placed on the fasting/refeeding protocol and from animals subjected to 2/3 partial hepatectomy did not reveal disorganization of the liver parenchyma or any other obvious changes in hepatocyte morphology between *c-myc^{fl/fl}* and *c-myc^{+/+} Alb-Cre* expressing mice (Figure 5).

Expression of members of the *c-myc/max/mad* network

We went on to explore whether the lack of an effect of reducing *c-myc* on hepatocyte proliferation, growth, and protein synthesis could be accounted for by compensatory induction of other *myc* family members or the c-Myc binding partner Max. We had previously found that *max* expression at both the RNA and protein level correlated with hepatocyte proliferation during rat liver development and that overexpression of *max* induced a shift in c-Myc localization from the nucleolus to the nucleus [15]. These data raise the possibility that compensatory induction of Max could increase c-Myc activity. Multiplex RNase protection assays were performed on total RNA isolated from 8 and 10 week old *c-myc^{fl/fl}* and *c-myc^{+/+} Alb-Cre* expressing animals of both sexes (Figure 6). Two of the *myc* family members, *B-myc* and *L-myc* were expressed in murine liver, while *N-myc* expression was below the level of detection in our assay. There was no difference in the expression of these family members or of *max* in *c-myc^{fl/fl}* compared to wild-type *c-myc* Alb-Cre expressing mice.

There is substantial overlap between the role of c-Myc and Wnt/β-catenin signaling in the regulation of postnatal liver development, hepatic organization, and liver regeneration [27]. In addition, c-myc is a downstream target of β-catenin [28]. Given the interaction between c-myc and β-catenin, we investigated whether deletion of *c-myc* is compensated by upregulation of β-catenin signaling. Immunohistochemical analysis for β-catenin was performed on liver sections from wild-type and *c-myc* deficient mice. No difference in the localization of β-catenin was observed between the two genotypes of mice. These results were confirmed by Western

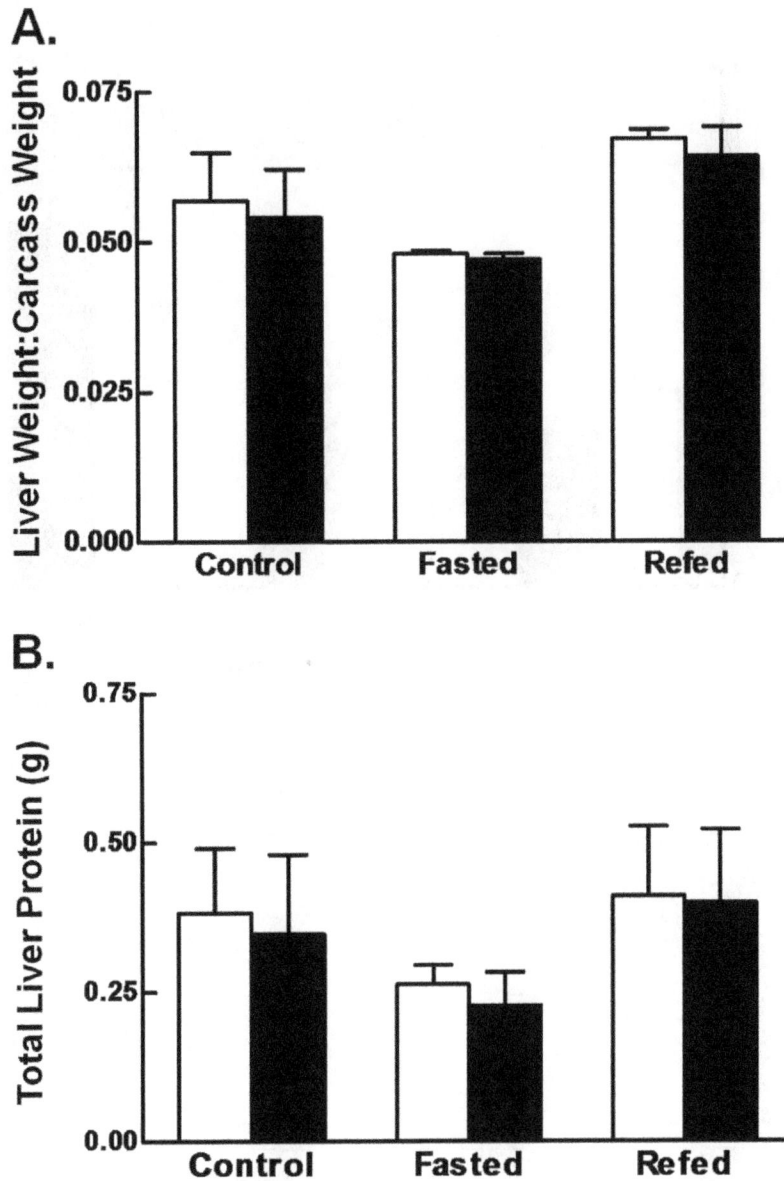

Figure 3 Effect of conditional *c-myc* deletion on liver growth following starvation. Male and female mice were fed ad libitum (control), fasted for 48 hr (fasted), or fasted for 48 hr then refed ad libitum for 24 hr (refed). A. The graph shows liver:carcass weight ratios for *c-myc*$^{+/+}$ (open bars) and *c-myc*$^{fl/fl}$ (closed bars) *Alb-Cre* expressing mice expressed as the mean + 1 SD. n ≥ 3 mice/group. B. Liver homogenates were prepared and protein concentration determined using the bichoninic acid method. Total liver protein was then calculated based on total liver weight. The graph shows total liver protein content for *c-myc*$^{+/+}$ (open bars) and *c-myc*$^{fl/fl}$ (closed bars) *Alb-Cre* expressing mice expressed as the mean + 1 SD. n ≥ 3 mice/group.

immunoblotting of nuclear and post-nuclear fractions prepared from liver of wild-type and *c-myc* deficient mice (data not shown).

Effect of *c-myc*$^{fl/fl}$ on Cre expression

Numerous studies using the *Alb*-Cre transgene to delete various genetic loci involved in hepatocyte proliferation, growth, and survival have reported recombination nearing 100% and complete ablation of the expression of the gene

of interest [29-31]. Given our results, which varied markedly from published experience, we investigated the expression and activity of the *Alb*-Cre transgene in *c-myc*$^{+/+}$ and *c-myc*$^{fl/fl}$ mice to ascertain whether floxing *c-myc* had an effect on the expression of the *Alb*-Cre transgene such that *c-myc* deletion would be impaired in our model. RNA was isolated from livers obtained from *c-myc*$^{+/+}$;*Alb-Cre*$^{+/+}$ and *c-myc*$^{fl/fl}$;*Alb-Cre*$^{+/+}$ animals at 4, 8, and 10 weeks of age. RT-qPCR was performed to assess *cre*

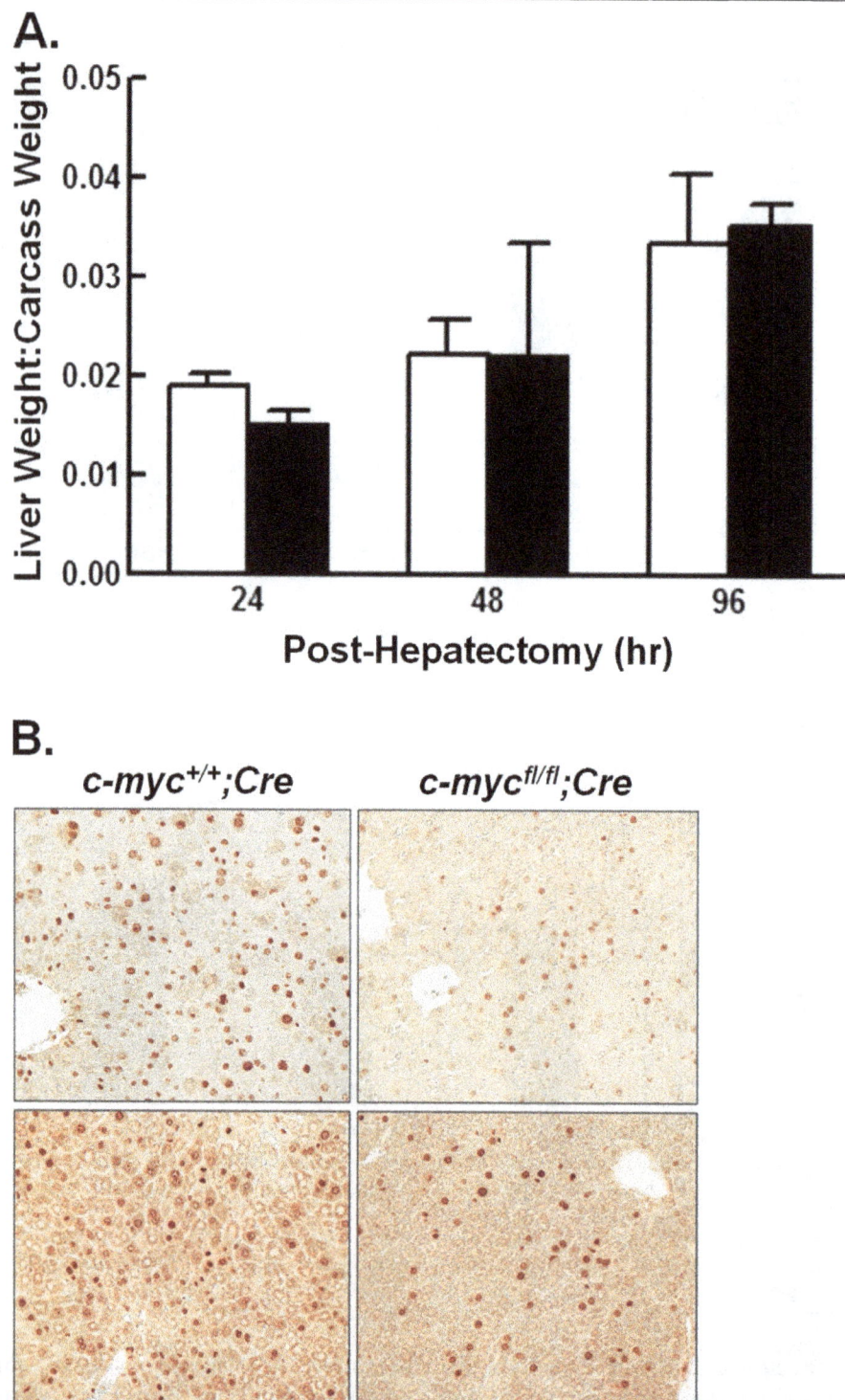

Figure 4 Effect of conditional *c-myc* deletion on liver regeneration. Male mice were subjected to 2/3 hepatectomy and assessed 24, 48, or 96 hr after resection. A. The graph shows liver:carcass weight ratio for *c-myc$^{+/+}$* (open bars) and *c-myc$^{fl/fl}$* (closed bars) *Alb-Cre* expressing mice. The data are expressed as the mean + 1 SD. n ≥ 3 mice/group. B. Hepatocyte proliferation in duplicate *c-myc$^{+/+}$* and *c-myc$^{fl/fl}$* *Alb-Cre* expressing mice 48 hr post-hepatectomy as assessed by Ki-67 immunohistochemistry. Representative 20× images are shown.

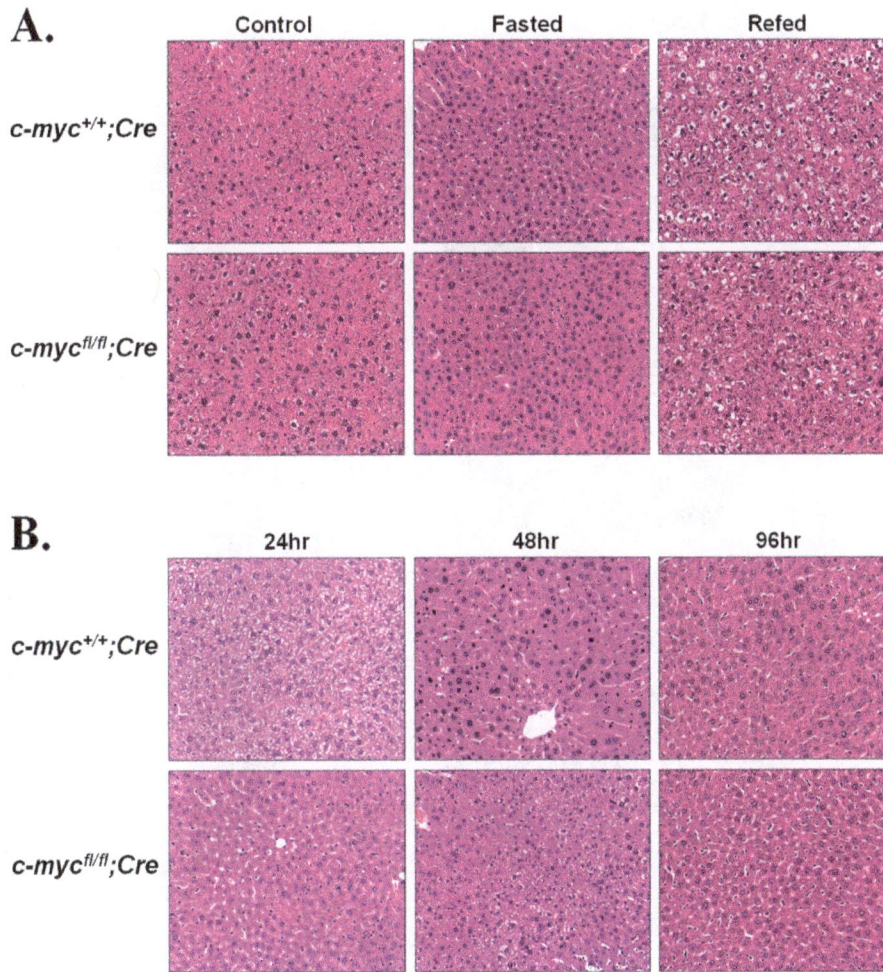

Figure 5 Effect of conditional *c-myc* deletion on parenchymal organization during fasting/refeeding and liver regeneration. Formalin fixed liver from male and female mice was processed and stained with H&E. Slides were scanned with an Aperio Scanscope CS and randomly selected representative areas with a scan zoom of 20 were acquired. A. Images (20×) obtained from control, 48 hr fasted, and 48 hr fasted followed by 24 hr refeeding *c-myc*$^{+/+}$ and *c-myc*$^{fl/fl}$ *Alb*-Cre expressing mice. B. Representative 20× images from *c-myc*$^{+/+}$ and *c-myc*$^{fl/fl}$ *Alb*-Cre expressing mice 24, 48, or 96 hr post-hepatectomy.

expression (Figure 7A). A statistically significant difference in *cre* expression was observed in *c-myc*$^{fl/fl}$ compared to *c-myc*$^{+/+}$ mice at 4 weeks of age suggesting that deletion of *c-myc* suppressed expression of the *Alb-Cre* transgene. At 8 and 10 weeks of age there was no statistically significant difference in *cre* expression between *c-myc*$^{fl/fl}$ and *c-myc*$^{+/+}$ mice. However, in comparison to 4-week old animals, *cre* expression in older mice varied considerably from animal-to-animal.

To ascertain whether the variation in *cre* expression correlated with the amount of c-*myc* we compared the relative abundance of *cre* and *c-myc* in individual *c-myc*$^{fl/fl}$;*cre*$^{+/+}$ mice at 4, 8, and 10 weeks (Figure 7B). This analysis revealed a significant association between floxing *c-myc* and the expression of *cre* (Spearman r = -0.6609, p = 0.0019).

We further characterized the pattern of Cre activity in our model by crossing our mice to the ROSA26 reporter line. The ROSA26 line has a lacZ gene that is expressed when an upstream stop codon is removed by Cre-mediated recombination. In order to study the effect of floxing *c-myc* on Cre activity, mice were further crossed to obtain *c-myc*$^{fl/fl}$;*Alb*-Cre;ROSA26 and *c-myc*$^{+/+}$;*Alb*-Cre;ROSA26 mice. Sections prepared from six-week old mice were stained for β-galactosidase activity using X-gal. Analysis revealed a wide pattern of LacZ-staining across 20× fields of individual sections in both genotypes of mice (Figure 8). In some fields, the majority of the hepatocytes displayed intense nuclear and cytoplasmic staining while other hepatocytes exhibited weak cytoplasmic staining. There were also fields where many of the hepatocytes appeared negative for Lac-Z staining.

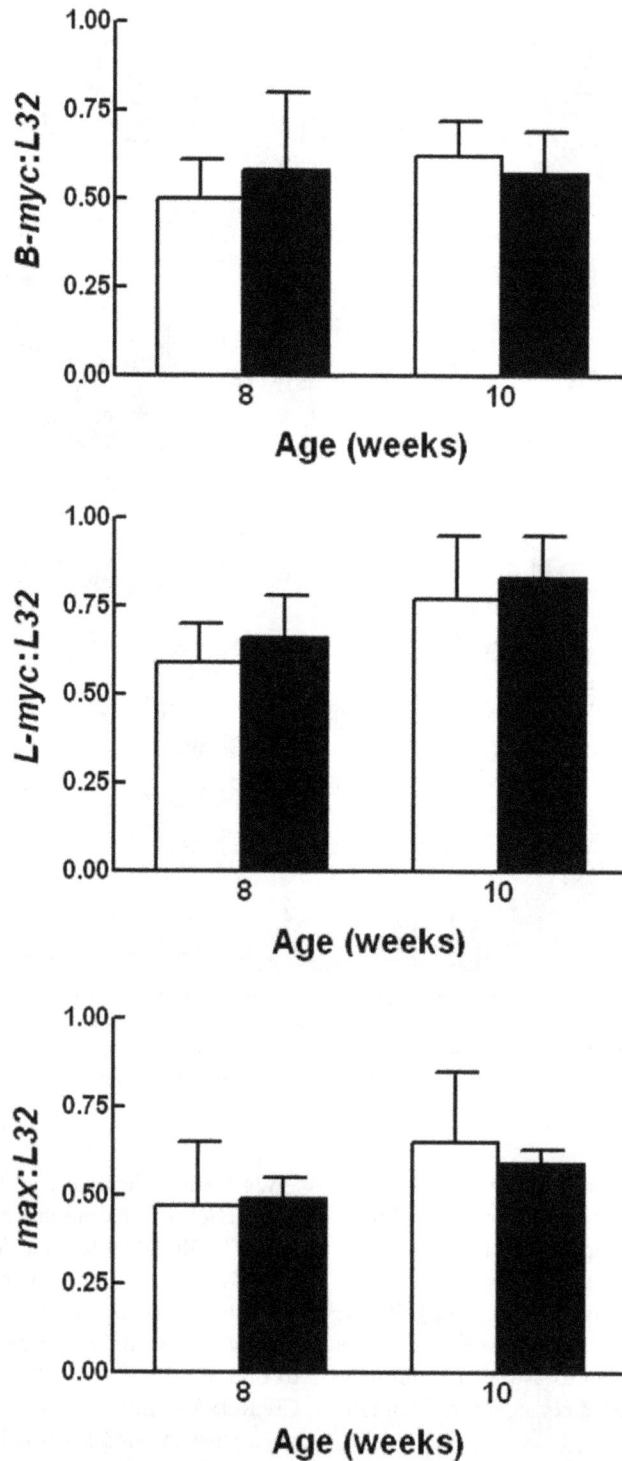

Figure 6 Expression of members of the *c-myc/max/mad* network in liver derived from male and female control and *c-myc* conditional knockout mice. Total liver RNA was isolated from triplicate *c-myc* wild-type (open bars) and *c-myc*$^{fl/fl}$ (closed bars) *Alb-Cre* expressing mice at 8 and 10 weeks of age and a multiprobe RNase protection assay performed. Expression levels of *B-myc*, *L-myc*, and *max* were quantified and normalized to the internal control *L32*. Data are expressed as mean + 1 SD.

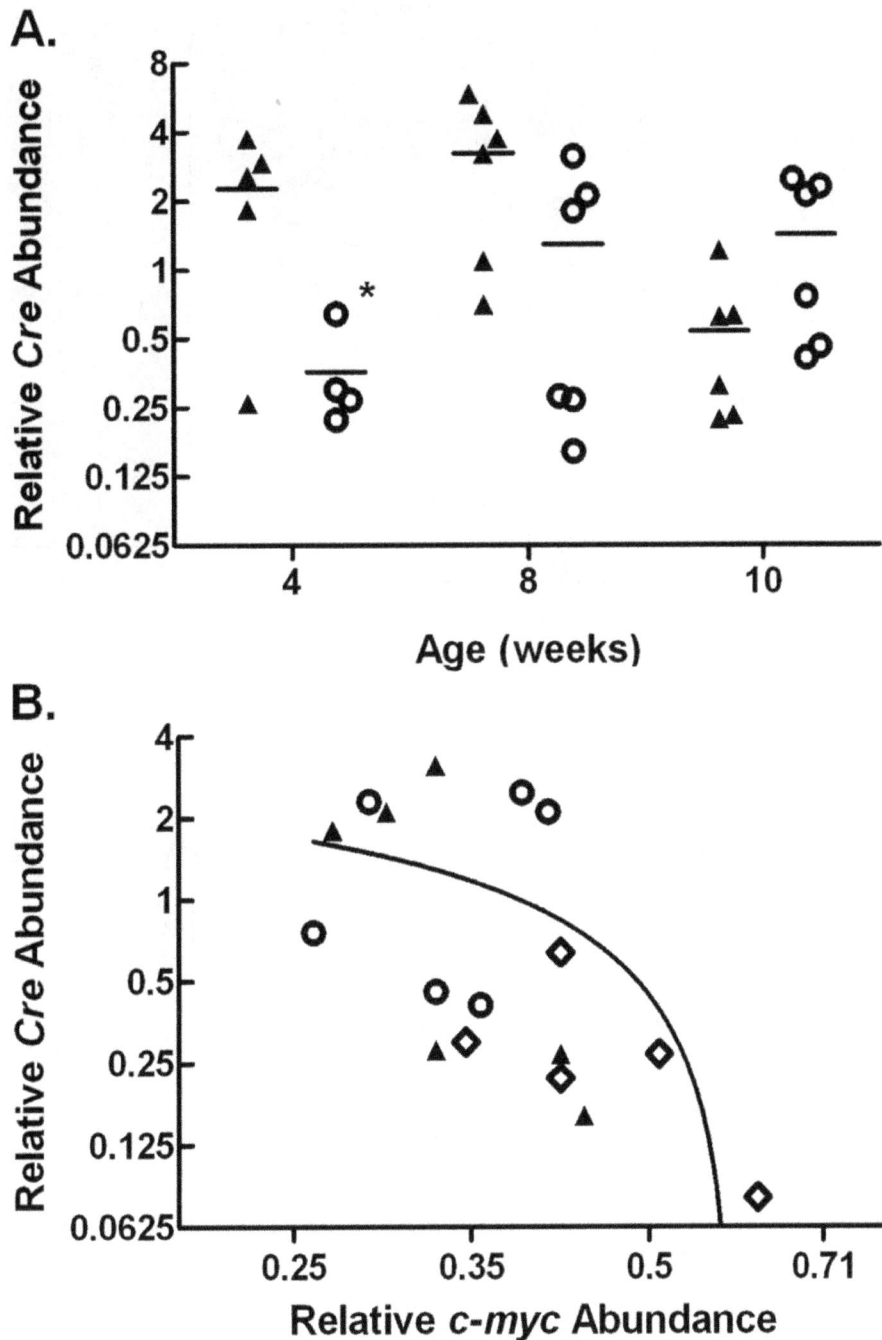

Figure 7 Cre expression in *c-myc* conditional knockout and control mice. A. Total liver RNA was isolated from male and female *c-myc*[+/+]; *Alb-Cre*[+/+] (▲) *and c-myc*[fl/fl];*Alb-Cre*[+/+] (○) mice and *cre* expression assessed using RT-qPCR. Data are shown as individual points with the mean. *, P = 0.0303 4 wk *c-myc*[fl/fl];*Alb-Cre*[+/+] vs control. B. The correlation between *cre* expression and *c-myc* abundance in *c-myc*[fl/fl];*Alb-Cre*[+/+] expressing mice at 4, 8 and 10 weeks of age. Data are expressed as individual points. ◊, 4 weeks; ▲, 8 weeks; ○, 10 weeks.

In light of the qualitative nature of the Lac-Z staining, we prepared liver homogenates from 6-8 week old mice and performed β-gal ELISA assays in order to quantitate Cre activity (data not shown). No difference in B-gal content was found in the *c-myc*[fl/fl];*Alb*-Cre;ROSA26 versus the *c-myc*[+/+];*Alb*-Cre;ROSA26 controls.

Discussion

The transcription factor c-Myc has long been assigned a prominent role in the synchronous hepatocyte proliferation that occurs during liver regeneration [9,11]. A series of *in vivo* studies performed in our laboratory characterizing the regulation of the *c-myc/max/mad*

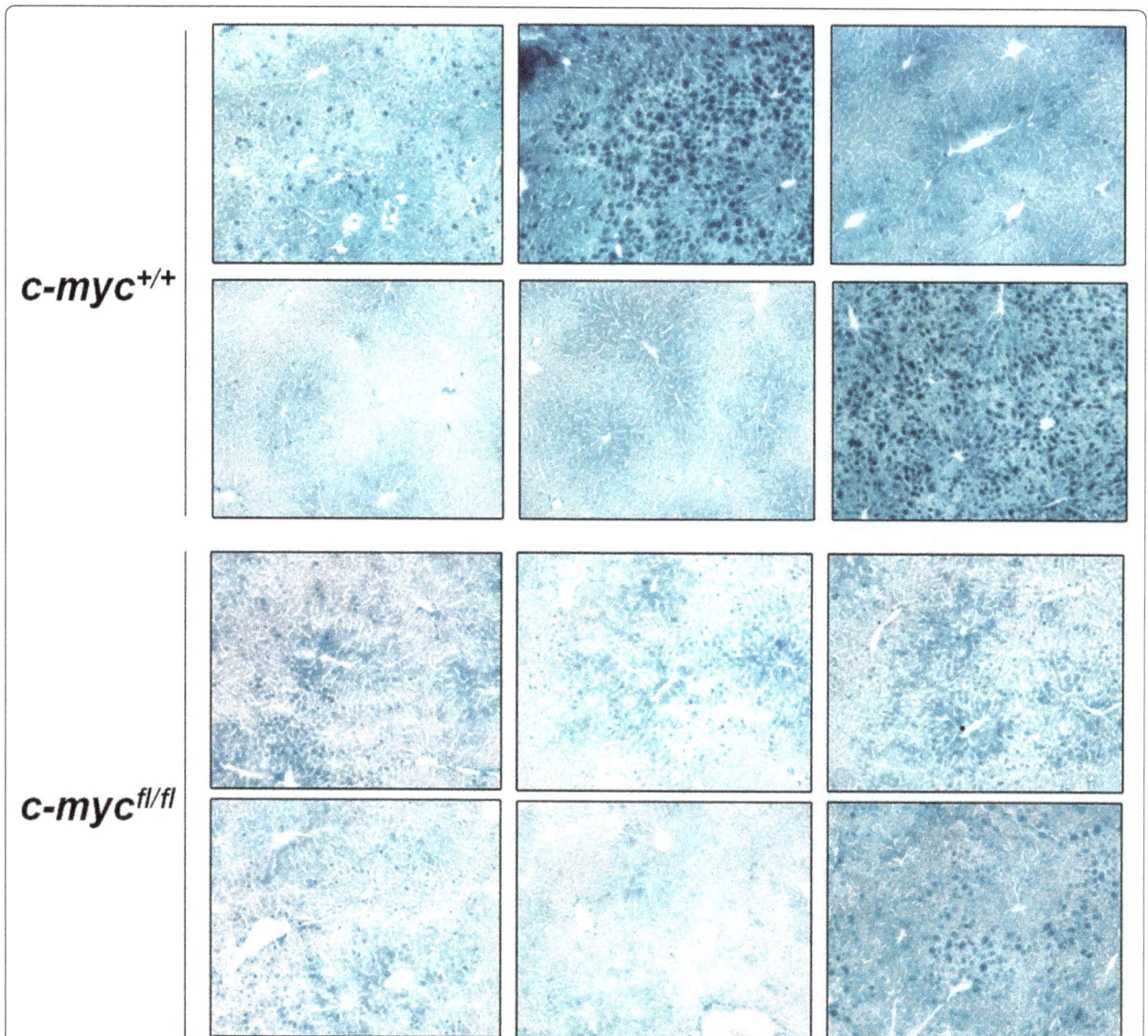

Figure 8 Cre activity in *c-myc* conditional knockout and control mice. Cre expressing *c-myc*[+/+] and *c-myc*[fl/fl] mice were crossed to mice carrying the Rosa26R allele to obtain *c-myc*[+/+];*Rosa;Alb*-Cre and *c-myc*[fl/fl];*Rosa;Alb*-Cre mice. Liver cyrosections (10 μm) from male and female mice were fixed and stained for Lac-Z. Photomicrographs of three 20x fields from individual sections acquired from *c-myc*[+/+];*Rosa;Alb*-Cre and *c-myc*[fl/fl]; *Rosa;Alb*-Cre mice are shown. All panels show images that are representative of the results obtained on multiple sections from at least 2 animals per group. The results were replicated in a duplicate experiment. The contrast was adjusted across the entire image to accurately reflect the appearance of the sections under the microscope.

network in fetal and adult liver revealed that c-Myc was present in quiescent adult hepatocytes and was localized to the nucleolus [16]. These studies led us to hypothesize a functional role for c-Myc in adult liver that was independent of its role in proliferation. In order to test this hypothesis, we generated a conditional knockout using floxed *c-myc* and *Albumin-Cre* mice. This approach led to significant reduction in *c-myc* expression one month after birth in *c-myc*[fl/fl];*Alb*-Cre expressing mice. We observed greater recombination efficiency in *c-myc*[fl/fl];*Alb*-Cre homozygous compared to

hemizygous animals. However, there was no difference in liver weight ratios during development in *c-myc*[fl/fl]; *Alb-Cre*[+/+] compared to *c-myc*[fl/fl];*Alb-Cre*[+] animals. As we did not observe differences in these two groups in regards to histology, liver regeneration or the recovery from fasting, the animals were grouped together for comparison with *c-myc* wild-type *Alb-Cre* expressing mice. There was a low level of residual *c-myc* that persisted in *c-myc*[fl/fl];*Alb-Cre* expressing livers even up to four months. This residual level may be a result of expression in nonparenchymal cells or a subset of hepatocytes in which the albumin promoter is not expressed. However, we were unable to exclude a low level of *c-myc* expression in the larger population of hepatocytes. Interestingly, floxed *c-myc* had an inhibitory effect on *Cre* expression in one month old mice. In contrast, in older animals *Cre* expression was extremely variable regardless of *c-myc* status. This variation may be a result of age-dependent silencing of the *Cre* transgene.

Variegation of transgene expression is a well documented phenomenon in many lines of transgenic mice [32-34] although the cause and mechanism is not known. In a mouse model where *lacZ* was driven by the *β-globin* promoter, there was a general tendency of decreased transgene expression with age [35]. In contrast to other reports on variable transgene expression, we observed a negative effect of our floxed gene on *Cre* recombinase expression. We speculate that this effect is a result of a selective pressure to retain *c-myc* in hepatocytes. It is possible that this selective effect could manifest itself in ways other than an effect on Cre expression.

There was no apparent phenotypic effect of significantly reducing *c-myc* in hepatocytes. The livers of *c-myc^{fl/fl}*;*Alb-Cre* expressing and control mice were of similar size and histology, consistent with the conclusion that *c-myc* is not required for hepatocyte proliferation during normal liver growth and maintenance. We used two models, partial hepatectomy and liver growth following refeeding to determine c-Myc function in the presence or absence of a proliferative stimulus. c-Myc has been considered to have a prominent role in the hepatocyte proliferation that occurs during liver regeneration. After partial hepatectomy there was a slight decrease in the number of hepatocytes in the cell cycle at 48 hr. However, no delay in the restoration of liver mass was observed, indicating that *c-myc* is not required for liver regeneration following 2/3 partial hepatectomy. While these studies were in progress, two conflicting reports were published on the effect of deleting *c-myc* on liver regeneration. Baena et al. found that deletion of *c-myc* resulted in impaired liver regeneration [36]. However, Li et al. reported a total restoration of liver mass by 7 days post-resection in mice where floxed *c-myc* was deleted using adenoviral Cre [37]. In contrast to our study and Li et al., where liver/body mass ratio was used as the outcome measurement for liver regeneration, Baena et al. used PCNA and Cyclin A content as an indirect measure of hepatocyte proliferation. Furthermore, the content of these proteins was only determined 2 day post-hepatectomy leaving it unclear whether liver regeneration would have been affected at later time points. Taken together, these studies indicate that *c-myc* is not essential for restoration of liver mass during regeneration.

In some systems, changes in *c-myc* content affect cell size without affecting cell proliferation [38]. In order to assess the function of c-Myc in a non-proliferative model of hepatocyte growth, mice were fasted for 48 hr followed by a 24 hr refeeding period. In accordance with our published data in the rat, a 48 hr fast resulted in decreased liver/body mass ratio and liver protein content while refeeding resulted in restoration of liver mass and protein despite a significant reduction in *c-myc*. c-Myc has been proposed to play a role in essential processes leading to hepatocyte growth, such as, ribosomal biogenesis and protein synthesis. Kim et al found that transient *c-myc* overexpression in mouse liver led to hepatocyte hypertrophy, the induction of ribosomal genes, and increased protein synthesis [12]. Our results indicate that protein synthesis and hepatocyte growth can occur in spite of a significant reduction in *c-myc*, raising the notion that overexpression of c-Myc may result in the activation of gene regulatory networks and pathways not normally controlled by c-Myc in adult hepatocytes.

Studies by Murphy et al. led to the conclusion that the level of *c-myc* expressed in a cell is crucial to its biological effect [39]. These studies used a mouse model where the activation of Cre recombinase results in the expression of a tamoxifen inducible MycER fusion protein with the amount of c-Myc expressed dependent on whether the mouse carried one or two MycER alleles. The authors report that modest increases in c-Myc can activate cellular proliferation while a higher threshold is needed to stimulate apoptosis. This study suggests that a high level of c-Myc may lead to the binding of a different set of target genes from those regulated by endogenous levels of c-Myc. This notion is further supported by studies on the role of c-Myc in hepatocarcinogenesis. Deregulation of c-Myc through gains in copy number, point mutations, and transactivation by viral proteins is observed in 30-60% of human hepatocellular carcinomas (HCC) [40,41]. Although its role in the development of human HCC is unclear, studies in transgenic mice have shown that overexpression of this oncogene results in increased hepatocyte proliferation, genomic instability and apoptosis. The paradoxical activation of cellular proliferation and growth in concert with apoptosis leads to the requirement of secondary mutations for tumor development [42,43].

Our studies do not rule out a subtle effect of deleting *c-myc* on other aspects of liver physiology. It is possible that *c-myc* deletion affects other pathways. c-Myc has been shown to regulate many genes involved in liver metabolism and can ameliorate the effects of diabetes on glucose metabolism in mice [25,44]. Regardless of potential effects on other pathways overall adult liver physiology appeared to be unaffected by *c-myc* deletion.

Studies performed to assess the requirement and function of c-Myc in other mature tissues suggest that the role of this protein in proliferation, growth, and other cellular processes is cell-type dependent. Deletion of *c-myc* in the hematopoietic lineage results in defective hematopoiesis and angiogenesis leading to embryonic lethality while there was no requirement for *c-myc* in endothelial cells [45]. Moreover, normal adult intestinal homeostasis occurs in the absence of *c-myc*, yet *c-myc* is required for the formation of intestinal crypts [46]. These studies lead to the conclusion that the *in vivo* targets of *c-myc* will vary based on cell type and developmental stage thus adding another layer of complexity to understanding the functional role of *c-myc*.

Conclusions

Our studies indicate that a reduction in hepatic *c-myc* does not affect normal postnatal liver growth and development. Furthermore, reducing this proto-oncogene does not affect the restoration of liver mass during liver regeneration or the restoration of liver protein following fasting. However, our studies do not rule out subtle effects of *c-myc* on liver metabolism or liver physiology. Decreasing *c-myc* correlated with a reduction in the expression of the *Albumin-Cre* transgene, suggesting a selective pressure to maintain *c-myc*. Furthermore, this pressure may prevent the complete deletion of hepatic *c-myc* by traditional conditional knockout strategies.

Acknowledgements

We thank Shu-Whei Tsai for assistance with the animal studies and Kate Brilliant for assistance with cryosections. We also thank Joan Boylan for helpful discussions and critical review of the manuscript. Support for this study was provided by National Institutes of Health grants R01HD24455 and R01HD35831 (to P.G.) and R01FM041690 (to JMS). JAS was supported by National Institutes of Health grant P20RR017695. Core facility support from the COBRE awards P20 RR015578 and P20 RR017695 is also gratefully acknowledged.

Author details

[1]Department of Pediatrics, Rhode Island Hospital and Brown University, Providence, RI 02903, USA. [2]Department of Molecular Biology, Cell Biology and Biochemistry, Brown University, Providence, RI 02912, USA. [3]Center for Genomics and Proteomics, Brown University, Providence, RI 02912, USA. [4]Department of Pathology, MacNeal Hospital, Berwyn, IL, USA.

Authors' contributions

JAS, JMS and PG conceived the study. JAS performed all practical aspects of the study. CS contributed to design and analysis of qPCR assays. The manuscript was prepared by JAS and PG. All authors read and approved the final manuscript.

Competing interests

The authors declare that they have no competing interests.

References

1. Mao DY, Watson JD, Yan PS, Barsyte-Lovejoy D, Khosravi F, Wong WW, et al: Analysis of Myc bound loci identified by CpG island arrays shows that Max is essential for Myc-dependent repression. *Curr Biol* 2003, 13:882-886.
2. O'Connell BC, Cheung AF, Simkevich CP, Tam W, Ren X, Mateyak MK, et al: A large scale genetic analysis of c-Myc-regulated gene expression patterns. *J Biol Chem* 2003, 278:12563-12573.
3. Grandori C, Cowley SM, James LP, Eisenman RN: The Myc/Max/Mad network and the transcriptional control of cell behavior. *Annu Rev Cell Dev Biol* 2000, 16:653-699.
4. Gregory MA, Xiao Q, Cornwall GA, Lutterbach B, Hann SR: B-Myc is preferentially expressed in hormonally-controlled tissues and inhibits cellular proliferation. *Oncogene* 2000, 19:4886-4895.
5. Prochownik EV: c-Myc as a therapeutic target in cancer. *Expert Rev Anticancer Ther* 2004, 4:289-302.
6. Lin CP, Liu JD, Chow JM, Liu CR, Liu HE: Small-molecule c-Myc inhibitor, 10058-F4, inhibits proliferation, downregulates human telomerase reverse transcriptase and enhances chemosensitivity in human hepatocellular carcinoma cells. *Anticancer Drugs* 2007, 18:161-170.
7. Ohgaki H, Sanderson ND, Ton P, Thorgeirsson SS: Molecular analyses of liver tumors in c-myc transgenic mice and c-myc and TGF-alpha double transgenic mice. *Cancer Lett* 1996, 106:43-49.
8. Collier JJ, Doan TT, Daniels MC, Schurr JR, Kolls JK, Scott DK: c-Myc is required for the glucose-mediated induction of metabolic enzyme genes. *J Biol Chem* 2003, 278:6588-6595.
9. Fausto N, Mead JE, Braun L, Thompson NL, Panzica M, Goyette M, et al: Proto-oncogene expression and growth factors during liver regeneration. *Symp Fundam Cancer Res* 1986, 39:69-86.
10. Steer CJ: Liver regeneration. *FASEB J* 1995, 9:1396-1400.
11. Thompson NL, Mead JE, Braun L, Goyette M, Shank PR, Fausto N: Sequential protooncogene expression during rat liver regeneration. *Cancer Res* 1986, 46:3111-3117.
12. Kim S, Li Q, Dang CV, Lee LA: Induction of ribosomal genes and hepatocyte hypertrophy by adenovirus-mediated expression of c-Myc in vivo. *Proc Natl Acad Sci USA* 2000, 97:11198-11202.
13. Riu E, Ferre T, Hidalgo A, Mas A, Franckhauser S, Otaegui P, et al: Overexpression of c-myc in the liver prevents obesity and insulin resistance. *FASEB J* 2003, 17:1715-1717.
14. Riu E, Bosch F, Valera A: Prevention of diabetic alterations in transgenic mice overexpressing Myc in the liver. *Proc Natl Acad Sci USA* 1996, 93:2198-2202.
15. Sanders JA, Gruppuso PA: Coordinated regulation of c-Myc and Max in rat liver development. *Am J Physiol Gastrointest Liver Physiol* 2006, 290: G145-G155.
16. Sanders JA, Gruppuso PA: Nucleolar localization of hepatic c-Myc: a potential mechanism for c-Myc regulation. *Biochim Biophys Acta* 2005, 1743:141-150.
17. de Alboran IM, O'Hagan RC, Gartner F, Malynn B, Davidson L, Rickert R, et al: Analysis of C-MYC function in normal cells via conditional gene-targeted mutation. *Immunity* 2001, 14:45-55.
18. Postic C, Shiota M, Niswender KD, Jetton TL, Chen Y, Moates JM, et al: Dual roles for glucokinase in glucose homeostasis as determined by liver and pancreatic beta cell-specific gene knock-outs using Cre recombinase. *J Biol Chem* 1999, 274:305-315.
19. Soriano P: Generalized lacZ expression with the ROSA26 Cre reporter strain. *Nat Genet* 1999, 21:70-71.
20. Higgins GM, Anderson RM: Restoration of the liver of the white rat following partial removal. *Arch Path Lab Med* 1931, 12:916-922.
21. de Alboran IM, Baena E, Martinez A: c-Myc-deficient B lymphocytes are resistant to spontaneous and induced cell death. *Cell Death Differ* 2004, 11:61-68.
22. Le Y, Sauer B: Conditional gene knockout using Cre recombinase. *Mol Biotechnol* 2001, 17:269-275.
23. Davis AC, Wims M, Spotts GD, Hann SR, Bradley A: A null c-myc mutation causes lethality before 10.5 days of gestation in homozygotes and reduced fertility in heterozygous female mice. *Genes Dev* 1993, 7:671.
24. Postic C, Magnuson MA: DNA excision in liver by an albumin-Cre transgene occurs progressively with age. *Genesis* 2000, 26:149-150.
25. Riu E, Ferre T, Mas A, Hidalgo A, Franckhauser S, Bosch F: Overexpression of c-myc in diabetic mice restores altered expression of the

transcription factor genes that regulate liver metabolism. *Biochem J* 2002, **368**:931-937.

26. Anand P, Gruppuso PA: **Rapamycin inhibits liver growth during refeeding in rats via control of ribosomal protein translation but not cap-dependent translation initiation.** *J Nutr* 2006, **136**:27-33.

27. Thompson MD, Monga SP: **WNT/beta-catenin signaling in liver health and disease.** *Hepatology* 2007, **45**:1298-1305.

28. He TC, Sparks AB, Rago C, Hermeking H, Zawel L, da Costa LT, *et al*: **Identification of c-MYC as a target of the APC pathway.** *Science* 1998, **281**:1509-1512.

29. Mayhew CN, Bosco EE, Fox SR, Okaya T, Tarapore P, Schwemberger SJ, *et al*: **Liver-specific pRB loss results in ectopic cell cycle entry and aberrant ploidy.** *Cancer Res* 2005, **65**:4568-4577.

30. Romero-Gallo J, Sozmen EG, Chytil A, Russell WE, Whitehead R, Parks WT, *et al*: **Inactivation of TGF-beta signaling in hepatocytes results in an increased proliferative response after partial hepatectomy.** *Oncogene* 2005, **24**:3028-3041.

31. Michael MD, Kulkarni RN, Postic C, Previs SF, Shulman GI, Magnuson MA, *et al*: **Loss of insulin signaling in hepatocytes leads to severe insulin resistance and progressive hepatic dysfunction.** *Mol Cell* 2000, **6**:87-97.

32. Schulz TJ, Glaubitz M, Kuhlow D, Thierbach R, Birringer M, Steinberg P, *et al*: **Variable expression of Cre recombinase transgenes precludes reliable prediction of tissue-specific gene disruption by tail-biopsy genotyping.** *PLoS One* 2007, **2**:e1013.

33. Garrick D, Sutherland H, Robertson G, Whitelaw E: **Variegated expression of a globin transgene correlates with chromatin accessibility but not methylation status.** *Nucleic Acids Res* 1996, **24**:4902-4909.

34. Dobie KW, Lee M, Fantes JA, Graham E, Clark AJ, Springbett A, *et al*: **Variegated transgene expression in mouse mammary gland is determined by the transgene integration locus.** *Proc Natl Acad Sci USA* 1996, **93**:6659-6664.

35. Robertson G, Garrick D, Wilson M, Martin DI, Whitelaw E: **Age-dependent silencing of globin transgenes in the mouse.** *Nucleic Acids Res* 1996, **24**:1465-1471.

36. Baena E, Gandarillas A, Vallespinos M, Zanet J, Bachs O, Redondo C, *et al*: **c-Myc regulates cell size and ploidy but is not essential for postnatal proliferation in liver.** *Proc Natl Acad Sci USA* 2005, **102**:7286-7291.

37. Li F, Xiang Y, Potter J, Dinavahi R, Dang CV, Lee LA: **Conditional deletion of c-myc does not impair liver regeneration.** *Cancer Res* 2006, **66**:5608-5612.

38. Zanet J, Pibre S, Jacquet C, Ramirez A, de Alboran IM, Gandarillas A: **Endogenous Myc controls mammalian epidermal cell size, hyperproliferation, endoreplication and stem cell amplification.** *J Cell Sci* 2005, **118**:1693-1704.

39. Murphy DJ, Junttila MR, Pouyet L, Karnezis A, Shchors K, Bui DA, *et al*: **Distinct thresholds govern Myc's biological output in vivo.** *Cancer Cell* 2008, **14**:447-457.

40. Schlaeger C, Longerich T, Schiller C, Bewerunge P, Mehrabi A, Toedt G, *et al*: **Etiology-dependent molecular mechanisms in human hepatocarcinogenesis.** *Hepatology* 2008, **47**:511-520.

41. Feitelson MA: **c-myc overexpression in hepatocarcinogenesis.** *Hum Pathol* 2004, **35**:1299-1302.

42. Calvisi DF, Thorgeirsson SS: **Molecular mechanisms of hepatocarcinogenesis in transgenic mouse models of liver cancer.** *Toxicol Pathol* 2005, **33**:181-184.

43. Cavin LG, Wang F, Factor VM, Kaur S, Venkatraman M, Thorgeirsson SS, *et al*: **Transforming growth factor-alpha inhibits the intrinsic pathway of c-Myc-induced apoptosis through activation of nuclear factor-kappaB in murine hepatocellular carcinomas.** *Mol Cancer Res* 2005, **3**:403-412.

44. Valera A, Pujol A, Gregori X, Riu E, Visa J, Bosch F: **Evidence from transgenic mice that myc regulates hepatic glycolysis.** *FASEB J* 1995, **9**:1067-1078.

45. He C, Hu H, Braren R, Fong SY, Trumpp A, Carlson TR, *et al*: **c-myc in the hematopoietic lineage is crucial for its angiogenic function in the mouse embryo.** *Development* 2008, **135**:2467-2477.

46. Bettess MD, Dubois N, Murphy MJ, Dubey C, Roger C, Robine S, *et al*: **c-Myc is required for the formation of intestinal crypts but dispensable for homeostasis of the adult intestinal epithelium.** *Mol Cell Biol* 2005, **25**:7868-7878.

2

Sympathoactivation and rho-kinase-dependent baroreflex function in experimental renovascular hypertension with reduced kidney mass

Rainer U Pliquett[1,2*], Sebastian Benkhoff[1], Oliver Jung[1,3] and Ralf P Brandes[1]

Abstract

Background: Dysregulation of the autonomic nervous system is frequent in subjects with cardiovascular disease. The contribution of different forms of renovascular hypertension and the mechanisms contributing to autonomic dysfunction in hypertension are incompletely understood. Here, murine models of renovascular hypertension with preserved (2-kidneys-1 clip, 2K1C) and reduced (1-kidney-1 clip, 1K1C) kidney mass were studied with regard to autonomic nervous system regulation (sympathetic tone: power-spectral analysis of systolic blood pressure; parasympathetic tone: power-spectral analysis of heart rate) and baroreflex sensitivity of heart rate by spontaneous, concomitant changes of systolic blood pressure and pulse interval. Involvement of the renin-angiotensin system and the rho-kinase pathway were determined by application of inhibitors.

Results: C57BL6N mice (6 to 11) with reduced kidney mass (1K1C) or with preserved kidney mass (2K1C) developed a similar degree of hypertension. In comparison to control mice, both models presented with a significantly increased sympathetic tone and lower baroreflex sensitivity of heart rate. However, only 2K1C animals had a lower parasympathetic tone, whereas urinary norepinephrine excretion was reduced in the 1K1C model. Rho kinase inhibition given to a subset of 1K1C and 2K1C animals improved baroreflex sensitivity of heart rate selectively in the 1K1C model. Rho kinase inhibition had no additional effects on autonomic nervous system in either model of renovascular hypertension and did not change the blood pressure. Blockade of AT1 receptors (in 2K1C animals) normalized the sympathetic tone, decreased resting heart rate, improved baroreflex sensitivity of heart rate and parasympathetic tone.

Conclusions: Regardless of residual renal mass, blood pressure and sympathetic tone are increased, whereas baroreflex sensitivity is depressed in murine models of renovascular hypertension. Reduced norepinephrine excretion and/or degradation might contribute to sympathoactivation in renovascular hypertension with reduced renal mass (1K1C). Overall, the study helps to direct research to optimize medical therapy of hypertension.

Keywords: Arterial hypertension, Sympathetic nervous system, Baroreflex, Irbesartan

Background

Nephrogenic arterial hypertension comprising renovascular and renoparenchymal aetiologies is increasingly prevalent [1]. Hypertensive patients with chronic kidney disease (CKD) are three times more likely to die within 8 years than hypertensive counterparts without CKD [2]. Regarding renovascular hypertension, revascularization strategies do not convey any benefit when compared to the best conservative therapy [3,4]. Angiotensin II-subtype-1 (AT1) receptor blockers [5] or angiotensin-converting enzyme (ACE) inhibitors [6] slow the progression of CKD, yet they are contraindicated in bilateral renal artery stenosis or in unilateral renal artery stenosis and (functional) single kidney situation. Given the constraints inherent to medical and interventional therapies of renovascular hypertension, novel therapeutic targets are still needed.

The autonomic nervous system is such a potential target. Baroreflex function is attenuated in renovascular disease, regardless of residual kidney mass [7]. On the basis

* Correspondence: rpliquett@endothel.de
[1]Institute for Cardiovascular Physiology, Vascular Research Centre, Fachbereich Medizin, Goethe University, Frankfurt (Main), Germany
[2]Department of Nephrology, Clinic of Internal Medicine 2, University Clinic Halle, Martin Luther University Halle-Wittenberg, Ernst-Grube-Str. 40, Halle (Saale) 06120, Germany
Full list of author information is available at the end of the article

of the effect of propranolol and atropine methyl nitrate on resting heart rate, an elevated sympathetic tone in models of renovascular hypertension with (1-kidney-one-clip; 1K1C) and without kidney-mass reduction (2-kidneys-one-clip; 2K1C) was identified [8,9]. Aside from heart-rate changes, muscle sympathetic nerve activity [10] and functional data like cold-pressor test [11] were not affected by propranolol. Therefore, additional surrogates of sympathetic tone are needed.

The pathomechanism of sympathoactivation in renovascular hypertension is unclear. In experimental renovascular hypertension with preserved kidney mass (2K1C), the renin-angiotensin-aldosterone system (RAAS) is found to be activated [12], and central nervous system effects of angiotensin II probably are the driving force of sympathoactivation [13]. In experimental renovascular hypertension with reduced kidney mass (1K1C), however, the RAAS is suppressed [12], and other sympathoactivating pathomechanisms must be operative.

The intracellular Rho A/Rho kinase system emerges as a novel target for the treatment of cardiovascular disease [14]. Rho A, a small GTPase, has numerous functions and is involved in cytoskeletal organization. Upon activation, Rho A interacts with and activates the Rho A-dependent kinase (ROCK). As a consequence endothelial nitric oxide synthase mRNA is destabilized and cellular contraction is initiated by means of calcium-sensitization [15] which also increases endothelial cell permeability [16].

Established Rho A/ROCK inhibitors are Fasudil but also statins, 3-hydroxy-3-methylglutaryl-Coenzyme A reductase inhibitors. Statins inhibit the formation of geranyl-geranylpyrophosphate, a prerequisite for RhoA membrane anchoring [14,17]. We have previously shown that simvastatin lowers sympathetic tone in experimental chronic heart failure, another condition characterized by sympathoexcitation [18,19]. Also ROCK inhibition (ROKI) by Fasudil was shown to improve baroreflex sensitivity in experimental chronic heart failure when given in to the intracerebroventricular space [20]. This effect was blunted by intracerebroventricular application of L-NAME, an inhibitor of endothelial nitric oxide synthase, suggesting direct central effects and a contribution of central nitric oxide in this process. The value of ROCK inhibition for the treatment of hypertension at large, however, is still unclear.

In the present study, we hypothesize that sympathoactivation is more pronounced in renovascular hypertension with preserved (2K1C) versus reduced (1K1C) kidney mass when using heart-rate independent surrogates of sympathetic tone. Sham surgery animals and irbesartan (Irb)-treated 2K1C animals were used as control groups. The AT1-receptor blocker treatment was used as a positive control for its sympathoinhibitory actions [21-24]. Secondly, we hypothesize that ROKI enhances

baroreflex sensitivity of heart rate in models of renovascular hypertension (1K1C; 2K1C) in analogy to the chronic-heart failure situation [20].

Methods

Animals

Male C57BL/6 N mice (6–11 per group, age: 10–12 weeks, Charles River, Sulzfeld, Germany) were housed in individual cages in a separate room under standard conditions (21°C, 12 h dark–light cycle), standard chow and drinking water ad libitum. Care was provided daily at the same time, body weight was taken weekly. All animal procedures and experiments adhered to the APS's Guiding Principles in the Care and Use of Vertebrate Animals in Research and Training. During surgeries, inhalational anaesthesia using a precision vaporizer with isoflurane (2% initially, 0.8–1% continuously in an oxygen stream of 0.2 l/min), and subcutaneous (SC) fentanyl (0.06 mg/kg) were used. Following surgeries, pain-relief medication buprenorphine (0.3 mg/kg SC), and antibiotic prophylaxis with ampicillin (50 mg/kg SC) were administered. After observing the animals for 4–6 weeks, mice were sacrificed (isoflurane anaesthesia, decapitation), and heart weight (absolute and relative to body weight) was determined. Ethical approval was obtained from local animal-care officials and the supervising federal authority (approval number: V54-19c20/15F28K2154 issued by Regierungspräsidium Darmstadt, Hesse, Germany).

Telemetric monitoring

Aortic blood pressure of unrestrained, conscious mice was monitored by telemetry (telemetry unit: TA11PA-C10, Data Sciences International, St. Paul, Minnesota, USA) attached to a femoral-artery catheter. For catheter placement, a 15 mm skin incision was made, and the left femoral artery and vein were separated using a non-serrated fine-tip forceps (Dumont°, Roboz Surgical Instrument Co. Inc., USA). The left femoral artery was tied off (PERMA-HAND° silk, Ethicon, USA) caudally of the superficial epigastric and superficial circumflex iliac artery. A second tie was placed 10 to 12 mm cranially and kept under tension to stop perfusion. A 90°-bent 26 gauge injection needle serving as a catheter introducer was inserted into the left common femoral artery right above the distal tie. The telemetry catheter was inserted and advanced to the proximal tie. After releasing the proximal tie temporarily, the catheter was further advanced into the lower aorta (below the renal artery) and secured by two knots. After freeing a subcutaneous pouch on the right flank, the transmitter unit connected to the intra-arterial catheter was inserted and 0.05 – 0.1 g gentamicin solution (3 mg/g) was applied before skin suture (4–0 Prolene, Ethicon, USA). Blood pressure readings were transmitted to a receiver placed below the mouse cage, digitized with a sampling rate of 1000 Hz and stored and analyzed on a workstation in a separate room. Systolic and diastolic blood pressures, pulse pressure and pulse intervals (defined as consecutive dP/dt) were extracted from aortic blood pressure waveforms using ART 4.2 Gold software (Data Sciences International; St. Paul, Minnesota, USA). One week later, the mice were randomized in a 1:2 fashion to sham surgery (normal controls) or unilateral renal-artery stenosis, i.e. the 2K1C model of hypertension with preserved kidney mass. There, a U-shaped metal clip (Exidel SA, Switzerland; width: 110 ± 0.07 μm) was implanted around the right renal artery as reported previously [12,25]. One week later, every second 2K1C mouse was subjected to nephrectomy of the non-clipped kidney yielding the 1K1C model of renovascular hypertension with reduced kidney mass.

Autonomic nervous system testing

After a two-week recovery period, a one-hour baseline recording was taken in the morning. Thereafter, intra-peritoneal injections of atropine-methyl nitrate (ATR, 2 mg/kg in 4 ml/kg saline, Sigma) [26] or metoprolol (MET, 1 mg/kg in 4 ml/kg saline; Sigma) were performed. ATR was used to block the parasympathetic component while MET was used to block the sympathetic component of the autonomic nervous system. After injection of either substance, another hour of continuous blood-pressure recording was performed. For each one-hour recording, the last 30 minutes were used for analysis. Mean heart rate and blood pressure were determined. In addition, consecutive, continuous one-minute series of digitized systolic blood pressure and pulse-interval data were linearly interpolated with an equidistant sampling interval of 0.05 s (20 Hz). Power spectral analysis of those systolic blood pressure and pulse intervals was performed using Fourier transformation (1024-point series corresponding to a 51.2-s period). Each spectral band obtained was a harmonic of 20/1024 Hz (0.019 Hz). The power spectral analysis of blood pressure and pulse intervals yielded intensities (units: $mmHg^2$ and ms^2) for a given spectral bandwidth. The cumulative intensity of the low-frequency band (0.15-0.6 Hz) of power spectrum of systolic blood pressure (LF-SBP) was regarded as a quantitative measure of sympathetic tone, whereas the cumulative intensity of the high-frequency band (2.5-5.0 Hz) of power spectrum of heart rate (HF-HRV) was considered as a quantitative measure of parasympathetic tone [26,27].

Power spectrum (high-frequency band: 1.0-5 Hz) of systolic blood pressure (HF-SBP) [28,29] and power spectrum (low-frequency band: 0.4-1.5 Hz) of heart rate (LF-HRV) were provided as supplemental data. With regard to sympathovagal balance, interpretation of HF-SBP data still remains inconclusive for the mouse model. However, in contrast to humans, LF-HRV is considered to be an alternative quantitative measure of parasympathetic tone in mice [30].

In addition, changes in resting heart rate after administration of metoprolol or atropine were determined. An overnight recovery was required after injection of either substance.

Baroreflex sensitivity

Baroreflex sensitivity was determined by the sequence technique [31] of concomitant changes of systolic blood pressure and pulse intervals (digitized, linearly interpolated) utilizing the Hemolab software (http://www.haraldstauss.com/HemoLab/HemoLab.php). Concomitant changes of systolic blood pressure (of at least 15 mmHg) and pulse intervals of at least 4 consecutive heart beats were correlated. For individual baroreflex curves, a correlation coefficient of at least 0.9 was mandated for analysis. In addition, a time delay of 0 seconds was chosen for analysis of concomitant blood-pressure and pulse-interval changes according to a previous study with murine models [32]. The average of at least 10 individual baroreflex slopes (linear portion of systolic blood pressure – pulse-interval relationship; unit: Δbpm/ΔmmHg) was considered as baroreflex sensitivity.

Urinary catecholamine assay

Mice were placed in metabolic cages (Tecniplast) for 24-hour urine collection. Urine was collected over 24 hours in a vial containing 30 μl HCl (0.5 mol/l), stored at –20°C. For analysis urinary norepinephrine, dopamine and epinephrine were determined by a radioimmunoassay method (LDN 3-CAT RIA, Labor Diagnostika Nord, Nordhorn, Germany).

Medical intervention

The AT1 receptor blocker irbesartan (Irb) was dissolved in water (c = 150 mg/l, projected dose: 30 mg/kg/d) and given to five 2K1C mice orally ad libitum. Drug uptake was recorded by weighing drinking bottles every 48 h. Likewise, the Rho-kinase inhibitor SAR407899A was given to 2K1C and 1K1C mice with the drinking water (c = 50 mg/l, projected dose: 10 mg/kg/d). The actual drug uptake is shown in Table 1. Experiments were carried out after 7 – 9 days

Table 1 Drug uptake with the drinking water (mg/kg/d) in renovascular-hypertension models: 2-kidney-1-clip, 1-kidney-1-clip

	2-kidneys-1-clip model of hypertension	1-kidney-1-clip model of hypertension	P
Rho-kinase inhibitor SAR407899A	10.5 ± 2.4	10.9 ± 3.5	ns
Irbesartan	26.8 ± 2.0	NA	NA

Statistical analysis was performed between groups.

on treatment and compared to normal controls and to 2K1C animals without treatment. Irbesartan and the Rho-kinase inhibitor SAR407899A were kindly provided by Sanofi-Aventis, Frankfurt/Main, Germany.

Statistics

Results are given as means ± one standard deviation. For inter-group comparisons with equal variances, one-way ANOVA/Newman-Keul post-hoc test or one- or two-tailed student's t-test were used, where appropriate. If the normality test failed, nonparametric tests (Kruskal Wallis test/Dunn's post-hoc test or – for two-groups - Mann–Whitney-U or Wilcoxon-matched pairs test) were used, where appropriate. A p < 0.05 was considered significant. Asterisks highlight significances (*p < 0.05; **p < 0.01; ***p < 0.001). Statistical analysis was carried out with Graphpad (La Jolla, California, USA).

Results

Characteristics of models of renovascular arterial hypertension (2K1C, 1K1C)

Pulse pressure, systolic and diastolic blood pressure were significantly elevated in both models (2K1C, 1K1C)

of renovascular hypertension as compared to controls (Figure 1, upper panel). Treatment with the Rho-kinase inhibitor SAR407899A did not affect blood pressure (data not shown). In comparison to controls, 1K1C animals also exhibited an increase in both absolute and relative heart weight. This difference in heart weight was not observed after ROKI (SAR407899A) treatment (Figure 1, lower panel). As the increase in heart weight indicates left-ventricular hypertrophy, this finding suggests that ROKI treatment attenuates 1K1C-associated left-ventricular hypertrophy.

Heart rate was not different among groups at baseline or following selective autonomic-nervous-system blockade with atropine (ATR) or metoprolol (MET) (Table 2). However, resting heart rate significantly increased in response to ATR in all groups. In the control group, ATR also increased the diastolic blood pressure. Neither pulse pressure nor systolic blood pressure were affected by ATR or MET in any group. To gauge autonomic nervous system effects of an AT1 blockade, Irb treatment was performed in 2K1C animals. Hemodynamic effects of Irb included a decrease of both systolic blood pressure and heart rate in 2K1C animals (Figure 2).

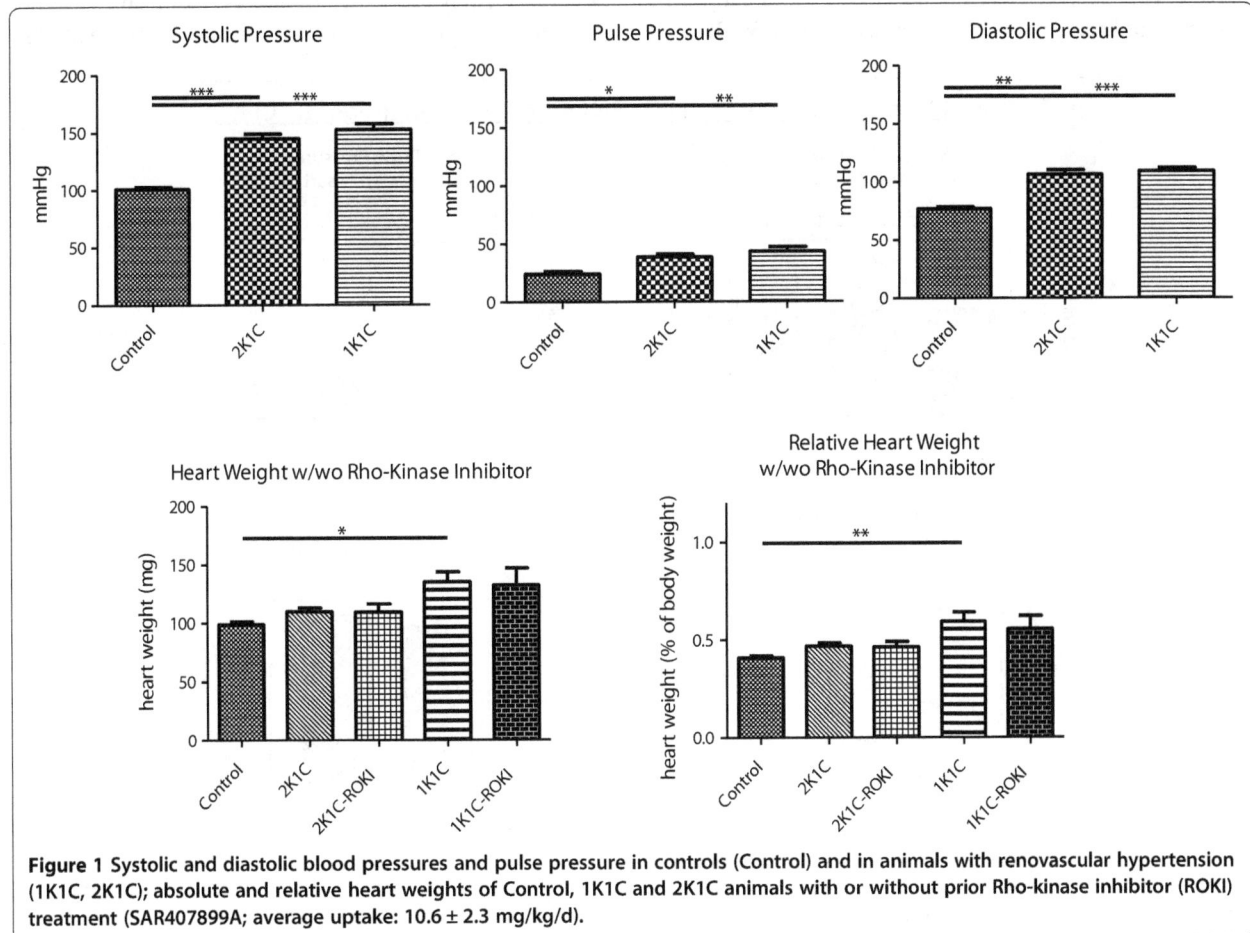

Figure 1 Systolic and diastolic blood pressures and pulse pressure in controls (Control) and in animals with renovascular hypertension (1K1C, 2K1C); absolute and relative heart weights of Control, 1K1C and 2K1C animals with or without prior Rho-kinase inhibitor (ROKI) treatment (SAR407899A; average uptake: 10.6 ± 2.3 mg/kg/d).

Table 2 Baseline characteristics of renovascular-hypertension models (2-kidney-1-clip, 1-kidney-1-clip), and of normal controls following sham-surgery

	Normal controls	2-kidneys-1-clip model of hypertension	1-kidney-1-clip model of hypertension	P
Heart rate (bpm)	455.3 ± 60.8	472.5 ± 54.9	463.6 ± 55.4	ns
Systolic blood pressure - baseline (mmHg)	100.9 ± 5.5	144.8 ± 13.0	152.3 ± 16.6	<0.0001
Diastolic blood pressure - baseline (mmHg)	76.7 ± 4.3	106.4 ± 12.7	109.2 ± 8.7	0.0001
Heart rate – after atropine (bpm)	559.8 ± 58.1	575.9 ± 82.5	604.4 ± 55.4	ns
Systolic blood pressure - after atropine (mmHg)	108.9 ± 6.6	152.7 ± 16.1	151.2 ± 15.3	<0.0001
Diastolic blood pressure - after atropine (mmHg)	85.9 ± 6.0	116.0 ± 11.9	111.2 ± 8.4	<0.0001
Heart rate – after metoprolol (bpm)	463.0 ± 74.0	513.8 ± 67.6	479.3 ± 49.4	ns
Systolic blood pressure - after metoprolol (mmHg)	100.2 ± 10.8	155.1 ± 14.9	151.1 ± 15.3	<0.0001
Diastolic blood pressure - after metoprolol (mmHg)	77.3 ± 9.2	114.1 ± 13.4	111.4 ± 10.5	<0.0001

Statistical analysis was performed among groups.

Baroreflex sensitivity of heart rate is attenuated in models of renovascular hypertension, irrespective of residual renal mass (2K1C, 1K1C)

In comparison to controls, baroreflex sensitivity of heart rate was significantly attenuated in both models of renovascular hypertension. Beta-1-adrenergic blockade with MET did not alter this difference (Figure 3A-B). Following ATR, baroreflex sensitivity of heart rate was blunted in all groups. AT1-receptor blockade with Irb restored baroreflex sensitivity of heart rate in 2K1C animals (Figure 3C-D).

Elevated sympathetic tone in both models of renovascular arterial hypertension (2K1C, 1K1C)

In comparison to controls, both models of renovascular hypertension (2K1C, 1K1C) presented with an elevated sympathetic nervous system tone as determined by power spectral analysis of systolic blood pressure. In 2K1C as well as in 1K1C animals, sympathoactivation persisted after ATR application (Figure 4A-B). In the 2K1C model, sympathetic tone was significantly higher without Irb and returned to normal levels with Irb

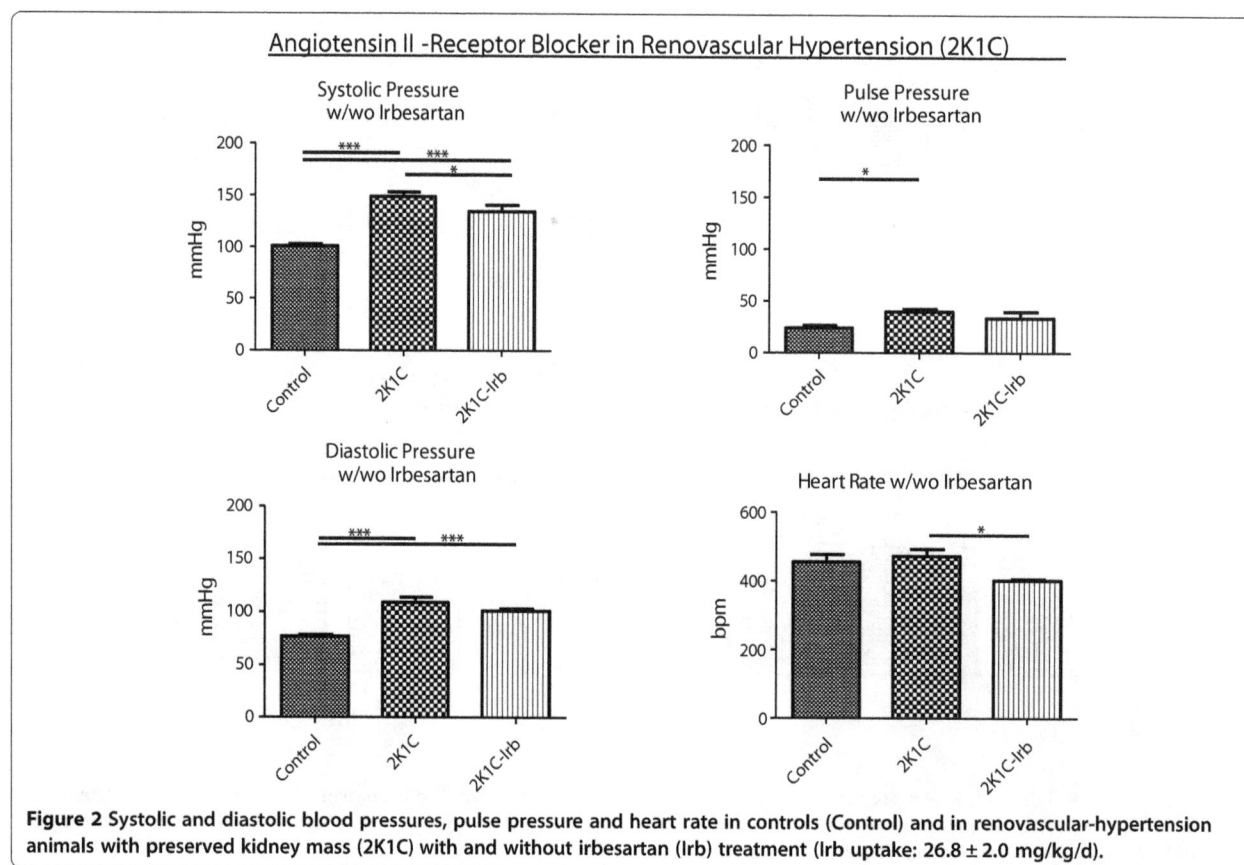

Figure 2 Systolic and diastolic blood pressures, pulse pressure and heart rate in controls (Control) and in renovascular-hypertension animals with preserved kidney mass (2K1C) with and without irbesartan (Irb) treatment (Irb uptake: 26.8 ± 2.0 mg/kg/d).

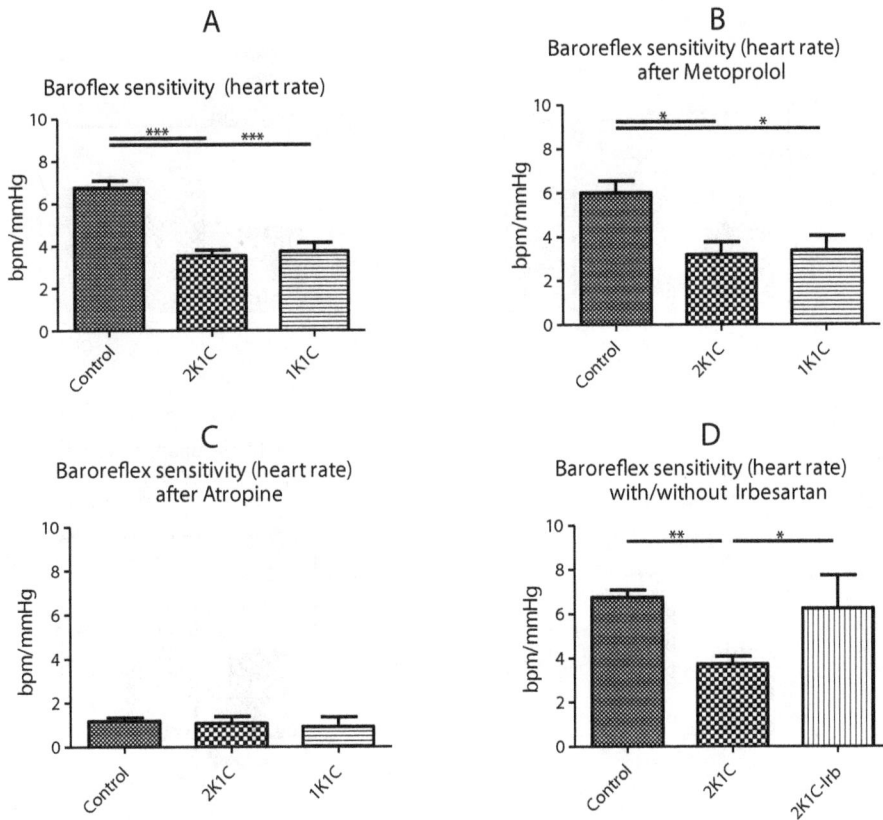

Figure 3 Baroreflex sensitivity of heart rate in controls (Control), 1K1C, and 2K1C animals (A); in Control, 1K1C, and 2K1C animals following MET (B); in Control, 1K1C, and 2K1C animals following ATR (C); in Control and in irbesartan (Irb)-treated and untreated 2K1C animals (D).

treatment. This effect was maintained after ATR injection (Figure 4C-D).

Parasympathetic tone is reduced in the model of renovascular hypertension with preserved kidney mass (2K1C)

Parasympathetic tone, as determined by the cumulative intensity of HF-HRV, was significantly attenuated in both models of renovascular hypertension. Beta-adrenergic blockade with MET confirmed the significant attenuation of parasympathetic tone in 2K1C animals. An AT1-receptor blockade with Irb prevented the significant attenuation of parasympathetic tone in comparison to controls (Figure 5, upper panel).

As an alternative assessment of parasympathetic tone, LV-HRV was determined (Table 3). Following metoprolol, LF-HRV data confirmed the suppression of parasympathetic tone in 2K1C animals in comparison to controls (p < 0.05 in post-hoc test). However, when using LF-HRV as a surrogate for parasympathetic tone, there was no significant change in parasympathetic tone

following AT1-receptor blockade in 2K1C animals (Table 4). In addition to the LF-HRV data, HF-SBP data is provided for all groups in Table 3 and Table 4.

Collectively, renovascular hypertension with preserved kidney mass (2K1C) associates with a lower parasympathetic tone when compared to normal controls, which is reversed, at least partly, by AT1 receptor blocker treatment.

Urinary catecholamines do not reflect sympathoexcitation in renovascular hypertension

Urinary norepinephrine excretion was significantly reduced in renovascular hypertension with reduced kidney mass (1K1C) when compared to normal controls (Figure 5, lower panel). In renovascular hypertension with preserved kidney mass, norepinephrine excretion was not different when compared to 1K1C animals or normal controls. This finding contrasts telemetric power spectral data of systolic blood pressure suggesting a state of sympathoactivation in both models of hypertension (1K1C, 2K1C), irrespective of residual kidney mass.

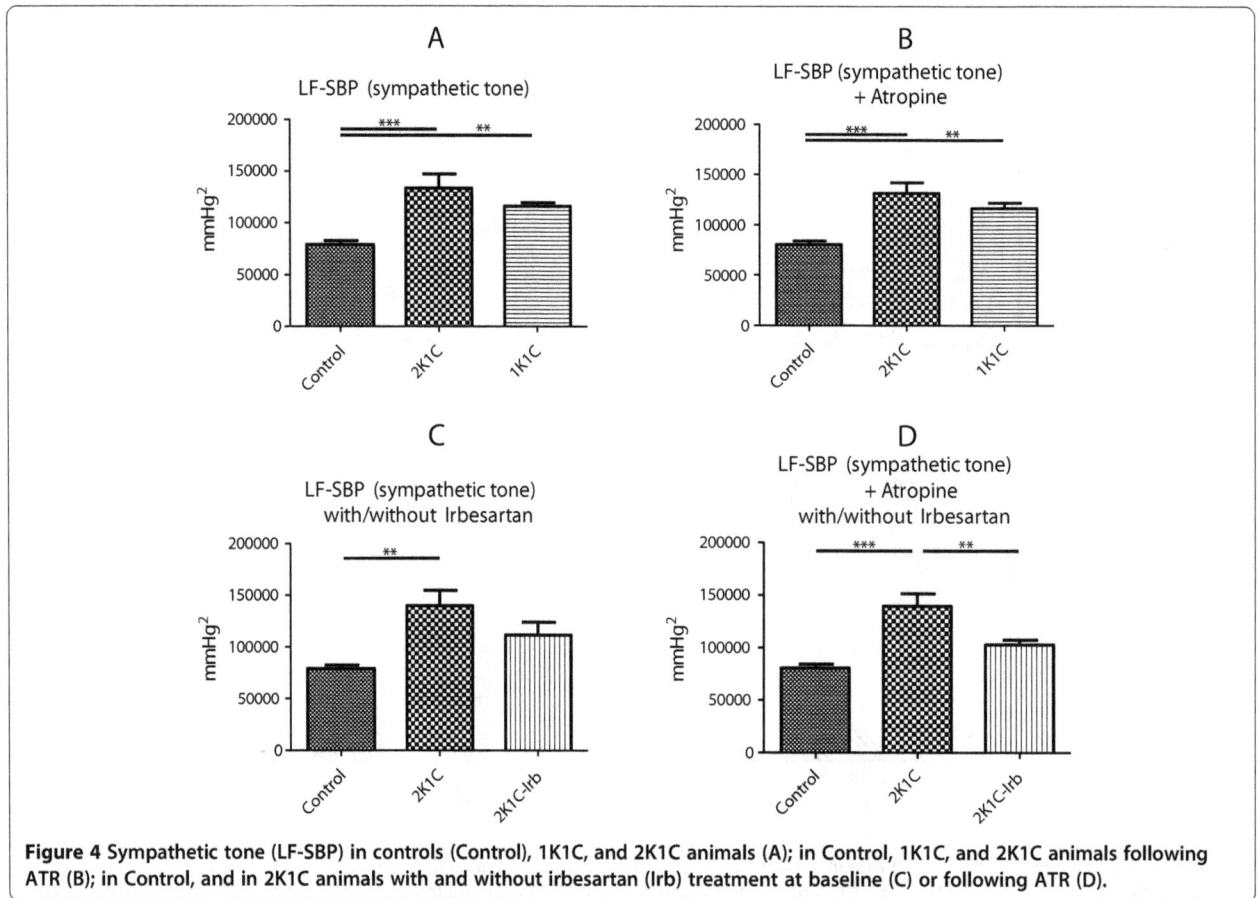

Figure 4 Sympathetic tone (LF-SBP) in controls (Control), 1K1C, and 2K1C animals (A); in Control, 1K1C, and 2K1C animals following ATR (B); in Control, and in 2K1C animals with and without irbesartan (Irb) treatment at baseline (C) or following ATR (D).

Rho-kinase inhibition improves baroreflex sensitivity of heart rate in renovascular hypertension with reduced kidney mass

As demonstrated in Figure 6, baroreflex sensitivity of heart rate was improved by ROKI treatment in renovascular hypertension with reduced renal mass (1K1C). In contrast, ROKI treatment led to an attenuation of baroreflex sensitivity of heart rate in renovascular hypertension with preserved kidney mass (2K1C). These differential treatment effects of SAR407899A did, however, not translate into alterations of sympathetic or parasympathetic tone (Figure 6).

Discussion

In this study, power spectral analysis of systolic blood pressure [26] and urinary catecholamines [33] were determined to gauge sympathetic tone. In addition, vagal tone was assessed using power spectral analysis of heart rate [26,30]. Slope data of concomitant, spontaneous pulse-interval and blood-pressure changes were gathered to estimate baroreflex function [31].

The results suggest that therapeutic interventions in renovascular hypertension may depend on residual renal mass. As shown for Rho-kinase inhibition, a beneficial

effect on baroreflex function only emerged in the 1K1C model, but not in the 2K1C model of renovascular hypertension. This finding may potentially be due to the oxidative stress in the 1K1C model which leads to a more profound Rho A/ROCK activation [34-36]. In addition, Rho-Kinase inhibition may increase nitric oxide availability in hypothalamic centres of baroreflex regulation similar to the heart failure situation [20] which, in turn, improves baroreflex sensitivity of heart rate. Although baroreflex sensitivity of heart rate improved upon Rho-kinase inhibition in the 1K1C model of hypertension, this change did not translate into a reduction of the sympathetic or an increase in parasympathetic tone. This observation was unexpected given that carotid baroreflex function and/or baroreflex-dependent central nervous system regulations affect both sympathetic and parasympathetic tone [37,38].

In renovascular hypertension with preserved kidney mass (2K1C model), AT1-receptor blockade improved baroreflex sensitivity of heart rate. These data are supported by observations in humans with "essential" hypertension [39]. In addition, in response to AT1 receptor blockade, sympathetic tone normalized in the 2K1C model of hypertension which is in line with previous

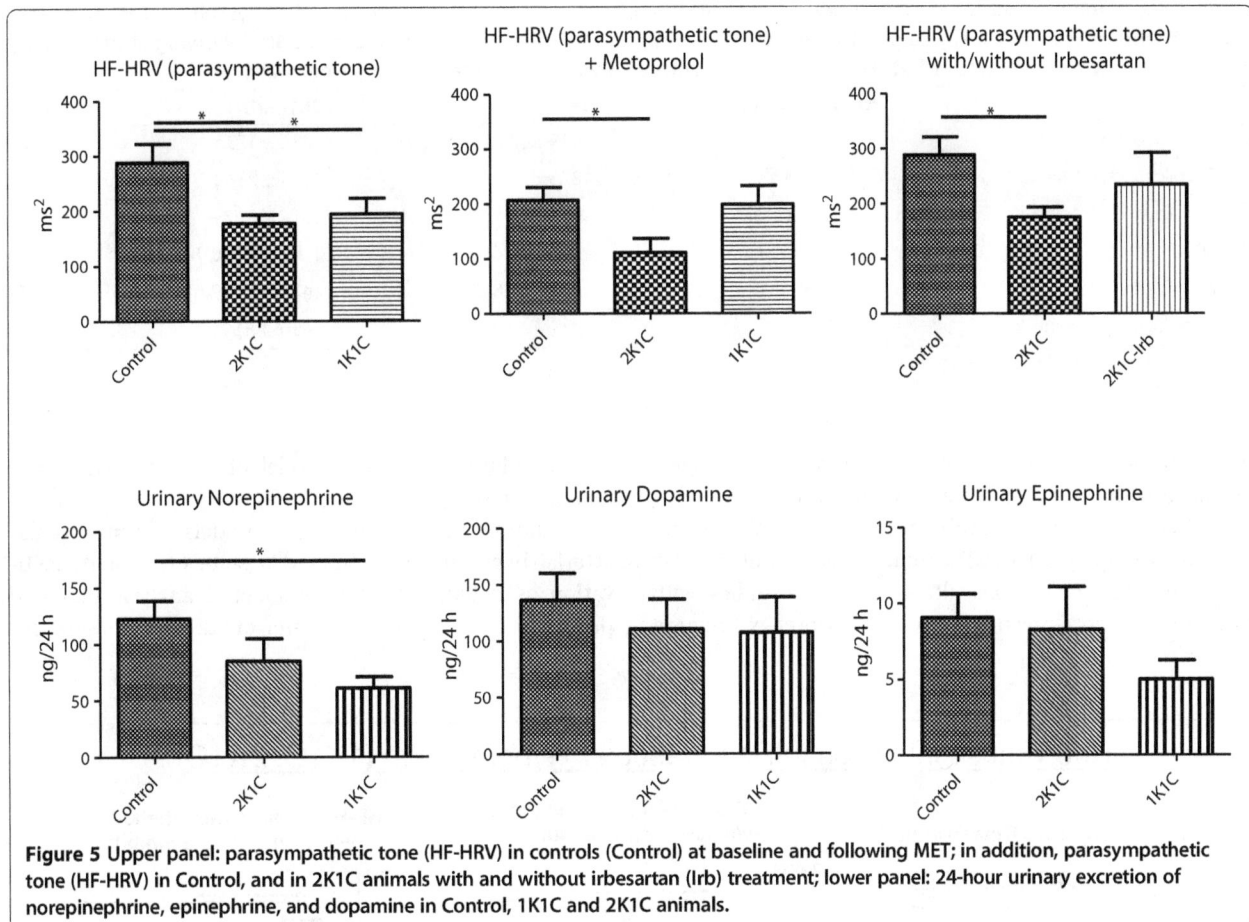

Figure 5 Upper panel: parasympathetic tone (HF-HRV) in controls (Control) at baseline and following MET; in addition, parasympathetic tone (HF-HRV) in Control, and in 2K1C animals with and without irbesartan (Irb) treatment; lower panel: 24-hour urinary excretion of norepinephrine, epinephrine, and dopamine in Control, 1K1C and 2K1C animals.

observations [40]. However, Rho-kinase inhibition was not shown to improve baroreflex sensitivity of heart rate in the 2K1C model. This difference to the 1K1C model may be due to lower nitric oxide availability in hypothalamic centres of baroreflex regulation in the 2K1C model of hypertension. Additional studies on the effect of Rho kinase inhibition are therefore needed to dissect the specific regulations of autonomic nervous system tone in different models of renovascular hypertension.

Concerning the parasympathetic tone, different results have been obtained for the renovascular hypertension models with and without reduced kidney mass (1K1C; 2K1C) as well. 2K1C animals showed a significantly depressed parasympathetic tone which persisted after beta-adrenergic blockade. As novel findings, AT1-receptor blockade with Irb significantly increased parasympathetic tone, decreased resting heart rate, and restored baroreflex sensitivity of heart rate in renovascular hypertension with preserved kidney mass (2K1C). Baroreflex and heart-rate data are in line with published evidence from experimental renoparenchymal hypertension [41]. Given the tremendous effect of baroreflex activating therapies in refractory

Table 3 Supplemental power spectral data, i.e. cumulative intensity of high-frequency band of systolic blood pressure (HF-SBP) and of low-frequency band of heart rate (LF-HRV), is shown in normal control animals following sham surgery as well as in hypertensive animals (2-kidney-1-clip (2K1C); 1-kidney-1-clip (1K1C))

	Normal controls	2K1C	1K1C	P
LF-HRV	411.1 ± 170.8	282.8 ± 125.2	298.9 ± 133.2	0.15
LF-HRV following Metoprolol	328.0 ± 103.3	174.7 ± 105.2	271.1 ± 90.2	< 0.05
LF-HRV following Atropine	151.0 ± 111.1	90.4 ± 43.7	86.2 ± 68.5	< 0.05
HF-SBP	103208 ± 12697	154311 ± 35205	159123 ± 24991	<0.001
HF-SBP following Metoprolol	102988 ± 12776	148740 ± 28677	165959 ± 31325	<0.001
HF-SBP following Atropine	134689 ± 25981	178285 ± 35102	189734 ± 30970	<0.01

Statistical analysis was performed among groups.

Table 4 Supplemental power spectral data, i.e. cumulative intensity of high-frequency band of systolic blood pressure (HF-SBP) and of low-frequency band of heart rate (LF-HRV), is shown in normal control animals following sham surgery and in hypertensive animals (2-kidney-1-clip (2K1C)) with and without irbesartan (Irb) treatment

	Normal controls	2K1C	2K1C-Irb	P
LF-HRV	411.1 ± 170.8	303.9 ± 128.1	328.0 ± 170.5	0.36
LF-HRV following Metoprolol	328.0 ± 103.3	187.3 ± 120.6	439.1 ± 237.3	0.07
LF-HRV following Atropine	151.0 ± 111.1	96.7 ± 52.0	131.7 ± 83.7	0.36
HF-SBP	103208 ± 12697	157333 ± 36560	134874 ± 35018	<0.01
HF-SBP following Metoprolol	102988 ± 12776	154627 ± 28676	147225 ± 32901	<0.01
HF-SBP following Atropine	134689 ± 25981	182574 ± 42032	165463 ± 59555	0.11

Statistical analysis was performed among groups.

hypertension [42], the beneficial role of AT1-receptor blockade with regard to baroreflex function deserves further attention in studies. In the present study, AT1 blockade was not applied to 1K1C animals because of the risk of kidney failure. Previous ultra-short term studies with losartan have not shown an improved baroreflex function in this volume-dependent model of renovascular hypertension (1K1C) [43].

As another main result, both models of renovascular arterial hypertension exhibited a state of sympathoactivation as detected by power spectral analysis of blood pressure. Thus, previous results obtained with selective

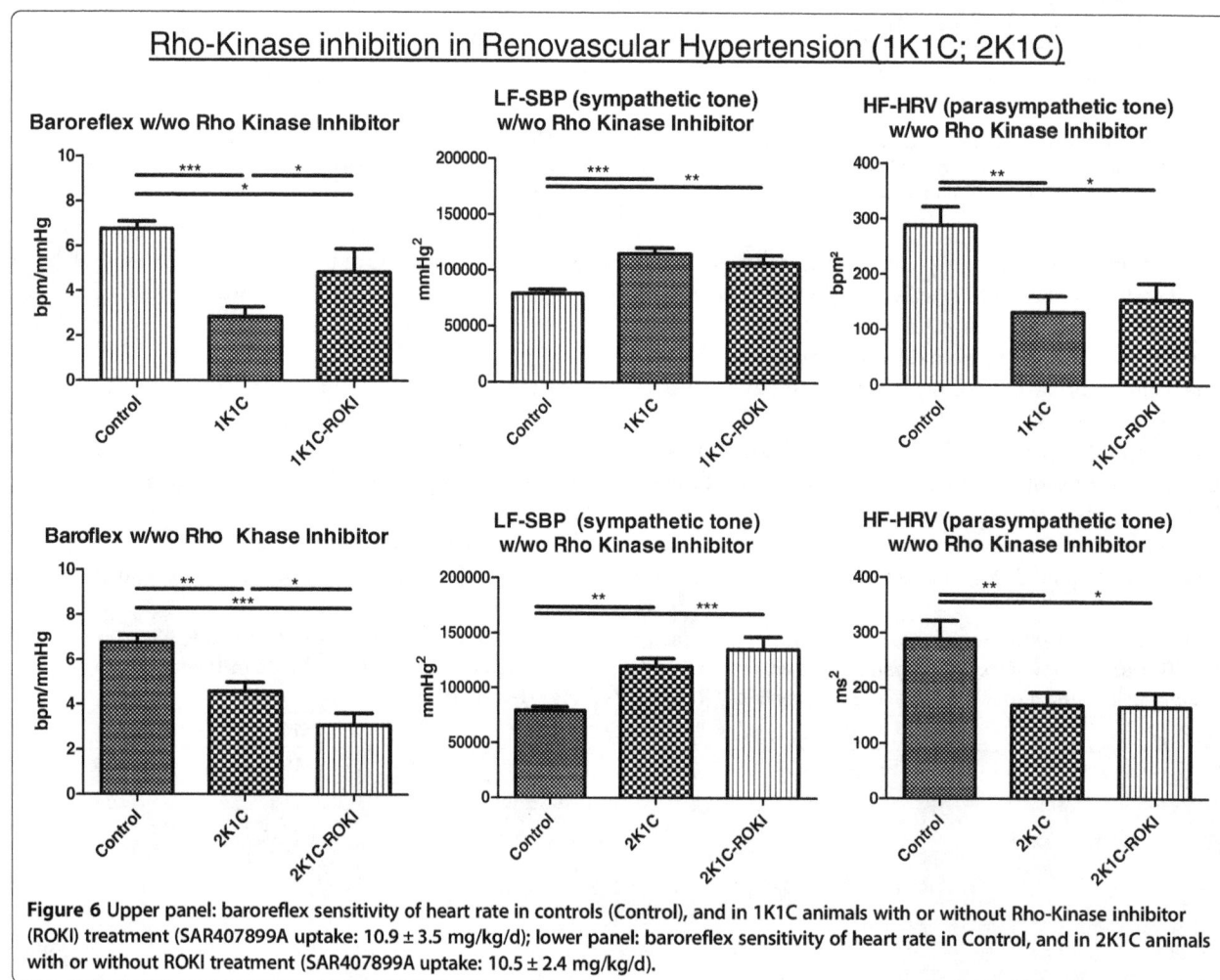

Figure 6 Upper panel: baroreflex sensitivity of heart rate in controls (Control), and in 1K1C animals with or without Rho-Kinase inhibitor (ROKI) treatment (SAR407899A uptake: 10.9 ± 3.5 mg/kg/d); lower panel: baroreflex sensitivity of heart rate in Control, and in 2K1C animals with or without ROKI treatment (SAR407899A uptake: 10.5 ± 2.4 mg/kg/d).

blockade (atropine and propranolol) experiments on heart rate were confirmed [8,9]. For renovascular hypertension with preserved kidney function (2K1C), a prevalent sympathoactivation was also reported in a recent study using the same methodology in rats as used in the present study [44]. Interestingly, in that study, baroreflex depression occurred almost instantaneously upon induction of Goldblatt hypertension (2K1C). In the present study, the level of sympathoactivation was similar between 1K1C and 2K1C animals, despite the different hormonal cause of hypertension [12] and the different volume state [45]. Apart from renovascular hypertension, a state of sympathoactivation was found in patients with "essential" arterial hypertension [46-49] and in chronic heart failure. In the latter, effects on the central nervous system by angiotensin II were postulated [50,51]. For the 1K1C model, the detailed mechanism of sympathoactivation, however, is still unclear. In 1K1C animals, renin release is known to be similar to normal controls [12]. Therefore, systemic RAAS activation cannot be a cause of sympathoactivation under this condition. However, the brain "ouabain" and/or the brain renin-angiotensin system may become pertinent for sympathoactivation in renovascular hypertension with reduced kidney mass possibly through a sodium-dependent mechanism [52]. In addition, kidney mass reduction and renal artery stenosis may reduce urinary norepinephrine excretion as shown here (Figure 6). Diminished excretion and/or attenuated catecholamine degradation in the kidney [53-55] may lead to catecholamine accumulation and, potentially, sympathoactivation. As a limitation of the present study, plasma catecholamines were not determined. Uremic toxins are unlikely to play a sympathoactivating role in the 1K1C model because glomerular filtration was shown to be reduced by only 30% [56].

Conclusions

As main results, sympathetic tone (with or without vagal blockade) was found to be increased, whereas baroreflex sensitivity of heart rate was depressed in models of renovascular hypertension, irrespective of residual renal mass. Differential results relate to parasympathetic tone (with or without beta 1-adrenergic blockade) that was depressed in the 2K1C model only. In addition, left ventricular hypertrophy was present in experimental renovascular hypertension with reduced renal mass (1K1C) only. Renal norepinephrine excretion was reduced in the 1K1C model exclusively. Hypothetically, renal reduced catecholamine excretion and/or impaired renal catecholamine degradation may be considered as mechanisms of sympathoactivation in the 1K1C model. Finally, Rho-kinase inhibition improved baroreflex function solely in experimental renovascular hypertension with reduced renal mass (1K1C), whereas AT1 blockade improved

baroreflex sensitivity of heart rate in renovascular hypertension with preserved kidney mass (2K1C). Taken together, Rho-kinase inhibition might be an additive strategy to improve survival in renovascular hypertension with reduced renal mass, whereas low-dose AT1 blockade might be a therapeutic choice in all other cases of renovascular hypertension.

Competing interests

The authors declare that they have no competing interests.

Authors' contributions

RUP made substantial contributions in study conception and design and the acquisition of data. He performed experiments and drafted the manuscript. SB and OJ collected data, performed experiments and provided substantial input in data interpretation and analysis. RPB conceived the study, contributed to study design and was involved in drafting the manuscript. All authors gave final approval to the version to be published.

Acknowledgements

The authors thank Günther Amrhein and Susanne Schütze for technical assistance. In addition, Dr. V. Gross, Mrs. I. Kamer (Max-Delbrück Centre, Berlin, Germany), Dr. I. H. Zucker (University of Nebraska, Medical Center, Omaha, NE, USA), associates of the laboratory of Jean-Luc Elghozi, Faculté de Médecine René Descartes, Paris, France, and H. Stauss (University of Iowa, IA, U.S.) helped in many ways in telemetry-related and data-analysis issues. The authors are grateful for the investigational drugs Irb and Rho-kinase inhibitor SAR407899A kindly provided by Sanofi, Frankfurt/Main, Germany. Lastly, RUP is grateful for the grant received by Deutsche Nierenstiftung 2008.

Author details

[1]Institute for Cardiovascular Physiology, Vascular Research Centre, Fachbereich Medizin, Goethe University, Frankfurt (Main), Germany. [2]Department of Nephrology, Clinic of Internal Medicine 2, University Clinic Halle, Martin Luther University Halle-Wittenberg, Ernst-Grube-Str. 40, Halle (Saale) 06120, Germany. [3]Department of Nephrology, Goethe University, Frankfurt (Main), Germany.

References

1. Coresh J, Selvin E, Stevens LA, Manzi J, Kusek JW, Eggers P, Van Lente F, Levey AS: Prevalence of chronic kidney disease in the United States. *JAMA: The Journal of the American Medical Association* 2007, **298**:2038–2047.
2. Shulman NB, Ford CE, Hall WD, Blaufox MD, Simon D, Langford HG, Schneider KA: Prognostic value of serum creatinine and effect of treatment of hypertension on renal function: results from the hypertension detection and follow-up program: the hypertension detection and follow-up program cooperative group. *Hypertension* 1989, **13**:I80–I93.
3. Cooper CJ, Murphy TP, Cutlip DE, Jamerson K, Henrich W, Reid DM, Cohen DJ, Matsumoto AH, Steffes M, Jaff MR, Prince MR, Lewis EF, Tuttle KR, Shapiro JI, Rundback JH, Massaro JM, D'Agostino RB Sr, Dworkin LD, CORAL Investigators: Stenting and medical therapy for atherosclerotic renal-artery stenosis. *N Engl J Med* 2013, **370**:13–22.
4. ASTRAL Investigators, Wheatley K, Ives N, Gray R, Kalra PA, Moss JG, Baigent C, Carr S, Chalmers N, Eadington D, Hamilton G, Lipkin G, Nicholson A, Scoble J: Revascularization versus medical therapy for renal-artery stenosis. *N Engl J Med* 2009, **361**:1953–1962.
5. Lewis EJ, Hunsicker LG, Clarke WR, Berl T, Pohl MA, Lewis JB, Ritz E, Atkins RC, Rohde R, Raz I, Collaborative Study Group: Renoprotective effect of the angiotensin-receptor antagonist irbesartan in patients with nephropathy due to type 2 diabetes. *N Engl J Med* 2001, **345**:851–860.
6. Lewis EJ, Hunsicker LG, Bain RP, Rohde RD: The effect of angiotensin-converting-enzyme inhibition on diabetic nephropathy: the collaborative study group. *N Engl J Med* 1993, **329**:1456–1462.

7.   Gao SA, Johansson M, Rundqvist B, Lambert G, Jensen G, Friberg P: **Reduced spontaneous baroreceptor sensitivity in patients with renovascular hypertension.** *J Hypertens* 2002, 20:111–116.

8.   Cabrai AM, Vasquez EC: **Time course of cardiac sympathetic and vagal tone changes in renovascular hypertensive rats.** *Am J Hypertens* 1991, 4:815–819.

9.   Borges GR, Salgado HC, Silva CA, Rossi MA, Prado CM, Fazan R: **Changes in hemodynamic and neurohumoral control cause cardiac damage in one-kidney, one-clip hypertensive mice.** *Am J Physiol Regul Integr Comp Physiol* 2008, 295:R1904–R1913.

10. Tank J, Diedrich A, Schroeder C, Stoffels M, Franke G, Sharma AM, Luft FC, Jordan J: **Limited effect of systemic + beta-blockade on sympathetic outflow.** *Hypertension* 2001, 38:1377–1381.

11. O'Connor DT, Preston RA: **Propranolol effects on autonomic function in hypertensive men.** *Clin Cardiol* 1982, 5:340–346.

12. Wiesel P, Mazzolai L, Nussberger J, Pedrazzini T: **Two-kidney, one clip and one-kidney, one clip hypertension in mice.** *Hypertension* 1997, 29:1025–1030.

13. McMullan S, Goodchild AK, Pilowsky PM: **Circulating angiotensin II attenuates the sympathetic baroreflex by reducing the barosensitivity of medullary cardiovascular neurones in the rat.** *J Physiol* 2007, 582:711–722.

14. Loirand G, Guérin P, Pacaud P: **Rho kinases in cardiovascular physiology and pathophysiology.** *Circ Res* 2006, 98:322–334.

15. Fukata Y, Amano M, Kaibuchi K: **Rho-rho-kinase pathway in smooth muscle contraction and cytoskeletal reorganization of non-muscle cells.** *Trends Pharmacol Sci* 2001, 22:32–39.

16. van Nieuw Amerongen GP, van DS, Vermeer MA, Collard JG, van HV: **Activation of RhoA by thrombin in endothelial hyperpermeability: role of Rho kinase and protein tyrosine kinases.** *Circ Res* 2000, 87:335–340.

17. Laufs U, Kilter H, Konkol C, Wassmann S, Bohm M, Nickenig G: **Impact of HMG CoA reductase inhibition on small GTPases in the heart.** *Cardiovasc Res* 2002, 53:911–920.

18. Pliquett RU, Cornish KG, Zucker IH: **Statin therapy restores sympathovagal balance in experimental heart failure.** *J Appl Physiol* 2003, 95:700–704.

19. Pliquett RU, Cornish KG, Peuler JD, Zucker IH: **Simvastatin normalizes autonomic neural control in experimental heart failure.** *Circulation* 2003, 107:2493–2498.

20. Haack KKV, Gao L, Schiller AM, Curry PL, Pellegrino PR, Zucker IH: **Central rho kinase inhibition restores baroreflex sensitivity and angiotensin II type 1 receptor protein imbalance in conscious rabbits with chronic heart failure.** *Hypertension* 2013, 61:723–729.

21. Balt JC, Mathy MJ, Pfaffendorf M, van Zwieten PA: **Sympatho-inhibitory actions of irbesartan in pithed spontaneously hypertensive and Wistar-Kyoto rats.** *Fundamental & Clinical Pharmacology* 2003, 17:83–91.

22. Nap A, Balt JC, Pfaffendorf M, Van Zwieten PA: **Sympatholytic properties of several AT1-receptor antagonists in the isolated rabbit thoracic aorta.** *J Hypertens* 2002, 20:1821–1828.

23. Ye S, Zhong H, Duong VN, Campese VM: **Losartan reduces central and peripheral sympathetic nerve activity in a rat model of neurogenic hypertension.** *Hypertension* 2002, 39:1101–1106.

24. Zhang J, Leenen FH: **AT(1) receptor blockers prevent sympathetic hyperactivity and hypertension by chronic ouabain and hypertonic saline.** *Am J Physiol Heart Circ Physiol* 2001, 280:H1318–H1323.

25. Jung O, Schreiber JG, Geiger H, Pedrazzini T, Busse R, Brandes RP: **gp91phox-containing NADPH oxidase mediates endothelial dysfunction in renovascular hypertension.** *Circulation* 2004, 109:1795–1801.

26. Baudrie V, Laude D, Elghozi JL: **Optimal frequency ranges for extracting information on cardiovascular autonomic control from the blood pressure and pulse interval spectrograms in mice.** *Am J Physiol Regul Integr Comp Physiol* 2007, 292:R904–R912.

27. Stauss HM: **Power spectral analysis in mice: what are the appropriate frequency bands?** *Am J Physiol Regul Integr Comp Physiol* 2007, 292:R902–R903.

28. Rodrigues FL, de OM, Salgado HC, Fazan R Jr: **Effect of baroreceptor denervation on the autonomic control of arterial pressure in conscious mice.** *Exp Physiol* 2011, 96:853–862.

29. Farah VM, Joaquim LF, Bernatova I, Morris M: **Acute and chronic stress influence blood pressure variability in mice.** *Physiol Behav* 2004, 83:135–142.

30. Tank J, Diedrich A, Szczech E, Luft FC, Jordan J: **Alpha-2 adrenergic transmission and human baroreflex regulation.** *Hypertension* 2004, 43:1035–1041.

31. Bertinieri G, Di RM, Cavallazzi A, Ferrari AU, Pedotti A, Mancia G: **A new approach to analysis of the arterial baroreflex.** *J Hypertens Suppl* 1985, 3:S79–S81.

32. Laude D, Baudrie V, Elghozi JL: **Applicability of recent methods used to estimate spontaneous baroreflex sensitivity to resting mice.** *Am J Physiol Regul Integr Comp Physiol* 2008, 294:R142–R150.

33. Silva P, Landsberg L, Besarab A: **Excretion and metabolism of catecholamines by the isolated perfused rat kidney.** *J Clin Invest* 1979, 64:850–857.

34. Bailey SR, Eid AH, Mitra S, Flavahan S, Flavahan NA: **Rho kinase mediates cold-induced constriction of cutaneous arteries: role of alpha2C-adrenoceptor translocation.** *Circ Res* 2004, 94:1367–1374.

35. Jin L, Ying Z, Webb RC: **Activation of Rho/Rho kinase signaling pathway by reactive oxygen species in rat aorta.** *Am J Physiol Heart Circ Physiol* 2004, 287:H1495–H1500.

36. Dobrian AD, Schriver SD, Prewitt RL: **Role of angiotensin II and free radicals in blood pressure regulation in a rat model of renal hypertension.** *Hypertension* 2001, 38:361–366.

37. Abdala AP, McBryde FD, Marina N, Hendy EB, Engelman ZJ, Fudim M, Desir GV: **Hypertension is critically dependent on the carotid body input in the spontaneously hypertensive rat.** *J Physiol* 2012, 590:4269–4277.

38. Kollai M, Jokkel G, Bonyhai I, Tomcsanyi J, Naszlady A: **Relation between baroreflex sensitivity and cardiac vagal tone in humans.** *Am J Physiol Heart Circ Physiol* 1994, 266:H21–H27.

39. Chern CM, Hsu HY, Hu HH, Chen YY, Hsu LC, Chao AC: **Effects of atenolol and losartan on baroreflex sensitivity and heart rate variability in uncomplicated essential hypertension.** *J Cardiovasc Pharmacol* 2006, 47:169–174.

40. Ramchandra R, Watson AMD, Hood SG, May CN: **Response of cardiac sympathetic nerve activity to intravenous irbesartan in heart failure.** *Am J Physiol Regul Integr Comp Physiol* 2010, 298:R1056–R1060.

41. Shang W, Han P, Yang C, Gu XW, Zhang W, Xu LP, Fu ST, Su DF, Xie HH: **Synergism of irbesartan and amlodipine on hemodynamic amelioration and organ protection in spontaneously hypertensive rats.** *Acta Pharmacol Sin* 2011, 32:1109–1115.

42. Alnima T, de Leeuw PW, Tan FES, Kroon AA: **Renal responses to long-term carotid baroreflex activation therapy in patients with drug-resistant hypertension.** *Hypertension* 2013, 61:1334–1339.

43. Farah VM, Moreira ED, Ushizima M, Cestari IA, Irigoyen MC, Krieger EM: **Acute AT1 receptor blockade does not improve the depressed baroreflex in rats with chronic renal hypertension.** *Braz J Med Biol Res* 2000, 33:1491–1496.

44. Oliveira-Sales EB, Toward MA, Campos RR, Paton JF: **Revealing the role of the autonomic nervous system in the development and maintenance of Goldblatt hypertension in rats.** *Auton Neurosci* 2014, 183:23–29.

45. Bahner U, Geiger H, Palkovits M, Ganten D, Klotz B, Heidland A: **Changes in the central ANF-system of renovascular hypertensive rats.** *Kidney Int* 1991, 39:33–38.

46. Esler M, Jennings G, Lambert G: **Noradrenaline release and the pathophysiology of primary human hypertension.** *Am J Hypertens* 1989, 2:140S–146S.

47. Goldstein DS: **Plasma catecholamines and essential hypertension: an analytical review.** *Hypertension* 1983, 5:86–99.

48. Yamada Y, Miyajima E, Tochikubo O, Matsukawa T, Ishii M: **Age-related changes in muscle sympathetic nerve activity in essential hypertension.** *Hypertension* 1989, 13:870–877.

49. Greenwood JP, Stoker JB, Mary DASG: **Single-unit sympathetic discharge: quantitative assessment in human hypertensive disease.** *Circulation* 1999, 100:1305–1310.

50. Zucker IH, Schultz HD, Patel KP, Wang W, Gao L: **Regulation of central angiotensin type 1 receptors and sympathetic outflow in heart failure.** *Am J Physiol Heart Circ Physiol* 2009, 297:H1557–H1566.

51. Zimmerman MC, Lazartigues E, Lang JA, Sinnayah P, Ahmad IM, Spitz DR, Davisson RL: **Superoxide mediates the actions of angiotensin II in the central nervous system.** *Circ Res* 2002, 91:1038–1045.

52. Huang BS, Leenen FHH: **Brain amiloride-sensitive Phe-Met-Arg-Phe-NH2-gated Na + channels and Na + –induced sympathoexcitation and hypertension.** *Hypertension* 2002, 39:557–561.

53. Xu J, Li G, Wang P, Velazquez H, Yao X, Li Y, Wu Y, Peixoto A, Crowley S, Desir GV: **Renalase is a novel, soluble monoamine oxidase that regulates cardiac function and blood pressure.** *J Clin Invest* 2005, 115:1275–1280.

3

The ΔF508-CFTR mutation inhibits wild-type CFTR processing and function when co-expressed in human airway epithelia and in mouse nasal mucosa

Torry A Tucker[1,2,4], James A Fortenberry[2], Akos Zsembery[1,2,3], Lisa M Schwiebert[1,2*] and Erik M Schwiebert[1,2,5*]

Abstract

Background: Rescue or correction of CFTR function in native epithelia is the ultimate goal of CF therapeutics development. Wild-type (WT) CFTR introduction and replacement is also of particular interest. Such therapies may be complicated by possible CFTR self-assembly into an oligomer or multimer.

Results: Surprisingly, functional CFTR assays in native airway epithelia showed that the most common CFTR mutant, ΔF508-CFTR (ΔF-CFTR), inhibits WT-CFTR when both forms are co-expressed. To examine more mechanistically, both forms of CFTR were transfected transiently in varying amounts into IB3-1 CF human airway epithelial cells and HEK-293 human embryonic kidney cells null for endogenous CFTR protein expression. Increasing amounts of ΔF-CFTR inhibited WT-CFTR protein processing and function in CF human airway epithelial cells but not in heterologous HEK-293 cells. Stably expressed ΔF-CFTR in clones of the non-CF human airway epithelial cell line, CALU-3, also showed reduction in cAMP-stimulated anion secretion and in WT-CFTR processing. An ultimate test of this dominant negative-like effect of ΔF-CFTR on WT-CFTR was the parallel study of two different CF mouse models: the ΔF-CFTR mouse and the bitransgenic CFTR mouse corrected in the gut but null in the lung and airways. WT/ΔF heterozygotes had an intermediate phenotype with regard to CFTR agonist responses in in vivo nasal potential difference (NPD) recordings and in Ussing chamber recordings of short-circuit current (ISC) in vitro on primary tracheal epithelial cells isolated from the same mice. In contrast, CFTR bitransgenic +/− heterozygotes had no difference in their responses versus +/+ wild-type mice.

Conclusions: Taken altogether, these data suggest that ΔF-CFTR and WT-CFTR co-assemble into an oligomeric macromolecular complex in native epithelia and share protein processing machinery and regulation at the level of the endoplasmic reticulum (ER). As a consequence, ΔF-CFTR slows WT-CFTR protein processing and limits its expression and function in the apical membrane of native airway epithelia. Implications of these data for the relative health of CF heterozygous carriers, for CFTR protein processing in native airway epithelia, and for the relative efficacy of different CF therapeutic approaches is significant and is discussed.

Keywords: Cystic fibrosis (CF), CFTR, Biogenesis, CF heterozygote, Oligomer, Chloride ion channels

* Correspondence: lschwieb@uab.edu; erik@discoverybiomed.com
[1]Departments of Cell Developmental and Integrative Biology, University of Alabama at Birmingham, 1918 University Blvd, Birmingham, AL 35294-0005, USA
[2]Gregory Fleming James Cystic Fibrosis (CF) Research Center, University of Alabama at Birmingham, 1918 University Blvd, Birmingham 35294-0005AL, USA
Full list of author information is available at the end of the article

Background

CF is a monogenic disorder, a rare misfolded protein disorder, and the most common autosomal recessive genetic disease found in the Caucasian population [1-3]. CF is caused by mutations in CFTR that lead to reduced surface expression and/or function of this cyclic AMP-regulated chloride (Cl⁻) channel among other airway, gastrointestinal and other epithelial tissue defects [1-4]. The most commonly occurring CF mutation is the ΔF508-CFTR (ΔF-CFTR) mutation that occurs in approximately 70-90% of the CF population worldwide [1-4]. This mutation causes a folding defect in the CFTR protein that causes ER retention of the majority of the ΔF-CFTR protein [1-6].

CF disease phenotype correlates better with *CFTR* genotype in the gastrointestinal (GI) tract, where secretion of pancreatic enzymes and bile along with salt, bicarbonate, and water is essential for function [4]. However, in the CF lung and airways, there is little correlation between *CFTR* genotype and lung and airways disease phenotype [4]. One ΔF-CFTR homozygous patient can have severe disease and another ΔF-CFTR homozygous patient can present a more mild disease; this is the rationale for CF siblings and twins genotype/phenotype correlation studies currently in progress [7,8]. This lack of correlation may be explained by: (a) secondary or modifier genes that protect or fail to protect an individual from CF lung and airways disease progression [7]; (b) additional genes that cause predisposition to CF lung and airways disease progression [7,8]; and/or (c) CFTR's known role as a regulator of other conductances and cellular processes [4]. Better understanding of ΔF-CFTR biology, physiology and lung and airways defects is critical, because the majority of the associated pathology and corresponding mortality of CF occurs in the pulmonary system.

One of the hypothesized and more viable methods to treat CF is by gene correction or protein replacement [9,10]. The goal is to introduce or replace the defective copy of CFTR with a functional wild-type (WT) copy that could generate a normal mRNA and a functional protein. Promising methods of introducing the WT-CFTR gene is via lipid- or virally-mediated transduction [9,10]. Barriers to these methods are currently being overcome [9,10]. One overwhelming problem is the lack of an animal model that displays the characteristic lung pathology seen in humans that a gene-bearing vector seeks to correct [9,10]; however, recent work on porcine and ferret animal models of CF is promising [11-13]. Work described herein introduces another concept that needs to be addressed in the context of these putative therapies: What if the mutant CFTR protein interacts with and affects the processing and function of the introduced WT-CFTR? A dominant negative-like effect of the endogenous ΔF-CFTR could also limit the effect of a WT-CFTR gene or protein correction or a CF corrector drug in a target cell.

Recent work has focused on examination of WT-CFTR and mutant CFTR biogenesis, trafficking, and functions within CFTR's native environment, the polarized airway epithelial cell. In this light, we published important methods on transient transfection of CFTR into non-polarized and polarized epithelial cells [14]. We also showed that WT-CFTR processing in epithelial cells is more efficient than first suggested in heterologous cell systems over-expressing CFTR [15]. In the context of this work, we observed curious results that led us to test the hypothesis that mutant forms of CFTR can interact with and inhibit WT-CFTR function in airway epithelial cells. We present results herein with *in vivo* and *in vitro* approaches that support the hypothesis that ΔF-CFTR inhibits WT-CFTR in a dominant negative-like manner when co-expressed together in the same epithelium.

This hypothesis is germane to two different fields of CF research. The former relates to whether defects or predispositions to dysfunction are found in the CF heterozygous carrier. The latter involves whether or not CFTR exists within an oligomeric protein complex in epithelial cells as a monomer or a multimer. Throughout the clinical study of endpoints in CF, partial defects or dysfunction in the CF heterozygous carrier have been observed. However, because the CF carrier does not present with full progressive CF disease in the GI tract or in the lung and airways and because genotypes were not fully defined in these older studies, CF carriers have not be studied deeply or as a full study group compared to homozygotes or WT controls. Heterozygous cell models are also not available for similar reasons. However, partial loss in the volume of sweat or in rate of secretion in response to agonists has been documented in CF heterozygotes versus WT controls [16,17], whereas CF homozygotes fail to respond to agonists. Graded differences in sweat [Cl⁻] amounts were observed that yielded three statistically different groups in a continuum between CF homozygote patients, CF heterozygote carriers, and WT controls. Clinical endpoints have noted statistically valid predispositions to pancreatitis, rhinitis and sinusitis, allergic bronchopulmonary aspergillosis, and airway hyper reactivity in CF heterozygotes [18-21]. The latter predisposition to airway reactivity has been studied for several decades and have driven asthma geneticists to document prevalence of CF gene mutations in populations with severe asthma prevalence [18]. Additional studies were found in our literature review, but only the subset cited above studied all three genotypes. Nevertheless, the listed observations above provided a compelling rationale for studying wild-type CFTR and mutant CFTR interaction as a possible cause of heterozygote dysfunction.

A multitude of studies focusing on CFTR protein biochemistry have concluded that CFTR is a monomer

[22-26]. However, this conclusion was supported by work largely performed in heterologous cell over-expression systems and was arrived at before the identification of CFTR binding partners at the N- and C-termini [27-34]. In particular, the identification of the PDZ-binding motif on the extreme C-terminal end of the carboxy-terminal tail and epithelial PDZ binding proteins such as EBP-50 (NHERF-1), E3-KARP (NHERF-2), CAP-70, and CAL among others have made many investigators re-think this conclusion [35-41]. This is particularly true in the context of the epithelial cell, where a single CFTR monomer could associate with a second CFTR monomer or with a larger number of CFTR monomers via PDZ-dependent contacts. Several investigators have shown that association with PDZ binding proteins affect CFTR Cl⁻ channel function, trafficking and localization [36-41]. Bear and colleagues have recently assessed the monomer versus multimer issue with CFTR expressed in different cell models and subjected the CFTR-enriched lysates to sucrose gradient analysis under non-denaturing and denaturing conditions [22]. Their conclusion was that CFTR existed as a monomer, as a dimer, and, possibly, in higher order multimers, but that a monomer was sufficient for Cl⁻ channel activity. Moreover, Naren and colleagues have shown in heterologous and epithelial cells that CFTR is a multimer that self-associates by a mechanism that does not appear to involve the PDZ motif in the C-terminus [23]. In addition, Cormet-Boyaka et al. characterized a trans-complementation mechanism where fragments of CFTR could rescue CFTR folding mutations [33]. They state that masking the mutated region of the CFTR polypeptide with a corresponding WT fragment could cause the mutant to escape the ER [32,33]. Zerhusen et al. showed that a CFTR concatemer acted in a similar manner to a single CFTR protein, arguing for possible cooperation of multiple CFTR proteins to form a functional channel [27]. In their discussion, these authors hint at the idea that mutant CFTR proteins could affect WT-CFTR [22,23,27,32,33]. The same has been studied recently for mdr P-glycoproteins, where monomeric and multimeric conclusions have been drawn [28]. Therefore, it is still an open question whether CFTR assembles as a multimer through: (a) self-association; (b) as an oligomeric complex; or (c) resides as a multimer within an oligomer. Nevertheless, there are compelling data from our laboratory and from others that multiple CFTR polypeptides can interact by either or both mechanisms in epithelial cells.

In the study herein, our data address both issues of heterozygote dysfunction and CFTR multimerization by assessing the dominant negative-like inhibition of WT-CFTR by ΔF-CFTR in human airway epithelial cells. Critically, the effect is specific to the ΔF-CFTR mutant. The results also speak to the need to overcome mutant CFTR effects on WT-CFTR introduced by emerging therapeutic methods. We show that ΔF-CFTR, when co-expressed with wild-type CFTR by multiple methods, inhibits WT-CFTR processing and, therefore, function in epithelial cells but not in heterologous cells.

Methods and materials
Cell culture
All cell culture substrates (plates, flasks, and filters supports) for epithelial cells were coated with 1:15 diluted Vitrogen 100 solution in Ca/Mg Free Dulbecco's PBS (Life Technologies/Invitrogen). The diluted Vitrogen solution is added, allowed 2–3 min to coat the substrate, and is then removed for air drying in a sterile hood. CALU-3 (a human non-CF submucosal airway serous cell line endogenously expressing CFTR) [42] and HEK293T (a human embryonic kidney heterologous cell model over-expressing the large T antigen to amplify cDNA expression) [43] were grown in Minimal Essential Medium (MEM) with 10% heat-inactivated fetal bovine serum (Life Technologies/Invitrogen), 6 ml of penicillin-streptomycin 100× solution (penicillin 100 U/ml and streptomycin 100 μg/ mg final; Life Technologies/Invitrogen), 6 ml of 200 mM L-glutamine 100X solution (2 mM Final; Life Technologies/Invitrogen), and 2 ml of fungizone solution (amphotericin B, 1 ug/ml final; Life Technologies/Invitrogen). The IB3-1 cell line (derived from a CF human bronchus expressing the ΔF508 and W1282X mutant forms of CFTR) was grown in LHC-8 media without gentamycin (Biofluids) supplemented with 5% heat-inactivated fetal bovine serum, 6 ml of penicillin-streptomycin 100x solution (penicillin 100 U/ml and streptomycin 100 μg/mg final), 6 ml of 200 mM L-glutamine 100X solution (2 mM final), and 2 ml of fungizone solution (amphotericin B, 1 ug/ml final).

Culture of polarized epithelial cell monolayers
CALU-3 non-CF human epithelial cells (parental, G418-resistant lacking mutant CFTR, and G418-resistant expressing mutant CFTR; see selection procedure below) were seeded onto coated 6.5 mm diameter polyester Transwell Filters (Corning-Costar, Corning, NY) at 1×10^6 cells per insert. For these cell monolayers, a measured transepithelial electrical resistance (R_{TE}) of > 2,000 $\Omega \cdot cm^2$ was achieved routinely and sufficient to perform the subsequent Ussing Chamber transepithelial Cl⁻ secretion assays.

Transient transfection of non-polarized epithelial cells
These methods have been published previously [14]. However, co-transfection of wild-type and mutant CFTR cDNAs was a novel feature of this study to simulate a "heterozygous" cell. The methods of LipofectAMINE PLUS-mediated transient transfection were similar; however, the DNA combinations were varied in the following

manner for a typical experiment presented below for cells grown in a 10 cm diameter coated culture plate:

- EV or Empty Vector = 6.75 µg of pcDNA 3.1 plasmid DNA devoid of CFTR cDNA
- WT-CFTR-bearing Vector = 0.75 µg (Balance "backfilled" with 6 µg of empty vector or EV)
- ΔF-CFTR-bearing Vector = 0.75 µg (Balance "backfilled" with 6 µg of EV).

Note below that the amount of ΔF-CFTR was increased in a titration to determine how much ΔF-CFTR vector needed to be transfected to make ΔF-CFTR protein that was equivalent to WT-CFTR because of the dramatically reduced protein half-life of this ER retention mutant [44,45]. Thus, in other transiently transfected cultures, a mixture of WT-CFTR and ΔF-CFTR-bearing vector was co-expressed in the same cells in the following mixtures:

- 1×WT with 1×ΔF = 0.75 µg WT, 0.75 µg ΔF, 5.25 µg EV
- 1×WT with 2×ΔF = 0.75 µg WT, 1.5 µg ΔF, 4.5 µg EV
- 1×WT with 4×ΔF = 0.75 µg WT, 3.0 µg ΔF, 3.0 µg EV
- 1×WT with 8×ΔF = 0.75 µg WT, 6.0 µg ΔF; 0 µg EV

These ratios were used for the IB3-1 CF and HEK-293 T cells transfected transiently. For G551D-CFTR experiments, the same amounts of G551D-CFTR bearing plasmid were used as a substitute for ΔF-CFTR. These DNA combinations were incubated with PLUS reagent in OptiMEM-1 serum-free medium for 15 min at room temperature. After the first incubation, LipofectAMINE reagent from a separate tube was mixed with the PLUS reagent-primed plasmid DNA combinations. The complete transfection cocktail was incubated for another 15 min at room temperature. During the incubation periods, the cells were washed 3X with Opti-MEM-1 medium to remove all serum and to sensitize the cells to the serum-free medium. After the final wash, the transfection cocktail was brought up to a final volume of 6 mls from a mixing volume of 1 ml. The cells were then incubated for 6 h at 37°C in the humified CO_2 incubator. After the 6-h incubation, the cells were washed 2× with Opti-MEM and 1× with FBS containing media to remove excess lipid-DNA complexes. The cells were re-fed 24 h after transfection and studied for CFTR biochemistry and function 48 h post-transfection.

Transient transfection of HEK293T heterologous cells

Similar methods were followed to those described above with the notable exception that Effectene reagent (Qiagen) was used for HEK293T cells [14]. This reagent was found to be toxic to all epithelial cell models but ideal for HEK-293 cells [14]. Surprisingly, there was minimal toxicity to HEK-293 cells while a transfection efficiency of 90-95% was routine. Enhancer reagent was added to OptiMEM-1 medium along with the same DNA combinations above. The mixture was incubated for 10 min at room temperature. After the initial incubation, 24 µl of Effectene reagent was added to each tube, followed by 10 min incubation at room temperature. During the incubations, the cells are washed 3× with Opti-MEM. After the final wash, all media is removed from the cells, and transfection cocktails are brought up to a 6 ml volume and added to the culture dishes. The cells were incubated in transfection cocktail for 4 h at 37°C in the humified CO_2 incubator. After the 4-h incubation, the cells were washed 2× with Opti-MEM and 1× with FBS containing media. The cells were re-fed 24 h after transfection and studied for CFTR biochemistry and function 48 h post-transfection.

Stable transfection and selection of "heterozygous" cells

Similar LipofectAMINE PLUS-based methods were used as above. Vector bearing ΔF508-CFTR cDNA was transiently transfected in combination with the pcDNA 3.1 vector with a G418-resistance gene cassette to confer antibiotic resistance into the non-CF airway epithelial cell lines, CALU-3. CALU-3 cells grow as 'islands' of cells that eventually grow and fuse together as a confluent monolayer. The cells were transfected as small islands dispersed throughout the culture dish. The cells were re-fed 24 h after transfection and cultures were allowed to grow until the islands grew much larger but were still not yet fused together as a confluent culture. After 7–10 days of culture as described above, MEM complete media was added that was also supplemented with 700 µg/ml of genetic in (G418) to select stably transfected CALU-3 cell islands. The cells were washed with PBS and fed G418-containing MEM complete medium every other day that was made fresh and filtered to keep G418 activity high in the cultures. The majority of the cell islands died; however, some cells within islands lived and began to form isolated colonies. These 'island colonies' were then selected using cloning rings (the reason for using 10 cm diameter dishes was that sterile cloning rings could be inserted by simply lifting the lid of the dish). The cloning rings were dipped in sterile, autoclaved vasoline gel to allow them to adhere to the bottom of the plate. Once these colonies grew to confluence within the cloning ring, the clonal 'island colony' was transferred to a 24 well plate for further expansion. They were then expanded further into flasks as well as frozen in micro-aliquots to have the earliest possible passage following selection cryopreserved.

Immunoprecipitation and phospholabeling of CFTR

Published methods were followed [15]. Cells were washed 1X with CaMg containing PBS. The cells were kept at 4°C during washes. The cells were subsequently lysed in "Radioimmunopreciptiation Assay" (RIPA) Buffer containing NP40 (1%), sodium deoxycholate (.5%), SDS (0.1% at pH 8.0), and sodium chloride (150 mM) supplemented with Protease Inhibitor Cocktail (Roche). Samples were homogenized and incubated for 30 min at 4°C. The lysates were then centrifuged at 14,000 g at 4°C for 20 min. The supernatants were then collected and protein concentrations calculated using the BCA Protein Assay Kit and a microplate reader. Immunoprecipitations were performed using Protein A Agarose and the anti-CFTR Ab targeted to the NBD-1/R region of CFTR (Bedwell/Collawn) with at least 800 ng of lysate supernatant. The supernatants were added to the Ab/Protein Agarose Solution and allowed to incubate at 4°C for 2 h or overnight on an end-over-end shaker (rotator). Samples were then centrifuged at 14,000 g for 2 min and the supernatant removed from the pelleted agarose beads. RIPA buffer (750 µl) was then added to the beads, centrifuged for 2 min at 14,000 g, and the supernatant removed. This was repeated 2 times. On the final wash, the pelleted beads were washed with 750 µl PKA Buffer. Two µl of PKA catalytic subunit and 10 µl $[\gamma^{-32}P]$ ATP were added to phosphorylate the bound CFTR to make it detectable with phosphor-imaging technology. The samples were then allowed to incubate for 45 min at 30°C. After the incubation, the cells were washed 3X with RIPA buffer at room temperature. Excess RIPA buffer was then removed from the beads. Thirty-five µl of 2X sample buffer with β-mercaptoethanol was added to the samples and incubated at 37°C for 15 min. Samples were then run on a 6% Tris Agarose gel at 150 V for 90 min, dried in a gel dryer, and analyzed on the PhosphorImager.

Voltohmeter open-circuit and ussing chamber short-circuit current measurements of monolayer electrical properties

R_{TE} was measured using the Millipore MilliCell ERS Voltohmeter that uses Ag-AgCl pelleted chopstick electrodes. The R_{TE} was monitored on a daily basis and was used as an indicator of the level of maturity of the monolayer. When monolayers had matured and reached a R_{TE} plateau (> 1,000-2,000 Ohms), Ussing chamber recordings of the short-circuit currents were performed. Ussing chamber experiments were performed as described previously [46]; however, they were designed to activate and monitor CFTR Cl⁻ currents in accordance with recent published studies. Recordings were performed in OptiMEM-1 reduced serum medium or in Ringers enriched with bicarbonate on CALU-3 non-CF airway epithelial cells grown as monolayers (a submucosal gland serous cell model with abundant endogenous CFTR expression) that were or were not stably transduced with ΔF508-CFTR. Amiloride (10 µM) was added to the apical solution to inhibit any residual ENaC-mediated Na⁺ currents which were negligible in these cell models grown under these conditions. Then, forskolin (2 µM) was added to both sides of the cell monolayers to increase cyclic AMP and stimulate CFTR Cl⁻ conductance. To maximally activate CFTR Cl⁻ conductance in these monolayers, genistein (50 µM) was added to both sides of the monolayer. In some experiments, glibenclamide (glyburide, 50 µM) was added to inhibit the CFTR-mediated Cl⁻ conductance (data not shown). Magnitude of the forskolin- and genistein-activated Cl⁻ conductance was compared statistically between parental or G418-resistant clones CALU-3 cells that lacked ΔF508-CFTR versus those that possessed ΔF508-CFTR.

SPQ halide fluorescence assay of halide transport

The SPQ assay was used to detect the amount of active CFTR Cl⁻ channels that are functional at the plasma membrane of the transiently transfected cells. It has been used previously by our laboratory in published papers [47]. The SPQ fluorescent dye is sensitive to halides, some of which quench the dye's fluorescence (iodide, chloride) and some of which do not (nitrate). The cells are seeded onto a glass coverslip. After a 24 h period, the cells were then transiently transfected with the CFTR cDNAs. Twenty-four hours after initiation of transfection, the cells were placed in media containing the SPQ dye (10 mg/ml) for overnight incubation. After another 24 h, the cover slips were taken and placed on the fluorescence scope (the cover slips actually form the bottom of the flow chamber). Twenty-five to 30 individual cells were selected based upon the intensity of their fluorescence, which denotes the efficiency of SPQ dye uptake. Their fluorescence is then measured and recorded. The SPQ fluorescence protocol is as follows. The cells were placed in the perfusion chamber and exposed to 3 different buffers: (1) NaI buffer (iodide enters the cells and quenches SPQ fluorescence; (2) NaNO₃ buffer (nitrate reverses this gradient and allows the iodide to passively diffuse out of the cells and unquenches the fluorescence); (3) NaNO₃ buffer with a cAMP agonist cocktail (100 µM isobutylmethylxanthine (IBMX), 10 µM forskolin, and 200 µM dibutyryl-cAMP, 8-bromo-cAMP or CPT-cAMP) to stimulate CFTR Cl⁻ conductance and stimulate additional iodide efflux from the cell; and (4) NaI buffer without agonists, to wash out and reverse agonist effects as well as re-quench SPQ fluorescence. The reversibility and re-quenching is also a good indicator of the viability of and level of dye within the cells throughout the entire experiment. The relative background for each cover slip was subtracted from the recorded arbitrary light unit measurements. The resultant data points are analyzed and plotted dependent upon the first recorded point which establishes the baseline.

Nasal potential difference (NPD) assays on two different cf mouse models

NPD assays were performed as described previously but were designed to specifically study and activate CFTR maximally. We performed experiments on all three *CFTR* genotypes in each mouse model. One mouse model was the ΔF508-CFTR mouse developed by Thomas and colleagues [48]. The second mouse model was the UNC knockout mouse that was corrected in the gastrointestinal tract by complementation with a fatty acid binding protein (FABP) promoter-driven *CFTR* construct. The lung and airways remain null for CFTR (a generous gift from Dr. Jeffrey Whitsett, M.D., Ph.D. to the UAB CF Center, [49]. Amiloride (50 μM) was added in a standard Lactated Ringers in step 1 of the assay to inhibit all Na^+ absorptive pathways. In the continued presence of amiloride, a low Cl^- (6 mM) solution was perfused to gauge Cl^- permeability of the nasal mucosa epithelium. Wild-type and heterozygous animals possessed a low Cl^- response, while homozygous animals did not. In the presence of amiloride and in a low Cl^- solution, adenosine and salbutamol (100 μM each) were added together to increase cyclic AMP maximally via their respective G protein-coupled receptors that engage adenyl cyclase. Isoproterenol (Isoprel™) or albuterol (salbutamol) alone were not enough to maximally stimulate CFTR. It was adenosine together with a β-adrenergic agonist that gave us consistent cyclic AMP induction of CFTR above and beyond the low Cl^- response. This modification was done based on the work of Clancy and colleagues on adenosine regulation of CFTR in mice and humans [50,51]. The change in PD, in the negative direction (hyperpolarization) during the low Cl^- phase and adenosine and salbutamol (cyclic AMP) phase of the recordings, was quantified from the strip-chart records. Ussing chamber assays were performed as described above on primary mouse tracheal epithelial cell monolayers derived from these mice.

MTE monolayer culture and ussing chamber analysis

After analysis of *in vivo* CFTR function by nasal PD in the three *CFTR* genotypes in each mouse model, tracheae were excised by surgery in anesthetized mice and were kept separated as to genotype. Tracheae were first washed in a CaMg-free PBS with 5X penicillin/streptomycin (500 U/ml penicillin, 500 μg/ml streptomycin). Tracheae were then washed in a series of dishes containing CaMg-free DMEM/F12 medium with 5X penicillin/streptomycin. Excess tissue was removed from the tracheae, and they were filleted open down the midline from the laryngeal cartilage to its base. The dissection was performed in the above DMEM/F12 Dissection

Medium. The filleted tracheae were then placed in CaMg-free DMEM/F12 medium with 2X penicillin/streptomycin and 1 μg/ml protease type XIV and 0.1 μg/ml DNase I on ice. The tracheae were digested at 4°C overnight in this Digestion Medium without agitation. After the 18 h overnight digestion in the cold, tracheae were inverted in the tubes 15X to maximally dissociate cells. FBS (20%) was then added to inactivate the enzymes, and the dissociated cells were placed into a separate tube on ice. The digested tracheae were then washed (with 15X tube inversion again) in mouse tracheal epithelial (MTE) cell Monolayer Maturation - CaMg-containing DMEM/F12 medium supplemented per 500 mls of medium with 20% FBS (Life Technologies, Certified and Heat-Inactivated), 2X Pen/Strep, 5 mls of L-glutamine (from 100X stock), 2 mls of hydrocortisone (from 10 ml stock solubilized in ethanol, Becton-Dickinson), 2 mls of endothelial cell growth supplement (ECGS from 10 ml stock, Becton-Dickinson), 2 mls of bovine pituitary extract (BPE from 10 ml stock, Becton-Dickinson), and 4 mls of insulin-transferrin-selenium (ITS from 20 ml stock, Becton-Dickinson). Washes were collected and placed on ice. Then, the tracheae were exposed to fresh Digestion Medium for 1 h at 37°C. After the second digestion, the tubes were inverted 15X, FBS (20%) was added to inactivate the enzymes, dissociated cells were collected in a separate tube, and washes with standard culture medium were performed as above. Four separate sets of tubes (two digestions, two washes) were centrifuged for 3–5 min to pellet any and all cells. Pellets were then obtained from all 4 phases of the MTE cell isolation. Then, cells were combined (still separated as to *CFTR* genotype), pelleted and resuspended in a minimal volume (50–100 μl per filter support). Four filter supports can be seeded per 1 trachea. Filter supports were coated with CellTak and with a 1:10 diluted Vitrogen 100 solution (in CaMg-free PBS) that also contained 1 mg human fibronectin (Becton-Dickinson) added into a 50 ml total volume one day prior to seeding. The cell seeding day was deemed Day 0. Cells were allowed to attach over an initial 3-day period with medium bathing both sides of the filter support. Then, on Day 3, medium was removed and only the basolateral (bottom) side of the filter support was fed to initiate air-fluid interface (AFI) culture. MTE monolayers were maintained in this way until leak of medium was no longer observed from the bottom to the top of the filter support. Visual inspection of the cells on the filter support when no leak was observed showed "doming" and "ridging" of a confluent monolayer. After this point in monolayer culture, R_{TE} and V_{TE} were monitored with a Voltohmeter (Millipore or World Precision Instruments). R_{TE} above 1,000 $\Omega \cdot cm^2$ and a significant negative V_{TE} were then measured on or after Days 8–10. We performed Ussing chamber analysis when the electrical parameters had plateaued in open-circuit measurements and did not increase further.

Statistics

Explanation of quantification and statistical analysis of the data generated in all assays was explained in the context of the specific methods presented above.

Results

Early Evidence of ΔF508-CFTR inhibition of wild-type CFTR function

As a collaborative effort among multiple authors and laboratories involved in this study, a study was published in which optimization of transient transfection of polarized epithelial cell monolayers was performed [14]. The founding context of this work was that CFTR biogenesis, trafficking and function would be best studied in its native environment, the polarized human airway epithelial cell. During these studies, we observed that ΔF-CFTR expression in epithelia inhibited WT-CFTR driven cyclic AMP-activated Cl⁻ channel activity, monolayer maturation, and regulation of chemokine release. These observations provided the rationale for designing and undertaking the studies described below.

Is the expression of wild-type cftr altered by co-expression of ΔF508-CFTR?

To determine whether the processing of WT-CFTR is affected by the presence of ΔF-CFTR, we co-expressed the WT and mutant forms of CFTR in IB3-1 CF human airway epithelial cells that are null for detectable endogenous CFTR protein (Figure 1A). Examination of immunoprecipitated and PKA-decorated proteins on a 6% SDS-PAGE gel showed that processing of a fixed amount of WT-CFTR was altered by increasing amounts of ΔF-CFTR. In native epithelia, CFTR is immunoprecipitated as two major forms. "C band" is a broad band between 160–180 kDa that is the maturely glycosylated form of CFTR that successfully traffics through the secretory pathway to the apical plasma membrane. C band is the only form found when exogenous WT-CFTR was expressed alone in IB3-1 cells. "B band" is a tighter immaturely glycosylated band between 140–150 kDa that is an ER form of CFTR. It is a single band in native epithelia and a doublet of bands in HEK-293 cells (see below). B band is the only band observed when exogenous ΔF-CFTR was expressed alone IB3-1 cells. In Figure 1A, as the amount of ΔF-CFTR cDNA was increased in the presence of a fixed amount of WT-CFTR cDNA, there was decreased processing of the C band of WT-CFTR protein. Inhibition of C band formation was most notable when 4-8-fold more ΔF-CFTR plasmid was co-transfected versus WT-CFTR (refer to both examples in Figure 1A for different examples of the same dominant negative-like effect. We speculate that this is due to the increased rate of degradation in the ER of ΔF-CFTR versus WT-CFTR [44,45]. However, when

the same co-transfection experiment was performed in the heterologous human embryonic kidney cell line, HEK-293 T, over-expression of ΔF-CFTR was without effect on WT-CFTR processing (Figure 1B). These results suggest that CFTR processing may be different in epithelial cells versus heterologous cells and that epithelial-specific accessory proteins may be essential for driving this ΔF-CFTR inhibitory interaction with WT-CFTR.

Is this dominant negative-like effect of ΔF508-CFTR on WT-CFTR dependent upon Its PDZ motif?

To assess specificity of this ΔF-CFTR/WT-CFTR interaction, we co-expressed ΔF-CFTR with a fixed amount of ΔTRL-CFTR, a CFTR variant lacking the C-terminal PDZ binding motif but that processes efficiently through the Golgi to the plasma membrane [52]. The CFTR PDZ motif is critical for CFTR interactions with PDZ binding proteins such as EBP50 (NHERF), E3KARP, CAP-70, CAL, etc., connects CFTR to larger macromolecular complexes in organelle and plasma membranes, and influences CFTR function [35-41,53]. In contrast to dominant negative-like effects on WT-CFTR by ΔF-CFTR, increasing amounts of ΔF-CFTR failed to affect the maturation of ΔTRL-CFTR in IB3-1 CF human airway epithelial cells (Figure 1C). Summary data is also presented from multiple experiments (Figure 1C). ΔF-CFTR was also without effect on ΔTRL-CFTR in HEK-293 T cells (data not shown). These results suggest that the PDZ motif of CFTR is critical to the inhibitory influence of ΔF-CFTR on WT-CFTR at the level of the ER.

Is this a specific and exclusive interaction between ΔF508-CFTR and WT-CFTR?

We wished to take addition steps to provide specificity and exclusivity for this macromolecular complex and PDZ motif-driven ΔF-CFTR/WT-CFTR inhibitory interaction, we expressed increasing amounts of G551D-CFTR with a fixed amount of WT-CFTR. We observed only accumulating amounts of C band that did not appear to saturate during the co-expression of this mutant and WT-CFTR (Figure 2A). It is important to underscore the fact that G551D-CFTR is not an ER retention mutant but rather is processed normally to the plasma membrane. Rather, G551D-CFTR is a dysfunctional Cl⁻ channel because ATP binding and gating to its NBDs is impaired. This is why the CFTR potentiator drug, VX-770 (ivacaftor, Kalydeco) [54] is markedly effective in G551D-CFTR patients, while the CF corrector drug, VX-809, corrects/rescues ΔF-CFTR from ER quality control and is without effect on G551D-CFTR patients [55,56]. We also wished to determine whether this dominant negative-like effect of ΔF-CFTR was not non-specific to other glycosylated membrane proteins. The epithelial

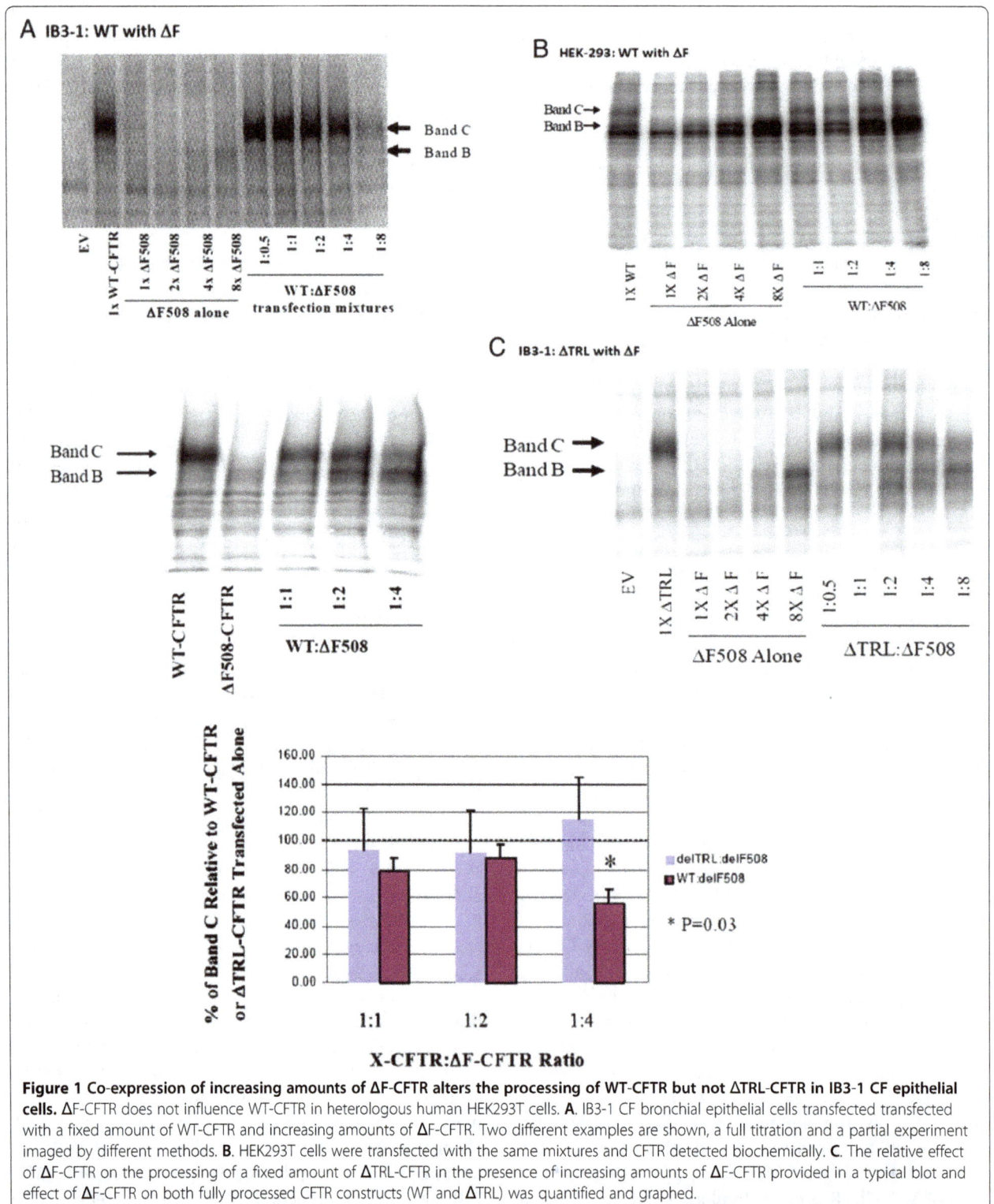

Figure 1 Co-expression of increasing amounts of ΔF-CFTR alters the processing of WT-CFTR but not ΔTRL-CFTR in IB3-1 CF epithelial cells. ΔF-CFTR does not influence WT-CFTR in heterologous human HEK293T cells. **A**. IB3-1 CF bronchial epithelial cells transfected transfected with a fixed amount of WT-CFTR and increasing amounts of ΔF-CFTR. Two different examples are shown, a full titration and a partial experiment imaged by different methods. **B**. HEK293T cells were transfected with the same mixtures and CFTR detected biochemically. **C**. The relative effect of ΔF-CFTR on the processing of a fixed amount of ΔTRL-CFTR in the presence of increasing amounts of ΔF-CFTR provided in a typical blot and effect of ΔF-CFTR on both fully processed CFTR constructs (WT and ΔTRL) was quantified and graphed.

$P2X_4$ purinergic receptor calcium entry channel also has immature (~40 kDa) and maturely glycosylated (60–65 kDa) forms and robust expression in both CF and non-CF human airway epithelial cells [57]. $P2X_4$ expression is robust in Western blot analysis and no difference in expression of either form of the receptor channel was observed with increasing amounts of ΔF508-CFTR plasmid expression (Figure 2B). These data, along with other internal controls above in Figure 1, suggest that ER stress is not a cause of ΔF-CFTR inhibition of WT-CFTR processing.

A

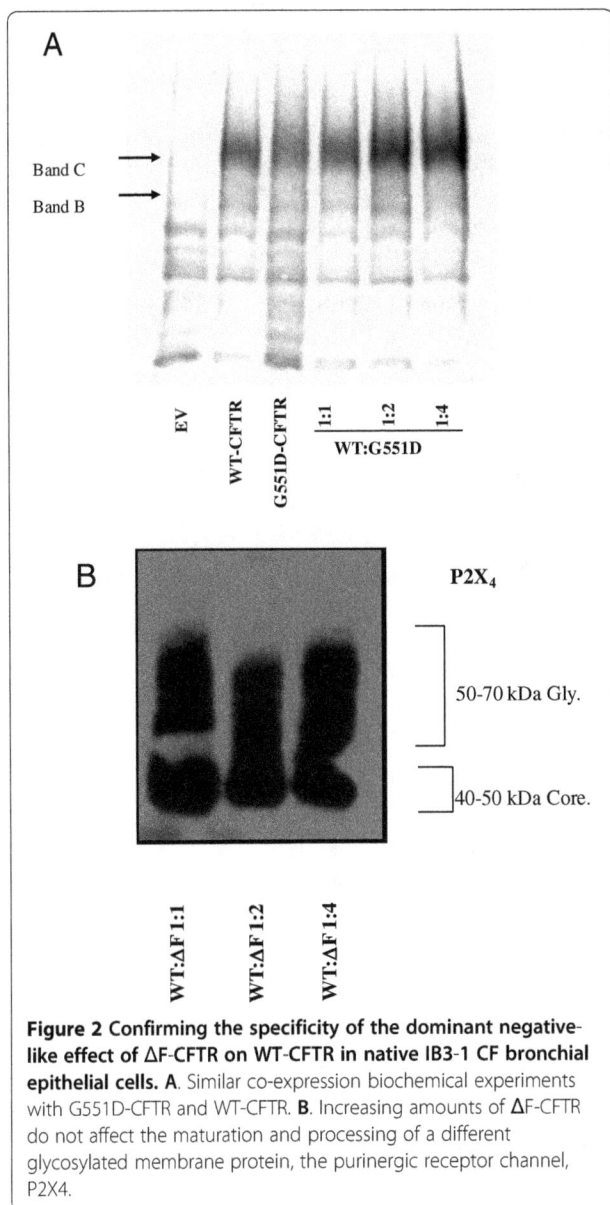

Band C

Band B

EV

WT-CFTR

G551D-CFTR

1:1 1:2 1:4

WT:G551D

B

P2X₄

50-70 kDa Gly.

40-50 kDa Core.

WT:ΔF 1:1

WT:ΔF 1:2

WT:ΔF 1:4

Figure 2 Confirming the specificity of the dominant negative-like effect of ΔF-CFTR on WT-CFTR in native IB3-1 CF bronchial epithelial cells. A. Similar co-expression biochemical experiments with G551D-CFTR and WT-CFTR. **B**. Increasing amounts of ΔF-CFTR do not affect the maturation and processing of a different glycosylated membrane protein, the purinergic receptor channel, P2X4.

Is the function of WT-CFTR altered by co-expression of ΔF-CFTR?

To complement the biochemical experiments above, we also assayed for CFTR Cl⁻ channel function with the SPQ halide efflux assay [47]. IB3-1 cells were co-transfected with increasing amounts of ΔF-CFTR versus a fixed amount of WT-CFTR as above. These cells were later incubated with the halide-sensitive dye, SPQ, overnight in medium prior to the experiment 2 days after transient transfection. Cover slips of transiently transfected cells were mounted into a perfusion chamber and bathed in sodium iodide (NaI) buffer to maintain quenching of SPQ fluorescence. First, the cells were challenged with $NaNO_3$ buffer, which dequenchs SPQ and assays for basal halide efflux which is augmented by WT-CFTR expression.

Second, a cocktail of cyclic AMP agonists (CPT-cAMP, 200 μM; forskolin, 2 μM; IBMX, 100 μM) was perfused into the chamber in $NaNO_3$ buffer to stimulate additional CFTR Cl⁻ channel activity (measured by increased halide efflux). Mock and ΔF-CFTR-expressing cells failed to respond to $NaNO_3$ buffer alone or to the cocktail of cyclic AMP agonists (Figure 3A). In contrast, WT-CFTR-transfected cells responded markedly to both $NaNO_3$ buffer alone or to the cyclic AMP cocktail (Figure 2A). However, in the co-expression experiments, increasing amounts of ΔF-CFTR inhibited wild-type CFTR activity in an apparent dose-dependent manner (Figure 3A). The functional assay showed complete inhibition with 4:1 ΔF-CFTR:WT-CFTR expression, while biochemical assays showed complete inhibition with 8:1 ΔF-CFTR:WT-CFTR expression. In contrast, similar experiments in the HEK-293 T system showed no inhibition of WT-CFTR with increasing amounts of ΔF-CFTR (Figure 3B). Taken together, these data suggests that ΔF-CFTR interacts with WT-CFTR during its processing and inhibits its functional expression in the plasma membrane in a dominant negative-like manner in human airway epithelial cells.

Are the processing and function of WT-CFTR altered by stable expression of ΔF-CFTR in a polarized non-CF human airway epithelial cell line that expresses endogenous CFTR?

One potential problem of the co-transfection and co-expression studies above was the necessity to transiently transfect with large quantities of plasmid DNA and to over-express ΔF-CFTR in order to inhibit WT-CFTR processing and function. Again, we speculate that this is likely necessary to overcome the increased rate of degradation of ΔF-CFTR protein versus WT-CFTR protein. However, to account for this issue and to approach this inhibitory interaction differently, we employed the well-characterized WT-CFTR-expressing airway epithelial cell line, CALU-3, and stably transfected ΔF-CFTR into it, generating several clones that were CF heterozygous cell lines. We also chose the CALU-3 cell line because of its high level of endogenous WT-CFTR expression and its ability for form polarized cell monolayers when grown on filter supports. Upon expansion and cryopreservation of the clones, CFTR biochemistry was performed. Parental CALU-3 cells expressed the C band form of CFTR almost exclusively (Figure 4A); all clones stably expressing ΔF-CFTR as an engineered heterozygous CF cell expressed both B band and C band forms and with reduced C band amounts in all clones. To assay for CFTR Cl⁻ channel function, we grew parental CALU-3 cells and ΔF-CFTR-expressing CALU-3 clones on permeable filter supports for Ussing chamber analysis of short-circuit current (I_{SC}). Monolayers with a transepithelial resistance (R_{TE}) at or above 1,000 $\Omega \cdot cm^2$ were used in these experiments. In all experiments (Figure 4B

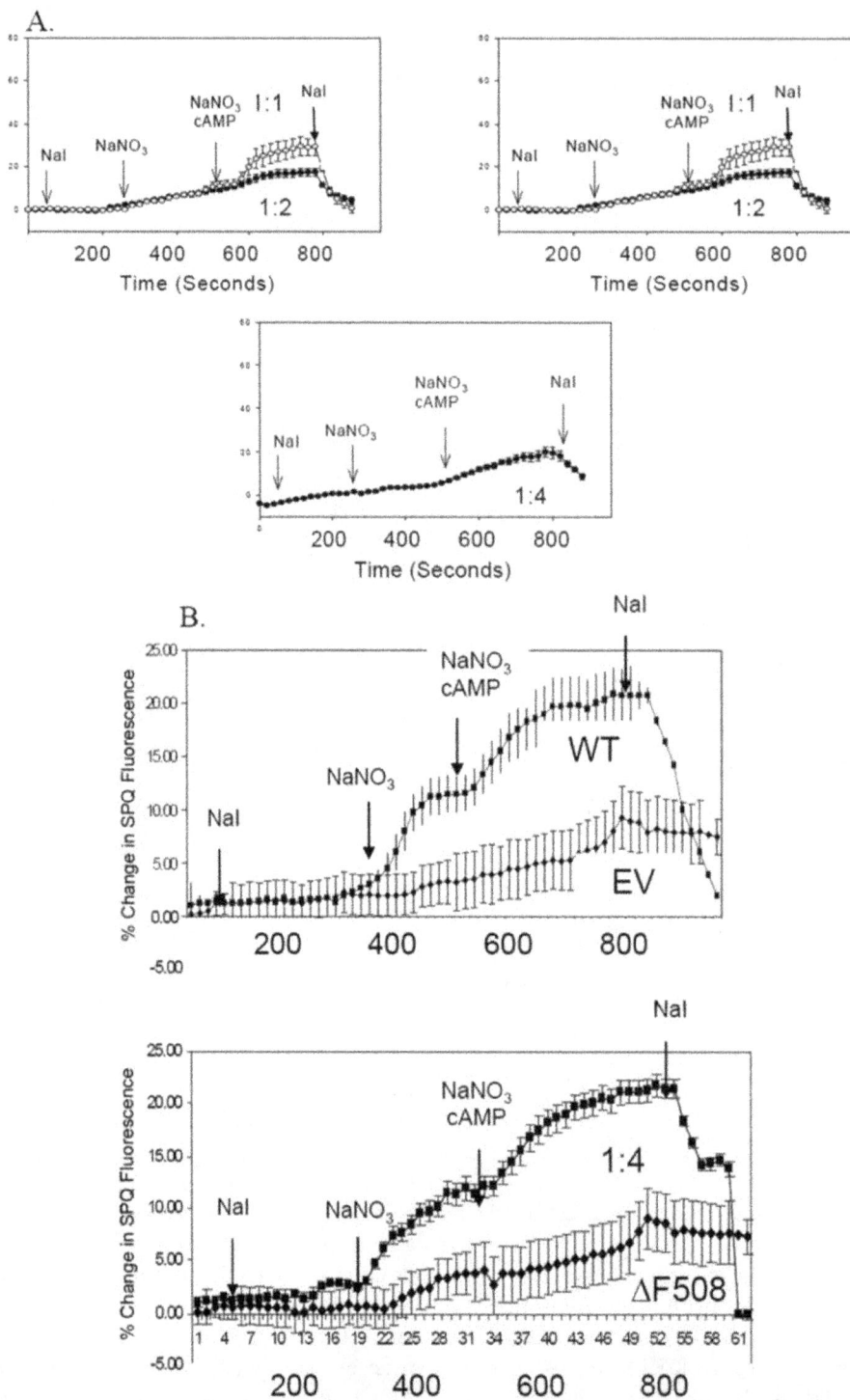

Figure 3 Co-expression of increasing amounts of ΔF-CFTR alters the function of WT-CFTR in IB3-1 CF epithelial cells but not in HEK293T cells. A. IB3-1 cells are seeded on Vitrogen coated coverslips and transiently transfect in the manner previously described in Figure 1. Twenty-four hours after transfection the cells are loaded with the halide sensitive dye, SPQ, overnight. The cells relative fluorescence is then measured while incubated in three different buffers: NaI, NaNO₃, and NaNO₃ with cAMP agonists, and then back into NaI. **B**. HEK293T cells were seeded on Vitrogen free coverslips and transfected, loaded, and measured as previously described in **A**.

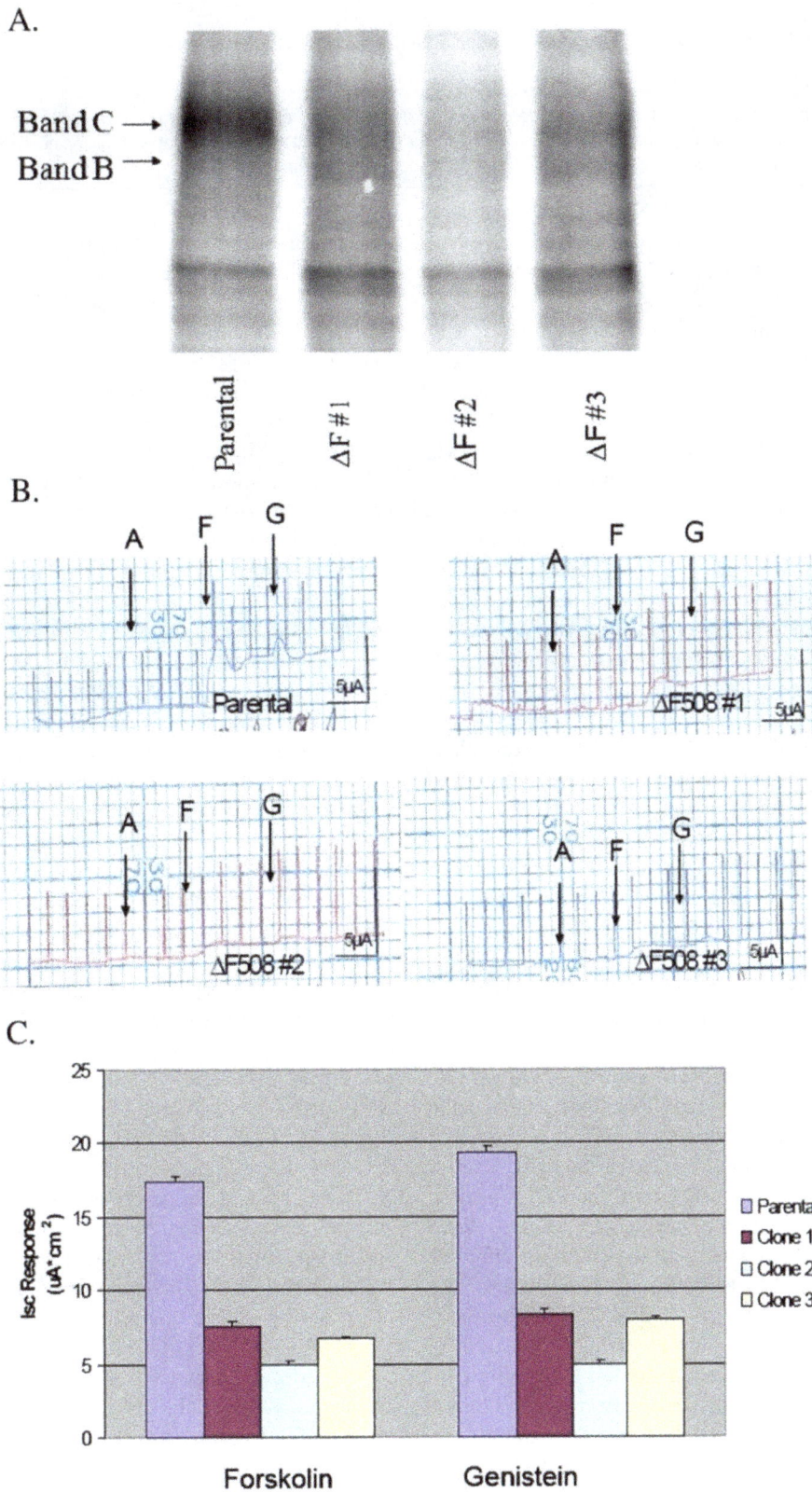

Figure 4 (See legend on next page.)

(See figure on previous page.)
Figure 4 Stable Transfection of ΔF508-CFTR into CALU-3 non-CF epithelial cells alters the processing and function of endogenous WT-CFTR. A. CFTR was IP'd from parental and stably transfected CALU-3 cells. The samples were then phosphorylated and resolved as described previously. **B.** Parental and stably transfected CALU-3 cells were seeded on 6.5 mm Vitrogen coated permeable filter supports. The CALU-3 monolayers were then allowed to reach a transepithelial resistance (R_{TE}) of 2,000 $\Omega \cdot cm^2$ or above prior to experimentation. I_{SC} is then measured in response to 10 μM amiloride, 20 μM forskolin and 50 μM genistein added apically via an Ussing chamber. Typical traces are shown. **C.** Summary analysis of parental and stably transfected CALU-3 cells I_{SC} response to agonists.

and C), amiloride (10 μM) was added to block any Na$^+$ absorption which is minimal in this epithelial cell model. Typical traces are shown for a parental CALU-3 cell monolayer and for multiple stable clones expressing ΔF-CFTR as an engineered heterozygous cell model co-expressing WT-CFTR and ΔF-CFTR endogenously. After amiloride pretreatment, forskolin (10 μM) was added to stimulate CFTR-dependent Cl$^-$ secretion via cyclic AMP. Then, genistein (50 μM) was added to open any and all remaining CFTR Cl$^-$ channels in the apical membrane. While parental CALU-3 cell monolayers responded with an averaged 5 μA to forskolin and an additional 1 μA to genistein in the presence of forskolin (Figure 4B), stable clones co-expressing both WT-CFTR and ΔF-CFTR endogenously responded only half as well or less so than parental cell monolayers. Figure 4C provides the summary data for this Ussing chamber analysis. Taken together, these data show that equivalent expression of WT-CFTR and ΔF5-CFTR endogenous to an airway epithelial cell leads to inhibition of WT-CFTR processing and, thus, function. Stable expression of both forms of CFTR also obviated the need to express more ΔF-CFTR in a transient transfection versus WT-CFTR to observe the same dominant negative-like effect.

Is the function of WT-CFTR altered by ΔF-CFTR in WT-CFTR/ΔF-CFTR heterozygous 'carrier' mice in vivo and in vitro?

In vitro results above suggested a dominant negative-like inhibition of WT-CFTR by ΔF-CFTR that was specific to this most common ER retention folding mutant and observed in native human airway epithelial cells. Studies of human patients populations, where the WT (normal), heterozygous carrier, and homozygous CF patients were analyzed as separate groups, has shown three different phenotypes for a given endpoint in past studies. We wished to confirm our *in vitro* studies with *in vivo* nasal potential difference (NPD) measurements in the ΔF508-CFTR mouse [48]. A previous argument explaining partial CF heterozygous defects was simply gene dilution (e.g., 1 copy or allele of WT-CFTR versus 2 copies). As such and in parallel, we performed NPD assays on a bitransgenic CF mouse model generously provided to our UAB CF Center Mouse Transgenic CORE by Dr. Jeffrey Whitsett. This model is a CFTR knockout mouse that is corrected in the gastrointestinal tract with a fatty

acid binding protein (FABP) promoter-driven *CFTR* construct [49]. In this bitransgenic mouse, however, the lung and airways remain null for *CFTR* in the CF (−/−) homozygous condition, the heterozygous mice have 1 allele of CFTR (+/−), and the WT mice have two alleles of CFTR (+/+). This is different from the ΔF-CFTR mouse, where the WT mice will be WT/WT, the heterozygotes will be WT/ΔF, and the homozygotes will be ΔF/ΔF.

Figure 5A shows typical NPD recordings from all 3 genotypes of the ΔF-CFTR mouse. Summary data that includes and illustrates results from all mice studied in shown in Figure 5B. Homozygous mice failed to respond to the low Cl$^-$ solution, indicating a lack of Cl$^-$ permeability in the nasal mucosa (Figure 5A and B). Homozygotes also failed to respond significantly to cyclic AMP agonists, adenosine (100 μM) and albuterol (salbutamol, 100 μM) (Figure 5A and B), although a small response was noted a subset of mice (Figure 5B). In contrast, WT mice within the ΔF-CFTR litters responded most vigorously to both the low Cl$^-$ maneuver and to the dual cyclic AMP agonists (Figures 5A and B). It should be noted that the inclusion of adenosine was essential for these studies, because Isoprel or salbutamol alone failed to elicit as large or as reproducible responses in the NPD assay. This modification was undertaken based on the work of our colleague and collaborator, Dr. JP Clancy et al., on adenosine regulation of CFTR [50,51]. Notably, the ΔF-CFTR heterozygous mice had an intermediate phenotype between WT mice and homozygous mice with regard to the low Cl$^-$ and cyclic AMP-induced responses (Figures 5A and B). Both hyperpolarization responses were significantly less than WT. These *in vivo* NPD data suggest that there is a decrement in CFTR Cl$^-$ channel activity in heterozygous ΔF-CFTR carrier mice versus WT mice when assessed across 6 different litters.

To derive closely paired *in vitro* data from these litters of ΔF-CFTR mice, tracheae were excised from these same mice in which CFTR NPD measurements were performed previously to isolate and establish mouse tracheal epithelial (MTE) cell monolayers grown on permeable filter supports in primary culture. Typical recordings of I_{SC} from all 3 genotypes from ΔF-CFTR mouse model are shown in Figure 6A. Summary data are shown in Figure 6B. As in *in vivo* NPD assays above, WT MTE monolayers gave the most vigorous response to forskolin and genistein, while heterozygous MTE

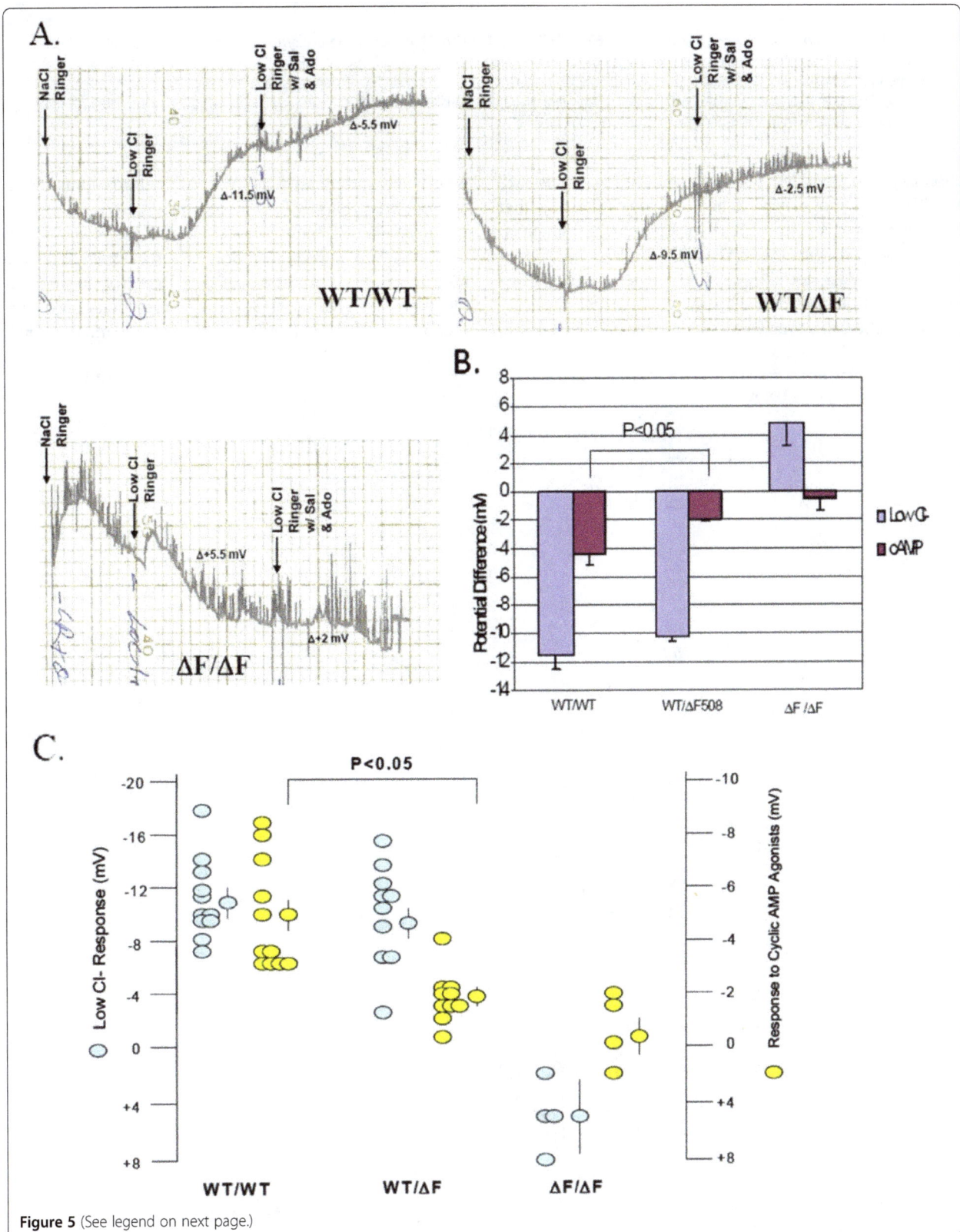

Figure 5 (See legend on next page.)

(See figure on previous page.)
Figure 5 Nasal Potential Difference is altered by ΔF508-CFTR in WT- CFTR/ΔF508-CFTR Heterozygous mice. A. Nasal Potential Difference Assays (NPD) were performed on the three genotypes of the ΔF508 mice: WT/WT, WT/ΔF, and ΔF/ΔF. NPD recordings were measured for each genotype in the presence of normal Ringer's solution, low Cl- ringer's solution, and then low Cl- Ringer's solution containing the cAMP agonist salbutamol (100 μM) and adenosine (100 μM). **B**. Summary data of the results illustrated in **A**. **C**. Scatterplot representation of the NPD measurements performed in the 3 genotypes of the ΔF508 mice.

monolayers responded less well and homozygous ΔF-CFTR MTE monolayers failed to respond altogether (Figure 6A and B). In a subset of recordings, glibenclamide (100 μM) inhibited the CFTR-mediated secretory Cl⁻ current (data not shown). Taken together, these data are similar to results derived from *in vivo* NPD measurements of the same mice and suggest that CFTR activity is partially attenuated in WT/ΔF heterozygous MTE monolayers versus WT/WT controls.

Our parallel CF mouse model was the *FABPxCFTR* gut-corrected UNC knockout mouse that remains null for the lung and airways. In this case, the WT controls in these litters have 2 WT *CFTR* alleles, the heterozygous mice have 1 copy of WT *CFTR*, and the homozygous mice are null

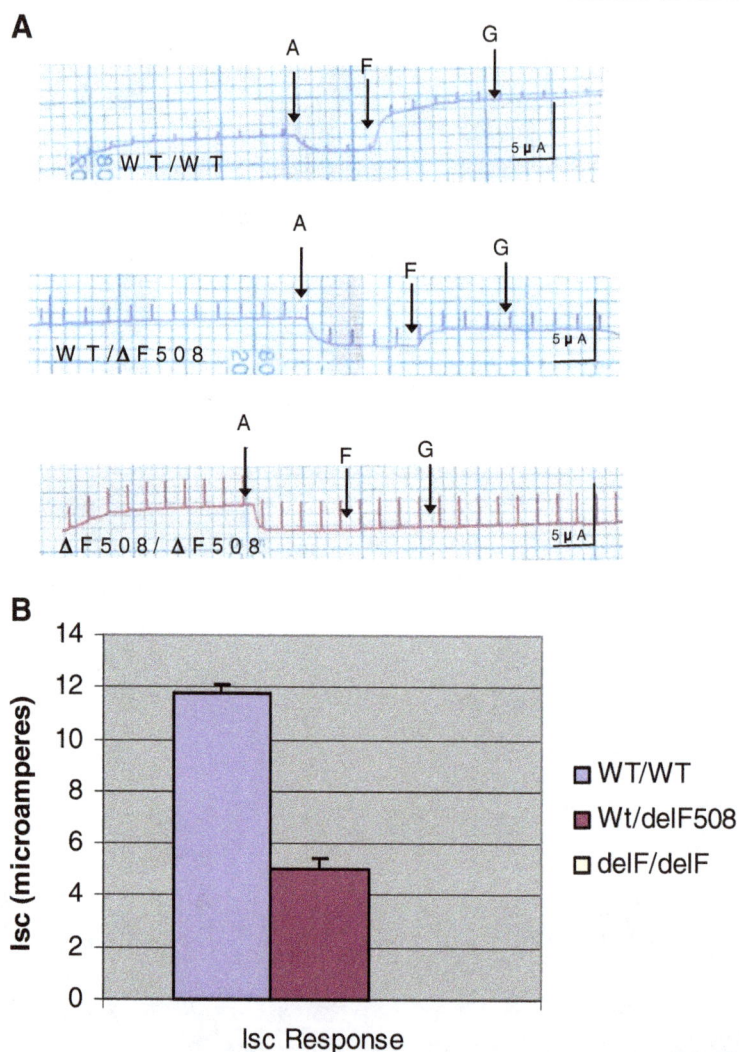

Figure 6 WT-CFTR function is altered by ΔF508-CFTR in WT-CFTR/ΔF508-CFTR heterozygous MTE A. Mouse tracheal epithelial cells (MTE) were seeded on Vitrogen coated filter inserts as previously described. On day three, the cells are grown in an air/liquid interface: media on the basolateral side but no media on the apical side. The R_{TE} of the MTE monolayers are allowed to reach 1000 Ω·cm² or above prior to experimentation The MTE monolayer I_{SC} current response to amiloride, forskolin, and genistein are then measured and record ed. **B.** Summary of the I_{SC} data of the three genotypes of the ΔF508 MTE monolayers. Homozygous cell monolayers failed to respond altogether and the summary I_{SC} response was equal to zero.

for *CFTR*. This is an important parallel study to the one above because ΔF-CFTR is not expressed in this mouse model. Figure 7A shows typical NPD recordings from all three *CFTR* genotypes in the Cincinnati bitransgenic mice. In this case, 1 copy of *CFTR* appeared sufficient for full function. There was no difference in low Cl⁻ or cyclic AMP agonist response between the WT and heterozygous mice (Figure 7A,B,C). Homozygous mice failed to respond to either maneuver (Figure 7A,B,C). Figure 7B is a scatterplot which represents the response of each mouse to low Cl⁻ and cAMP agonists segregated to genotype. Results from all mice are shown in the summary data (Figure 7C).

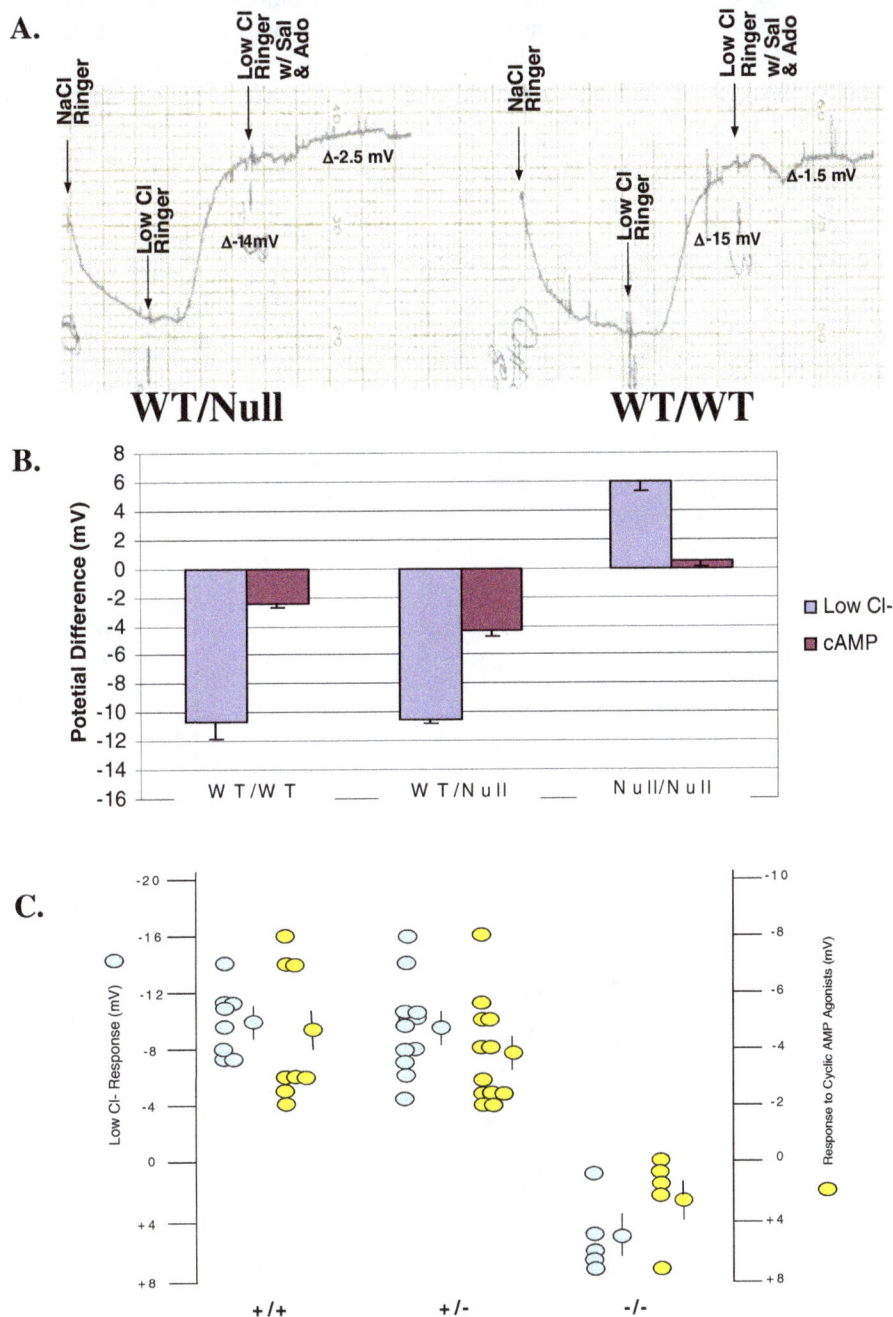

Figure 7 WT-CFTR function is not affected by the null CFTR allele in the Cincinnati WT-CFTR/Null mice. A. Nasal Potential Difference Assays (NPD) were performed on the three genotypes of the mice: WT/WT, WT/null, and null/null. NPD recordings were measured for each genotype in the presence of normal Ringer's solution, low Cl⁻ ringer's solution, and then low Cl⁻ Ringer's solution containing the cAMP agonist salbutamol (100 µM) and adenosine (100 µM). **B**. Summary data of the results illustrated in **A**. **C**. Scatterplot which represents the NPD response of each mouse to low Cl⁻ and cAMP agonists segregated to genotype.

These data suggested that 1 *CFTR* allele is enough for full function in an epithelium and in the absence of the ΔF *CFTR* mutation.

We then established MTE monolayers from tracheae of the same mice in the Cincinnati bitransgenic mouse litters. Figure 8A shows representative I_{SC} traces, Figure 8B shows the summary data, and Figure 8C is a scatterplot which represents the response of each mouse to low Cl⁻ and cAMP agonists segregated to genotype. Again, WT and heterozygous MTE monolayers had a similar response to both forskolin and genistein. Homozygous MTE monolayers did not respond to either agonist. Taken together, it is important to note that there is no decrement in overall WT-CFTR function when the number of CFTR alleles is reduced from 2 to 1, suggesting again that ΔF-CFTR is a dominant negative inhibitor of WT-CFTR in airway epithelia.

Discussion

The results indicate that ΔF-CFTR alters the processing and function of WT-CFTR in a dominant negative manner when co-expressed in a CF human airway epithelial cell. This dominant negative effect required CFTR's PDZ-

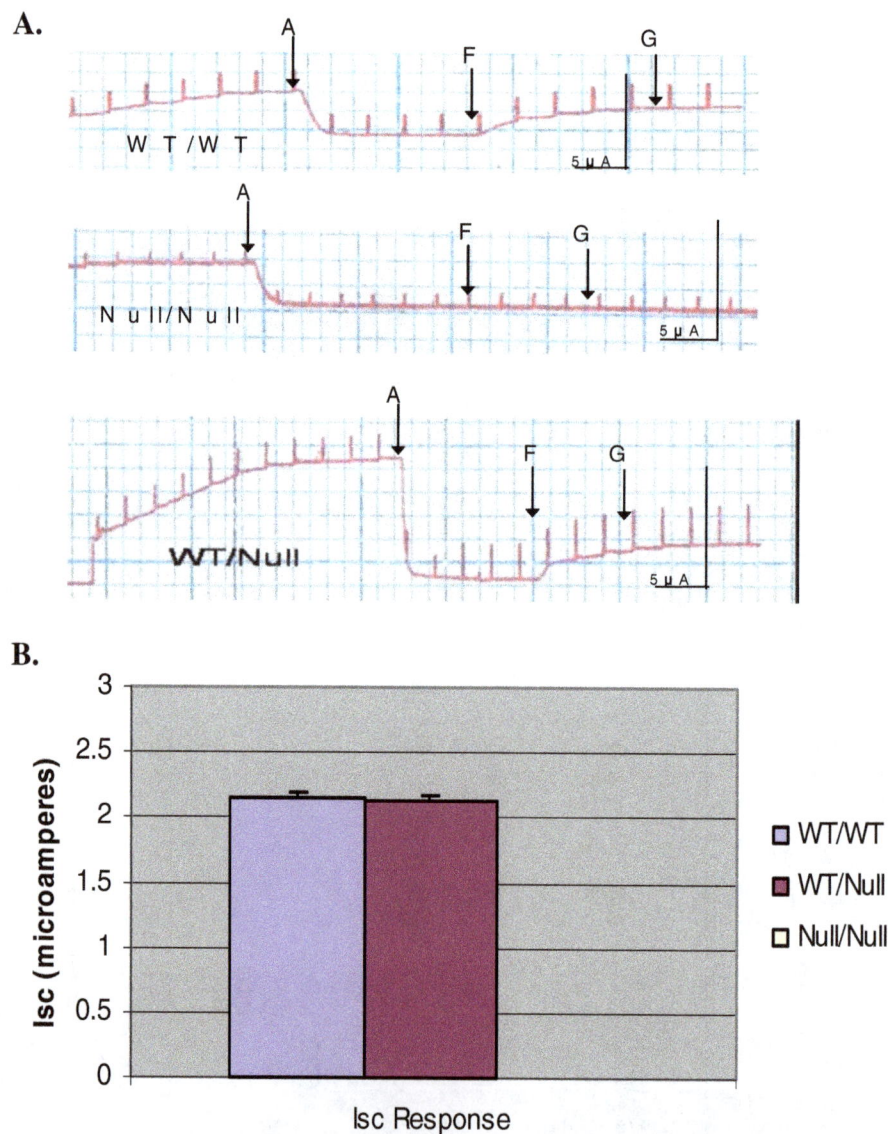

Figure 8 WT-CFTR function is not altered by the null CFTR allele in the Cincinnati WT-CFTR/null MTE. A. Mouse tracheal epithelial cells (MTE) were seeded on Vitrogen coated filter inserts as previously described. On day three, the cells are grown in an air/liquid interface: media on the basolateral side but no media on the apical side. The R_{TE} of the MTE monolayers are allowed to reach 1000 Ω•cm² or above prior to experimentation The MTE monolayer I_{SC} current response to amiloride, forskolin, and genistein are then measured and recorded. **B.** Summary of the I_{SC} data of the three genotypes of the bitransgenic MTE monolayers.

binding motif on its C-terminal end. Such an effect of ΔF-CFTR on WT-CFTR could be conferred theoretically by direct protein-protein interaction within a CFTR dimer or multimer, the association of and regulation by accessory proteins (i.e., PDZ binding proteins) for processing, trafficking and function, and/or the association of and regulation by necessary ER chaperones for protein folding.

With these three main biochemical factors impacting upon CFTR biology in native epithelia, we present a single unifying hypothesis to defend this effect in native epithelia. First and foremost, this hypothesis is driven by the fact that our observations hold in native epithelia. Throughout our collective work over the last 15 years, we continue to champion the idea that CFTR functions differently and is processed differently in native human epithelial cell platforms versus non-human or human heterologous cell platforms. CFTR is a limited copy mRNA and protein in native epithelia. Given the copious data on CFTR monomer versus dimer versus larger multimer, we are inclined to agree that CFTR is a monomer; however, that does not mean that CFTR cannot be multimeric in nature. Our central hypothesis speaks to this idea and is predicated on the finding that CFTR resides in a large macromolecular signaling complex that is driven in part by its C-terminal PDZ binding motif. The importance of the PDZ motif has been supported mainly by data generated in native and polarized epithelial cell platforms. There is also evidence in native epithelia for PDZ-interacting proteins being involved in processing and trafficking of CFTR [35-41,53]. Following on these suppositions in a logical manner, ER resident chaperones and the supportive cytoskeleton would be involved actively in the folding and placement of the multiple proteins within this CFTR-resident macromolecular complex. Our hypothesis also assumes that multiple copies (at least 2 copies) of the CFTR protein are processed at the ER, trafficked through the Golgi, and functional at the apical plasma membrane within such a large complex. With similar supportive logic and assuming multiple copies of CFTR per complex and likely multiple complexes within each vesicle as cargo, a ΔF-CFTR copy would attract chaperones that would identify the folding defect and attempt to retain this misfolded ΔF-CFTR protein and associated proteins. More than one ΔF-CFTR protein copy would amplify such attempted ER retention. If copies of WT-CFTR are also present within this large complex, they would be retained, snared or 'caught up in' this delF-CFTR retention in other parts of the large complex. Finally, we believe that this dominant negative effect would occur ahead of either Golgi-driven trafficking to the plasma membrane or non-traditional GRASP dependent trafficking that do not involve the complex Golgi apparatus [58,59].

There are a number of proteins that are associated with CFTR that could influence a dominant negative inhibition of WT-CFTR by ΔF-CFTR. Two classes of epithelial-specific accessory proteins likely involved are ER resident chaperones and the PDZ binding proteins. The heat shock family of proteins (HSP) is known to associate with CFTR at the level of the ER as a key group of CFTR chaperones. All members of this family have ATPase activity that is directly linked to their ability to associate/disassociate with their protein substrate. Potential candidates include HSP90, HSP70 and its cognate HSC70 in conjunction with HSP40 and CHIP [60-67]. Recently, Balch and coworkers identified a 'chaperone trap' for CFTR that included HSP40, HSP70 and HSP90 [67]. The latter HSP is known to interact with both WT-CFTR and ΔF-CFTR and exists in a dimeric state. A CFTR dimer could conceivably form through an HSP90 dimer at least transiently during CFTR biogenesis in the ER. HSP70 is a less studied protein in CF; however, it does bind CFTR. Its cognate relative, HSC70, is better understood. HSC70 mediates CFTR degradation in the ER through its interaction with HSP40 and CHIP [64]. HSC70's association with CFTR and other protein substrates is regulated by its fellow chaperone, Hdj-2, an HSP40 family member [64]. In addition, CHIP, as a co-chaperone, binds the HSC70/Hdj-2 complex via one of three tetratricopeptide repeat (TRP) domains. This interaction inhibits the ATPase activity induced by Hdj-2 on HSC 70 and prolongs the interaction of CHIP with HSC70 and with the nascent CFTR peptide. Moreover, CHIP has 3 TRP domains and could bind at least 3 CFTR/HSC70/Hdj-2 complexes [64] and target all to the degradation pathway if one or more of the CFTR polypeptides being processed bore the ΔF-CFTR.

The second class of proteins likely involved in the dominant negative interaction are the PDZ binding domain family of proteins that have the class 1 PDZ domains which recognizes the QDTRL sequence in the end of the CFTR C terminus. Candidates include CAL, EBP50/NHERF-1, E3KARP, and CAP70 that likely influence both trafficking and anchoring of membrane proteins like CFTR and that may be more deeply involved in the ER processing than described previously [35-41,53]. CAL or CFTR-associated ligand is a Golgi resident PDZ protein which can prevent CFTR from reaching the plasma membrane. CAL has only one PDZ domain but exist in a homomultimeric state and could tether multiple CFTR polypeptides together. EBP-50, ezrin-binding protein 50 or Na/H exchange regulatory factor 1 (NHERF-1) has two PDZ binding domains which could, in theory, tether nascent ΔF-CFTR and WT-CFTR polypeptides together if co-expressed in the ER. CAP70, CFTR-associating protein 70, has 4 PDZ domains and 3 of those domains bind CFTR with significant affinity in the order, 3 > 1 > 4. This protein could also bind up to three CFTR molecules and transport them to the cell surface or divert the three "tethered" proteins to the degradation pathway if one or two of the three CFTR polypeptides possessed the ΔF-CFTR mutation. We hypothesize that chaperones, co-chaperones, and PDZ binding proteins resident in the ER may all play a significant role in the ΔF-CFTR/WT-CFTR inhibitory interaction during processing in airway epithelia.

Our finding and the associated CFTR biology in native epithelial cells has profound implications regarding the development of efficient therapeutic methods to correct or replace ΔF-CFTR *in vivo*. Although the understanding of CFTR biology has advanced significantly in recent years, there is much still poorly understood regarding the processing and function of CFTR in native epithelial cells. A primary and fundamental problem which still exists in the field is a lack in the understanding of how epithelial CFTR is processed, what the exact nature of CFTR's stoichiometry is, and what epithelial accessory proteins interact with epithelial CFTR in the ER, in the Golgi and other organelles, and at the plasma membrane. The discovery and development of CF corrector drugs such as Vertex's VX-809 being examined in CF clinical trials currently is also influenced by this biology and the concept of a ΔF-CFTR dominant negative inhibition of WT-CFTR when expressed together within an epithelial cell [55,56]. An uncorrected ΔF-CFTR could conceivably still inhibit a corrected ΔF-CFTR in a similar dominant negative manner.

There was a premise within the CF research community that only 10% of cells along the CF airway or a 10% correction of ΔF-CFTR within a given CF cell would be sufficient for a successful therapy. A 10-20% level of correction was achieved with VX-809 in a recent published study [55]. However, VX-809 itself does not appear potent or effective enough as a single drug in recent clinical trials; it was disappointing by itself in a combination trial with the CFTR potentiator drug, VX-770 (ivacaftor, Kalydeco™) in ΔF-CFTR homozygous patients. It is now felt that a 50% level of correction is a better benchmark that is equivalent to 27°C reduced temperature correction in a biochemical correction assay. This also approaches the CF heterozygous condition where a carrier would have 50% of the functional CFTR than a normal or WT individual. This level may need to be the new benchmark for a ΔF-CFTR correction therapy. While many members in the CF field have been resistant to the concept that the CF heterozygote may harbor dysfunction since CF heterozygotes do not display a fully developed CF disease phenotype, correction of a ΔF-CFTR bearing homozygote to a ΔF-CFTR bearing heterozygote would control CF disease. Our work also suggests that more research should be done addressing both the CF patient and the heterozygotic CF carrier in contrast to the normal or non-CF WT controls. One

suggestion from these studies is that WT mice, CF heterozygous mice, and CF homozygous mice, especially within ΔF-CFTR mouse models, should be studied as three separate experimental groups in the future. In particular, these three experimental groups may be informative to the study of CFTR biology and its influence on other epithelial cell functions.

Conclusions

Taken together, ΔF-CFTR inhibition of WT-CFTR during protein processing in the ER of native CF human bronchial epithelial cells explains CF-like disease symptoms but not fully developed CF disease in CF heterozygous carriers, the majority of whom are WT/ΔF carriers in the overall population. Attainment of CF heterozygote level of function with CF corrector drugs and other strategies would also serve as a critical benchmark for CF therapy in the near future. Finally, we propose that both ER-resident chaperones and PDZ-binding proteins likely play critical roles in CFTR-driven multimeric, oligomeric and/or macromolecular complex formation that provide a suitable environment for ΔF-CFTR dominant negative inhibition of WT-CFTR processing and, thus, trafficking and function.

Competing interests
These studies were purely basic science in nature. There are no competing or non-competing financial interests related to this work.

Authors' contributions
All authors warrant authorship as outlined by BioMedCentral guidelines. TAT was the main driver of this study and made the initial observation of a dominant negative-like effect of delF508-CFTR on wild-type CFTR expression and function when optimizing lipid-based transient transfection methods on polarized and non-polarized airway and other epithelial cell cultures. This study was highly controversial several years ago when it was performed because of the debates over CFTR monomer versus multimer, over disease phenotypes in CF heterozygotes, over differences in CFTR protein processing in epithelial versus heterologous cells, etc. It remains so. AZ assisted TAT on the SPQ and Ussing chamber functional assays. JAF assisted TAT, AZ and EMS on the NPD recordings in the two different CF mouse models on behalf of the UAB CF Center. MD, LF and DMB assisted the program in CF mouse strain breeding and husbandry. EMS and LMS are collaborators and were involved in supervision of the overall study. All authors read and approved the final manuscript.

Acknowledgments
We thank the Department of Cell Developmental and Integrative Biology for infrastructure support in the accomplishment of this important study. In particular, we thank Drs. Karoly Varga, Zsuzsanna Bebok and Jim Collawn for advice about biochemical methods of CFTR detection. We also thank the Gregory Fleming James Cystic Fibrosis Center and its Transgenic Mouse, Ussing Chamber Electrophysiology and Nasal Potential Difference Measurement Cores within the Center's Research Development Center and its P30 Translational and Research Core Centers for the collective support. Multiple NIH grants from the NIDDK and NHLBI for EMS, LMS, and DMB are also cited for critical support for this study.
We also thank the Gregory Fleming James Cystic Fibrosis Center and its Transgenic Mouse, Ussing Chamber Electrophysiology and Nasal Potential Difference Measurement Cores within the Center's Research Development

Center and its P30 Translational and Research Core Centers for the collective support. In particular, we thank Drs. Ming Du and David M. Bedwell and the Transgenic Mouse Core for extensive animal husbandry for the numerous nasal PD measurements made for this study. Multiple past NIH grants from the NIDDK and NHLBI for EMS and LMS are also cited for critical support for this study.

Author details
[1]Departments of Cell Developmental and Integrative Biology, University of Alabama at Birmingham, 1918 University Blvd, Birmingham, AL 35294-0005, USA. [2]Gregory Fleming James Cystic Fibrosis (CF) Research Center, University of Alabama at Birmingham, 1918 University Blvd, Birmingham 35294-0005AL, USA. [3]Department of Experimental Human Physiology, Semmelweis University, Budapest, Hungary. [4]Department of Biochemistry, University of Texas Health Sciences Center at Tyler, Tyler, TX, USA. [5]DiscoveryBioMed, Inc, Birmingham, AL, USA.

References

1. Riordan JR, Rommens JM, Kerem B, Alon N, Rozmahel R, Grzelczak Z, Zielenski J, Lok S, Plavsic N, Chou JL, *et al*: **Identification of the cystic fibrosis gene: cloning and characterization of complementary DNA.** *Science* 1989, **245**:1066–1073.
2. Rommens JM, Iannuzzi MC, Kerem B, Drumm ML, Melmer G, Dean M, Rozmahel R, Cole JL, Kennedy D, Hidaka N, *et al*: **Identification of the cystic fibrosis gene: chromosome walking and jumping.** *Science* 1989, **245**:1059–1065.
3. Kerem B, Rommens JM, Buchanan JA, Markiewicz D, Cox TK, Chakravarti A, Buchwald M, Tsui LC: **Identification of the cystic fibrosis gene: genetic analysis.** *Science* 1989, **245**:1073–1080.
4. Schwiebert EM, Benos DJ, Egan ME, Stutts MJ, Guggino WB: **CFTR is a conductance regulator as well as a chloride channel.** *Phys Rev* 1999, **79**:S145–S166.
5. Lukacs GL, Verkman AS: **CFTR: Folding, misfolding, and correcting the deltaF508 conformational defect.** *Trends Mol Med* 2012, **18**(2):81–91.
6. Guggino WB, Stanton BA: **New insights into cystic fibrosis: Molecular switches that regulate CFTR.** *Nat Rev Mol Cell Biol* 2006, **7**(6):426–436.
7. Salvatore F, Scudiero O, Castaldo G: **Genotype-phenotype correlation in cystic fibrosis: the role of modifier genes.** *Am J Med Genet* 2002, **111**:88–95.
8. Rowntree RK, Harris A: **The phenotypic consequences of CFTR mutations.** *Ann Hum Genet* 2003, **67**:471–485.
9. Oceandy D, McMorran BJ, Smith SN, Schreiber R, Kunzelmann K, Alton EWFW, Hume DA, Wainwright BJ: **Gene complementation of airway epithelium in the cystic fibrosis mouse is necessary and sufficient to correct the pathogen clearance and inflammatory abnormalities.** *Human Mol Genet* 2002, **11**(9):1059–1067.
10. Driskell RA, Engelhardt JF: **Current status of gene therapy for inherited lung diseases.** *Annu Rev Physiol* 2003, **65**:585–612.
11. Stoltz DA, *et al*: **Cystic fibrosis pigs develop lung disease and exhibit defective bacterial eradication at birth.** *Sci Transl Med* 2010, **2**(29):29–31.
12. Sun X, *et al*: **Disease phenotype of a ferret CFTR-knockout model of cystic fibrosis.** *J Clin Invest* 2011, **120**(9):3149–3160.
13. Keiser NW, Engelhardt JF: **New animal models of cystic fibrosis: What are they teaching us?** *Curr Opin Pulm Med* 2011, **17**(6):478–483.
14. Tucker TA, Varga K, Bebok Z, Zsembery A, McCarty NA, Collawn JF, Schwiebert EM, Schwiebert LM: **Transient transfection of polarized epithelial monolayers with CFTR and reporter genes using efficacious lipids.** *Am J Physiol Cell Physiol* 2003, **284**:C791–C804.
15. Varga K, Jurkuvenaite A, Wakefield J, Hong JS, Guimbellot JS, Venglarik CJ, Niraj A, Mazur M, Sorscher EJ, Collawn JF, Bebok Z: **Efficient intracellular processing of the endogenous cystic fibrosis transmembrane conductance regulator in epithelial cell lines.** *J Biol Chem* 2004, **279**:22578–22584.
16. Behm JK, Hagiwara G, Lewiston NJ, Quinton PM, Wine JJ: **Hyposecretion of beta-adrenergically induced sweating in cystic fibrosis heterozygotes.** *Pediatr Res* 1987, **22**:271–276.
17. Davis PB: **Physiologic implications of the autonomic aberrations in cystic fibrosis.** *Horm Metab Res* 1986, **18**:217–220.
18. Dahl M, Tybjaerg-Hansen A, Lange P, Nordestgaard BG: **DeltaF508 heterozygosity in cystic fibrosis and susceptibility to asthma.** *Lancet* 1998, **351**:1911–1913.
19. Miller PW, Hamosh A, Macek M Jr, Greenberger PA, MacLean J, Walden SM, Slavin RG, Cutting GR: **Cystic fibrosis transmembrane conductance regulator (CFTR) gene mutations in allergic bronchopulmonary aspergillosis.** *Am J Hum Genet* 1996, **59**:45–51.
20. Coste A, Girodon E, Louis S, Pruliere-Escabasse V, Goossens M, Peynegre R, Escudier E: **Atypical sinusitis in adults must lead to looking for cystic fibrosis and primary ciliary dyskinesia.** *Laryngoscope* 2004, **114**:839–843.
21. Steagall WK, Elmer HL, Brady KG, Kelley TJ: **Cystic fibrosis transmembrane conductance regulator-dependent regulation of epithelial inducible nitric oxide synthase expression.** *Am J Respir Cell Mol Biol* 2000, **22**:45–50.
22. Bear CE LIC, Kartner N, Bridges RJ, Jensen TJ, Ramjeesingh M, Riordan JR: **Cl⁻ channel activity in Xenopus oocytes expressing the cystic fibrosis gene.** *Cell* 1992, **68**:809–818.
23. Li C, Roy K, Dandridge K, Naren AP: **Molecular assembly of cystic fibrosis transmembrane conductance regulator in plasma membrane.** *J Biol Chem* 2004, **279**:24673–24684.
24. Ramjeesingh M, Ugwu F, Li C, Dhani S, Huan LJ, Wang Y, Bear CE: **Dimeric cystic fibrosis transmembrane conductance regulator exists in the plasma membrane.** *Biochem J* 2003, **375**:633–641.
25. Chen JH, Chang XB, Aleksandrov AA, Riordan JR: **CFTR is a monomer: biochemical and functional evidence.** *J Membr Biol* 2002, **188**:55–71.
26. Eskandari S, Wright EM, Kreman M, Starace DM, Zampighi GA: **Structural analysis of cloned plasma membrane proteins by freeze-fracture electron microscopy.** *Proc Natl Acad Sci USA* 1998, **95**:11235–11240.
27. Zerhusen B, Zhao J, Xie J, Davis PB, Ma J: **A single conductance pore for chloride ions formed by two cystic fibrosis transmembrane conductance regulator molecules.** *J Biol Chem* 1999, **274**:7627–7630.
28. Boscoboinik D, Debanne MT, Stafford AR, Jung CY, Gupta RS, Epand RM: **Dimerization of the P-glycoprotein in membranes.** *Biochim Biophys Acta* 1990, **1027**:225–228.
29. Wang S, Yue H, Derin RB, Guggino WB, Li M: **Accessory protein facilitated CFTR-CFTR interaction, a molecular mechanism to potentiate the chloride channel activity.** *Cell* 2000, **103**:169–179.
30. Raghuram V, Mak DD, Foskett JK: **Regulation of cystic fibrosis transmembrane conductance regulator single-channel gating by bivalent PDZ-domain-mediated interaction.** *Proc Natl Acad Sci USA* 2001, **98**:1300–1305.
31. Lukacs GL, Chang XB, Bear C, Kartner N, Mohamed A, Riordan JR, Grinstein S: **The delta F508 mutation decreases the stability of cystic fibrosis transmembrane conductance regulator in the plasma membrane. Determination of functional half-lives on transfected cells.** *J Biol Chem* 1993, **268**:1592–1598.
32. Clarke LL, Gawenis LR, Hwang TC, Walker NM, Gruis DB, Price EM: **A domain mimic increases DeltaF508 CFTR trafficking and restores cAMP-stimulated anion secretion in cystic fibrosis epithelia.** *Am J Physiol Cell Physiol* 2004, **287**:C192–C199.
33. Cormet-Boyaka E, Jablonsky M, Naren AP, Jackson PL, Muccio DD, Kirk KL: **Rescuing cystic fibrosis transmembrane conductance regulator (CFTR) processing mutants by transcomplementation.** *Proc Natl Acad Sci USA* 2004, **101**:8221–8226.
34. Heda GD, Tanwani M, Marino CR: **The Delta F508 mutation shortens the biochemical half-life of plasma membrane CFTR in polarized epithelial cells.** *Am J Physiol Cell Physiol* 2001, **280**:C166–C174.
35. He J, Bellini M, Xu J, Castleberry AM, Hall RA: **Interaction with CAL inhibits beta-1-adrenergic receptor surface expression.** *J Biol Chem* 2004, **279**:50190–50196.
36. Cheng J, Moyer BD, Milewski M, Loffing J, Ikeda M, Mickle JE, Cutting GR, Li M, Stanton BA, Guggino WB: **A Golgi-associated PDZ domain protein modulates cystic fibrosis transmembrane regulator plasma membrane expression.** *J Biol Chem* 2002, **277**:3520–3529.
37. Swiatecka-Urban A, Duhaime M, Coutermarsh B, Karlson KH, Collawn J, Milewski M, Cutting GR, Guggino WB, Langford G, Stanton BA: **PDZ domain interaction controls the endocytic recycling of the cystic fibrosis transmembrane conductance regulator.** *J Biol Chem* 2002, **277**:40099–40105.
38. Cheng J, Cebotaru V, Cebotaru L, Guggino WB: **Syntaxin 6 and CAL mediate the degradation of the CFTR.** *Mol Biol Cell* 2010, **21**(7):1178–1187.
39. Cushing PR, Fellows A, Villone D, Boisguerin P, Madden DR: **The relative binding affinities of PDZ partners for CFTR: a biochemical basis for efficient endocytic recycling.** *Biochemistry* 2008, **47**(38):10084–10098.

40. Tandon C, De Lisle RC, Boulatnikov I, Naik PK: **Interaction of carboxyl-terminal peptides of cystolic-tail of apactin with PDZ domains of NHERF/EBP50 and PDZK-1/CAP70.** *Mol Cell Biochem* 2007, **302**(1–2):157–167.

41. Lee JH, Richter W, Namkung W, Kim KH, Kim E, Conti M, Lee MG: **Dynamic regulation of cystic fibrosis transmembrane conductance regulator by competitive interactions of molecular adaptors.** *J Biol Chem* 2007, **282**(14):10414–10422.

42. Cuthbert AW, MacVinish LJ: **Mechanisms of anion secretion in Calu-3 human airway epithelial cells by 7,8-benzoquinoline.** *Br J Pharmacol* 2003, **140**:81–90.

43. Xiao YF, Wright SN, Wang GK, Morgan JP, Leaf A: **Fatty acids suppress voltage-gated Na^+ currents in HEK293t cells transfected with the alpha-subunit of the human cardiac Na^+ channel.** *Proc Natl Acad Sci USA* 1998, **95**:2680–2685.

44. Ward CL, Kopito RR: **Intracellular turnover of cystic fibrosis transmembrane conductance regulator. Inefficient processing and rapid degradation of wild-type and mutant proteins.** *J Biol Chem* 1994, **269**:25710–25718.

45. Jensen TJ, Loo MA, Pind S, Williams DB, Goldberg AL, Riordan JR: **Multiple proteolytic systems, including the proteasome, contribute to CFTR processing.** *Cell* 1995, **83**:129–135.

46. Li H, Sheppard DN, Hug MJ: **Transepithelial electrical measurements with the Ussing chamber.** *J Cyst Fibros* 2004, **2**:123–126.

47. Braunstein GM, Zsembery A, Tucker TA, Schwiebert EM: **Purinergic signaling underlies CFTR control of human airway epithelial cell volume.** *J Cyst Fibros* 2004, **3**:109–117.

48. Zeiher BG, Eichwald E, Zabner J, Smith JJ, Puga AP, McCray PB Jr, Capecchi MR, Welsh MJ, Thomas KR: **A mouse model for the delta F508 allele of cystic fibrosis.** *J Clin Invest* 1995, **96**:2051–2064.

49. Snouwaert JN, Brigman KK, Latour AM, Malouf NN, Boucher RC: **An animal model for cystic fibrosis made by gene targeting.** *Science* 1992, **257**:1083–1088.

50. Hentchel-Franks K, Lozano D, Eubanks-Tarn V, Cobb B, Fan L, Oster R, Sorscher E, Clancy JP: **Activation of airway Cl⁻ secretion in human subjects by adenosine.** *Am J Respir Cell Mol Biol* 2004, **31**:140–146.

51. Cobb BR, Ruiz F, King CM, Fortenberry J, Greer H, Kovacs T, Sorscher EJ, Clancy JP: **A(2) adenosine receptors regulate CFTR through PKA and PLA (2).** *Am J Physiol Lung Cell Mol Physiol* 2002, **282**:L12–L25.

52. Moyer BD, Denton J, Karlson KH, Reynolds D, Wang S, Mickle JE, Milewski M, Cutting GR, Guggino WB, Li M, Stanton BA: **A PDZ-interacting domain in CFTR is an apical membrane polarization signal.** *J Clin Invest* 1999, **104**(10):1353–1361.

53. Li C, Naren AP: **Analysis of CFTR interactome in macromolecular complexes.** *Methods Mol Biol* 2011, **741**:255–270.

54. Accurso FJ, *et al*: **Effect of VX-770 in persons with cystic fibrosis and the G551D-CFTR mutation.** *N Engl J Med* 2010, **363**(21):1991–2003.

55. Van Goor F, *et al*: **Correction of the delF508-CFTR protein processing defect in vitro by investigational drug VX-809.** *Proc Natl Acad Sci USA* 2011, **108**(46):18843–18848.

56. Clancy JP, *et al*: **Results of a Phase IIa study of VX-809, an investigational CFTR corrector compound, in subjected with cystic fibrosis homozygous for the delF508-CFTR mutation.** *Thorax* 2010, **67**(1):12–18.

57. Schwiebert LM, Rice WC, Kudlow BA, Taylor AL, Schwiebert EM: **Extracellular ATP signaling and P2X nucleotide receptors in monolayers of primary human vascular endothelial cells.** *Am J Physiol Cell Physiol* 2002, **282**:C289–C301.

58. Gee HY, Noh SH, Tang BL, Kim KH, Lee MG: **Rescue of deltaF508-CFTR trafficking via a GRASP-dependent unconventional secretion pathway.** *Cell* 2011, **146**(5):746–760.

59. Yoo JS, Moyer BD, Bennykh S, Yoo HM, Riordan JR, Balch WE: **Non-conventional trafficking of the cystic fibrosis transmembrane conductance regulator through the early secretory pathway.** *J Biol Chem* 2002, **277**(13):11401–11409.

60. Rubenstein RC, Lyons BM: **Sodium 4-phenylbutyrate downregulates HSC70 expression by facilitating mRNA degradation.** *Am J Physiol Lung Cell Mol Physiol* 2001, **281**:L43–L51.

61. Gebauer M, Zeiner M, Gehring U: **Proteins interacting with the molecular chaperone hsp70/hsc70: physical associations and effects on refolding activity.** *FEBS Lett* 1997, **417**:109–113.

62. Choo-Kang LR, Zeitlin PL: **Induction of HSP70 promotes DeltaF508 CFTR trafficking.** *Am J Physiol Lung Cell Mol Physiol* 2001, **281**:L58–L68.

63. Meacham GC, Patterson C, Zhang W, Younger JM, Cyr DM: **The Hsc70 co-chaperone CHIP targets immature CFTR for proteasomal degradation.** *Nat Cell Biol* 2001, **3**:100–105.

64. Meacham GC, Lu Z, King S, Sorscher E, Tousson A, Cyr DM: **The Hdj-2/Hsc70 chaperone pair facilitates early steps in CFTR biogenesis.** *EMBO J* 1999, **18**:1492–1505.

65. Loo MA, Jensen TJ, Cui L, Chang XB, Riordan JR: **Perturbation of Hsp90 interaction with nascent CFTR prevents its maturation and accelerates its degradation by the proteasome.** *EMBO J* 1998, **17**:6879–6887.

66. Wang X, Koulov AV, Kellner WA, Riordan JR, Balch WE: **Chemical and biological folding contribute to temperature-sensitive deltaF508-CFTR trafficking.** *Traffic* 2008, **9**(11):1878–1893.

67. Coppinger JA, Hutt DM, Razvi A, Koulov AV, Pankow S, Yates JR 3rd, Balch WE: **A chaperone trap contributes to the onset of cystic fibrosis.** *PLoS One* 2012, **7**(5):e37682. May 31 Epub ahead of print.

Quinine controls body weight gain without affecting food intake in male C57BL6 mice

Philippe Cettour-Rose[1], Carole Bezençon[1], Christian Darimont[1], Johannes le Coutre[1,2] and Sami Damak[1*]

Abstract

Background: Quinine is a natural molecule commonly used as a flavouring agent in tonic water. Diet supplementation with quinine leads to decreased body weight and food intake in rats. Quinine is an *in vitro* inhibitor of Trpm5, a cation channel expressed in taste bud cells, the gastrointestinal tract and pancreas. The objective of this work is to determine the effect of diet supplementation with quinine on body weight and body composition in male mice, to investigate its mechanism of action, and whether the effect is mediated through Trpm5.

Results: Compared with mice consuming AIN, a regular balanced diet, mice consuming AIN diet supplemented with 0.1% quinine gained less weight (2.89 ± 0.30 g vs 5.39 ± 0.50 g) and less fat mass (2.22 ± 0.26 g vs 4.33 ± 0.43 g) after 13 weeks of diet, and had lower blood glucose and plasma triglycerides. There was no difference in food intake between the mice consuming quinine supplemented diet and those consuming control diet. Trpm5 knockout mice gained less fat mass than wild-type mice. There was a trend for a diet-genotype interaction for body weight and body weight gain, with the effect of quinine less pronounced in the Trpm5 KO than in the WT background. Faecal weight, energy and lipid contents were higher in quinine fed mice compared to regular AIN fed mice and in Trpm5 KO mice compared to wild type mice.

Conclusion: Quinine contributes to weight control in male C57BL6 mice without affecting food intake. A partial contribution of Trpm5 to quinine dependent body weight control is suggested.

Keywords: Obesity, Food intake, Fat, Body composition, Gastrointestinal tract

Background

Quinine is a natural molecule extracted from the bark of the cinchona tree commonly used as a flavoring agent in tonic water and bitter lemon and, at higher doses, for the treatment of some forms of malaria. Consumption of quinine by rats strongly reduces food intake and body weight [1-7]. The decrease in food intake was initially attributed to the intense bitter taste of quinine but it was later shown that diminished food intake is observed with rats consuming a diet supplemented with quinine, but not with a diet supplemented with iso-bitter sucrose octaacetate, suggesting that palatability is not the only cause of decreased food intake in rats consuming quinine in the diet [1]. Furthermore it is unclear from the rat experiments whether there is a direct effect of quinine on body weight, independently of food intake. Quinine was recently shown to inhibit the activity of Trpm5 [8] a

calcium activated cation channel expressed in the taste buds [9], gastrointestinal tract [10], pancreas [11] and other hollow organs, involved in taste signaling and glucose homeostasis. Here we present evidence that quinine controls body weight independently of food intake in male C57BL6 mice and investigate its mechanism of action, including a possible role of Trpm5 in mediating the effect of quinine on body weight control.

Results

Initially we planned to use encapsulated quinine to mask its bitterness and eliminate any potential impact on food intake caused by unpalatable diet. During the course of optimising the encapsulation procedure, we found that C57BL6 mice consume equal amounts of regular diet or non-encapsulated quinine supplemented diet (data not shown). Therefore the encapsulation approach was dropped and all subsequent experiments were carried out with regular, non encapsulated quinine.

* Correspondence: sami.damak@rdls.nestle.com
[1]Nestlé Research Center, Vers-chez-les-Blanc, Lausanne 1000, Switzerland
Full list of author information is available at the end of the article

Quinine fed mice gain less body weight and fat mass than mice on a regular diet (study 1)

We supplemented a regular balanced diet (AIN) of wild type male mice with quinine, and measured their body weight and fat mass for 13 weeks. We tested quinine concentrations of 0.01%, which is the highest concentration allowed in drinks for human consumption, and 0.1%. Compared with wild type mice consuming regular diet (WT control), wild-type mice consuming 0.1% quinine supplemented diet (WT quinine) had lower body weight ($p < 0.05$, Figure 1A) and lower fat mass ($p < 0.01$) (Figure 1B), whereas there was no significant difference in lean mass between WT control and WT quinine (Figure 1C). WT quinine mice gained less weight (2.89 ± 0.30 g vs 5.39 ± 0.50 g $p < 0.001$, Figure 1D), less fat mass (2.22 ± 0.26 g vs $4.33 \pm$ 0.43 g $p < 0.001$, Figure 1E) and less lean mass (1.07 ± 0.18 g vs 1.82 ± 0.20 g $p < 0.05$) than WT control mice. There was no significant difference in body weight, fat mass or lean mass between WT control and WT mice consuming 0.01% quinine (Figure 1).

Food intake is not different between quinine fed mice and mice fed a regular diet (study 1)

There was no significant difference in cumulative food intake between the WT control mice, WT quinine mice, and mice fed a diet supplemented with 0.01% quinine (238 ± 3.5 g, 235 ± 3.2 g, 248 ± 4.8 g, respectively, Figure 2A). A preliminary experiment showed that the percentage of waste was very small, and real daily food intake (measured food intake minus waste) was not

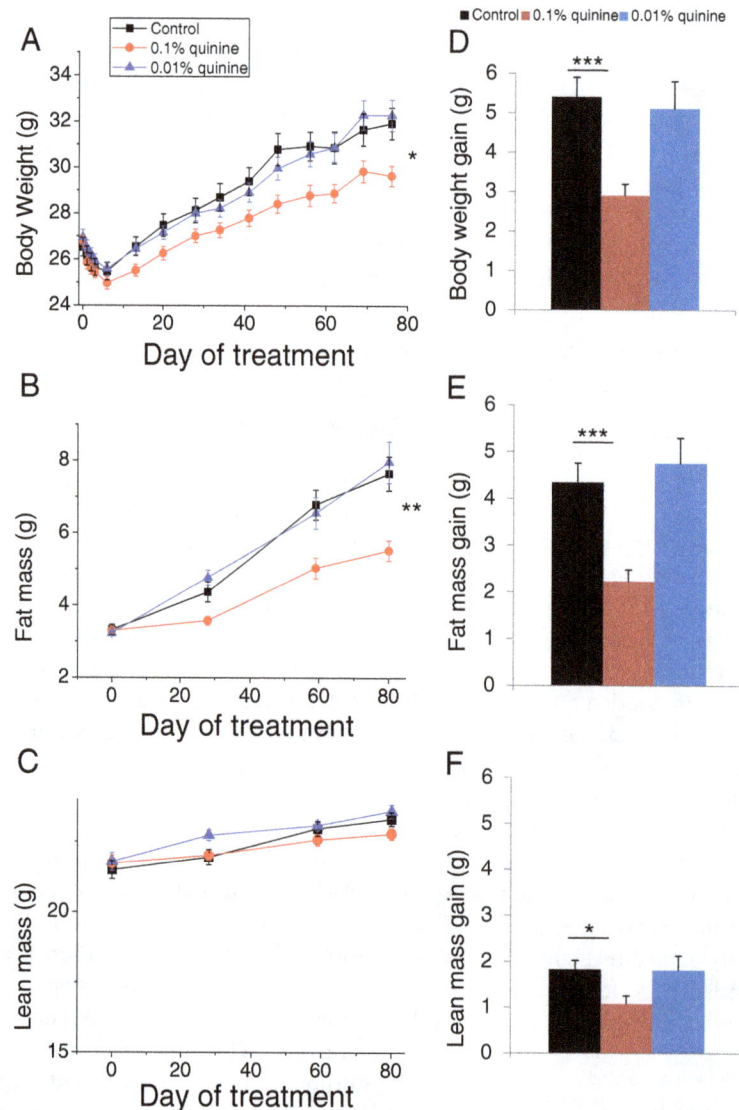

Figure 1 Body weight, fat and lean mass of WT mice on control diet, diet + 0.1% quinine, or diet + 0.01% quinine, showing lower body weight and fat mass gains with 0.1% quinine but not with 0.01% quinine, compared to regular diet. * $p < 0.05$, **$p < 0.01$, ***$p < 0.001$.

significantly different between groups, although there was a trend for increased real food intake by animals fed quinine supplemented diets (Figure 2B). When given the choice between two diets with or without quinine (Study 5), wild type mice avoid the quinine containing diet in favour of the regular diet, demonstrating aversion for the bitter taste of quinine (Figure 1C). In contrast, when given only one choice, mice consume the same amounts of regular or quinine supplemented diet (Figure 2B). Thus the decreased body weight and fat mass gains observed in the WT quinine mice are not caused by diminished intake of unpalatable food.

Metabolic parameters are improved by treatment with quinine (study 1)

Compared with WT control mice, blood glucose and plasma triglycerides were lower in WT quinine mice (p < 0.005, and p < 0.01, respectively, Figure 3). Blood glucose was lower in Trpm5 KO mice than in control (Study 2, p < 0.05). There was no significant difference in plasma free fatty acids and insulin between WT control and WT quinine mice (Figure 3).

Effect of diet supplementation with 0.1% quinine on body weight and body composition of wild type and Trpm5 knockout mice (study 2)

Since quinine inhibits Trpm5 *in vitro*, in this experiment we investigated whether the effect of quinine on body weight and body composition was mediated through Trpm5. To this effect, we measured body weight and composition of WT control, WT quinine, Trpm5 KO mice with regular AIN diet (KO control) and Trpm5 KO mice with 0.1% quinine supplemented AIN diet (KO quinine) and compared the effect of genotype (WT vs KO), diet (control vs quinine) and genotype*diet interaction. The means for body weight gain and fat mass gain for each group are given in Table 1. There was a significant effect of diet on body weight repeated measurements and gain (control > quinine, p < 0.01), but no effect of genotype. There was a significant effect of diet on fat mass repeated measurements and gain (Control > quinine, p < 0.001). There was a significant effect of genotype on fat mass gain (WT > KO, p < 0.05). There was a trend for an interaction diet*genotype for repeated measurements of body weight (p = 0.10) and body weight gain (p = 0.12) (Figure 4). These data confirm the effect of quinine on body weight and fat mass found in study 1. Trpm5 KO mice gain less fat mass than WT animals. The diet*genotype interaction trend suggests that part of the effect of quinine on body weight and fat mass may be Trpm5-dependent. There was no significant effect of genotype or diet on lean mass gain (Values in Table 1).

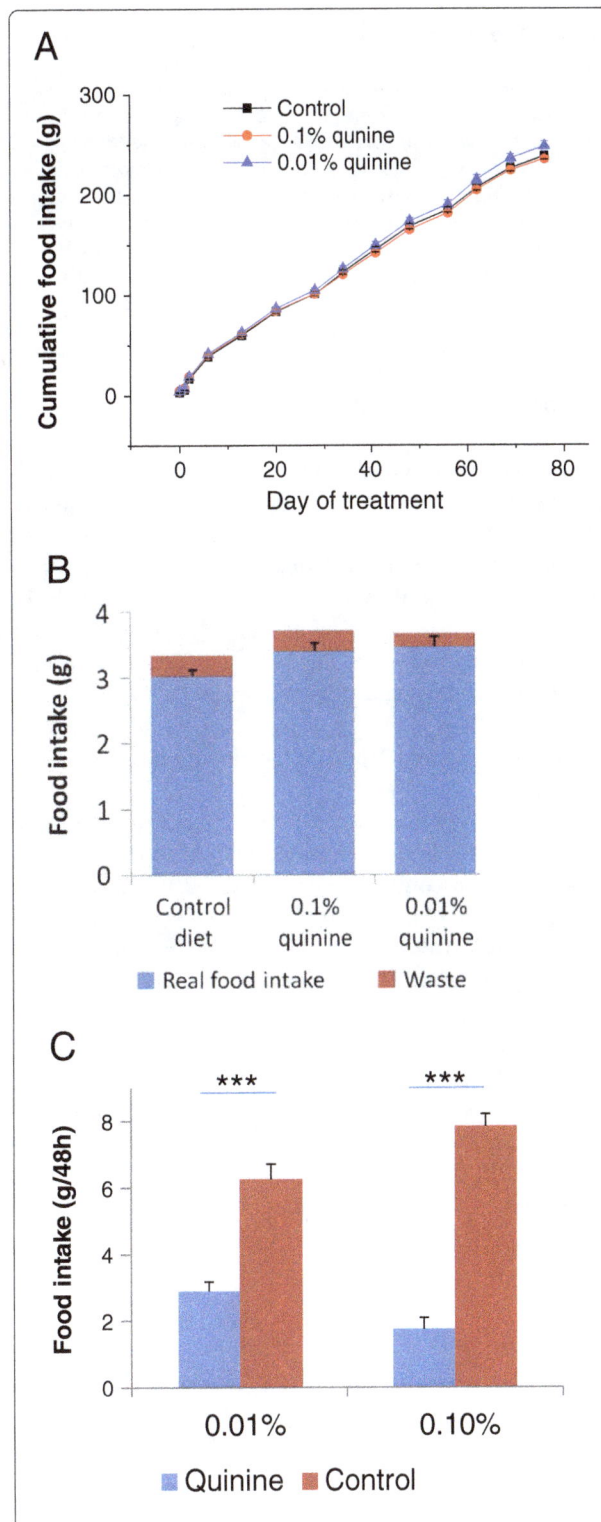

Figure 2 Food intake of WT mice on AIN diet with or without quinine. A. Cumulative food intake of mice on control AIN diet, AIN diet + 0.1% quinine, or AIN diet + 0.01 % quinine, showing no difference between any of the groups. **B**. Daily real food intake and food waste of wild type mice consuming AIN diet, or AIN diet supplemented with 0.1% or 0.01% quinine. Real food intake was calculated by subtracting waste from measured food intake. There is no significant difference between groups with different diets. There is a trend for increased real food intake by animals fed quinine supplemented diets. **C**. Diet preference tests, comparing AIN diet and AIN diet supplemented with either 0.01% or 0.1% quinine, showing aversion for the quinine supplemented diets.

Mice do not regain weight after removal of quinine (study 2)

After 13 weeks of consuming a diet supplemented with quinine, mice were switched to a control diet for 4 weeks. During that period there was no significant effect on weight gain of diet and a strong trend for genotype (p = 0.087) with no significant interaction (values in Table 1). Thus quinine treated mice do not regain weight after being switched to regular diet, whereas Trpm5 KO mice tend to gain less weight than WT mice.

Effect of quinine and Trpm5 KO on energy balance (study 2)

Faeces from WT control, WT quinine, KO control and KO quinine mice were collected and their total energy, fat and protein contents were measured (Figure 5). The amount of dried faeces per 24 h, faecal energy per gram of faeces, faecal energy per 24 h, faecal free fatty acids, faecal triglycerides, and faecal cholesterol were higher in mice receiving the quinine supplemented diet than those on control diet (Figure 5). The amount of dried faeces per 24 h, faecal energy per 24 h, faecal free fatty acids, and faecal cholesterol were higher in Trpm5 KO mice than in control mice (Figure 5). Phospholipids were not detectable in the faeces. There was no significant effect of genotype or diet on faecal nitrogen content. There

was no genotype*diet interaction for any of those parameters.

The effect of quinine on fat mass gain is small and short lived in diet-induced obese mice fed a high fat diet (study 3)

The aim of this experiment was to determine if supplementation of the diet of obese mice with quinine would lead to weight loss. Diet-induced obese mice were fed a 45% fat diet with or without supplementation with 0.1% quinine for 12 weeks. WT quinine mice gained less weight than WT control mice, but fat mass was lower in WT quinine mice only after 6 weeks of exposure to the experimental diet (p < 0.05, Figure 6). At week 11, there was no significant difference in fat mass. Lean mass was lower in quinine-treated mice at week 6 and week 11 (p < 0.01 and p < 0.05, respectively). Cumulative food intake was lower in mice fed quinine supplemented high fat diet than in control (177 ± 2.4 g vs 189 ± 3.1 g p < 0.05). Thus when high fat diet is used, the effect of quinine on fat mass is small, short lived and caused at least in part by diminished food intake.

Twenty four-hour energy expenditure and activity are not different between WT control, WT quinine, and KO control mice (study 4)

Twenty four-hour energy expenditure, respiratory quotient and activity were measured after mice were fed the experimental diets for two weeks and did not differ between WT control, WT quinine and KO control fed AIN (Figure 7) or high fat diet (not shown).

Markers of hepatic toxicity and of systemic inflammation are normal in quinine-fed mice (study 1)

To rule out the possibility that the diminished body weight gain observed in the quinine fed animals was caused by liver toxicity or general inflammation, we measured plasma liver enzymes and cytokines. Plasma

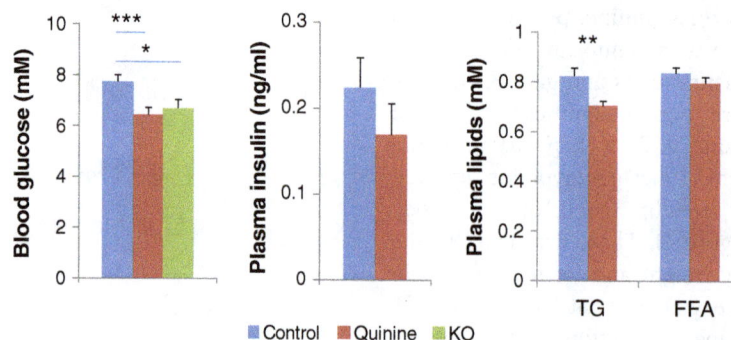

■ Control ■ Quinine ■ KO

Figure 3 Blood glucose, plasma insulin, triglycerides (TG), and free fatty acids (FFA) from 0.1% quinine fed (quinine) and control diet fed (control) WT mice, and from Trpm5 KO mice fed a control diet (KO) for blood glucose. Blood glucose is more elevated in the control than in quinine or Trpm5 KO mice. There is no difference in plasma insulin between control and quinine. TG, but not FFA are more elevated in control than in quinine. * p < 0.05, **p < 0.01, ***p < 0.001.

Table 1 Results of study 2, showing means ± SEM for gains in body weight, fat mass, lean mass and body weight after quinine removal from the diet in the four experimental groups of mice

	Body weight gain (g)	Fat mass gain (g)	Lean mass gain (g)	Body weight gain after quinine removal (g)
WT control	4.90 ± 0.63	3.35 ± 0.46	1.19 ± 0.14	2.14 ± 0.22
WT quinine	2.86 ± 0.31	1.61 ± 0.21	0.66 ± 0.19	2.00 ± 0.28
KO control	3.84 ± 0.33	2.19 ± 0.38	1.13 ± 0.30	1.39 ± 0.36
KO quinine	3.12 ± 0.28	1.38 ± 0.23	1.38 ± 0.31	1.78 ± 0.24

aspartate-amino-transferase (AST) and alanine-amino-transferase (ALT), which are elevated in case of hepatic toxicity, were within normal range in mice fed a diet containing 0.1% quinine and not significantly different from control (AST: 47.2 ± 1.5 U/L and 43.2 ± 1 U/L; ALT 20.9 ± 1.6 U/L and 18.2 ± 0.7 U/L for control and quinine, respectively).

Two mice in the control group and one mouse in the quinine fed group had elevated INF-γ, IL-10, IL-12p70, and IL-6, suggesting that those three mice had systemic inflammation (Figure 8). For all other mice the levels of IL-1β, IL-12p70, INF-γ, IL-6, and TNF-α were either undetectable, in most cases, or slightly above the detection threshold. The levels of KC and IL-10 were detectable above threshold in all mice, with no significant

difference between control and quinine (medians for control and quinine, respectively, KC: 86 pg/ml and 74 pg/ml; IL-10: 19 pg/ml and 13 pg/ml).

Together these data show that there is no evidence of liver toxicity or systemic inflammation associated with quinine supplemented diet.

Discussion

In this study, we tested the effect of quinine on mouse body weight and body composition and investigated possible mechanisms, including the role of Trpm5. Mice consuming a balanced diet supplemented with 0.1% quinine gained less fat mass than mice on a regular diet and maintained this difference at least for one month after quinine was removed from the diet.

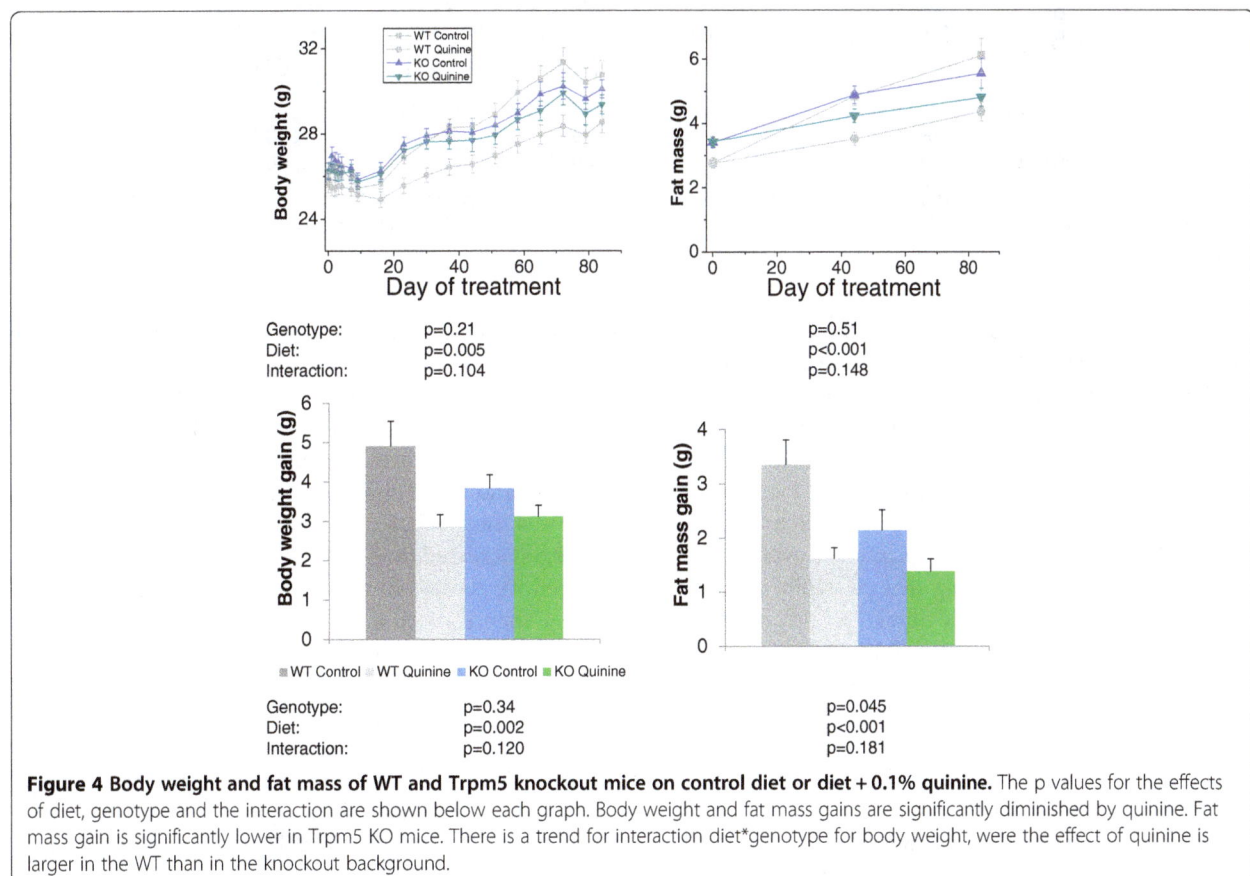

Figure 4 Body weight and fat mass of WT and Trpm5 knockout mice on control diet or diet + 0.1% quinine. The p values for the effects of diet, genotype and the interaction are shown below each graph. Body weight and fat mass gains are significantly diminished by quinine. Fat mass gain is significantly lower in Trpm5 KO mice. There is a trend for interaction diet*genotype for body weight, were the effect of quinine is larger in the WT than in the knockout background.

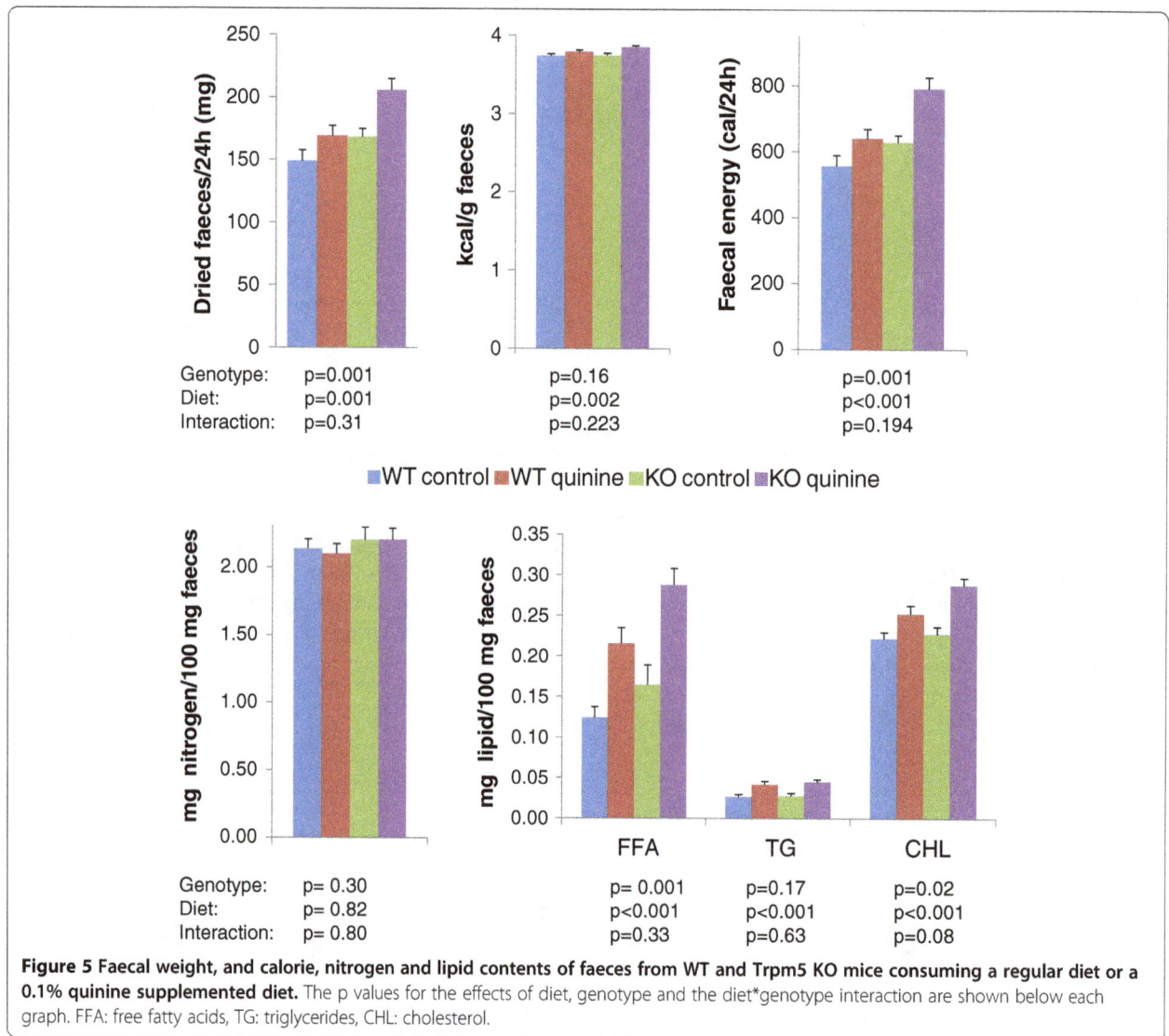

Figure 5 Faecal weight, and calorie, nitrogen and lipid contents of faeces from WT and Trpm5 KO mice consuming a regular diet or a 0.1% quinine supplemented diet. The p values for the effects of diet, genotype and the diet*genotype interaction are shown below each graph. FFA: free fatty acids, TG: triglycerides, CHL: cholesterol.

Previous experiments investigating the role of quinine in food intake and body weight were conducted using rats [1-7]. Quinine has an intense bitter taste to humans and is aversive to rodents. Adding quinine to the diet of rats results in a large decrease in food intake accompanied by diminished body weight. The decrease in food intake is observed with rats consuming a diet supplemented with quinine, but not with a diet supplemented with iso-bitter sucrose octaacetate, suggesting that palatability is not the only cause of decreased food intake in rats consuming quinine in the diet [1]. Our results differ from those obtained with rats in that food intake was not diminished in mice consuming quinine supplemented diet compared to those consuming regular diet. In preliminary experiments we found that when given the choice between two diets with or without 0.1% quinine, wild type mice avoid the quinine containing diet in favour of the regular diet, demonstrating aversion for the bitter taste of quinine. In contrast, when given only one choice, mice consume the same amounts of regular or quinine supplemented diet. Food intake was carefully measured in studies 1–4 and the results were consistent for all the studies where AIN diet was used. We also measured waste in a separate experiment and found that it was minimal, and real food intake was not affected by addition of quinine. Thus, whereas decreased food intake explains part of the quinine induced weight loss in rats, it does not in regular diet fed mice. Rats are more likely to decrease their food intake because of palatability than mice.

Smaller gain in body weight and fat mass may be caused by increased energy expenditure, due to increased metabolism or activity, or decreased nutrient ingestion and/or absorption. We found an increase of total faeces, faecal energy and lipid content in the quinine treated mice compared to mice on control diet. There was no difference in protein content. Faecal carbohydrate content cannot be

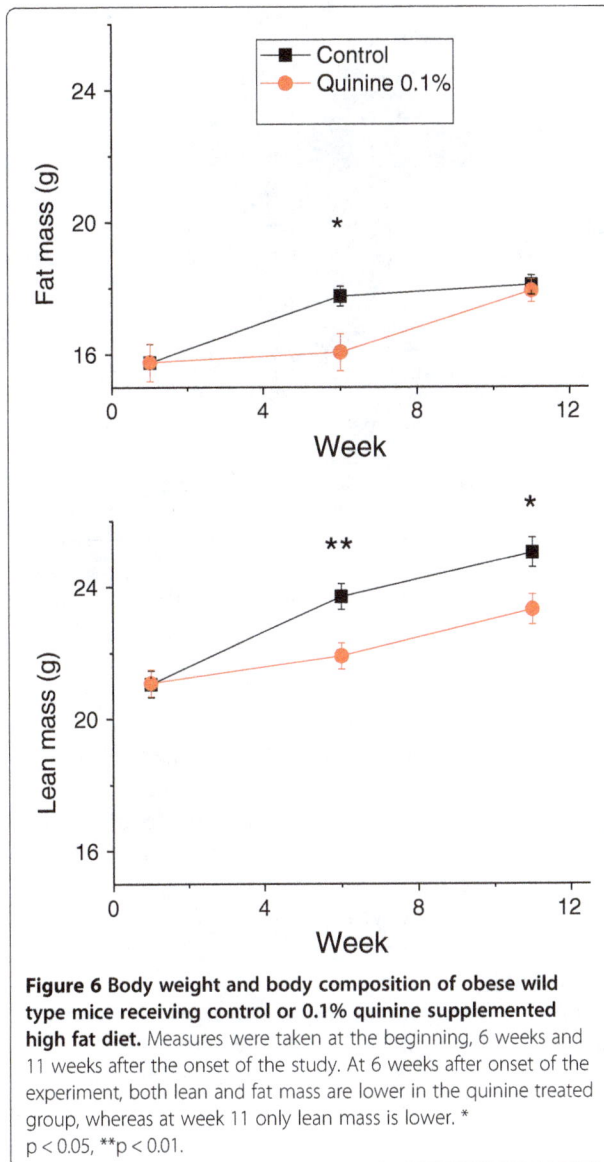

Figure 6 Body weight and body composition of obese wild type mice receiving control or 0.1% quinine supplemented high fat diet. Measures were taken at the beginning, 6 weeks and 11 weeks after the onset of the study. At 6 weeks after onset of the experiment, both lean and fat mass are lower in the quinine treated group, whereas at week 11 only lean mass is lower. * $p < 0.05$, **$p < 0.01$.

absorption rather than energy expenditure. All mice, including quinine fed animals, looked healthy without any signs of distress during the experiment. There were no biological signs of liver toxicity, and biological signs of systemic inflammation were found in two mice in the control group and one mouse fed quinine. Thus, it is unlikely that insults to visceral organs may have accounted for the diminished weight gain observed in quinine fed mice.

Quinine-fed mice did not regain weight during a 4-week follow up period after quinine-containing diet was replaced with a regular AIN diet. This fact is of clinical relevance. If quinine were to be investigated as a body weight control measure in humans, it may not be necessary to provide it on a continuous basis.

Is the effect of quinine on body weight and body composition Trpm5 dependent? For body weight and body weight gain there is a trend for an interaction genotype-diet, with a clear effect of quinine on WT type and a very small non significant effect on the knockout. This trend suggests the existence of a Trpm5 and quinine-dependent mechanism of body weight and fat mass gain prevention. Total faeces, caloric and lipid faecal contents are increased by quinine treatment both in the KO and WT backgrounds (no interaction diet-genotype) indicating that they represent Trpm5-independent quinine-dependent mechanisms of body weight control. Quinine is likely to act on multiple targets, including possibly Trpm5, bitter taste receptors [13], which are expressed in the gastrointestinal tract [14], potassium channels [15,16] or by direct activation of G-proteins [17].

What is then the Trpm5-dependent mechanism of diminished body weight gain? Trpm5 is expressed in the taste buds [9], gastrointestinal tract [10], pancreas [11] and other hollow organs. In the gastrointestinal tract Trpm5 is expressed in solitary cells disseminated throughout the gut, some of which also co-express T1rs, the receptors for sweet and *umami* tastes, suggesting that they might be chemosensory cells. Intestinal Trpm5 expressing cells produce endogenous opioids (β-endorphin and Met-enkephalin) and uroguanylin, and they secrete β-endorphin in response to various stimuli, particularly hypertonic stimuli, in a Trpm5-dependent fashion [18]. Opioids are well known to inhibit intestinal motility. It is tempting to speculate that inactivation of Trpm5 by gene knockout leads to increased intestinal motility through diminished release of β-endorphin thereby reducing intestinal nutrient uptake. Consistent with this hypothesis increased faecal weight, and faecal caloric and lipid contents are found in Trpm5 KO mice compared to wild type mice, although the differences are less marked as with quinine versus control. Given that the Trpm5-dependent prevention of weight gain takes place over a very long period, it is understandable that its underlying physiological changes are subtle. Quinine,

directly measured since sugars are converted in the colon by the gut microflora into short chain fatty acids [12]. The largest contribution to faecal lipid difference between quinine treated and control mice was from free fatty acids, suggesting that absorption of fatty acids, not digestion of triglycerides is deregulated by quinine treatment. The 24 h faecal weight is larger in quinine fed mice than in mice fed regular diet. The difference (~20 mg) cannot be accounted for by the difference in lipid content, as the difference in faecal FFA between quinine fed mice and control diet fed mice is only ~0.1 mg. The bulk of the difference in faecal weight most likely results from differences in the amount of undigested starch. Indirect calorimetry and measurement of activity showed no difference between WT control, WT quinine and KO control. Altogether these data suggest that quinine administration deregulates intestinal nutrient

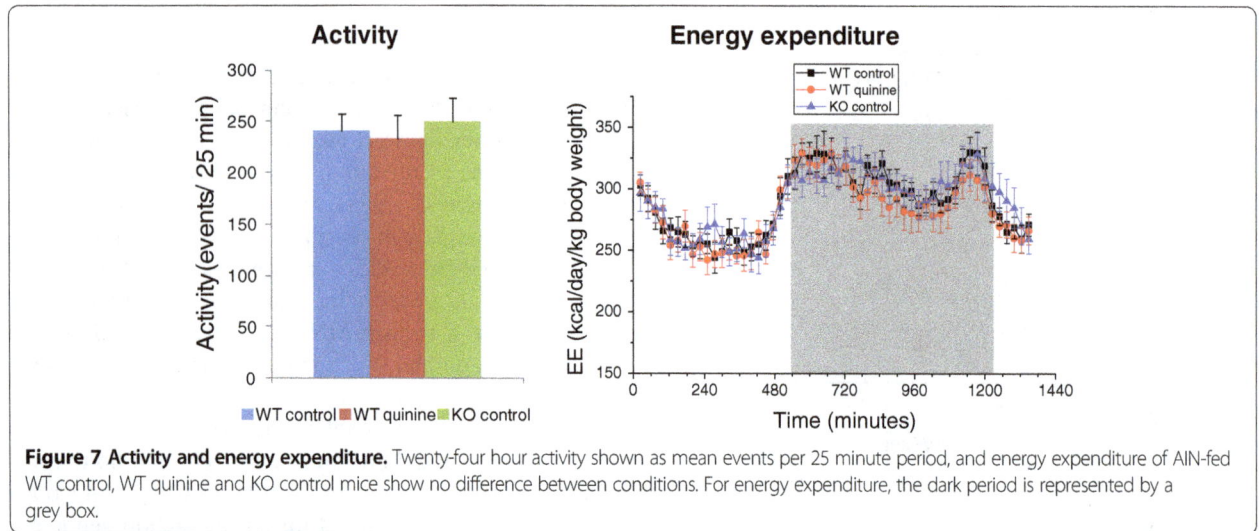

Figure 7 Activity and energy expenditure. Twenty-four hour activity shown as mean events per 25 minute period, and energy expenditure of AIN-fed WT control, WT quinine and KO control mice show no difference between conditions. For energy expenditure, the dark period is represented by a grey box.

on the other hand decreases gastrointestinal transit [19] and therefore would increase faecal weight, energy and lipids through a mechanism independent of Trpm5 inhibition.

Quinine mediated control of body weight and fat mass is clearly observed in mice fed a balanced diet (AIN) but is less clear when mice are fed high fat diet and interpretation of the results is confounded by lower food intake in the quinine group. Mice fed high fat diet overeat because of the palatability of fat, and this overeating may have been smaller in the quinine group because of bitterness.

Conclusion
Our data show that quinine contributes to the control of body weight and fat mass without impacting food intake in male mice fed a balanced diet and therefore may

constitute a novel tool for the fight against the obesity epidemic.

Methods
Animals
All experiments were conducted according to Swiss animal experimentation laws and guidelines and were approved by an internal animal experimentation ethics committee and by the Veterinary Office of the Canton de Vaud. Mice were maintained at 22 degrees C with a 12 h dark-12 h light cycle.

Study design
Study 1: body weight and body composition of wild-type mice consuming quinine supplemented diet
Wild type C57BL6/J male mice three months old at the beginning of the experiment were used. They were fed a balanced semi synthetic diet (AIN 93 G, 64% calories from carbohydrates, 20% from proteins, 16% from fat, Diet # D10012G, Research Diets, New Brunswick, NJ, USA) with or without different doses of quinine, for 13 weeks. Three groups of 20 mice each were studied: A. Wild type fed AIN 93 G diet; B. Wild type fed AIN 93 G diet supplemented with 0.1% quinine HCl; C. Wild type fed AIN 93 G diet supplemented with 0.01% quinine HCl. 0.01% quinine corresponds to the maximal concentration allowed in drinks for human consumption. Groups were matched for fat mass assessed by NMR at the beginning of the study.

Body weight, food and fluid intake were measured weekly throughout the study. Body composition was measured at the beginning of the study, and on week 4, 8 and 12. At the end of week 13, mice were fasted for 6 hours, a drop of blood was collected by making a small incision in the tail vein, from which blood glucose was measured, then the mice were anesthetised with 3% isoflorane and blood was

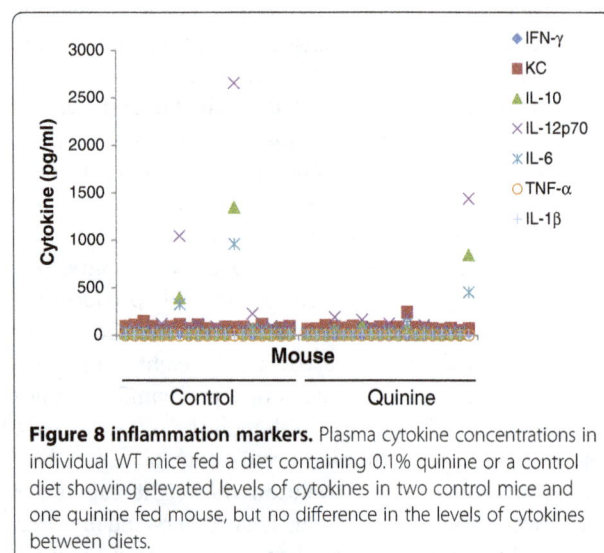

Figure 8 inflammation markers. Plasma cytokine concentrations in individual WT mice fed a diet containing 0.1% quinine or a control diet showing elevated levels of cytokines in two control mice and one quinine fed mouse, but no difference in the levels of cytokines between diets.

collected from the abdominal aorta for measurement of plasma insulin, aspartate-amino-transferase (AST), alanine-amino-transferase (ALT), pro-inflammatory cytokines, free fatty acids and triglycerides.

Study 2: body weight and body composition of WT and Trpm5 KO mice consuming quinine supplemented diet

The aims of this study were to: 1. confirming the results of Study 1; 2. determine if the effect of quinine on body weight was mediated by Trpm5; 3. Investigate the effect of quinine on energy intake; 4. Determine if mice regain weight once quinine is removed from the diet.

Wild type and Trpm5 KO male mice three months old at the beginning of the experiment were used. Trpm5 knockout (KO) mice (obtained from Deltagen, San Mateo, CA, USA) were described in [20]. The KO mice were backcrossed for six generations into C57BL6/J background. Mice were fed a balanced semi synthetic diet (AIN 93 G) with or without 0.1% quinine for 13 weeks. In order to determine if the effect on body weight persists when the mice are no longer fed quinine, all mice were fed AIN 93 G without quinine after the initial 13-week trial for an additional 4 weeks. Four groups of 15 male mice each were studied: A. Wild type C57BL6/J fed AIN 93 G diet (WT control); B. Wild type C57BL6/J fed AIN 93 G diet supplemented with 0.1% quinine HCl (WT quinine); C. Trpm5 KO fed AIN 93 G diet (KO control); D. Trpm5 KO fed AIN 93 G diet supplemented with 0.1% quinine HCl (KO quinine). Groups A and C were matched with groups B and D, respectively, for fat mass and body weight at the beginning of the study.

Body weight, food and fluid intake were measured weekly throughout the study. Body composition was measured at the beginning of the study, on week 7 and on week 13. On weeks 1, 7 and 13, mice were placed on a grid above a piece of cardboard covering the bottom of the cage for 72 hours. The faeces were separated from food crumbs and powder, and collected daily for measurement of weight, macronutrient content and direct calorimetry. On week 13 blood glucose was measured from a drop of blood collected by making a small incision in the tail vein.

Study 3: body weight and body composition of wild-type obese mice consuming quinine supplemented high fat diet

The aim of this experiment was to determine if supplementation with quinine of the diet of obese mice would lead to weight loss. Seven-week old wild type male C57BL6/J mice were fed a diet with 60% calories from fat (research diets D12492) for 9 weeks to make them obese. They were then fed a 45% high fat diet (research Diets D12451) for one week in order to maintain their weight and to get habituated to the 45% fat diet. Then one group of 19 mice continued to be fed 45% high fat diet (control), and the other group of 19 mice was fed 45% high fat diet containing 0.1% quinine-HCl for 12 weeks. Groups were matched for fat mass assessed by NMR at the beginning of the study.

Body weight, food and fluid intake were measured weekly throughout the study. Body composition was measured at the beginning of the study, and on week 6 and 11.

Study 4: energy expenditure and activity

Three groups of 10 male mice 3 month old and weight matched, were tested: A. Wild type mice without quinine, B. Wild type mice with 0.1% quinine HCl, C. Trpm5 KO mice without quinine.

Mice were fed a balanced diet (AIN-93 G) with or without 0.1% quinine HCl for two weeks, then were fed high fat diet (60% energy from fat, Research Diets #12492) with or without 0.1% quinine HCl for two weeks. Energy expenditure was measured after each two-week period; the mice were placed into metabolic cages for a 24-hour acclimation period then VO_2, VCO_2, respiratory quotient (RQ) and activity were measured over 24 hours using an Oxylet system (Panlab, Barcelona, Spain) with O_2 and CO_2 sensors, coupled to a SEDACOM infrared system to measure activity. Respiratory quotient (RQ) is the ratio of carbon dioxide production to oxygen consumption. Energy expenditure was calculated using the Weir equation (EE = $1.44 \times VO_2 \times (3.815 + 1.23 \times RQ)$).

Study 5: two diet preference tests

Two groups of 8 male 3-month old C57BL6/J mice were tested. Every mouse received two diets, AIN-93 G and AIN-93 G supplemented with 0.01% quinine HCl (Group A) or with 0.1% quinine HCl (Group B). The two diets were placed on the cage lid, separated by the water bottle. The positions of the diets were switched after 24 hours. The diets were weighed at the beginning of the experiment, and 24 h and 48 hours later. The amount consumed from each diet were calculated and compared by paired Student T-tests.

Body composition

Body composition was determined in duplicate using an EchoMRI-900 Body Composition Analyzer (Echo Medical System, LLC, Houston, TX, USA).

Food intake

Food intake was calculated by weighing the diet and subtracting the weight at the end of the measured period from that at the beginning. Spillage of food on the bottom of the cage was collected and weighed to ensure the quality of food intake measurements.

In a preliminary experiment, we measured food waste by wild-type C57BL6/J mice consuming AIN diet, AIN diet + 0.1% quinine HCl or AIN diet +0.01% quinine HCl, 7 male mice each. Mice were placed on a grid above a piece of cardboard covering the bottom of the cage for 72 h. Food powder and pellet crumbs were separated from faeces and weighed.

Analysis of faecal contents

Mice were placed on a grid for 72 h and faeces were collected every 24 hours at the bottom of the cages which were covered with a piece of absorbent cardboard to minimise contamination of the faeces by urine. Faeces collected during a 24 h period were vacuum oven-dried (50°C, 24 hours) and weighed.

For measurement of caloric contents, the dried material was turned into powder with a mortar. The powder was compacted into two pellets using a Pellet Press 2811 (Parr Instrument Company, Moline, IL, USA). The dried materials were added to 0.4 g benzoic acid and burned in a 6100 Oxygen Bomb Calorimeter (Parr Instrument Company) to measure their caloric content. Measurements were done in duplicate.

For measurement of nitrogen content, 2 mg of dried and homogenised faeces were placed in a sealed capsule and inserted into an elemental analyser (CHNS-932, Leco, St Joseph, MI, USA) and combusted at 1000°C in presence of oxygen. The total contents of N in the sample were quantitatively converted to N_2 and subsequently determined by measurement of the thermal conductivity after separation of the gaseous components. Measurements were done in quadruplicate.

Faecal lipids were measured as described [21]. Briefly, lipids were extracted from 100 mg of dried faeces with 2 ml chloroform-methanol 2:1. The organic phase was recovered and 1 ml of water was added to it. Following a second centrifugation, the organic phase was recovered and evaporated under N_2 for 30 min and resuspended in 500 μl 1% Triton X 100 in Chloroform, evaporated under N_2 for 10 min and resuspended in 500 μl water. The following commercial kits were used for the measurement of lipids, according to the manufacturer's protocol: NEFA HR (2), Wako, Osaka, Japan, for free fatty acids; TG PAP 150, BioMerieux, Marcy l'Etoile, France for triglycerides; LabAssay Cholesterol, Wako, for cholesterol, LabAssay Phospholipids, Wako, for phospholipids.

Blood parameters

Mice were food deprived for six hours, then glucose was measured from a drop of blood obtained from an incision of the tail vein, using a glucometer (Ascensia Elite, Bayer, Germany). The measures were done in duplicate.

After measurement of glucose, the mice were anesthetised with 3% isoflorane and blood was collected from the aorta for the remaining measurements using commercial kits (NEFA HR (2), Wako, for free fatty acids; TG PAP 150, BioMerieux, Marcy l'Etoile, France for triglycerides; Ultra Sensitive Mouse Insulin ELISA Kit, Crystal Chem, Downers Grove, IL, USA, for insulin, and Roche reagents, Meylan, France for ALT and AST) according to the manufacturer's protocol. Cytokines were measured using a multiplex immunoassay (Meso Scale Discovery, Gaithersburg, MD, USA). The cytokines included in the multiplex assay are Interleukin (IL)-1β, IL-12p70, Interferon-γ (INF-γ), IL-6, keratinocyte chemoattractant (KC), IL-10, and Tumour Necrosis Factor-α (TNF-α)

Statistical analysis
Studies 1, 3 and 4
For all parameters except body weight, fat mass and lean mass, the data were analysed with the General Linear Model univariate of the statistics program SPSS with the measured parameter as a within-subject factor and diet as a between subject factor. When more than two groups were compared and a significant difference was found, a *post hoc* Tukey test was performed to determine which groups differ.

For body weight, fat mass and lean mass, the data were analyzed with the General Linear Model Repeated Measures of the statistics program SPSS with the measured parameter as a within-subject factor and diet as a between subject factor. When more than two groups were compared and a significant difference was found, a *post hoc* Tukey test was performed to determine which groups differ.

For each cytokine the non-parametric Mann Whitney test was used to assess the difference between control and quinine fed mice and the results are presented as medians.

Study 2
The data were analyzed with the General Linear Model of the statistics program SPSS with the measured parameter as a within-subject factor and diet and genotype as between subject factors. The interaction diet*genotype was also analyzed.

Data are presented as mean ± SEM. A p value <0.05 was considered significant.

Competing interests

All of the authors are, or were, employees of Nestec Ltd, which is a subsidiary of Nestlé Ltd. and provides professional assistance, research, and consulting services for food, dietary, dietetic, and pharmaceutical products of interest to Nestlé Ltd. No other conflicts of interest are reported. The study was funded by Nestec Ltd.

Authors' contribution
The authors' responsibilities were as follows: CD, JleC, SD: designed the study; PCR and CB: organized and executed the trials; SD, CD and JleC: interpreted the data, wrote and edited the manuscript. All authors red and approved the final manuscript.

Acknowledgements
The authors thank the staff of the Nestlé Research Center animal facility for excellent animal care and assistance with experiments, Manuel Oliveira for the measurement of cytokines and Corinne Ammon Zufferey for the measurement of liver enzymes. This work was supported by internal funds from Nestec S.A.

Author details
[1]Nestlé Research Center, Vers-chez-les-Blanc, Lausanne 1000, Switzerland.
[2]Organization for Interdisciplinary Research Projects, The University of Tokyo, Tokyo, Japan.

References

1. Heybach JP, Boyle PC: Dietary quinine reduces body weight and food intake independent of aversive taste. *Physiol Behav* 1982, **29**:1171–1173.
2. King BM, Grossman SP: Effects of chronic quinine-adulteration of the water supply on food and fluid intake and body weight in lean and obese hypothalamic hyperphagic rats. *Physiol Behav* 1979, **22**:1203–1206.
3. Kratz CM, Levitsky DA: Post-ingestive effects of quinine on intake of nutritive and non-nutritive substances. *Physiol Behav* 1978, **21**:851–854.
4. Kratz CM, Levitsky DA, Lustick SL: Long term effects of quinine on food intake and body weight in the rat. *Physiol Behav* 1978, **21**:321–324.
5. Kratz CM, Levitsky DA, Lustick S: Differential effects of quinine and sucrose octa acetate on food intake in the rat. *Physiol Behav* 1978, **20**:665–667.
6. Oku J, Bray GA, Fisler JS: Effects of oral and parenteral quinine on rats with ventromedial hypothalamic knife-cut obesity. *Metabolism* 1984, **33**:538–544.
7. Peck JW: Rats drinking quinine- or caffeine-adulterated water defend lean body weights against caloric and osmotic stress. *Physiol Behav* 1978, **21**:599–607.
8. Talavera K, Yasumatsu K, Yoshida R, Margolskee RF, Voets T, Ninomiya Y, *et al*: The taste transduction channel TRPM5 is a locus for bitter-sweet taste interactions. *FASEB J* 2008, **22**:1343–1355.
9. Perez CA, Huang L, Rong M, Kozak JA, Preuss AK, Zhang H, *et al*: A transient receptor potential channel expressed in taste receptor cells. *Nat Neurosci* 2002, **5**:1169–1176.
10. Bezençon C, le Coutre J, Damak S: Taste-signaling proteins are coexpressed in solitary intestinal epithelial cells. *Chem Senses* 2006, **32**:41–49.
11. Brixel LR, Monteilh-Zoller MK, Ingenbrandt CS, Fleig A, Penner R, Enklaar T, *et al*: TRPM5 regulates glucose-stimulated insulin secretion. *Pflugers Arch* 2010, **460**:69–76.
12. Cummings JH: Colonic absorption: the importance of short chain fatty acids in man. *Scand J Gastroenterol Suppl* 1984, **93**:89–99.
13. Meyerhof W, Batram C, Kuhn C, Brockhoff A, Chudoba E, Bufe B, *et al*: The molecular receptive ranges of human TAS2R bitter taste receptors. *Chem Senses* 2010, **35**:157–170.
14. Wu SV, Rozengurt N, Yang M, Young SH, Sinnett-Smith J, Rozengurt E: Expression of bitter taste receptors of the T2R family in the gastrointestinal tract and enteroendocrine STC-1 cells. *Proc Natl Acad Sci U S A* 2002, **99**:2392–2397.
15. Bokvist K, Rorsman P, Smith PA: Block of ATP-regulated and Ca2 (+)-activated K + channels in mouse pancreatic beta-cells by external tetraethylammonium and quinine. *J Physiol* 1990, **423**:327–342.
16. Fatherazi S, Cook DL: Specificity of tetraethylammonium and quinine for three K channels in insulin-secreting cells. *J Membr Biol* 1991, **120**:105–114.
17. Naim M, Seifert R, Nurnberg B, Grunbaum L, Schultz G: Some taste substances are direct activators of G-proteins. *Biochem J* 1994, **297**(Pt 3):451–454.
18. Kokrashvili Z, Rodriguez D, Yevshayeva V, Zhou H, Margolskee RF, Mosinger B: Release of endogenous opioids from duodenal enteroendocrine cells requires Trpm5. *Gastroenterology* 2009, **137**:598–606.
19. Santos FA, Rao VS: Quinine-induced inhibition of gastrointestinal transit in mice: possible involvement of endogenous opioids. *Eur J Pharmacol* 1999, **364**:193–197.
20. Riera CE, Vogel H, Simon SA, Damak S, le Coutre J: Sensory attributes of complex tasting divalent salts are mediated by TRPM5 and TRPV1 channels. *J Neurosci* 2009, **29**:2654–2662.
21. Mataki C, Magnier BC, Houten SM, Annicotte JS, Argmann C, Thomas C, *et al*: Compromised intestinal lipid absorption in mice with a liver-specific deficiency of liver receptor homolog 1. *Mol Cell Biol* 2007, **27**:8330–8339.

5

Cardiac responses to elevated seawater temperature in Atlantic salmon

Sven Martin Jørgensen[1], Vicente Castro[2], Aleksei Krasnov[1], Jacob Torgersen[1], Gerrit Timmerhaus[1], Ernst Morten Hevrøy[3], Tom Johnny Hansen[4], Sissel Susort[5], Olav Breck[6] and Harald Takle[1,2]*

Abstract

Background: Atlantic salmon aquaculture operations in the Northern hemisphere experience large seasonal fluctuations in seawater temperature. With summer temperatures often peaking around 18-20°C there is growing concern about the effects on fish health and performance. Since the heart has a major role in the physiological plasticity and acclimation to different thermal conditions in fish, we wanted to investigate how three and eight weeks exposure of adult Atlantic salmon to 19°C, previously shown to significantly reduce growth performance, affected expression of relevant genes and proteins in cardiac tissues under experimental conditions.

Results: Transcriptional responses in cardiac tissues after three and eight weeks exposure to 19°C (compared to thermal preference, 14°C) were analyzed with cDNA microarrays and validated by expression analysis of selected genes and proteins using real-time qPCR and immunofluorescence microscopy. Up-regulation of heat shock proteins and cell signaling genes may indicate involvement of the unfolded protein response in long-term acclimation to elevated temperature. Increased immunofluorescence staining of inducible nitric oxide synthase in spongy and compact myocardium as well as increased staining of vascular endothelial growth factor in epicardium could reflect induced vascularization and vasodilation, possibly related to increased oxygen demand. Increased staining of collagen I in the compact myocardium of 19°C fish may be indicative of a remodeling of connective tissue with long-term warm acclimation. Finally, higher abundance of transcripts for genes involved in innate cellular immunity and lower abundance of transcripts for humoral immune components implied altered immune competence in response to elevated temperature.

Conclusions: Long-term exposure of Atlantic salmon to 19°C resulted in cardiac gene and protein expression changes indicating that the unfolded protein response, vascularization, remodeling of connective tissue and altered innate immune responses were part of the cardiac acclimation or response to elevated temperature.

Keywords: Temperature, Thermal acclimation, Cardiac tissue, Gene expression, Microarray, Immunofluorescence microscopy, iNOS, VEGF, Collagen I, Immune response

Background

Environmental temperature has been termed the master abiotic factor which controls and limits all biochemical, physiological and life history activities in teleost fishes [1]. The thermal optimum for different species have been extensively studied, representing the temperature where the difference between routine and maximum metabolic rates is greatest; i.e. the aerobic scope is at its maximum [2]. For Atlantic salmon (*Salmo salar* L.), optimum temperature for growth in sea has been found to occur at 13-15°C [3], with upper critical temperatures around 22°C [4]. In response to natural temperature fluctuations outside of the thermal tolerance window, fish respond by behavioral, biochemical and physiological modifications in order to maintain cellular homeostasis and physiological performance [5,6]. As the key organ supplying oxygen and fuels to the circulatory system for energy production, the heart has a major role in the physiological plasticity and acclimation to different thermal conditions in fish, showing alterations in cardiorespiratory performance, myocardial morphology and expression and phosphorylation of structural genes and proteins [7-10]. The occurrence of a

* Correspondence: harald.takle@nofima.no
[1]Nofima AS, P.O. Box 210, N-1431 Ås, Norway
[2]AVS Chile S.A., Casilla 300, Puerto Varas, Chile
Full list of author information is available at the end of the article

thermal optimum (T_{opt}) for cardiovascular function is reflected by different salmonid species having different T_{opt} for maximum oxygen uptake, aerobic scope and critical swimming speed [11,12]. At temperatures below and above T_{opt} the scope for aerobic metabolism will decline until a critical temperature (T_{crit}) is reached, where no aerobic activity can be performed besides routine metabolism [1]. In salmonids, the decreased aerobic scope observed with increasing temperatures above T_{opt} is associated with a limited oxygen supply suggested to be caused by a failure in maximum cardiac output to increase above T_{opt} [13]. Acclimation to high temperatures has been associated with cardiac remodeling of tissue composition and morphology [10], which is assumed to compensate for the decreased power-generating ability [14]. The nitric oxide synthase (NOS) system is another important inter- and intracellular regulator of cardiac function and oxygen supply in fish [15], and in long-term warm acclimated eel (*Anguilla anguilla*) inhibition of NO production significantly reduced the Frank-Starling response [16]. Another interesting yet poorly understood aspect of cardiac responses to temperature increase in fish is the effects on hematological and immunological responses, which may have a significant impact on the health and disease performance of Atlantic salmon in aquaculture, since heart is a target organ for several harmful viral pathogens [17,18].

In Atlantic salmon aquaculture in the Northern hemisphere, fish are exposed to large seasonal fluctuations in seawater temperature. Peak summer temperatures around 18-20°C are regularly experienced at production sites in the western and southern regions of Norway, causing concerns regarding the possible negative impact on productivity, fish performance and welfare. We recently reported that long-term exposure (56 days, simulating a warm water period in aquaculture) of adult (~2 kg) Atlantic salmon to 19°C under controlled conditions significantly reduced growth performance when compared to fish reared at 14°C, a difference driven by a 50% reduction in feed intake [19]. The objective of the present study was to investigate effects of such temperature increase on molecular responses in cardiac tissues from the same experimental fish. To achieve this, cDNA microarray screening and single gene expression validation with real-time qPCR were employed to evaluate transcriptional changes after 21 days (simulating a short warm water period) and 56 days (simulating a long warm water period) thermal acclimation. In addition, expression of selected proteins of interest were analysed with immunofluorescence microscopy in cardiac tissues after long-term thermal acclimation.

Methods
Temperature challenge trial
The experimental design is described in detail elsewhere [19]. This study used half of the groups; those fed the standard diet (L34). In brief, 170 adult (~1.6 kg) immature Atlantic salmon of the Norwegian salmon procreation strain (NLA) were randomly selected from sea cages and distributed into six 5.3 m³ light-gray round tanks (3 m diameter × 0.75 m water depth, temperature 14°C) at Matre Research Station, Matre (61°N), Norway. After 50 days acclimation period all fish were weighed (average body weight 2.0 ± 0.4 kg), and the temperature in three of the tanks was increased to 19°C at a rate of 1°C per day, while the three remaining tanks were kept at 14°C. Fish were reared under simulated natural photoperiod in 35 g L^{-1} seawater and oxygen level was kept constant on 90% saturation (measured continuously in the water outlet) by adding oxygen-supersaturated seawater (350% saturation). Fish were fed by automatic feeders that were adjusted daily to maintain 10% in excess. Feed which were not eaten were collected in an outlet trap. Feed was offered between 8 and 9 am and between 1 and 2 pm. To standardize sampling, all fish were fed *ad libitum* exactly four hours before sampling. Individually sampled fish (3 per tank, N = 9) were killed by a blow to the head and weights and fork lengths were measured to the nearest g and nearest 0.5 cm at the start, 21 days, and 56 days after commencement of the temperature increase. On days 0, 21 and 56, heart samples were collected from all sampled individuals under sterile conditions and divided in two; one half was flash-frozen in liquid nitrogen and stored at -80°C for gene expression analyses while the other half was fixed in 4% paraformaldehyde for immunofluorescence microscopy. The trial was approved by The National Animal Research Authority according to the 'European Convention for the Protection of Vertebrate Animals used for Experimental and other Scientific Purposes' (EST 123).

RNA extraction
Sampled hearts for gene expression analyses were stored at -80°C prior to RNA extraction. Standardized tissue sections of 10 mg (equal mix of ventricle and atrium) were prepared under sterile/RNase-free conditions and transferred directly to 1 ml chilled TRIzol (Invitrogen, Carlsbad, CA, USA) in 2 ml tubes with screw caps (Precellys°24, Bertin Technologies, Orléans, France). Two steel beads (2 mm diameter) were added to each tube and the tissue was homogenized in a Precellys°24 homogenizer for two times 25 sec at 5000 rounds per minute with a break of 5 sec between rounds. RNA was extracted from the homogenized tissues using PureLink RNA Mini kits according to the protocol for TRIzol-homogenized samples (Invitrogen). The concentration of extracted total RNA was measured using NanoDrop 1000 Spectrometer (Thermo Scientific, Waltham, MA, USA), while RNA integrity was determined using Agilent 2100 Bioanalyzer with RNA Nano kits (Agilent Technologies, Santa Clara,

CA, USA). Only samples with a RNA integrity number (RIN) of 8 or higher were accepted.

Microarray analysis

Two microarrays were used for screening of transcriptional responses to high temperature (19°C) at both 21 and 56 days after temperature was raised from control (14°C). Each control and high temperature group consisted of a pool of 9 fish randomly selected from triplicate tanks per each time point. The salmonid fish cDNA microarray SFA2.0 (GEO Omnibus GPL6154) includes 1,800 genes, each printed in six spot replicates. Synthesis of cDNA and hybridizations were carried out as previously described [20]. In brief, samples with 10 μg RNA in each were labeled with Cy3-dUTP (reference control, 14°C groups) and Cy5-dUTP (test, 19°C groups) (Amersham Biosciences, UK) during cDNA synthesis using the SuperScript III reverse transcriptase kit (Invitrogen). After hybridization, slides were washed in $0.5 \times$ SSC/0.1% SDS (15 min), $0.5 \times$ SSC/0.01% SDS (15 min), and twice in $0.06 \times$ SSC (3 min each) at room temperature in dim lighting with gentle agitation. Slides were dried using ArrayIt® Microarray High-Speed Centrifuge. Scanning was performed with GenePix 4100A microarray scanner (Molecular Devices, CA, USA) at 5 μm resolution and with manually adjusted laser power to ensure an overall intensity ratio close to unity between Cy3 and Cy5 channels, and with minimal saturation of features. Images were processed with GenePix Pro 6.0 software. Spots were filtered by criterion $(I - B)/(SI + SB) \geq 0.6$, where I and B are mean signal and background intensities and SI and SB are standard deviations, respectively. Low-quality spots were excluded from analyses and genes with less than three high-quality spots on a slide were discarded. After subtraction of median background from median signal intensities and Lowess normalization, differential expression was assessed by difference of the mean $\log_2$-ER (expression ratios, high versus control temperature groups) from zero (six spot replicates per each gene; Student's t-test, p < 0.01). Complete data are provided in the GEO Omnibus (accession number GSE53908). Genes with $\log_2$-ER > 0.4 in at least one time point and common functional annotation according to the STARS program [21] were considered for interpretation in the Results section.

Quantitative real-time RT-PCR (qPCR)

Experiments were conducted according to the MIQE guidelines [22]. Synthesis of cDNA was performed on 0.2 μg DNAse-treated total RNA (Turbo DNA-free™, Ambion, Austin, TX, USA) using the TaqMan® Gold Reverse Transcription kit (Applied Biosystems, Foster City, CA, USA) in 25 μl reactions with random hexamer priming according to manufacturer's protocol. Complementary DNA was stored undiluted at -80°C in aliquots

to avoid repeated freeze-thawing. To avoid risk for presence of residual DNA contamination, control reactions without RT were tested and qPCR primers were designed to span introns when possible. Oligonucleotide primers for genes of Atlantic salmon were designed with the program eprimer3 from the EMBOSS program package (version 5.0.0, http://emboss.sourceforge.net/). Amplicon size was set to 80-200 and melting temperature to 59-61°C. Primers were purchased from Invitrogen (Table 1). *In silico* analysis of gene targets was performed using the STARS program for BLAST and sequence alignments. PCR amplicon size and specificity were confirmed by gel electrophoresis and melting curve analysis (Tm calling; LightCycler®480, Roche Diagnostics, Mannheim, Germany). QPCR was conducted in duplicate reactions as previously described [23]. Cycle threshold (C_T) values were calculated using the fit point method. Duplicate measurements that differed more than 0.5 C_T values were removed and reanalyzed. For relative quantification, the mean of duplicates was used. Relative gene expression ratios of test samples versus the average of the normalized controls (14°C) were calculated according to the Pfaffl method [24] with normalization using the following reference genes: *NADH dehydrogenase (ubiquinone) 1 beta subcomplex 19 kDa* and *SEC13-like protein* (used for all genes except HSP70),

Table 1 Genes and primer sequences used for qPCR analyses

Gene	Dir.	Primer sequence (5'-3')	GenBank acc. no.
HSP70[1]	F	TGACGTGTCCATCCTGACCAT	BT043589.1
	R	CTGAAGAGGTCGGAACACATCTC	
PGC1A[2]	F	GTCAATATGGCAACGAGGCTTC	FJ710605
	R	TCGAATGAAGGCAATCCGTC	
CPT1[3]	F	TCCCACATCATCCCCTTCAACT	AM230810
	R	TGTCCCTGAAGTGAGCCAGCT	
HBB[4]	F	ACAAACGTCAACATGGTCGACTGG	EG897325.1
	R	TCTTTCCCCACAGGCCTACGAT	
HBA[5]	F	AAGGCAGATGTCGTCGGTGCT	CK883845.1
	R	CAGCCCAGTGGGAGAAGTAGGTCTT	
CD8A[6]	F	CGTCTACAGCTGTGCATCAATCAA	AY693391
	R	GGCTGTGGTCATTGGTGTAGTC	
SEC13[7]	F	AGTGGGCCTGTATCAGCGACGT	EG882700.1
	R	ATCACTGCTCGTTCGTCGCTCC	
NDUFB8[8]	F	TCTGTCGCTGGGAGGAGAAGGA	DW532752.1
	R	GTCCAGGCAGGTCCGATACTCTGT	
EF1A[9]	F	CACCACCGGCCATCTGATCTACAA	AF321836
	R	TCAGCAGCCTCCTTCTCGAACTTC	

Complete gene names: [1]Heat shock protein 70, [2]Peroxisome proliferator-activated receptor gamma, coactivator 1, [3]Carnitine palmitoyltransferase 1, [4]Hemoglobin beta chain, [5]Hemoglobin alpha chain, [6]CD8 alpha T cell glycoprotein, [7]SEC13-like protein, [8]NADH dehydrogenase (ubiquinone) 1 beta subcomplex, 8, 19 kDa, [9]Elongation factor 1 alpha.

or *elongation factor 1 alpha* (used for HSP70 only). All reference genes were validated using the BestKeeper software [25]. The efficiency of the PCR reactions was estimated for all primer pairs by six times 1:5 dilution series of a cDNA mix of all used samples. Efficiency values were estimated by using the LightCycler® 480 Software (version 1.5.0.39). Differences in gene expression ratios (log$_2$-transformed values) between groups were assessed by two-sided pairwise t-tests with pooled standard deviation and p-value adjustment according to Holm (stats-package in R version 3.0.2 (http://cran.r-project.org).

Immunofluorescence microscopy

Hearts were fixed in 4% PFA (paraformaldehyde) and dehydrated in increasing ethanol concentrations prior to paraffin embedding and sectioning (7 μM). After paraffin removal and dehydration, microwave facilitated antigen retrieval was conducted in 10 mM Tris-Hcl (pH = 10) for 10 min. Permeabilization was achieved with 1% Triton X100 for 10 min before 2 hrs blocking in 5% dry milk dissolved in 1 × PBST. Primary antibodies used were rabbit polyclonal antibodies against salmon collagen type I (BioLogo, Kiel, Germany), human/mouse inducible nitric oxide synthase, iNOS (Thermo Fisher Scientific Inc., Rockford, USA) and human/mouse vascular endothelial growth factor, VEGF (147: sc-507, Santa Cruz Biotechnology Inc., Heidelberg, Germany). All were tested for reactivity and specificity in Atlantic salmon [26-28]. Primary antibodies were diluted to a concentration of 5-10 μg/ml in 1 × PBST with 2% dry milk and 1% DMSO. After overnight incubation at 4°C, the sections were washed thoroughly in 1 × PBST and incubated with Alexa conjugated secondary antibodies (Invitrogen) diluted 1:200 for 2 hrs at room temperature. As controls, secondary antibody only was used giving negative results. Final 1 × PBST washes were carried out before mounting and microscopy. All images were captured using a Zeiss Axioplan Z1 and post processed using the Zeiss Axiovison software and Corel Draw. Similar exposure and image manipulation settings were applied to the images to enable comparison between treatments and replicates. A total of three fish (three sections per heart) from each temperature and time point was analyzed. The whole tissue was inspected and one representative image was captured for each section (presented in Figures 1, 2 and 3). For quantification of iNOS expression, the average number of positive cells ± SEM in spongy myocardium (showing the most prominent staining differences between temperature groups) from all fish was calculated with Zeiss Axiovison software from two field of views per fish (25× objective). For quantification of VEGF expression, the average number of positively stained cells ± SEM along the entire epicardium from all fish was similarly calculated (two field of

views, 25× objective) and expressed as number of positive cells per mm epicardium. Expression of collagen I between temperature groups was presented as LUT (Look-Up Table) images showing fluorescence intensities of representative sections.

Results

A salmonid cDNA microarray was used to examine temperature effects on cardiac (ventricle) gene expression in adult Atlantic salmon exposed to 19°C (simulating peak summer temperature in Norwegian Atlantic salmon aquaculture) for 21 days (short-term acclimation) and 56 days (long-term acclimation). Temperature affected expression of 11.6% of the genes, of which 52 genes were up-regulated and 156 genes were down-regulated (expression ratio >1.3/log$_2$ expression ratio >0.4, 19°C versus 14°C) in at least one time point. These were further grouped according to functional annotation as shown in Table 2, which provided a fundament for supportive analysis on selected genes and proteins using real-time qPCR and immunofluorescence microscopy. Up-regulated features included seven genes involved in cell signaling responses to a diverse array of cellular perturbations such as heat stress and unfolded protein response, among them *hsp47, hsp90, mapk13, junB* (Table 2) and *hsp70* (qPCR; Figure 1A). Immunofluorescence microscopy of iNOS indicated staining of a higher number of cells and at stronger levels in the compact and spongy myocardium after 56 days at 19°C in comparison to control temperature (Figure 2). Immunostaining of VEGF indicated increased and more evenly distributed staining of cells along the epicardium in 19°C fish in comparison to controls, where VEGF was localised in epicardial foci (Figure 3). VEGF labelling was not seen in the compact and spongy muscle layers. Microarray genes coding for structural myocardial proteins showed coordinated down-regulation in fish reared at 19°C compared to 14°C at both time points (Table 2), including different transcripts for myosin, actin and troponin. Among genes regulating extracellular matrix, metalloproteinase genes, involved in degradation of extracellular matrix, was up-regulated whereas several transcripts for collagens were down-regulated with elevated temperature at both time points (Table 2). In contrast, immunostaining of collagen I indicated increased expression in the epicardium and compact myocardium of 19°C versus 14°C fish, while no staining was observed in the spongy layer at either temperature (Figure 4). In regard to energy metabolism, mitochondrial electron transport chain genes such as *NADH-ubiquinone oxidoreductase 15 kDa subunit, cytochromes b/c/c1/c2* and *ATP synthase* were down-regulated with elevated temperature at both time points (Table 2). In addition, genes for cardiac fatty acid oxidation showed significant up-regulation

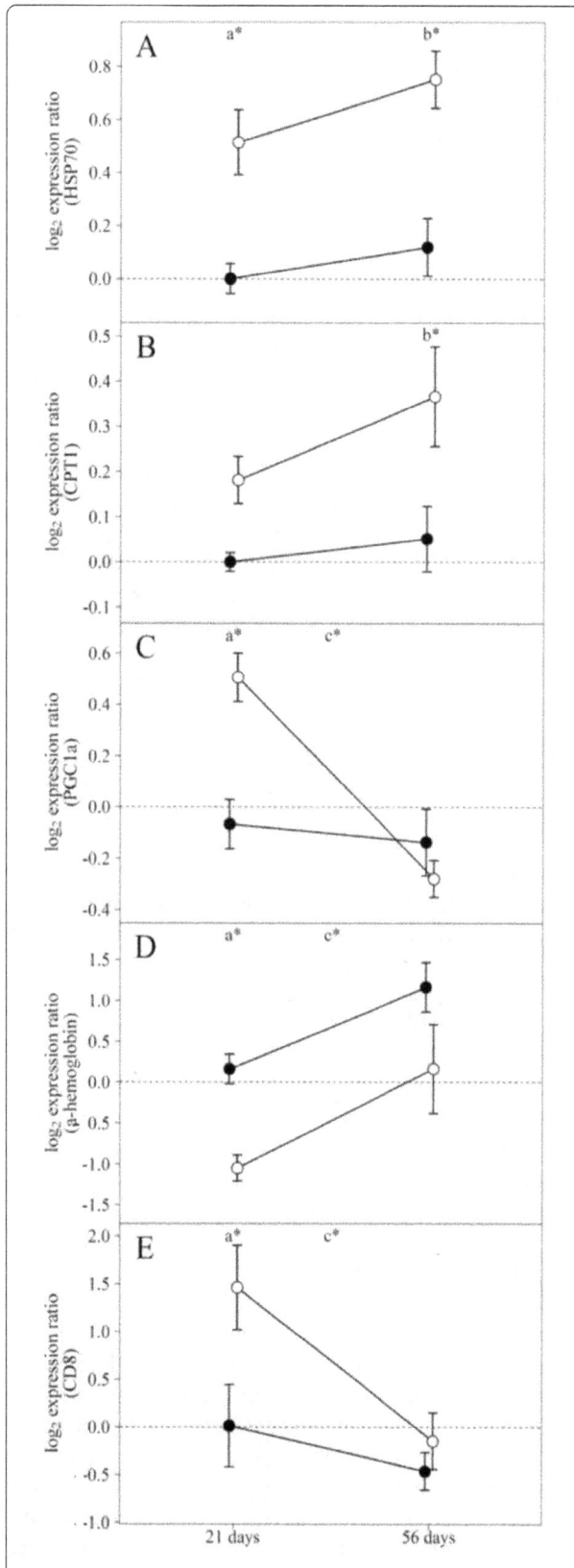

Figure 1 Cardiac expression of selected genes in fish reared under normal and elevated temperature. Relative mRNA transcription levels of **A)** *heat shock protein 70, HSP70;* **B)** *carnitine palmitoyltransferase 1, CPT1;* **C)** *peroxisome proliferator-activated receptor (PPAR)γ coactivator 1a, PGC1a;* **D)** *a-hemoglobin;* **E)** T cell antigen *CD8 alpha* in fish reared at normal (14°C, filled circles) and elevated (19°C, open circles) temperature for 21 and 56 days. Data are mean log$_2$ expression ratio ± SEM relative to the average of normalized controls (14°C, 21 days), real-time qPCR. Statistical differences (adjusted p-value < 0.05; pairwise t-tests of the four groups, N = 9) are indicated between temperatures (21 days: a*, 56 days: b*) and time points for 19°C fish (c*).

in 19°C fish, including *carnitine palmitoyltransferase (CPT)1* after 56 days (Figure 1B) and *peroxisome proliferator-activated receptor (PPAR)γ coactivator (PGC) 1α* after 21 days (Figure 1C). Genes involved in oxygen transport and the heme biosynthetic pathway, including several transcripts for *α/β-hemoglobin* and *d-aminolevulinate synthase*, were down-regulated in 19°C fish after 21 and 56 days (Table 2 and Figure 1D). Microarray results indicated that expression of immune-related genes were influenced by the temperature elevation, through down-regulation of genes encoding humoral components of the innate immune system (complement factors, chemokines and receptors, the serine protease activator *cathepsin C-3* and *annexin A1*). In contrast, genes coding for cellular components were up-regulated, such as *CD9 antigen, high affinity IgG Fc receptor I precursor, tyrosine-protein kinase BTK, gamma-interferon inducible lysosomal thiol reductase* (Table 2) and the T cell antigen *CD8 alpha* (Figure 1E).

Discussion

Seasonal fluctuations in seawater temperature are naturally occurring in the aquaculture of Atlantic salmon. Particularly in the summer months, western and southern regions of Norway experience temperature increments above thermal preference (15°C [3,29,30]) peaking around 18-20°C. In a recent study we observed significantly reduced feed intake, growth performance and endogenous energy storage in large (~2 kg) Atlantic salmon after long-term exposure to 19°C under controlled conditions [19]. This poor performance was linked to suppressed endocrine appetite regulation, leading to a negative energy homeostasis with depleted lipid stores in muscle and whole carcass. Based on these findings and the same experimental fish, the current study aimed to further understand how the chronic temperature elevation affected molecular processes at the levels of gene and protein expression in the heart, as a key organ for thermal plasticity and acclimation in salmonids [31,32].

Among genes that were strongly up-regulated with elevated temperature, it was not surprising to find several chaperones and other genes involved in the unfolded protein response. This included three heat shock proteins

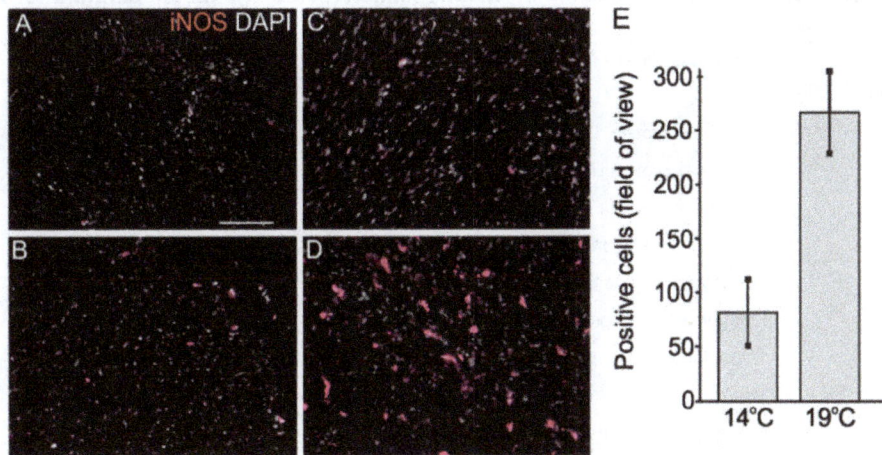

Figure 2 Inducible nitric oxide synthase (iNOS) expression in cardiac tissues of fish reared under normal and elevated temperature.
Immunofluorescence staining of iNOS (red color) and DAPI nuclear counterstain (white color) in cardiac tissues of fish reared for 56 days at normal temperature (14°C, upper panels) and high temperature (19°C, lower panels). At 14°C iNOS is expressed at low levels and in a few cells in the compact (**A**) and spongy (**B**) myocardium. At 19°C iNOS is expressed in a higher number of cells in the compact myocardium (**C**), and strong staining of individual myocytes is observed in the spongy myocardium (**D**). Panels **A-D** show one representative micrograph of three sections examined per fish from a total of three fish per temperature group. The 40 μm scale bar in panel **A** applies to all panels in the figure. **E**: Average number of positive cells ± SEM in spongy myocardium, calculated using a larger field of view (25× objective).

(HSPs), which are among the most studied proteins in the general response to a variety of stressors and perturbations in mammals and fish [33]. Although their use as suitable indicators of stressed states in fish has been disputed [34], synthesis of HSPs to maintain proper folding/refolding of proteins has been shown highly expensive for the organism [35]. In spite of a severely compromised energy homeostasis in the experimental fish, the sustained induced transcription of HSPs over time could indicate a need for chaperone activity and the unfolded protein response during cardiac acclimation to the elevated temperature.

The nitric oxide synthase system is an important inter- and intracellular regulator of mechanical performance and oxygen supply in the fish heart [15], and iNOS is exclusively expressed in ventricular cardiomyocytes under basal condition and after LPS stimulation [36]. Although the physiological and pathophysiological regulation of the NOS/NO system is very complex and only partly understood in fish, studies have shown that NOS

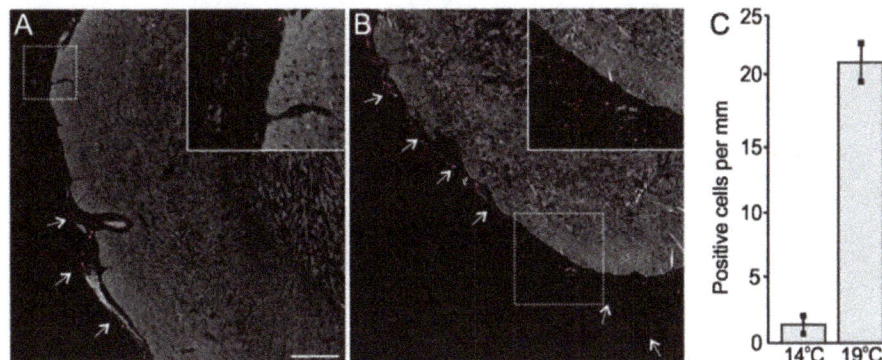

Figure 3 Vascular endothelial growth factor (VEGF) expression in cardiac tissues of fish reared under normal and elevated temperature.
Immunofluorescence staining of VEGF (red color) in cardiac tissues of fish reared for 56 days at control temperature (14°C, **A**) and elevated temperature (19°C, **B**). **A**: VEGF positive cells (arrows) are mainly located around already existing epicardial vasculature at 14°C. **B**: VEGF positive cells (arrows) are evenly distributed along the entire epicardium at 19°C. Panels **A-B** show one representative micrograph of three sections examined per fish from a total of three fish per temperature group, with one representative region per group shown at higher magnification (inset). The 400 μm scale bar in panel **A** applies to both panels in the figure. **C**: Average number of positive cells per mm epicardium ± SEM, calculated using a larger field of view (25× objective).

Table 2 Functional categories and genes regulated in Atlantic salmon reared at high temperature for 21 and 56 days identified from microarray analysis

Probe number	Name (best blast hit)	Day 21	Day 56
Unfolded protein response			
CA356940	Heat shock protein 47 kDa	1,15	1,35
CA373890	Heat shock protein HSP 90-beta-1	0,66	0,67
EST1-3A_F08	Heat shock protein HSP 90-beta-2	0,83	0,80
EXOB1_E03	Eukaryotic translation initiation factor 3 subunit 5	0,55	0,30
EXOB1_E08	Eukaryotic translation initiation factor 3 subunit 6-1	0,44	0,35
CA382570	Mitogen-activated protein kinase 13	0,29	0,57
EST1-3A_H06	Transcription factor jun-B-1	0,43	1,02
CA368716	Membrane-bound transcription factor site 2 protease	0,58	0,36
CA378435	Protein phosphatase 2C delta isoform	0,62	0,23
Tissue remodeling and cytoskeleton			
est03c04	Matrix metalloproteinase-9	0,34	0,51
EXOB3_H01	Matrix metalloproteinase-13	0,47	0,81
CA378743	Fibronectin precursor	0,44	0,29
utu04c11	Collagen alpha 1(I) chain-2	-0,32	-0,95
HK0003_C02	Collagen alpha 1(I) chain-1	-0,16	-0,51
utu02b11	Collagen a3(I)-2	-0,29	-0,56
utu02a06	Collagen a3(I)-1	-0,22	-0,41
HKT0001_B03	Alpha 2 type I collagen-1	-0,54	-0,91
HK0003_E07	Myosin light chain 2-1	-0,50	-0,73
utu02c02	Myosin heavy chain 1-1	-0,51	-0,54
utu04f06	Myosin heavy chain 1-2	-0,64	-0,95
HK0002_F05	Myosin heavy chain, fetal	-0,56	-0,50
HK0002_B06	Troponin T-3	-0,81	-0,67
HK0003_D01	Troponin C-1	-0,71	-0,17
HKT0001_E07	Actin, alpha 1	-0,39	-0,71
utu04d04	Actin, alpha 4	-0,13	-0,67
utu04f08	Actin, alpha 5	-0,58	-1,27
HK0003_C08	Parvalbumin alpha-2	-0,78	-0,65
est01e10	Tolloid-like protein (nephrosin)-1	-0,74	-0,47
Energy metabolism			
HKT0001_H05	Cytochrome b-3	0,32	0,41
utu02b07	Cytochrome c oxidase subunit II	0,59	0,44
HK0001_G02	ATP synthase beta chain-2	-0,43	-0,71
HK0002_G02	Creatine kinase, sarcomeric mitochondrial precursor	-0,41	-0,63
est03a08	Cytochrome c-1	-0,66	-0,99
HK0003_B03	Cytochrome c-2	-0,91	-1,16
EXOB1_C10	Cytochrome P450 2 K4-2	-0,94	-1,39
HK0002_A12	NADH-ubiquinone oxidoreductase 15 kDa subunit	-0,45	-0,43
Heme biosynthesis			
EXOB2_B10	Hemoglobin beta chain Omy 30073	-0,54	-1,64
HST0001_C04	Hemoglobin alpha chain Omy 11839	-0,96	-1,56
EXOB4_H06	Alpha-globin 1-3 Omy 8146	-0,76	-1,41

Table 2 Functional categories and genes regulated in Atlantic salmon reared at high temperature for 21 and 56 days identified from microarray analysis *(Continued)*

HST0001_C02	Alpha-globin I-1 Omy 11839	-0,18	-0,97
utu01e09	Embryonic alpha-type globin2 + collagen alpha 2(1)	-0,43	-0,68
HST0001_D08	Beta-globin Omy 9744	-0,79	-1,06
est01g04	5-aminolevulinate synthase	0,08	-0,52
CA381045	Aminolevulinate, delta-, synthase 1	-0,84	-1,23
HK0001_D09	Cytochrome P450 2 F1	-0,87	-1,15
Immune response			
EXOB1_F11	CD9	0,45	0,36
CA388403	CD9-like	0,20	0,54
CA378736	Tyrosine-protein kinase BTK	0,44	0,29
CA382425	B-cell translocation gene 1-2	0,49	0,42
EXOB4_C11	High affinity immunoglobulin γ Fc receptor I precursor	0,47	0,39
CA362806	Gamma-interferon inducible lysosomal thiol reductase	0,51	0,17
CA355488	Tapasin-2	0,40	0,45
CA373659	Mannan-binding lectin serine protease 2-2	0,25	0,46
ENH2_B05	Acute phase protein	0,41	0,53
CA370329	Lysozyme C precursor	0,87	0,61
CA362419	Complement component C6	0,47	0,40
HK0001_F01	Complement factor H-1	-0,82	-0,73
CA370696	Complement control protein factor I-B	-0,71	0,23
EXOB1_E12	Serine protease-like protein-3	-0,34	-0,53
EST1-3A_A09	Serine protease-like protein-2	-0,42	-0,65
EXOB3_B01	Cathepsin C-3	-0,90	-1,30
CA377504	Cold autoinflammatory syndrome 1 protein	-0,81	-0,62
HK0002_G10	T-cell receptor α chain V region HPB-MLT precursor (Fr)	-0,91	-0,52
CA372428	Leukotriene B4 receptor 1	-1,11	-0,82
HK0002_G11	Myristoylated alanine-rich protein kinase C substrate	-1,07	-0,87
EXOB2_G01	Leukocyte cell-derived chemotaxin 2	-0,97	-0,86
CA343700	CXC chemokine receptor transcript variant B	-0,52	-0,88
CA361151	Annexin A1-2	-0,58	-0,47

Expression values are $\log_2$-expression ratios (19°C versus 14°C) from analysis of pooled heart samples (per temperature treatment: 3 fish per triplicate tanks, n = 9).

influences cardiac inotropy (i.e. cardiac output) of salmon [37] and the red-blooded icefish *T. bernacchii* [36], which was also sensitive to acute temperature change [16]. Our results showing increased immunofluorescence staining of iNOS in compact and spongy myocardium may be a further indication of an involvement in the thermal acclimation or response to increased temperature. NO has also been shown to induce vasodilation and reduce coronary resistance under hypoxia in salmonids [38]. In this process, VEGF is another important regulator which promotes proliferation and migration of endothelial cells in the formation of new blood vessels under cardiac physiological and pathological conditions [39]. Whether the induced expression of VEGF and iNOS in our study reflected increased vascularization and/or vasodilation to

compensate for increased oxygen demand with elevated temperature should be subject to further study. In this regard, the lower abundance of several transcripts for heme biosynthesis and ATP production/energy metabolism after short- and long-term exposure to elevated temperature could also indicate that oxygen transport/uptake and possibly aerobic metabolism was affected.

A fundamental mode for increasing oxygen carrying capacity in vertebrates is by increasing the cardiac output. In salmonids, several studies have suggested that a limitation at the level of the heart is the primary cause of limited oxygen supply with increasing temperature because maximum cardiac output fails to increase above thermal optimum [13]. Furthermore, acclimation to high temperatures has been associated with increased thickness

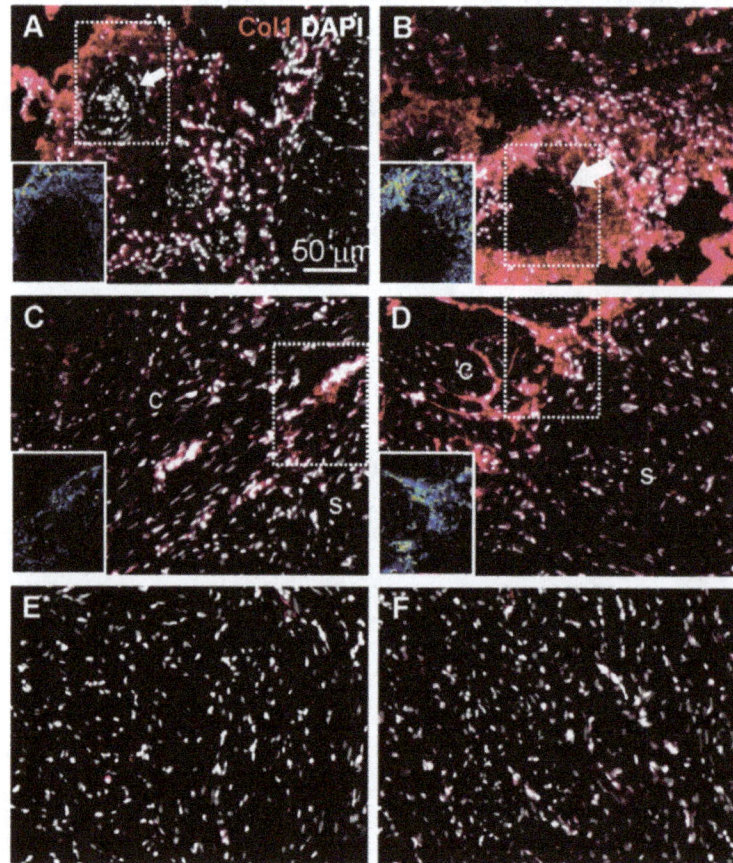

Figure 4 Collagen I expression in cardiac tissues of fish reared at normal and elevated temperature. Immunofluorescence staining of collagen I (red color) and DAPI nuclear counterstain (white color) in cardiac tissues of fish reared for 56 days at 14°C (left panels, **A**, **C**, **E**) and 19°C (right panels, **B**, **D**, **F**). **A**: Collagen I is abundant in the epicardium and vasculature (arrow) at 14°C. **B**: Increased signal intensity is observed at 19°C. **C**: At 14°C collagen I is expressed in cell clusters in the compact (c) but not in the spongy (s) myocardium. **D**: At 19°C collagen I is strongly expressed in larger structures resembling connective tissue of the compact (c) but not in the spongy (s) myocardium. **E-F**: Cells in the spongy myocardium show weak staining at both temperatures. Fluorescence intensities are shown as LUT (Look-Up Table) images in panels **A-D** (inset). Panels show one representative micrograph of three sections examined per fish from a total of three fish per temperature group. The 50 μm scale bar in panel **A** applies to all panels in the figure.

of the compact myocardium, which is assumed to compensate for the decreased power-generating ability [14] or simply reflecting an increased activity level at higher temperatures [40]. A recent study with warm-acclimated rainbow trout also reported that the increased thickness of the compact layer was associated with reduced connective tissue, however this was only observed for male and not female fish [10]. Correspondingly, we observed lower abundance of collagen mRNA with high temperature, however effects of sex was not determined. On the contrary, immunostaining demonstrated increased deposition of collagen I in large bundles exclusively in the compact myocardium at high temperature. This discrepancy between protein and transcript levels of collagen could be methodology based, since gene expression was measured in total RNA extracted from the whole myocardium (both spongy and compact layers) whereas immunofluorescence detection of collagen showed increased staining with

temperature only in the compact myocardium, which typically comprises 30-50% of the heart in athletic fishes [7]. In fact, Klaiman *et al.* [10] reported reduction in muscle bundle area in spongy myocardium with warm acclimation, thus lower collagen gene expression levels could simply reflect altered proportions of compartments with increased temperature. Pointing in the same direction, we also observed substantially lower transcript levels of several cytoskeleton genes including actin, myosin and troponin after short- and long-term acclimation. In view of the severely compromised growth performance and energy homeostasis of the fish in this study after long-term high temperature, implications of the compact myocardium increase in collagen I protein expression on cardiac function and possibly fibrosis should be further studied. Reduced mitochondrial capacity above thermal optimum has been demonstrated for fish [41]. Interestingly, we found significantly higher mRNA levels of CPT1 (after 56 days) and

PGC1α (after 21 days) in fish kept at 19°C. It could be speculated whether this was a tissue response in order to balance the overall energetic status, a notion supported from reduced hepatic beta-oxidation in the same fish [19].

High temperature affected cardiac expression of important immune-related genes. The salmon heart is an immune-relevant organ in the sense that it represents a major replication site for several viral pathogens of high importance [17,18]. Common for these diseases is the strong inflammation of the myocardium which coincides with a strong activation of a CD8 T cell response [18,23,42]. Consequently, given the temperature-induced gene expression of cellular immune components including CD8 alpha in the present study, it may be speculated if high seawater temperatures can further elevate myocardial inflammation during infection and thus represent a relevant risk factor affecting disease outcome. It has been proposed that low environmental temperature diminishes the humoral immune response, since primary antibody response has been found to be either dampened or retarded at lower temperatures [43,44]. Here, we report that expression of some genes involved in the innate humoral immune response were down-regulated with high temperature. At the same time, a suite of genes representing cellular components were up-regulated, including some involved in B- and T-cell development. Our understanding of immunological effects of elevated temperatures in fish is far from complete, but studies have shown significant hematological modulation in response to thermal acclimation in salmonids [45-47]. A study with rainbow trout reported induced complement lytic activity and opsonization capacity with increased temperature in rainbow trout [48], which could agree with our finding of temperature-induced gene expression of *complement C6*, a part of the membrane attack complex. Another aspect relates to whether our observed regulation of cardiac innate immune response genes is ascribed to the temperature increase *per se* or (re)allocation of resources in view of the negative growth performance and energy homeostasis of the fish. This is a subject that should deserve attention in future research.

Conclusions

This study provides new knowledge on the molecular responses of cardiac tissues during long-term exposure to elevated seawater temperature reflective of the peak summer temperatures experienced in Atlantic salmon aquaculture. We report temperature-induced changes in expression of genes and proteins indicating that the unfolded protein response, vascularization and remodeling of connective tissue as well as altered innate immune responses were affected during cardiac acclimation to elevated temperature.

Competing interests
The authors declare that they have no competing interests.

Authors' contributions
SMJ designed and performed the microarray studies together with AK, and participated in samplings, data interpretation and wrote the manuscript together with VC, who also performed qPCR gene expression studies together with GT. AK were responsible for microarray data processing and analysis as well as revision of the manuscript. JT conducted immunofluorescence microscopy. HT obtained funding, planned and coordinated the experimental fish study and participated in samplings together with EMH, TJH, SS and OB, and also revised the manuscript. All authors read and approved the final manuscript.

Acknowledgements
The study was supported by the Research Council of Norway, grant nos. 187306/S40 and 225219/E40, and The Norwegian Seafood Research Fund (FHF) grant no. 900870. We wish to thank Katrine Hånes Kirste and Hege Munck for laboratory assistance.

Author details
[1]Nofima AS, P.O. Box 210, N-1431 Ås, Norway. [2]AVS Chile S.A., Casilla 300, Puerto Varas, Chile. [3]National Institute of Nutrition and Seafood Research (NIFES), P.O. Box 2029, N-5817 Bergen, Nordnes, Norway. [4]Institute of Marine Research, Matre Research Station, N-5984 Matredal, Norway. [5]Skretting Norway AS, P.O. Box 319, Sentrum N-4002 Stavanger, Norway. [6]Marine Harvest Norway AS, Sandviksbodene 78, N-5035 Bergen, Norway.

References
1. Brett JR: Energetic responses of salmon to temperature. A study of some thermal relations in the physiology and freshwater ecology of sockeye salmon (*Oncorhynchus nerka*). *Am Zool* 1971, **11**:99–113.
2. Fry FEJ: The effect of environmental factors on the physiology of fish. In *Fish Physiology*. Edited by Hoar WD, Randall DJ. New York: Academic; 1971.
3. Handeland SO, Bjornsson BT, Arnesen AM, Stefansson SO: Seawater adaptation and growth of post-smolt Atlantic salmon (*Salmo salar*) of wild and farmed strains. *Aquaculture* 2003, **220**(1–4):367–384.
4. Jonsson B, Jonsson N: A review of the likely effects of climate change on anadromous Atlantic salmon *Salmo salar* and brown trout *Salmo trutta*, with particular reference to water temperature and flow. *J Fish Biol* 2009, **75**(10):2381–2447.
5. Claireaux G, Webber DM, Lagardere JP, Kerr SR: Influence of water temperature and oxygenation on the aerobic metabolic scope of Atlantic cod (*Gadus morhua*). *J Sea Res* 2000, **44**(3–4):257–265.
6. Farrell AP, Richards JJ: Defining hypoxia: an integrative synthesis of the responses of fish to hypoxia. In *Hypoxia*. Edited by Richards JG, Farrell AP, Brauner CJ. Burlington: Academic; 2009.
7. Farrell AP, Eliason EJ, Sandblom E, Clark TD: Fish cardiorespiratory physiology in an era of climate change. *Can J Zool* 2009, **87**(10):835–851.
8. Goldspink G: Adaptation of fish to different environmental-temperature by qualitative and quantitative changes in gene-expression. *J Thermal Biol* 1995, **20**(1–2):167–174.
9. Hazel JR, Prosser CL: Molecular mechanisms of temperature compensation in poikilotherms. *Physiol Rev* 1974, **54**(3):620–677.
10. Klaiman JM, Fenna AJ, Shiels HA, Macri J, Gillis TE: Cardiac remodeling in fish: strategies to maintain heart function during temperature change. *Plos One* 2011, **6**(9):e24464.
11. Lee CG, Farrell AP, Lotto A, MacNutt MJ, Hinch SG, Healey MC: The effect of temperature on swimming performance and oxygen consumption in adult sockeye (*Oncorhynchus nerka*) and coho (*O-kisutch*) salmon stocks. *J Exp Biol* 2003, **206**(18):3239–3251.
12. Gamperl AK, Farrell AP: Cardiac plasticity in fishes: environmental influences and intraspecific differences. *J Exp Biol* 2004, **207**(15):2539–2550.
13. Steinhausen MF, Sandblom E, Eliason EJ, Verhille C, Farrell AP: The effect of acute temperature increases on the cardiorespiratory performance of resting and swimming sockeye salmon (Oncorhynchus nerka). *J Exp Biol* 2008, **211**(24):3915–3926.

14. Farrell AP, Gamperl AK, Hicks JMT, Shiels HA, Jain KE: **Maximum cardiac performance of rainbow trout (Oncorhynchus mykiss) at temperatures approaching their upper lethal limit.** *J Exp Biol* 1996, 199(3):663–672.

15. Tota B, Amelio D, Pellegrino D, Ip YK, Cerra MC: **NO modulation of myocardial performance in fish hearts.** *Comp Biochem Phys A* 2005, 142(2):164–177.

16. Amelio D, Garofalo F, Capria C, Tota B, Imbrogno S: **Effects of temperature on the nitric oxide-dependent modulation of the Frank-Starling mechanism: the fish heart as a case study.** *Comp Biochem Phys A* 2013, 164(2):356–362.

17. Haugland O, Mikalsen AB, Nilsen P, Lindmo K, Thu BJ, Eliassen TM, Roos N, Rode M, Evensen O: **Cardiomyopathy syndrome of Atlantic salmon (Salmo salar L.) is caused by a double-stranded RNA virus of the Totiviridae family.** *J Virol* 2011, 85(11):5275–5286.

18. Mikalsen AB, Haugland O, Rode M, Solbakk IT, Evensen O: **Atlantic salmon reovirus lifection causes a CD8 T cell myocarditis in Atlantic salmon (Salmo salar L.).** *Plos One* 2012, 7(6):e37269.

19. Hevroy EM, Waagbo R, Torstensen BE, Takle H, Stubhaug I, Jorgensen SM, Torgersen T, Tvenning L, Susort S, Breck O, Hansen T: **Ghrelin is involved in voluntary anorexia in Atlantic salmon raised at elevated sea temperatures.** *Gen Comp Endocrinol* 2012, 175(1):118–134.

20. Schiotz BL, Jorgensen SM, Rexroad C, Gjoen T, Krasnov A: **Transcriptomic analysis of responses to infectious salmon anemia virus infection in macrophage-like cells.** *Virus Res* 2008, 136(1–2):65–74.

21. Krasnov A, Timmerhaus G, Afanasyev S, Jorgensen SM: **Development and assessment of oligonucleotide microarrays for Atlantic salmon (Salmo salar L.).** *Comp Biochem Physiol Part D Genomics Proteomics* 2011, 6(1):31–38.

22. Bustin SA, Benes V, Garson JA, Hellemans J, Huggett J, Kubista M, Mueller R, Nolan T, Pfaffl MW, Shipley GL, Vandesompele J, Wittwer CT: **The MIQE guidelines: minimum information for publication of quantitative real-time PCR experiments.** *Clin Chem* 2009, 55(4):611–622.

23. Timmerhaus G, Krasnov A, Nilsen P, Alarcon M, Afanasyev S, Rode M, Takle H, Jorgensen SM: **Transcriptome profiling of immune responses to cardiomyopathy syndrome (CMS) in Atlantic salmon.** *BMC Genomics* 2011, 12:459.

24. Pfaffl MW, Horgan GW, Dempfle L: **Relative expression software tool (REST (c)) for group-wise comparison and statistical analysis of relative expression results in real-time PCR.** *Nucleic Acids Res* 2002, 30(9):e36.

25. Pfaffl MW, Tichopad A, Prgomet C, Neuvians TP: **Determination of stable housekeeping genes, differentially regulated target genes and sample integrity: BestKeeper - Excel-based tool using pair-wise correlations.** *Biotechnol Lett* 2004, 26(6):509–515.

26. Ebbesson LE, Tipsmark CK, Holmqvist B, Nilsen T, Andersson E, Stefansson SO, Madsen SS: **Nitric oxide synthase in the gill of Atlantic salmon: colocalization with and inhibition of Na+, K + -ATPase.** *J Exp Biol* 2005, 208(6):1011–1017.

27. Vuori KAM, Soitamo A, Vuorinen PJ, Nikinmaa M: **Baltic salmon (Salmo salar) yolk-sac fry mortality is associated with disturbances in the function of hypoxia-inducible transcription factor (HIF-1 alpha) and consecutive gene expression.** *Aquat Toxicol* 2004, 68(4):301–313.

28. Ytteborg E, Torgersen JS, Pedersen ME, Helland SJ, Grisdale-Helland B, Takle H: **Exercise induced mechano-sensing and Substance P mediated bone modeling in Atlantic salmon.** *Bone* 2013, 53(1):259–268.

29. Handeland SO, Imsland AK, Stefansson SO: **The effect of temperature and fish size on growth, feed intake, food conversion efficiency and stomach evacuation rate of Atlantic salmon post-smolts.** *Aquaculture* 2008, 283(1–4):36–42.

30. Hevroy EM, Hunskar C, de Gelder S, Shimizu M, Waagbo R, Breck O, Takle H, Sussort S, Hansen T: **GH-IGF system regulation of attenuated muscle growth and lipolysis in Atlantic salmon reared at elevated sea temperatures.** *J Comp Physiol B-Biochem Syst Environ Physiol* 2013, 183(2):243–259.

31. Anttila K, Casselman MT, Schulte PM, Farrell AP: **Optimum temperature in juvenile salmonids: connecting subcellular indicators to tissue function and whole-organism thermal optimum.** *Physiol Biochem Zool* 2013, 86(2):245–256.

32. Anttila K, Dhillon RS, Boulding EG, Farrell AP, Glebe BD, Elliott JAK, Wolters WR, Schulte PM: **Variation in temperature tolerance among families of Atlantic salmon (Salmo salar) is associated with hypoxia tolerance, ventricle size and myoglobin level.** *J Exp Biol* 2013, 216(7):1183–1190.

33. Iwama GK, Vijayan MM, Forsyth RB, Ackerman PA: **Heat shock proteins and physiological stress in fish.** *Am Zool* 1999, 39(6):901–909.

34. Iwama GK, Afonso LOB, Todgham A, Ackerman P, Nakano K: **Are hsps suitable for indicating stressed states in fish?** *J Exp Biol* 2004, 207(1):15–19.

35. Houlihan DF: **Protein turnover in ectotherms and its relationship to energetics.** In *Advances in comparative and environmental physiology*. Edited by Gilles R. Berlin: Springer; 1991.

36. Garofalo F, Amelio D, Cerra MC, Tota B, Sidell BD, Pellegrino D: **Morphological and physiological study of the cardiac NOS/NO system in the Antarctic (Hb(-)/Mb(-)) icefish Chaenocephalus aceratus and in the red-blooded Trematomus bernacchii.** *Nitric Oxide-Biol Ch* 2009, 20(2):69–78.

37. Gattuso A, Mazza R, Imbrogno S, Sverdrup A, Tota B, Nylund A: **Cardiac performance in Salmo salar with infectious salmon anaemia (ISA): putative role of nitric oxide.** *Dis Aquat Organ* 2002, 52(1):11–20.

38. Agnisola C: **Role of nitric oxide in the control of coronary resistance in teleosts.** *Comp Biochem Phys A* 2005, 142(2):178–187.

39. Yancopoulos GD, Davis S, Gale NW, Rudge JS, Wiegand SJ, Holash J: **Vascular-specific growth factors and blood vessel formation.** *Nature* 2000, 407(6801):242–248.

40. Farrell AP, Hammons AM, Graham MS, Tibbits GF: **Cardiac growth in rainbow trout, Salmo gardnieri.** *Can J Zool* 1988, 66(11):2368–2373.

41. Portner HO, Lannig G: **Oxygen and capacity limited thermal tolerance.** In *Hypoxia*. Edited by Richards JG, Farrell AP, Brauner CJ. Burlington: Academic; 2009.

42. Timmerhaus G, Krasnov A, Takle H, Afanasyev S, Nilsen P, Rode M, Jorgensen SM: **Comparison of Atlantic salmon individuals with different outcomes of cardiomyopathy syndrome (CMS).** *BMC Genomics* 2012, 13:205.

43. Avtalion RR: **Temperature effect on antibody production and immunological memory, in carp (Cyprinus carpio) immunized against bovine serum albumin (BSA).** *Immunology* 1969, 17(6):927–931.

44. Rijkers GT, Frederixwolters EMH, Vanmuiswinkel WB: **The immune-system of cyprinid fish - kinetics and temperature-dependence of antibody-producing cells in carp (Cyprinus carpio).** *Immunology* 1980, 41(1):91–97.

45. Hardie LJ, Fletcher TC, Secombes CJ: **Effect of temperature on macrophage activation and the production of macrophage activating factor by rainbow-trout (Oncorhynchus mykiss) leukocytes.** *Dev Comp Immunol* 1994, 18(1):57–66.

46. Houston AH, Dobric N, Kahurananga R: **The nature of hematological response in fish - Studies on rainbow trout Oncorhynchus mykiss exposed to simulated winter, spring and summer conditions.** *Fish Physiol Biochem* 1996, 15(4):339–347.

47. Pettersen EF, Bjorlow I, Hagland TJ, Wergeland HI: **Effect of seawater temperature on leucocyte populations in Atlantic salmon post-smolts.** *Vet Immunol Immunopathol* 2005, 106(1–2):65–76.

48. Nikoskelainen S, Bylund G, Lilius EM: **Effect of environmental temperature on rainbow trout (Oncorhynchus mykiss) innate immunity.** *Dev Comp Immunol* 2004, 28(6):581–592.

6

Interleukin-1 beta: a potential link between stress and the development of visceral obesity

Kristin J Speaker and Monika Fleshner[*]

Abstract

Background: A disproportionate amount of body fat within the abdominal cavity, otherwise known as visceral obesity, best predicts the negative health outcomes associated with high levels body fat. Growing evidence suggests that repeated activation of the stress response can favor visceral fat deposition and that visceral obesity may induce low-grade, systemic inflammation which is etiologically linked to the pathogenesis of obesity related diseases such as cardiovascular disease and type 2 diabetes. While the obesity epidemic has fueled considerable interest in these obesity-related inflammatory diseases, surprisingly little research is currently focused on understanding the functions of inflammatory proteins in healthy, non-obese white adipose tissue (WAT) and their possible role in modulating stress-induced shifts in body fat distribution.

Hypothesis: The current review presents evidence in support the novel hypothesis that stress-evoked interleukin-1 beta (IL-1β) signaling within subcutaneous adipose tissue, when repeatedly induced, contributes toward the development of visceral obesity. It is suggested that because acute stressor exposure differentially increases IL-1β levels within subcutaneous adipose relative to visceral adipose tissue in otherwise healthy, non-obese rats, repeated induction of this response may impair the ability of subcutaneous adipose tissue to uptake energy substrates, synthesize and retain triglycerides, and/or adapt to positive energy balance via hyperplasia. Consequently, circulating energy substrates may be disproportionately shunted to visceral adipose tissue for storage, thus driving the development of visceral obesity.

Conclusions: This review establishes the following key points: 1) body fat distribution outweighs the importance of total body fat when predicting obesity-related disease risk; 2) repeated exposure to stress can drive the development of visceral obesity independent of changes in body weight; 3) because of the heterogeneity of WAT composition and function, an accurate understanding of WAT responses requires sampling multiple WAT depots; 4) acute, non-pathogenic stressor exposure increases WAT IL-1β concentrations in a depot specific manner suggesting an adaptive, metabolic role for this cytokine; however, when repeated, stress-induced IL-1β in non-visceral WAT may result in functional impairments that drive the development of stress-induced visceral obesity.

Background

Advances in our understanding of the etiology of weight gain and the regulation of energy homeostasis have greatly contributed toward the widespread efforts to combat obesity. While it has become increasingly apparent that disproportionate amounts of visceral white adipose tissue (WAT) and a low-grade inflammatory state contribute to the pathogenesis of obesity [1-5] the mechanisms that regulate the distribution of body fat and the functions of inflammatory proteins in healthy, non-obese WAT remain

unclear. Interestingly, stressor exposure and immunity have both been found to impact metabolism and to be linked to the development of visceral obesity [5-13]. Despite this evidence, little attention has been paid to the metabolic effects of cytokines in healthy, non-obese adipose tissue or the potential effects of repeated stress on WAT function. Herein we present new data that inflammatory proteins are elevated by non-pathogenic stress resulting in depot-specific shifts in the local cytokine milieu of non-obese WAT [14] supporting the hypothesis that the immune system may play a role in the regulation of body fat distribution through depot specific immune-metabolic interactions. This review presents evidence that

* Correspondence: fleshner@colorado.edu
Department of Integrative Physiology, University of Colorado at Boulder, 1725 Pleasant Street, Boulder Colorado 80309, USA

repeated exposure to stress contributes to the development of visceral obesity and that stress-induced cytokine production may play an integral role in this maladaptive effect. We begin by arguing that body fat distribution outweighs the importance of total body fat followed by a discussion of stress-induced visceral obesity. We then present data in support of the hypothesis that acute, stress-induced shifts in non-visceral WAT cytokines serve adaptive functions that become maladaptive when repeated. More specifically, we hypothesize that stress-evoked elevations impair the ability of non-visceral WAT to uptake, resynthesize and retain lipids, and/or to expand in the face of positive energy balance and that these cytokine-driven impairments consequently contribute to the development of visceral obesity.

Body fat distribution and obesity-related disease risk

Obesity, or excess WAT, affects more than 33 % of the American population today [15] but is excess body fat really bad for you? Although studies demonstrate that chronic non-communicable diseases such as type 2 diabetes and cardiovascular disease coincide with the rise in obesity not all forms of obesity are associated with metabolic syndrome and chronic-disease development [16-19]. What's more, current epidemiological research suggests that the way in which WAT is distributed throughout the body is a better predictor of obesity-related disease risk than total body fat mass [1-4]. Numerous studies have demonstrated that obesity-related health risk in humans is strongly correlated with an increased ratio of visceral fat mass relative to non-visceral fat mass (i.e. increased anthropometric measures such as waist-circumference and waist-to-hip ratios) suggesting that this is a maladaptive body fat distribution reflective of visceral obesity [20-22]. A worldwide case–control study done by Yusuf et al. (2005), for example, demonstrated that the waist-to-hip circumference ratio - an indirect estimate of visceral obesity - far exceeds Body Mass Index (BMI = body weight (kg)/height (m)^2) in its association with myocardial infarction risk [1]. Evidence also conversely demonstrates that a reduced ratio of visceral fat mass relative to non-visceral fat mass is correlated with reduced disease risk [23,24]. Furthermore, while a disproportionate accumulation of visceral WAT is correlated with chronic low-grade inflammation and pathogenesis, the opposite appears to be true for disproportionate amounts of non-visceral WAT [3,25-27]. Manolopoulos et al. (2010) recently reviewed the protective properties of gluteofemoral fat in humans (i.e. WAT stored in the thighs and hips) suggesting that these non-visceral, subcutaneous fat depots act as a 'metabolic sink' for the daily influx and long term storage of dietary lipids [26]. In other words, to the degree it can effectively uptake circulating energy substrates such as lipids

and glucose, resynthesize and retain triglycerides (the storage form of energy in WAT) and expand in response to positive energy balance, non-visceral WAT - or subcutaneous WAT in humans - is thought to protect against the development of visceral obesity. Collectively these studies corroborate epidemiological evidence further demonstrating that body fat distribution outweighs the importance of total body fat when predicting obesity-related disease risk. What factors, then, lead to the disproportionate accumulation of visceral body fat?

Visceral obesity: the stress hypothesis

As with any long-term physiological response, the development of visceral obesity occurs as a result of complex interactions between genetic and environmental factors [28]. A summary of factors known to affect body fat distribution is presented in Table 1.

Notably, life stress, or the real or imagined experience of an adverse event [44] negatively impacts nearly all of the factors associated with the development of visceral obesity (Table 1). For example, high levels of life stress are linked to poor dietary habits [45], addictive behaviors such as smoking and alcohol consumption [46-48], a low socio-economic status [8], and an increased prevalence of mood disorders such as depression and anxiety [49].

The notion that visceral obesity may be a physiological adaptation to chronic or repeated stress first came to fruition in the early 1980s through the clinical research of Per Björntorp [50,51]. Along with collaborator Roland Rosmond, Björntorp observed that individuals with low economic status who were repeatedly subjected to psychosocial and economic stressors developed both perturbations in hypothalamic-pituitary-adrenal (HPA) axis function and increased visceral adiposity [42,50]. Björntorp and Rosmond accordingly hypothesized that disproportionate gains in visceral fat mass may be due to an increase in HPA axis activity induced by repeated

Table 1 Factors associated with the development of visceral obesity

Factor	Association	Reference
Genetics	Ethnicity, hypothalamic genetic disorders, etc.	[28-32]
Age	↑ Age → ↑ WC (Age > 60 → ↑ WC)	[33,34]
Sex	Male WC > Female WC	[33]
Physical Activity Status	↑ Physical Activity Status → ↓ WC	[35,36]
Dietary Composition	↑ Fat/Fructose content → ↑ WHR	[37-39]
Smoking	↑ Smoking → ↑ WHR	[8,40]
Alcohol Consumption	↑ Alcohol consumption → ↑ WHR	[8,41]
Socio-Economic Status	↓ Socio-Economic Status → ↑ WHR	[8,42]
Stress-related Mood Disorders	↑ Depression/Anxiety → ↑ WHR	[8,43]

Abbreviations: *WC*, waist-circumference; *WHR*, waist-to-hip circumference ratio.

exposure to stressors. Their subsequent work laid the foundation for stress-induced visceral obesity by demonstrating that: (a) the HPA axis is finely tuned to and in connection with an individual's real or perceived environment [9,52]; (b) frequent, repeated activation of the HPA axis often leads to dysregulated HPA activity as evidence by low diurnal variability with elevated and/or sustained glucocorticoid responses to an acute stressor and/or a dampened negative feedback response stress following an injection of dexamethasone (a glucocorticoid agonist) [9,53,54]; and (c) dysregulation of the HPA axis is positively correlated with visceral obesity [9].

Additional support for the stress hypothesis can be found in epidemiological studies demonstrating a correlation between waist-to-hip circumference ratio, low socio-economic status (i.e. low income and/or low education level) [15,55] and job stress [42,56]. Elevated waist-to-hip circumference ratios are also associated with stress-related mood disorders such as anxiety and depression [57]. Potential causative factors in the observed association between stress and visceral obesity include increased glucocorticoid activity in WAT depots [58], excessive vulnerability to the external environment due to the sustained and uncontrollable stress of poverty and/or threatening social pressures [59-61], and - due to their low cost and high palatability - increased consumption of foods that are high in fat and/or glycemic load and of a low nutritional value [45,60,61]. In spite of these correlative observations the pathogenic mechanisms linking stress with a central redistribution of body fat remain unclear. This is likely due to the fact that accurate assessment of visceral fat mass in humans can only be done through scan-based systems such as computed tomography and magnetic resonance imaging. Because they allow for the precise quantification of visceral fat mass through dissection, however, animal models serve as effective tools for investigating stress-induced visceral obesity [62,63].

Animal models of chronic stress include repeated exposure to physical restraint [64], conditioned fear [65], foot or tail-shock [66], novel or loud noises [64], social stress [67,68], or a combination of multiple stressors. In support of the stress hypothesis, animals exposed to chronic social stress often display maladaptive changes in their body fat distribution though this is rarely detected in the face of body weight gain [63,64]. Contrary to the high degree of body weight variability reported in chronically stressed humans [69] animals normally reduce their total body weight in response to repeated stressor exposure because they eat less in combination with the metabolic demands of the stress response [62,63,67]. Although these data superficially contradict the stress hypothesis, upon proper quantification of body fat distribution, chronically stressed animals often demonstrate a maladaptive shift in the distribution of their body fat stores irrespective of changes in body weight [67,70-74]. The development of visceral obesity may therefore not always be detected in animals exposed to repeated stress because a) visceral versus non-visceral fat depots remain unclearly defined; b) body fat distribution is assessed inconsistently or improperly and/or c) the lack of standardization with regard to the palatability of the diet. These inconsistent results highlight the importance of properly assessing and defining body fat distribution - not just total adiposity or individual fat pad weights - when evaluating the effects of stressor exposure on the development of visceral obesity.

Clarifying the assessment of body fat distribution: visceral versus non-visceral WAT

Although it is widely accepted that body composition is defined as the mass of total body fat relative to total body weight, the definition of body fat distribution remains unclear in the literature. Most agree that it is quantified as the ratio of visceral fat mass relative to non-visceral fat mass or total body fat mass [29]; the ambiguities lay within the conflicting opinions about the depots that constitute visceral WAT [58].

Based upon their anatomical location, WAT depots are heterogeneous in their innervation pattern [75-77], composition [78-81] and function [81-83]. The predominant storage locations of WAT in mammals are the subcutaneous depots located between the epidermis and muscle and the intra-abdominal depots found within the peritoneal cavity [29]. For the intra-abdominal depots - which include the omental, mesenteric, gonadal, retroperitoneal and perirenal depots - further distinctions are made in reference to the circulatory system into which they drain [84]. Explicitly, the omental and mesenteric depots drain directly into the portal venous system while the gonadal, retroperitoneal, and perirenal depots drain into the general venous circulation [84,85]. Because of this quintessential distinction the omental and mesenteric depots are considered to be true visceral WAT; the subcutaneous depots and remaining intra-abdominal depots (gonadal, retroperitoneal, perirenal) thus constitute non-visceral WAT [84-86]. When visceral WAT mass is clearly defined as portal draining WAT, body fat distribution emerges as a quantifiable ratio of visceral WAT mass, or the weight of the omental and mesenteric depots, relative to non-visceral WAT mass (total body fat mass - visceral mass). By clearly defining visceral vs. non-visceral WAT, shifts in body fat distribution can now be quantified as changes in the ratio between visceral and non-visceral fat mass. Using this definition, visceral obesity becomes the point at which the ratio of visceral to non-visceral WAT becomes pathogenic, or associated with disease, and the development of visceral obesity the process whereby visceral WAT depots dispro-portionately expand relative to non-visceral WAT.

Despite the emergent importance of accurately asses-sing body fat distribution and understanding the etiology of visceral obesity, the bulk of obesity-related research remains focused on the causes and consequences of ex-cessive body fat mass irrespective of its distribution. For example, it is clear that positive energy balance (energy input > energy expenditure) results in body fat gain and that factors affecting the energy balance equation con-tribute to the development or prevention of obesity [45,87,88]. It is also widely accepted that a state of low-grade systemic inflammation accompanies obesity-related diseases though whether low-grade systemic in-flammation is a cause or consequence of obesity-related diseases remains unclear and highly debated [89]. In spite of the wealth of knowledge regarding the causes and consequences of general obesity, however, very little is currently understood about the mechanisms control-ling the regional storage of excess energy or the func-tions cytokines serve in healthy, non-obese WAT. The subsequent sections of this review therefore present evi-dence in support of the novel hypothesis that the devel-opment of visceral obesity may be due to impairments in subcutaneous/non-visceral adipose function and that repeated stressor exposure may exert these effects through local, depot specific induction of cytokines.

A novel mechanistic hypothesis for the development of visceral obesity

A maladaptive shift in body fat distribution does not re-quire fat mass gain; it can occur in the face of weight sta-bility or even weight loss. In other words, the development of visceral obesity can occur in one of three ways: 1) vis-ceral fat mass expands to a greater relative extent than non-visceral fat mass, 2) non-visceral fat mass atrophies to a greater relative extent than visceral fat mass, or 3) a combination of the above. Changes in body fat distribution are consequently independent of total body fat mass and regulated by distinct mechanisms [50].

Ironically, despite the fact that body fat distribution is affected by both gains and/or losses in visceral and non-visceral adiposity, mechanistic research has focused on the pathways through which stress-induced perturba-tions in steroid hormone production impact visceral fat mass [6-12]. For that reason, little light has been shed upon the potential mechanisms whereby repeated stres-sor exposure impacts non-visceral fat mass and function. Considering non-visceral WAT protects against visceral obesity relative to its effectiveness as a storage depot [26], it is essential to consider the possibility that stress-induced visceral obesity occurs through a combination of maladaptive visceral and non-visceral effects.

Visceral obesity is marked by impaired subcutaneous adipose tissue function

In healthy mammals, non-visceral WAT depots comprise the majority of total body fat. Consequently, impairments in non-visceral WAT function can significantly impact lipid deposition in ectopic or visceral depots. In other words, to properly act as a metabolic 'sink' or buffer against excess energy storage in alternative locations, non-visceral adipose tissue must be able to effectively uptake circulating energy substrates, (re)synthesize, store and re-tain triglyceride molecules, and expand in response to positive energy balance [26]. If any of these buffering func-tions (uptake, synthesis, storage, retention, expansion) be-come impaired, the effectiveness of the tissue to buffer excess energy is subsequently compromised. The potential for deposition in the visceral depots thus increases as en-ergy substrates are shunted to alternative storage locations. In fact, data demonstrate that the capacity of subcutane-ous adipose tissue to uptake energy and grow is inversely associated with visceral obesity [90].

In healthy non-obese humans, Rebuffe-Scrive et al. (1988) demonstrated that both fat cell size and lipopro-tein lipase (LPL) activity (the enzyme which regulates the uptake of lipids from the bloodstream) were higher in femoral, non-visceral adipocytes than in abdominal adi-pocytes [90]. They further established that the difference in LPL activity between the abdominal and femoral depots was lost with the development of visceral obesity, but not with the development of non-visceral, lower body obesity [90]. Explicitly, a maladaptive shift in body fat distribution was marked by an increase in abdominal adipocyte LPL activity and a decrease in LPL activity in subcutaneous, femoral adipocytes [90]. Furthermore, Stanhope et al. (2011) recently demonstrated that a fruc-tose laden diet increased visceral adipose deposition due to a dampened subcutaneous LPL response to fructose based meals [91]. The authors hypothesized these obser-vations were due to the fact that subcutaneous LPL acti-vation is significantly more sensitive to insulin than visceral LPL [92] and fructose produces a dampened in-sulin response relative to glucose [91]. Thus, considering the lipogenic function of LPL, these data strongly suggest that the development of visceral obesity is directly due to a reduction in the ability of subcutaneous adipose tis-sue to uptake circulating lipids as determined by LPL ac-tivity and local adipocyte insulin sensitivity. Healthy, non-obese organisms have visceral adipose tissue that expands predominantly via adipocyte hypertrophy - the mature adipocytes get larger - whereas their non-visceral and/or subcutaneous adipose tissue expands predomin-antly via hyperplasia, or the process whereby new, ma-ture adipocytes are formed [82,93,94]. In contrast, viscerally obese organisms have subcutaneous depots that dis-play dampened hyperplasia potential. A series of studies by

Peinado et al. (2010) and Miranda et al. (2008) demonstrated that in lean individuals, lamin A and lamin C - essential proteins for preadipocyte differentiation - are typically over-expressed in the stroma-vascular cell fraction (i.e. non-adipocyte) of subcutaneous adipose tissue relative to visceral adipose tissue and this over-expression is lost when an individual becomes viscerally obese [95,96]. These data are highlighted because evidence suggests when a mature adipocyte reaches a certain size - as determined by its location - it signals the production of new adipocytes [97]. This process, termed adipogenesis, is tightly regulated by numerous factors and requires the commitment, proliferation and differentiation of resident preadipocytes [98]. If adipogenesis is impaired within subcutaneous adipose tissue its ability to adapt in the face of sustained, positive energy balance diminishes. Collectively these studies link visceral obesity to dysregulated subcutaneous WAT function suggesting this depot may play a pivotal role in the development of visceral obesity (Figure 1). We finish this review with evidence supporting the hypothesis that repeated stress-induced shifts in the cytokine milieu of non-visceral WAT impair subcutaneous function which contributes to the development of visceral obesity.

Stress induced IL-1β: a potential link between stress and the development of visceral obesity

Adipose tissue is comprised of a multitude of cells such as preadipocytes, mature adipocytes, mast cells, endothelial cells, fibroblasts and numerous types of immune cells [80,99]. Recent findings suggest that the cross-talk between resident immune cells and adipocytes modulates adipocyte metabolism, preadipocyte differentiation [100,101] and innate immune function [13]. The link between immunity and adipose metabolism was pioneered in the late 1980s by Besedovsky and colleagues who demonstrated that cytokines such as IL-1β were capable of inducing endocrine and metabolic changes within the body [102]. More recent work demonstrates that both preadipocytes and mature adipocytes express innate immune receptors and respond to endotoxin stimulation with the production of cytokines, chemokines and adipokines [103]. Resident adipose tissue immune cells have also been shown to act as local metabolic regulators through the release of factors that alter adipocyte metabolism and differentiation [100,104,105]. Moreover, changes in the number and proportion of circulating lymphocytes [106,107] coupled with a rise in systemic inflammatory markers (i.e. cytokines and acute phase proteins [66,106,107]) illustrates that the immune system actively responds to acute stressor exposure [108]. Collectively these studies demonstrate that the immune system and adipose metabolism are tightly linked, each contributing to the function of the other and that activation of the stress response serves as a pathway whereby immune-metabolic cross-talk is initiated. What's more, we have recent data demonstrating that inflammatory proteins in WAT are directly affected by stressor exposure in a depot specific manner.

Acute stressor exposure affects WAT cytokine concentrations

Healthy, non-obese rats, exposed to an acute stressor (tail shock) have elevated inflammatory protein concentrations

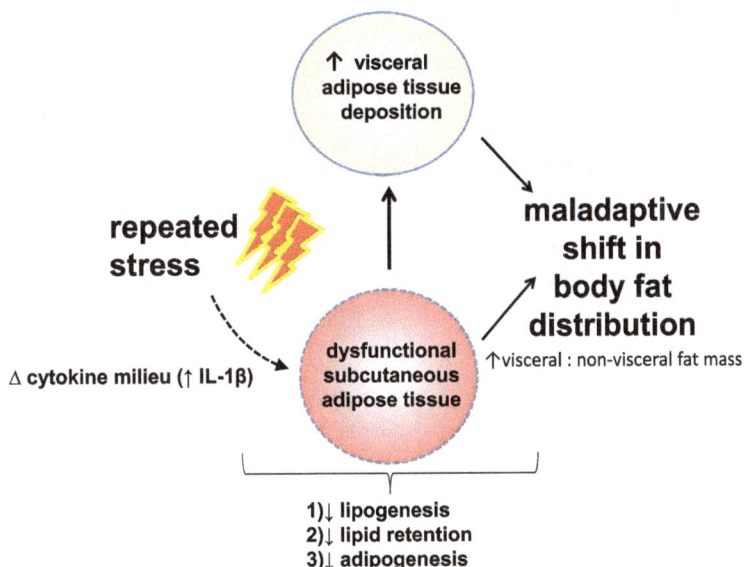

Figure 1 Stress-induced impairments in subcutaneous WAT function contribute to the development of visceral obesity. Exposure to acute stress alters local WAT IL-1β content in a depot specific manner. This depot specific response, when repeated, may lead to a maladaptive shift in the milieu of inflammatory proteins found within subcutaneous adipose tissue such that its ability to properly function becomes impaired. Consequently, circulating lipids are shunted towards to visceral adipose resulting in the development of visceral obesity as marked by a maladaptive shift in body fat distribution or an increase in the ratio of visceral to non-visceral fat mass.

in WAT [14]. Our lab has measured increases in IL- 1β (IL-1β), tumor necrosis factor-alpha (TNF-α), and interleukin-1 receptor antagonist (IL-1RA). Importantly only the IL-1β protein was affected in a depot selective fashion. More explicitly, stressor exposure increased IL-1β 5-fold in subcutaneous but not visceral WAT (Figure 2). We have therefore chosen to focus on IL-1β as a potential link between repeated stress and the development of visceral obesity. Within this framework, the data presented in Figure 2 lead to two important questions: 1) what is the functional significance of a regionally specific increase in subcutaneous IL-1β following acute stressor exposure and 2) how might repeated activation of this response play a role in the development of visceral obesity? Whereas the acute activation of this response likely serves beneficial functions, we hypothesize that repeated induction of this depot specific response may dampen the ability of non-visceral adipose tissue to absorb, retain lipids and/or expand via hyperplasia. Consequently visceral adipose deposition is increased, thus yielding potential mechanisms whereby stress-induced IL-1β signaling may affect body fat distribution. These hypotheses are further discussed in the final sections of this review.

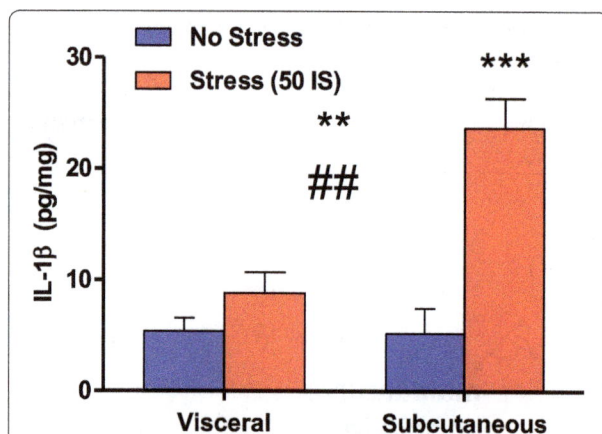

Figure 2 IL-1β response to acute stressor exposure in visceral and subcutaneous WAT. Effect of acute stressor exposure on the IL-1β protein content of visceral (omental) and subcutaneous (inguinal) WAT in healthy, non-obese rats. 21 week old male F344 rats were exposed to 50 inescapable 1.5 mA tail shocks (stress, n = 24) or remained in their home cages (no stress, n = 26). Rats were sacrificed immediately following stressor exposure. Approximately 0.3 g of omental and subcutaneous WAT depots were harvested, spot frozen in liquid nitrogen and processed via homogenization in a RIPA lysis buffer. IL-1β protein analysis (pg IL-1β per mg total WAT protein) was done via ELISA (R&D Systems Minneapolis, MN). Effect of depot on IL-1β concentration F(1,46) = 15.751, **P < 0.001. Effect of stress on IL-1β content: F(1,46) = 28.461, ***P < 0.0001. Depot by stress interaction: F(3,44) = 13.312, ##P < 0.001. Values represent group means + standard error of measurement. All experiment protocols were approved by the Animal Care and Use Committee of the University of Colorado at Boulder.

Potential adaptive functions of the acute IL-1β stress response in non-visceral adipose tissue

Elevations of inflammatory proteins in response to acute stressor exposure is part of the adaptive stress response and likely functions both locally (i.e. within tissues and organs) and systemically [109]. Cytokines such as IL-1β are best known for their role as immune modulators but they also affect local tissue functions such as adipose metabolism [100,110] suggesting that an acute, stress-induced rise in subcutaneous IL-1β content serves multiple functions within WAT. Given that this stress-induced IL-1β response occurs in the absence of a pathogen and in the WAT of healthy, non-obese rats, this cytokine may serve a non-traditional, metabolic function rather than acting as a traditional pro-inflammatory protein.

IL-1β is synthesized as a biologically inactive pro-protein following the activation and translocation of a transcription factor such as nuclear factor-kappa beta (NF-κB) [111,112]. Following activating signals that remain debated, pro-IL-1β is loaded onto a multi-protein platform called an inflammasome where it is cleaved by the IL-1β converting enzyme (caspase-1), converted into the mature form of IL-1β and released from the cell [112-114]. Because the cleavage of pro-IL-1β is thought to be followed by immediate release from its cellular source [115,116] and the ELISA kit (R&D Systems, Minneapolis, MN) used to quantify our preliminary data detects the mature form of the IL-1β protein [117], it is suggested that the measurable increase in WAT IL-1β reflects the release of mature IL-1β into the extracellular milieu of the tissue. In support of this theory, we have data demonstrating that the IL-1β measured in non-visceral WAT is not due to blood found in the tissue. Briefly, compared to non-perfused animals, rats exposed to tail shock and saline perfused (to remove blood from tissues) had equal increases in IL-1β content in their subcutaneous WAT (data not shown). Combined with evidence that the protein does not diffuse passively through the vascular endothelium [106,118] these data strongly suggest that IL-1β serves an autocrine and/or paracrine role within WAT [119]. Furthermore, since the primary functions of WAT are to store energy and act as an endocrine organ, stress-induced IL-1β signaling likely affects the metabolic and/or endocrine functions of WAT; however, because WAT also contains immune cells, mast cells, endothelial cells, preadipocytes and fibroblasts, IL-1β may also modulate a host of other functions. We therefore hypothesize that the stress-induced release of IL-1β within non-visceral WAT may serve metabolic and/or immunological functions that act in concert to fuel the high-energy demands of stress and promote host survival. The following are 4 ways in which stress-induced IL-1β could have these effects in non-visceral WAT.

Potentiates lipolysis in mature adipocytes

Multiple studies demonstrate that IL-1β has stimulating effect on lipolysis, or the liberation of free fatty acids and glycerol from mature adipocytes [120-123]. Stress induced free fatty acid release provides an oxidative fuel source for potentially active muscles and glycerol as a substrate for gluconeogenesis for the maintenance of blood glucose. IL-1β promotes lipolysis indirectly by reducing the production and/or activity of proteins that suppress lipolysis such as the lipid droplet-associated fat specific protein 27 (FSP27) [124] and lipoprotein lipase [120,125,126]. Reports have also shown that IL1β is able to induce changes in leptin secretion [127,128] which potentiates lipolysis through its inhibitory actions on insulin [129].

Potentiates stress-induced leptin release

We have preliminary data that acute stressor exposure induces leptin release both locally and systemically as marked by an increase in WAT and blood leptin concentrations (data not shown). Since leptin secreting adipocytes predominantly exist in the large, non-visceral, subcutaneous depots [130] and acute IL-1β signaling induces leptin secretion [127,128], stress-induced IL-1β in non-visceral WAT depots may potentiate leptin release. Leptin may subsequently act centrally to inhibit food intake, stimulate metabolic rate, and/or peripherally inhibit insulin action in adipocytes [129] - all of which would be appropriate and adaptive responses to an acute stressor. Moreover, leptin-suppressed insulin action in adipocytes would attenuate lipogenesis and/or potentiate lipolysis in non-visceral WAT demonstrating a potential mechanism for the regulation of body fat distribution.

Potentiates glucocorticoid activity

Evidence also suggests that, through its stimulating effect on the 11-beta hydroxysteroid dehydrogenase type 1 (11β-HSD1) enzyme which converts inactive glucocorticoids into their active form, IL-1β may indirectly increase local glucocorticoid activity [131,132]. This could consequentially serve beneficial metabolic and immunological functions in non-visceral WAT. For example, given that subcutaneous adipose tissue has a lower density of glucocorticoid receptors relative to visceral adipose tissue [11,133], subcutaneous-specific increases in glucocorticoid activity would help negate this difference. Metabolically this would be advantageous because glucocorticoids and insulin - both of which are released following acute stressor exposure relative to the severity of the stressor and the palatability of the diet available to the stressed subject [45] - are synergistic; glucocorticoids help insulin to promote lipid uptake and storage [134,135]. Increased depot specific/non-visceral, post-stress lipogenesis could then protect against visceral

obesity by reinstating and maintaining the mass of the non-visceral depots. (Note: Because circulating levels of glucose and free fatty acids are tightly regulated, stress induced energy substrates must be removed from the blood either via utilization or uptake and re-storage. The term 'post-stress lipogenesis', therefore, refers to the process of removing stress-induced substrates from the blood for storage as triglycerides within WAT. Hence, following stress, the WAT depots with the highest lipogenic potential will serve as the primary re-deposition sites for unused substrates.)

Second, the presence of IL-1β in sub-dermal tissues such as subcutaneous WAT may immunologically "prime" the organism to effectively and efficiently combat a sub-dermal infection and/or injury [30,136]. In this case, potentiated glucocorticoid signaling in these depots would serve to boost the anti-inflammatory effects of glucocorticoids thus ensuring efficient regulation of stress-induced immune responses. Briefly, IL-1β acts as a pro-inflammatory protein by activating the transcription factor nuclear factor-kappa beta (NF-kβ) which initiates the synthesis of inflammatory proteins. In the case of a non-pathogenic stressor such as tail shock, a tightly regulated innate immune response would benefit the organism not only by conserving energy - an activated immune system can be metabolically demanding [137] - but by preserving the life and function of innate immune cells such as neutrophils and monocytes.

Promotes lipogenesis in resident macrophage cell membranes

IL-1β signaling may also play a critical role in the regulation of lipogenesis in the lipid bilayer of macrophage cell membranes. Im et al. (2011) demonstrated that macrophages from mice that don't express sterol regulatory element binding protein-1a ((SREBP-1a) a nutrient sensing transcription factor) failed to activate lipogenesis and the release of IL-1β following a lipopolysaccharide challenge suggesting that IL-1β plays a central role in the link between lipid metabolism and the innate immune response [138].

These data also suggest that resident WAT macrophages are a cellular source of stress- induced IL-1β and that the SREBP-1a transcription factor may be involved in the sensing and transducing of the nutrient changes associated with acute stress in the local WAT environment. Moreover, Altintas et al. (2011) recently explored the distribution of mast cells and resident macrophages in subcutaneous and visceral fat of mice and found that resident macrophages were more prevalent than mast cells in lean WAT demonstrating that healthy, non-obese WAT does, in fact, contain resident macrophages [80]. Our lab also has data demonstrating that the highest concentration of basal and stress-induced IL- 1β lay within the stromal-vascular fraction of WAT (Figure 3).

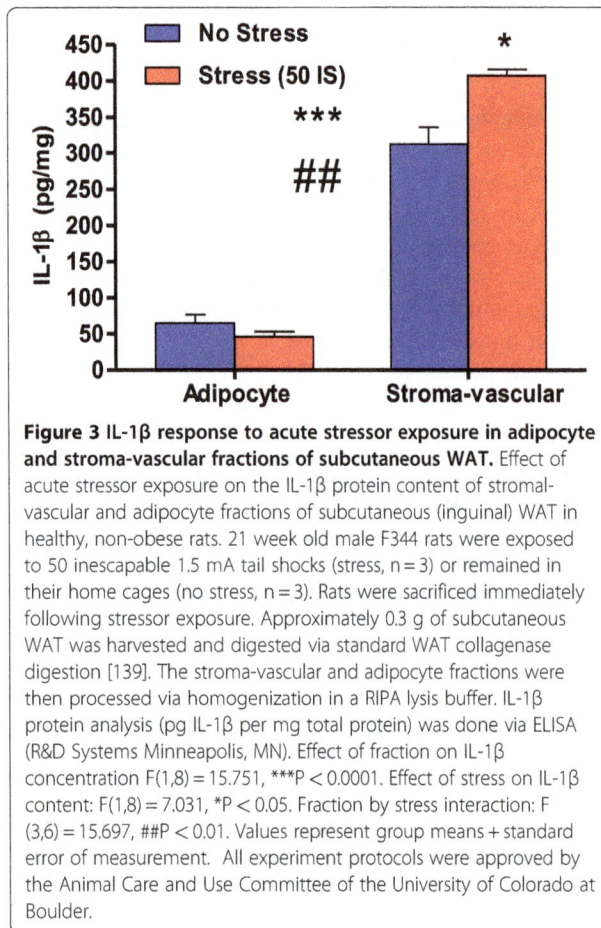

Figure 3 IL-1β response to acute stressor exposure in adipocyte and stroma-vascular fractions of subcutaneous WAT. Effect of acute stressor exposure on the IL-1β protein content of stromal-vascular and adipocyte fractions of subcutaneous (inguinal) WAT in healthy, non-obese rats. 21 week old male F344 rats were exposed to 50 inescapable 1.5 mA tail shocks (stress, n = 3) or remained in their home cages (no stress, n = 3). Rats were sacrificed immediately following stressor exposure. Approximately 0.3 g of subcutaneous WAT was harvested and digested via standard WAT collagenase digestion [139]. The stroma-vascular and adipocyte fractions were then processed via homogenization in a RIPA lysis buffer. IL-1β protein analysis (pg IL-1β per mg total protein) was done via ELISA (R&D Systems Minneapolis, MN). Effect of fraction on IL-1β concentration F(1,8) = 15.751, ***P < 0.0001. Effect of stress on IL-1β content: F(1,8) = 7.031, *P < 0.05. Fraction by stress interaction: F (3,6) = 15.697, ##P < 0.01. Values represent group means + standard error of measurement. All experiment protocols were approved by the Animal Care and Use Committee of the University of Colorado at Boulder.

These data, however, do not reveal that resident macrophages per se are the cellular source of stress-induced IL- 1β. More work is necessary to determine the precise cellular sources of stress-induced IL-1β as other cells found in the stromal-vascular fraction of WAT likely contribute to the stress-induced IL-1β pool.

In summary, following acute stressor exposure, depot specific induction of IL-1β release may serve adaptive functions including potentiated lipolysis, leptin release and glucocorticoid activity. While a short-lived rise in subcutaneous WAT IL-1β is likely beneficial in nature, we propose the opposite holds true when repeatedly induced [105,109]. Hence the final section of this review presents evidence suggesting that repeated exposure to IL-1β in subcutaneous WAT may elicit maladaptive effects that could collectively contribute to the development of visceral obesity.

Potential IL-1β related mechanisms whereby repeated stressor exposure induces a maladaptive shift in body fat distribution

Lipogenesis, or the process of removing energy substrates from the bloodstream and synthesizing them into a triglyceride molecule (i.e. three free fatty acids attached to a glycerol backbone), is the foundation upon which WAT stores and retains energy. The process of cleaving triglyceride molecules and liberating them as free fatty acids for energy utilization is termed lipolysis. The balance between these two processes, or lipolytic flux, determines the mean size of the mature adipocytes within the depot [76].

The protective nature and function of non-visceral adipose tissue is associated with its ability to uptake circulating energy substrate, synthesize and/or retain triglyceride [26] and to expand via hyperplasia during prolonged positive energy balance [139]. Conversely, the pathogenic nature of visceral adipose is related to its ability to expand via hypertrophy and/or hyperplasia. Dysfunction of WAT therefore implies that its lipogenic and/or adipogenic abilities become maladaptive relative to its location. Interestingly, recent data demonstrate that the local milieu of inflammatory proteins modulates lipid uptake and release [100] suggesting that inflammatory proteins such as IL-1β may impact body fat distribution through the sum of their local effects on adipose metabolism. Evidence also demonstrates that viscerally obese subjects have subcutaneous adipose tissue that is marked by decreased expression of lipogenic and adipogenic proteins [26,140-143]. In spite of this evidence, no clear mechanisms have been proposed to date for the means whereby these impairments occur. While it is possible that repeated stressor exposure may drive visceral fat expansion by increasing the capability of visceral WAT to expand via hypertrophy and/or hyperplasia, we pose that repeated stress-induced IL-1β signaling negatively affects subcutaneous adipose tissue by dampening its lipogenic and/or adipogenic function. We offer evidence for the following hypothetical mechanisms, each of which, through their negative affect on subcutaneous WAT function, could contribute to the development of visceral obesity (Figure 4). Notably, repeated stressor exposure also induces variations in glucose-homeostasis [144], however, further discussion on this topic is beyond the scope of this review.

Impaired lipogenesis

The capacity of adipose tissue to absorb circulating lipids is regulated by the local expression and activity of LPL [145]. Because LPL activity is known to vary between adipose depots, it is thought to play a major role in regulating the distribution of fat deposition [29]. As Rebuffe-Scrive et al. (1988) and Stanhope et al. (2011) have described, the development of visceral obesity is marked by a decrease in LPL activity in subcutaneous adipose tissue [90]. Interestingly, separate studies demonstrate not only that IL-1β signaling directly decreases the activity of the LPL enzyme [120,122,146] but that repeated exposure to the protein also reduces insulin sensitivity

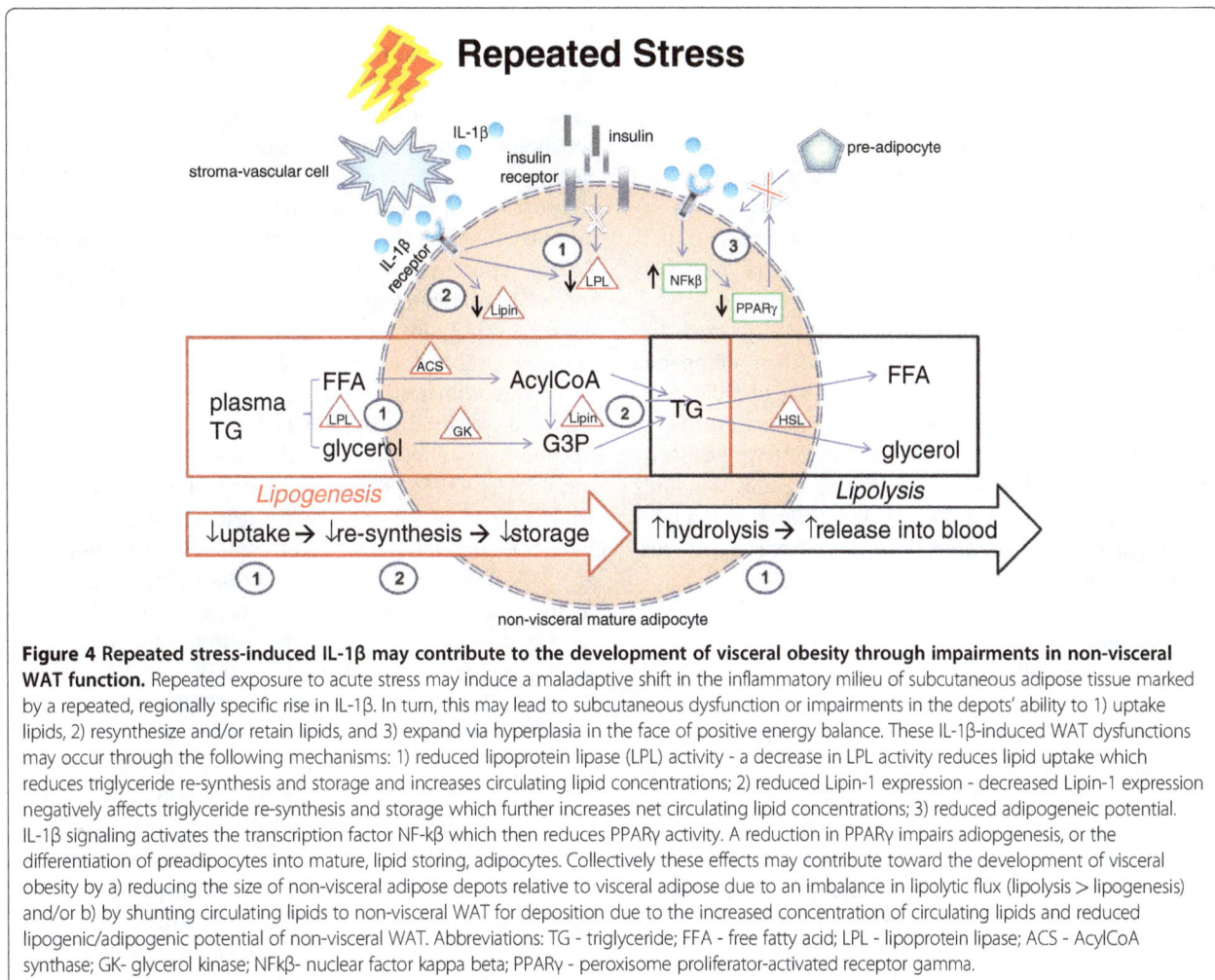

Figure 4 Repeated stress-induced IL-1β may contribute to the development of visceral obesity through impairments in non-visceral WAT function. Repeated exposure to acute stress may induce a maladaptive shift in the inflammatory milieu of subcutaneous adipose tissue marked by a repeated, regionally specific rise in IL-1β. In turn, this may lead to subcutaneous dysfunction or impairments in the depots' ability to 1) uptake lipids, 2) resynthesize and/or retain lipids, and 3) expand via hyperplasia in the face of positive energy balance. These IL-1β-induced WAT dysfunctions may occur through the following mechanisms: 1) reduced lipoprotein lipase (LPL) activity - a decrease in LPL activity reduces lipid uptake which reduces triglyceride re-synthesis and storage and increases circulating lipid concentrations; 2) reduced Lipin-1 expression - decreased Lipin-1 expression negatively affects triglyceride re-synthesis and storage which further increases net circulating lipid concentrations; 3) reduced adipogeneic potential. IL-1β signaling activates the transcription factor NF-kβ which then reduces PPARγ activity. A reduction in PPARγ impairs adiopgenesis, or the differentiation of preadipocytes into mature, lipid storing, adipocytes. Collectively these effects may contribute toward the development of visceral obesity by a) reducing the size of non-visceral adipose depots relative to visceral adipose due to an imbalance in lipolytic flux (lipolysis > lipogenesis) and/or b) by shunting circulating lipids to non-visceral WAT for deposition due to the increased concentration of circulating lipids and reduced lipogenic/adipogenic potential of non-visceral WAT. Abbreviations: TG - triglyceride; FFA - free fatty acid; LPL - lipoprotein lipase; ACS - AcylCoA synthase; GK- glycerol kinase; NFkβ- nuclear factor kappa beta; PPARγ - peroxisome proliferator-activated receptor gamma.

[121,147,148]. These data are important because LPL activity is largely under the control of insulin demonstrating that IL-1β can directly and indirectly affect the activity of LPL [144,149]. IL-1β is also known to induce leptin secretion which further reduces insulin signaling in adipocytes. The decrease in lipoprotein lipase activity found in the subcutaneous adipose of viscerally obese subjects may be therefore be due to impaired insulin signaling induced by repeated IL-1β signaling in chronically stressed, subcutaneous adipose tissue. It is important to state, however, that IL-1β's effects on insulin signaling and leptin secretion appear to be time-dependent; an acute rise in IL-1β has little to no effect on insulin sensitivity and potentiates leptin secretion whereas repeated or sustained exposure to the cytokine impairs insulin signaling and leptin secretion [121,127,146,147,150]. These data highlight the significance of short-term versus repeated or sustained IL-1β signaling and illustrate its potentially maladaptive effect on adipocyte function.

Mature adipocyte as well as lipid droplet size - adipocyte size is directly correlated to the size of its lipid droplets

[151] - have also been shown to modulate local adipose metabolism. Ranjit et al. (2011) recently demonstrated that the lipolytic action of IL-1β is accompanied by a marked decrease in lipid droplet size and the expression of lipid droplet-associated fat specific protein 27 (FSP27 - a lipolytic suppressor) in mouse adipocytes [124]. On the other hand, Boivin et al. (2007) examined adipocytes from omental and subcutaneous WAT of 33 men ranging in BMI from 24.6 to 79.1 kg/m2 and found no differences in basal or isoproterenol induced lipolysis values between the depots across waist circumference tertiles [152]. The authors speculate, however, that this could be partly explained by the fact that differences in adipocyte size are important determinants of regional differences in adipose metabolism and their subject's adipocytes were similar in size both between depots and across waist circumference [152]. Thus, through its potential effect on lipid droplet size, these data substantiate the hypothesis that IL-1β may play a role in the regulation of regionally-specific lipolytic responses to stress.

Evidence also suggests that IL-1β may dampen the ability of an adipocyte to resynthesize triglyceride molecules. Lu et al. (2008) examined the impact of IL-1β on the regulation of Lipin-1 expression and activity - an essential enzyme for triglyceride synthesis - and found that the expression of Lipin-1 was suppressed by IL-1β in cultured 3T3-L1 adipocytes and in mouse adipose tissue [123]. These data therefore suggest that repeated depot specific IL-1β signaling could contribute to a reduction in triglyceride synthesis thus reducing its buffering capacity while promoting the release of free fatty acids into the circulation.

Finally, in the case of sustained IL-1β and glucocorticoid signaling - the consequence of which is dampened insulin signaling - the acute benefit of site-specific post-stress lipogenesis becomes lost. In other words, if repeated stressor exposure reduces the buffering capacity of the non-visceral depots by impairing insulin signaling, LPL activity, and Lipin-1 expression it follows that a consequential increase in visceral and/or ectopic fat deposition would occur.

Impaired lipid retention

While acute mobilization of fatty acids from WAT is adaptive for energy mobilization during acute stress, if lipolysis is not equally opposed by post-stress lipogenesis, dissolution of the depot occurs. Lipid re-synthesis and retention in non-visceral WAT, therefore, is essential for the prevention visceral obesity. The ability of subcutaneous adipose tissue to retain lipids depends on the degree to which it is signaled to undergo lipolysis. As presented earlier, evidence suggests that IL-1β may both directly [83-85] and indirectly promote lipolysis. When unmatched by lipogenesis due to a decrease in LPL activity, insulin signaling, or Lipin-1 activity, atrophy of the subcutaneous depot occurs. These data therefore suggest that stress-induced IL-1β may lead to the development of visceral obesity by impeding the ability of subcutaneous adipose tissue to effectively uptake energy substrate and to re-synthesize and retain triglyceride molecules.

Impaired adipogenesis

Expansion of a WAT depot occurs through hypertrophy of mature adipocytes and/or through hyperplasia. The creation of new, mature adipocytes, or adipogenesis, involves the replication and differentiation of preadipocyte cells into mature, lipid storing adipoctyes and recent data demonstrate that the degree to which mature adipocytes can be formed depends upon the phenotype of the preadipocyte found within the depot [79,153]. Isakson et al. (2009) have further established that the phenotype of resident preadipocytes can be changed based on the composition of the inflammatory proteins found in the depot [142]. Moreover, whereas healthy, non-obese omental WAT contains preadipocytes with a reduced capacity for replication and differentiation [79], the preferred modality for healthy subcutaneous WAT expansion is through adipogenesis [82,94,154]. Because non-visceral depots constitute the bulk of total body fat mass, it therefore follows that a diminutive reduction in the adipogenic potential of subcutaneous WAT would negatively affect body fat distribution [82,93,94,139]. In support of our hypothesis that IL-1β could dampen the adipogenic potential of subcutaneous WAT, Lu et al. (2010) reported that the presence of as little as 5.0 pg/mL of IL-1β (equivalent to basal concentrations in visceral rat WAT) in the culture medium of 3T3-L1 preadipocytes inhibited adipogenesis [155]. Lu et al. (2010) further demonstrated that preadipocyte differentiation was also impaired upstream of IL-1β at the level of NF-κB due to its effect on the adipogenic transcription factor, PPARγ [155]. These data support other studies in which a rise in NF-κB activity leads to a reduction in PPARγ expression/activity and impairments in adipogenesis [156,157]. In this manner stress-induced IL-1β signaling could drive ectopic lipid deposition and visceral fat expansion by reducing the adipogenic potential of subcutaneous WAT. Contrary to this postulation, however, are data from Weise et al. (2008) suggesting that IL-1β stimulates the expression of tissue inhibitor of metalloproteinase (TIMP)-1, a protein thought to promote preadipocyte differentiation [158] and shown to be elevated in the serum of viscerally obese subjects [159]. Though Weise et al. (2008) demonstrated increased TIMP-1 secretion from mature 3T3-L1 adipocyte cells, concentrations of 0.5-20.0 ng/mL of IL-1β were required to induce this response [160] which may be outside of the physiological range for WAT. For example, as shown in Figure 2, stressed subcutaneous WAT concentrations rose to only 0.02 ng/mg total tissue. In addition, Weise et al. (2008) failed to demonstrate that IL-1β induced TIMP-1 synthesis leads to an increase in preadipocyte differentiation [160]. Consequently, the physiological relevance of their in vivo data in this study is unclear.

Finally, because glucocorticoid activation and signaling is known to stimulate early preadipocyte differentiation [161], an IL-1β induced rise in glucocorticoid activity seemingly contradicts the hypothesis that repeated exposure to IL-1β impairs the adiopogenic potential of adipose tissue. Interestingly, however, a transgenic study done by Masuzaki et al. (2001) demonstrated that depot specific increases in 11β-HSD1 activity did not, in fact, stimulate the differentiation of preadipocytes in either subcutaneous or visceral adipose tissue [12]. Instead, gains in adiposity instigated through transgenic overexpression of the enzyme were predominantly due to hypertrophy of the visceral adipocytes [12] suggesting that the effects of this enzyme are site dependent. While the authors speculated that exaggerated visceral fat deposition was due to enhanced glucocorticoid receptor expression, they did not provide a reason for the lack of hyperplasia found in the depots [12]. Although inflammatory proteins were not assessed in this study, our data along with the aforementioned studies [155,156] suggest that a rise in IL-1β activity and/or the activity of its primary transcription factor NF-κB may be involved in modulating the site specific effects of 11β-HSD1 and/or glucocorticoids on preadipocyte differentiation and adipocyte metabolism.

Despite conflicting evidence it is clear that sustained impairment of subcutaneous expansion or an increase in the capacity of visceral preadipocytes to expand or replicate in the face of positive energy balance could have momentous consequences on body fat distribution. As to which of these maladaptive events occurs first and where, though, remains unclear. Current data demonstrate that the inherent differences among the phenotypes of cells found within WAT depots contribute toward the interdepot variations seen in response to intrinsic and extrinsic stimuli such as IL-1β. Future research must therefore aim to understand the unique and adaptive functions of WAT and WAT proteins relative to time and depot location.

Conclusions

In closing, stressors are an unavoidable fact of life for every organism. Our apparent inability to adaptively minimize and cope with stressors, coupled with a highly palatable/contemporary diet, has contributed to the development of a viscerally obese population [162]. While there is substantial evidence to support the idea that chronic stress is associated with disproportionate gains in visceral adiposity, the mechanisms whereby this selective deposition pattern occurs remain unclear. What is more, many of the studies that have investigated the potential effects of chronic stressor exposure on visceral obesity have failed to accurately assess body fat distribution, making an accurate characterization of its effects difficult to decipher.

Recent evidence suggests that local inflammatory proteins modulate adipocyte function and may therefore play a role in the regulation of body fat distribution. We present new data that acute stressor exposure increases the concentration of mature IL-1β within subcutaneous white adipose tissue to a significantly greater extent than in visceral white adipose tissue of healthy, non-obese rats. Acutely, the rise in this inflammatory protein likely serves beneficial functions such as increased lipolysis, increased leptin secretion and potentiated glucocorticoid signaling. However, if IL-1β signaling is sustained through repeated stressor exposure it could contribute to gains in visceral fat mass by reducing the ability of the subcutaneous adipose tissue to uptake, synthesize and retain triglyceride, and/or expand via hyperplasia in the

face of positive energy balance. Further exploration of these novel hypotheses promises to expand our understanding of the adaptive functions of inflammatory proteins in healthy, non-obese adipose tissue and the mechanisms through which subcutaneous adipose tissue function may contribute to the regulation of body fat distribution and the development of visceral obesity. If local cross-talk between the innate and metabolic systems contributes to the development of visceral obesity, understanding the mechanisms whereby this occurs could lead to the development of therapeutic targets for the prevention of visceral obesity, the metabolic syndrome, and its associated diseases.

Competing interests
The authors declare no competing interests.

Acknowledgements
We gratefully acknowledge the support of our funding source, DARPA, ESR. We would also like to thank Dr. Benjamin Greenwood and Dr. Teresa Foley for their assistance in editing this manuscript, Dr. Paul Strong and Tom Maslanik, M.S. for their assistance with experimental procedures and Dr. Bente Pedersen for her informative and encouraging feedback.

Authors' contributions
KJS and MF were responsible for manuscript and figure preparation. KJS collected and analyzed the data. Both authors have read and approved the final version of this manuscript.

References
1. Yusuf S, Hawken S, Ounpuu S, Bautista L, Franzosi MG, Commerford P, Lang CC, Rumboldt Z, Onen CL, Lisheng L, et al: Obesity and the risk of myocardial infarction in 27,000 participants from 52 countries: a case–control study. Lancet 2005, 366:1640–1649.
2. Canoy D, Boekholdt SM, Wareham N, Luben R, Welch A, Bingham S, Buchan I, Day N, Khaw KT: Body fat distribution and risk of coronary heart disease in men and women in the European Prospective Investigation Into Cancer and Nutrition in Norfolk cohort: a population-based prospective study. Circulation 2007, 116:2933–2943.
3. Canoy D, Wareham N, Luben R, Welch A, Bingham S, Day N, Khaw KT: Serum lipid concentration in relation to anthropometric indices of central and peripheral fat distribution in 20,021 British men and women: results from the EPIC-Norfolk population-based cohort study. Atherosclerosis 2006, 189:420–427.
4. Bjorntorp P: Abdominal fat distribution and disease: an overview of epidemiological data. Ann Med 1992, 24:15–18.
5. Gleeson M, Bishop NC, Stensel DJ, Lindley MR, Mastana SS, Nimmo MA: The anti-inflammatory effects of exercise: mechanisms and implications for the prevention and treatment of disease. Nat Rev Immunol 2011, 11:607–615.
6. Bjorntorp P: Hormonal regulation of visceral adipose tissue. Growth Horm IGF Res 1998, 8(Suppl B):15–17.
7. Bjorntorp P: The regulation of adipose tissue distribution in humans. Int J Obes Relat Metab Disord 1996, 20:291–302.
8. Bjorntorp P: Do stress reactions cause abdominal obesity and comorbidities? Obes Rev 2001, 2:73–86.
9. Rosmond R, Dallman MF, Bjorntorp P: Stress-related cortisol secretion in men: relationships with abdominal obesity and endocrine, metabolic and hemodynamic abnormalities. J Clin Endocrinol Metab 1998, 83:1853–1859.
10. Kyrou I, Chrousos GP, Tsigos C: Stress, visceral obesity, and metabolic complications. Ann N Y Acad Sci 2006, 1083:77–110.
11. Rebuffe-Scrive M, Lundholm K, Bjorntorp P: Glucocorticoid hormone binding to human adipose tissue. Eur J Clin Invest 1985, 15:267–271.

12. Masuzaki H, Paterson J, Shinyama H, Morton NM, Mullins JJ, Seckl JR, Flier JS: A transgenic model of visceral obesity and the metabolic syndrome. *Science* 2001, **294:**2166–2170.

13. Mathis D, Shoelson SE: **Immunometabolism: an emerging frontier.** *Nat Rev Immunol* 2011, **11:**81.

14. Speaker KJ SA, Herrera J, Cox S, Strong P, Greenwood B, Fleshner M: Investigation of complex stressor exposure on metabolic and inflammatory proteins in plasma and white adipose tissue. *Brain, Behavior and Immmunity* 2011, 25:S233–S234.

15. Flegal KM, Carroll MD, Ogden CL, Curtin LR: **Prevalence and trends in obesity among US adults, 1999–2008.** *JAMA* 2010, **303:**235–241.

16. Kloting N, Fasshauer M, Dietrich A, Kovacs P, Schon MR, Kern M, Stumvoll M, Bluher M: **Insulin-sensitive obesity.** *Am J Physiol Endocrinol Metab* 2010, **299:**E506–E515.

17. Carey DG, Jenkins AB, Campbell LV, Freund J, Chisholm DJ: **Abdominal fat and insulin resistance in normal and overweight women: Direct measurements reveal a strong relationship in subjects at both low and high risk of NIDDM.** *Diabetes* 1996, **45:**633–638.

18. Karelis AD, St-Pierre DH, Conus F, Rabasa-Lhoret R, Poehlman ET: **Metabolic and body composition factors in subgroups of obesity: what do we know?** *J Clin Endocrinol Metab* 2004, **89:**2569–2575.

19. Ferrannini E, Natali A, Bell P, Cavallo-Perin P, Lalic N, Mingrone G: **Insulin resistance and hypersecretion in obesity. European Group for the Study of Insulin Resistance (EGIR).** *J Clin Invest* 1997, **100:**1166–1173.

20. Bjorntorp P: **Body fat distribution, insulin resistance, and metabolic diseases.** *Nutrition* 1997, **13:**795–803.

21. Fujimoto WY, Bergstrom RW, Boyko EJ, Chen KW, Kahn SE, Leonetti DL, McNeely MJ, Newell LL, Shofer JB, Tsunehara CH, Wahl PW: **Preventing diabetes–applying pathophysiological and epidemiological evidence.** *Br J Nutr* 2000, **84**(Suppl 2):S173–S176.

22. Cnop M, Landchild MJ, Vidal J, Havel PJ, Knowles NG, Carr DR, Wang F, Hull RL, Boyko EJ, Retzlaff BM, et al: **The concurrent accumulation of intraabdominal and subcutaneous fat explains the association between insulin resistance and plasma leptin concentrations: distinct metabolic effects of two fat compartments.** *Diabetes* 2002, **51:**1005–1015.

23. Thorne A, Lonnqvist F, Apelman J, Hellers G, Arner P: **A pilot study of long- term effects of a novel obesity treatment: omentectomy in connection with adjustable gastric banding.** *Int J Obes Relat Metab Disord* 2002, **26:**193–199.

24. Despres JP, Lemieux I: **Abdominal obesity and metabolic syndrome.** *Nature* 2006, **444:**881–887.

25. Kissebah AH, Krakower GR: **Regional adiposity and morbidity.** *Physiol Rev* 1994, **74:**761–811.

26. Manolopoulos KN, Karpe F, Frayn KN: **Gluteofemoral body fat as a determinant of metabolic health.** *Int J Obes (Lond)* 2010, **34:**949–959.

27. Tanko LB, Bagger YZ, Alexandersen P, Larsen PJ, Christiansen C: **Peripheral adiposity exhibits an independent dominant antiatherogenic effect in elderly women.** *Circulation* 2003, **107:**1626–1631.

28. Bjorntorp P: **Thrifty genes and human obesity. Are we chasing ghosts?** *Lancet* 2001, **358:**1006–1008.

29. Abate N, Garg A: **Heterogeneity in adipose tissue metabolism: causes, implications and management of regional adiposity.** *Prog Lipid Res* 1995, **34:**53–70.

30. Klein J, Permana PA, Owecki M, Chaldakov GN, Bohm M, Hausman G, Lapiere CM, Atanassova P, Sowinski J, Fasshauer M, et al: **What are subcutaneous adipocytes really good for?** *Exp Dermatol* 2007, **16:**45–70.

31. Kopelman PG: **Obesity as a medical problem.** *Nature* 2000, **404:**635–643.

32. Stevens J, Katz EG, Huxley RR: **Associations between gender, age and waist circumference.** *Eur J Clin Nutr* 2010, **64:**6–15.

33. Kuk JL, Saunders TJ, Davidson LE, Ross R: **Age-related changes in total and regional fat distribution.** *Ageing Res Rev* 2009, **8:**339–348.

34. Wong SL, Katzmarzyk P, Nichaman MZ, Church TS, Blair SN, Ross R: **Cardiorespiratory fitness is associated with lower abdominal fat independent of body mass index.** *Med Sci Sports Exerc* 2004, **36:**286–291.

35. Ross R, Dagnone D, Jones PJ, Smith H, Paddags A, Hudson R, Janssen I: **Reduction in obesity and related comorbid conditions after diet-induced weight loss or exercise-induced weight loss in men. A randomized, controlled trial.** *Ann Intern Med* 2000, **133:**92–103.

36. George V, Tremblay A, Despres JP, Leblanc C, Bouchard C: **Effect of dietary fat content on total and regional adiposity in men and women.** *Int J Obes* 1990, **14:**1085–1094.

37. Stanhope KL, Havel PJ: **Fructose consumption: considerations for future research on its effects on adipose distribution, lipid metabolism, and insulin sensitivity in humans.** *J Nutr* 2009, **139:**1236S–1241S.

38. Stanhope KL: **Role of Fructose-Containing Sugars in the Epidemics of Obesity and Metabolic Syndrome.** *Annu Rev Med* 2012, **63:**329–343.

39. Chiolero A, Faeh D, Paccaud F, Cornuz J: **Consequences of smoking for body weight, body fat distribution, and insulin resistance.** *Am J Clin Nutr* 2008, **87:**801–809.

40. Larsson B, Svardsudd K, Welin L, Wilhelmsen L, Bjorntorp P, Tibblin G: **Abdominal adipose tissue distribution, obesity, and risk of cardiovascular disease and death: 13 year follow up of participants in the study of men born in 1913.** *Br Med J (Clin Res Ed)* 1984, **288:**1401–1404.

41. Rosmond R: **Aetiology of obesity: a striving after wind?** *Obes Rev* 2004, **5:**177–181.

42. Rosmond R, Bjorntorp P: **Psychosocial and socio-economic factors in women and their relationship to obesity and regional body fat distribution.** *Int J Obes Relat Metab Disord* 1999, **23:**138–145.

43. Pilgaard L, Lund P, Rasmussen JG, Fink T, Zachar V: **Comparative analysis of highly defined proteases for the isolation of adipose tissue-derived stem cells.** *Regen Med* 2008, **3:**705–715.

44. Maier SF, Watkins LR: **Role of the medial prefrontal cortex in coping and resilience.** *Brain Res* 2010, **1355:**52–60.

45. Dallman MF, Pecoraro N, Akana SF, La Fleur SE, Gomez F, Houshyar H, Bell ME, Bhatnagar S, Laugero KD, Manalo S: **Chronic stress and obesity: a new view of "comfort food".** *Proc Natl Acad Sci U S A* 2003, **100:**11696–11701.

46. Gunn RC: **Smoking clinic failures and recent life stress.** *Addict Behav* 1983, **8:**83–87.

47. Cooper ML, Russell M, Skinner JB, Frone MR, Mudar P: **Stress and alcohol use: moderating effects of gender, coping, and alcohol expectancies.** *J Abnorm Psychol* 1992, **101:**139–152.

48. Brady KT, Sonne SC: **The role of stress in alcohol use, alcoholism treatment, and relapse.** *Alcohol Res Health* 1999, **23:**263–271.

49. van Praag HM: **Can stress cause depression?** *World J Biol Psychiatry* 2005, **6** (Suppl 2):5–22.

50. Bjorntorp PA: **Overweight is risking fate.** *Best Practice & Research Clinical Endocrinology & Metabolism* 1999, **13:**47–69.

51. Rosmond R: **Contribution of stress to the development of the metabolic syndrome. In memory of Per Bjorntorp (1931–2003).** *Lakartidningen* 2004, **101:**1371–1375.

52. Smyth J, Ockenfels MC, Porter L, Kirschbaum C, Hellhammer DH, Stone AA: **Stressors and mood measured on a momentary basis are associated with salivary cortisol secretion.** *Psychoneuroendocrinology* 1998, **23:**353–370.

53. Bjorntorp P, Holm G, Rosmond R: **Hypothalamic arousal, insulin resistance and Type 2 diabetes mellitus.** *Diabet Med* 1999, **16:**373–383.

54. Bjorntorp P, Holm G, Rosmond R: **Neuroendocrine disorders cause stress-related disease. "Civilization syndrome" is a growing health problem.** *Lakartidningen* 1999, **96:**893–896.

55. Kuczmarski RJ, Flegal KM, Campbell SM, Johnson CL: **Increasing prevalence of overweight among US adults. The National Health and Nutrition Examination Surveys, 1960 to 1991.** *JAMA* 1994, **272:**205–211.

56. Kalia M: **Assessing the economic impact of stress–the modern day hidden epidemic.** *Metabolism* 2002, **51:**49–53.

57. Wing RR, Marcus MD, Epstein LH, Jawad A: **A "family-based" approach to the treatment of obese type II diabetic patients.** *J Consult Clin Psychol* 1991, **59:**156–162.

58. Wajchenberg BL: **Subcutaneous and visceral adipose tissue: their relation to the metabolic syndrome.** *Endocr Rev* 2000, **21:**697–738.

59. Dickerson SS, Gruenewald TL, Kemeny ME: **When the social self is threatened: shame, physiology, and health.** *J Pers* 2004, **72:**1191–1216.

60. Adam TC, Epel ES: **Stress, eating and the reward system.** *Physiol Behav* 2007, **91:**449–458.

61. Drewnowski A, Specter SE: **Poverty and obesity: the role of energy density and energy costs.** *Am J Clin Nutr* 2004, **79:**6–16.

62. Coccurello R, D'Amato FR, Moles A: **Chronic social stress, hedonism and vulnerability to obesity: lessons from rodents.** *Neurosci Biobehav Rev* 2009, **33:**537–550.

63. Tamashiro KL, Nguyen MM, Sakai RR: **Social stress: from rodents to primates.** *Front Neuroendocrinol* 2005, **26:**27–40.

64. Day HE, Nebel S, Sasse S, Campeau S: **Inhibition of the central extended amygdala by loud noise and restraint stress.** *Eur J Neurosci* 2005, **21:**441–454.

65. Thompson RS, Strong PV, Fleshner M: **Physiological Consequences of Repeated Exposures to Conditioned Fear.** *Behavior Sciences* 2012, **2**(2):57–78.

66. Johnson JD, Campisi J, Sharkey CM, Kennedy SL, Nickerson M, Greenwood BN, Fleshner M: **Catecholamines mediate stress-induced increases in peripheral and central inflammatory cytokines.** *Neuroscience* 2005, **135:**1295–1307.

67. Ricart-Jane D, Cejudo-Martin P, Peinado-Onsurbe J, Lopez-Tejero MD, Llobera M: **Changes in lipoprotein lipase modulate tissue energy supply during stress.** *J Appl Physiol* 2005, **99:**1343–1351.

68. Solomon MB, Jankord R, Flak JN, Herman JP, Solomon MB, Jankord R, Flak JN, Herman JP: **Chronic stress, energy balance and adiposity in female rats.** *Physiol Behav* 2010, **102:**84–90.

69. Epel E, Jimenez S, Brownell K, Stroud L, Stoney C, Niaura R: **Are stress eaters at risk for the metabolic syndrome?** *Ann N Y Acad Sci* 2004, **1032:**208–210.

70. Tamashiro KL, Hegeman MA, Nguyen MM, Melhorn SJ, Ma LY, Woods SC, Sakai RR: **Dynamic body weight and body composition changes in response to subordination stress.** *Physiol Behav* 2007, **91:**440–448.

71. Tamashiro KL, Nguyen MM, Ostrander MM, Gardner SR, Ma LY, Woods SC, Sakai RR: **Social stress and recovery: implications for body weight and body composition.** *Am J Physiol Regul Integr Comp Physiol* 2007, **293:** R1864–R1874.

72. Jayo JM, Shively CA, Kaplan JR, Manuck SB: **Effects of exercise and stress on body fat distribution in male cynomolgus monkeys.** *Int J Obes Relat Metab Disord* 1993, **17:**597–604.

73. Shively CA, Clarkson TB: **Regional obesity and coronary artery atherosclerosis in females: a non-human primate model.** *Acta Med Scand Suppl* 1988, **723:**71–78.

74. Shively CA, Clarkson TB: **Social status and coronary artery atherosclerosis in female monkeys.** *Arterioscler Thromb* 1994, **14:**721–726.

75. Youngstrom TG, Bartness TJ: **Catecholaminergic innervation of white adipose tissue in Siberian hamsters.** *Am J Physiol* 1995, **268:**R744–R751.

76. Rebuffe-Scrive M: **Neuroregulation of adipose tissue: molecular and hormonal mechanisms.** *Int J Obes* 1991, **15**(Suppl 2):83–86.

77. Bartness TJ, Bamshad M: **Innervation of mammalian white adipose tissue: implications for the regulation of total body fat.** *Am J Physiol* 1998, **275:** R1399–R1411.

78. Toyoda M, Matsubara Y, Lin K, Sugimachi K, Furue M: **Characterization and comparison of adipose tissue-derived cells from human subcutaneous and omental adipose tissues.** *Cell Biochem Funct* 2009, **27:**440–447.

79. Tchkonia T, Tchoukalova YD, Giorgadze N, Pirtskhalava T, Karagiannides I, Forse RA, Koo A, Stevenson M, Chinnappan D, Cartwright A, *et al*: **Abundance of two human preadipocyte subtypes with distinct capacities for replication, adipogenesis, and apoptosis varies among fat depots.** *Am J Physiol Endocrinol Metab* 2005, **288:**E267–E277.

80. Altintas MM, Azad A, Nayer B, Contreras G, Zaias J, Faul C, Reiser J, Nayer A: **Mast cells, macrophages, and crown-like structures distinguish subcutaneous from visceral fat in mice.** *J Lipid Res* 2011, **52:**480–488.

81. Tchkonia T, Giorgadze N, Pirtskhalava T, Thomou T, DePonte M, Koo A, Forse RA, Chinnappan D, Martin-Ruiz C, von Zglinicki T, Kirkland JL: **Fat depotspecific characteristics are retained in strains derived from single human preadipocytes.** *Diabetes* 2006, **55:**2571–2578.

82. Joe AW, Yi L, Even Y, Vogl AW, Rossi FM: **Depot-specific differences in adipogenic progenitor abundance and proliferative response to high-fat diet.** *Stem Cells* 2009, **27:**2563–2570.

83. Roca-Rivada A, Alonso J, Al-Massadi O, Castelao C, Peinado JR, Seoane LM, Casanueva FF, Pardo M: **Secretome analysis of rat adipose tissues shows location-specific roles for each depot type.** *J Proteomics* 2011, **74:**1068–1079.

84. Bjorntorp P: **"Portal" adipose tissue as a generator of risk factors for cardiovascular disease and diabetes.** *Arteriosclerosis* 1990, **10:**493–496.

85. Catalano KJ, Stefanovski D, Bergman RN: **Critical role of the mesenteric depot versus other intra-abdominal adipose depots in the development of insulin resistance in young rats.** *Diabetes* 2010, **59:**1416–1423.

86. Frayn KN: **Visceral fat and insulin resistance–causative or correlative?** *Br J Nutr* 2000, **83**(Suppl 1):S71–S77.

87. Khnychenko LK, Sapronov NS: **Role stress on obesity and energy balance.** *Usp Fiziol Nauk* 2010, **41:**64–71.

88. Araujo EP, Torsoni MA, Velloso LA: **Hypothalamic inflammation and obesity.** *Vitam Horm* 2010, **82:**129–143.

89. Balistreri CR, Caruso C, Candore G: **The role of adipose tissue and adipokines in obesity-related inflammatory diseases.** *Mediators Inflamm* 2010, **2010:**802078.

90. Rebuffe-Scrive M, Krotkiewski M, Elfverson J, Bjorntorp P: **Muscle and adipose tissue morphology and metabolism in Cushing's syndrome.** *J Clin Endocrinol Metab* 1988, **67:**1122–1128.

91. Stanhope KL, Griffen SC, Bremer AA, Vink RG, Schaefer EJ, Nakajima K, Schwarz JM, Beysen C, Berglund L, Keim NL, Havel PJ: **Metabolic responses to prolonged consumption of glucose- and fructose-sweetened beverages are not associated with postprandial or 24-h glucose and insulin excursions.** *Am J Clin Nutr* 2011, **94:**112–119.

92. Fried SK, Russell CD, Grauso NL, Brolin RE: **Lipoprotein lipase regulation by insulin and glucocorticoid in subcutaneous and omental adipose tissues of obese women and men.** *J Clin Invest* 1993, **92:**2191–2198.

93. DiGirolamo M, Fine JB, Tagra K, Rossmanith R: **Qualitative regional differences in adipose tissue growth and cellularity in male Wistar rats fed ad libitum.** *Am J Physiol* 1998, **274:**R1460–R1467.

94. Einstein FH, Atzmon G, Yang XM, Ma XH, Rincon M, Rudin E, Muzumdar R, Barzilai N: **Differential responses of visceral and subcutaneous fat depots to nutrients.** *Diabetes* 2005, **54:**672–678.

95. Peinado JR, Jimenez-Gomez Y, Pulido MR, Ortega-Bellido M, Diaz-Lopez C, Padillo FJ, Lopez-Miranda J, Vazquez-Martinez R, Malagon MM: **The stromal-vascular fraction of adipose tissue contributes to major differences between subcutaneous and visceral fat depots.** *Proteomics* 2010, **10:**3356–3366.

96. Miranda M, Chacon MR, Gutierrez C, Vilarrasa N, Gomez JM, Caubet E, Megiam A, Vendrell J: **LMNA mRNA expression is altered in human obesity and type 2 diabetes.** *Obesity (Silver Spring)* 2008, **16:**1742–1748.

97. Faust IM, Johnson PR, Stern JS, Hirsch J: **Diet-induced adipocyte number increase in adult rats: a new model of obesity.** *Am J Physiol* 1978, **235:**E279–E286.

98. Ntambi JM, Young-Cheul K: **Adipocyte differentiation and gene expression.** *J Nutr* 2000, **130:**3122S–3126S.

99. Caspar-Bauguil S, Cousin B, Bour S, Castiella L, Penicaud L, Carpene C: **Adipose tissue lymphocytes: types and roles.** *J Physiol Biochem* 2009, **65:**423–436.

100. Permana PA, Menge C, Reaven PD: **Macrophage-secreted factors induce adipocyte inflammation and insulin resistance.** *Biochem Biophys Res Commun* 2006, **341:**507–514.

101. Suganami T, Nishida J, Ogawa Y: **A paracrine loop between adipocytes and macrophages aggravates inflammatory changes: role of free fatty acids andtumor necrosis factor alpha.** *Arterioscler Thromb Vasc Biol* 2005, **25:**2062–2068.

102. Besedovsky H, del Rey A, Sorkin E, Dinarello CA: **Immunoregulatory feedback between interleukin-1 and glucocorticoid hormones.** *Science* 1986, **233:**652–654.

103. Kopp A, Buechler C, Neumeier M, Weigert J, Aslanidis C, Scholmerich J, Schaffler A: **Innate immunity and adipocyte function: ligand-specific activation of multiple Toll-like receptors modulates cytokine, adipokine, and chemokine secretion in adipocytes.** *Obesity (Silver Spring)* 2009, **17:**648–656.

104. Juge-Aubry CE, Henrichot E, Meier CA: **Adipose tissue: a regulator of inflammation.** *Best Pract Res Clin Endocrinol Metab* 2005, **19:**547–566.

105. Black PH: **The inflammatory consequences of psychologic stress: relationship to insulin resistance, obesity, atherosclerosis and diabetes mellitus, type II.** *Med Hypotheses* 2006, **67:**879–891.

106. Steptoe A, Hamer M, Chida Y: **The effects of acute psychological stress on circulating inflammatory factors in humans: a review and meta-analysis.** *Brain Behav Immun* 2007, **21:**901–912.

107. Segerstrom SC, Miller GE: **Psychological stress and the human immune system: a meta-analytic study of 30 years of inquiry.** *Psychol Bull* 2004, **130:**601–630.

108. Pedersen BK, Hoffman-Goetz L: **Exercise and the immune system: regulation, integration, and adaptation.** *Physiol Rev* 2000, **80:**1055–1081.

109. Moraska A, Campisi J, Nguyen KT, Maier SF, Watkins LR, Fleshner M: **Elevated IL-1beta contributes to antibody suppression produced by stress.** *J Appl Physiol* 2002, **93:**207–215.

110. Coppack SW: **Pro-inflammatory cytokines and adipose tissue.** *Proc Nutr Soc* 2001, **60:**349–356.

111. Rubartelli A, Cozzolino F, Talio M, Sitia R: **A novel secretory pathway for interleukin-1 beta, a protein lacking a signal sequence.** *EMBO J* 1990, **9:**1503–1510.

112. Eder C: **Mechanisms of interleukin-1beta release.** *Immunobiology* 2009, **214:**543–553.

113. Petrilli V, Dostert C, Muruve DA, Tschopp J: **The inflammasome: a danger sensing complex triggering innate immunity.** *Curr Opin Immunol* 2007, **19**:615–622.

114. Pedra JH, Cassel SL, Sutterwala FS: **Sensing pathogens and danger signals by the inflammasome.** *Curr Opin Immunol* 2009, **21**:10–16.

115. Singer II, Scott S, Chin J, Bayne EK, Limjuco G, Weidner J, Miller DK, Chapman K, Kostura MJ: **The interleukin-1 beta-converting enzyme (ICE) is localized on the external cell surface membranes and in the cytoplasmic ground substance of human monocytes by immuno-electron microscopy.** *J Exp Med* 1995, **182**:1447–1459.

116. Watkins LR, Hansen MK, Nguyen KT, Lee JE, Maier SF: **Dynamic regulation of the proinflammatory cytokine, interleukin-1beta: molecular biology for non-molecular biologists.** *Life Sci* 1999, **65**:449–481.

117. Dinarello CA: **ELISA kits based on monoclonal antibodies do not measure total IL-1 beta synthesis.** *J Immunol Methods* 1992, **148**:255–259.

118. Patterson SM, Matthews KA, Allen MT, Owens JF: **Stress-induced hemoconcentration of blood cells and lipids in healthy women during acute psychological stress.** *Health Psychol* 1995, **14**:319–324.

119. Waki H, Tontonoz P: **Endocrine functions of adipose tissue.** *Annu Rev Pathol* 2007, **2**:31–56.

120. Doerrler W, Feingold KR, Grunfeld C: **Cytokines induce catabolic effects in cultured adipocytes by multiple mechanisms.** *Cytokine* 1994, **6**:478–484.

121. Lagathu C, Yvan-Charvet L, Bastard JP, Maachi M, Quignard-Boulange A, Capeau J, Caron M: **Long-term treatment with interleukin-1beta induces insulin resistance in murine and human adipocytes.** *Diabetologia* 2006, **49**:2162–2173.

122. Hardardottir I, Doerrler W, Feingold KR, Grunfeld C: **Cytokines stimulate lipolysis and decrease lipoprotein lipase activity in cultured fat cells by a prostaglandin independent mechanism.** *Biochem Biophys Res Commun* 1992, **186**:237–243.

123. Lu B, Lu Y, Moser AH, Shigenaga JK, Grunfeld C, Feingold KR: **LPS and proinflammatory cytokines decrease lipin-1 in mouse adipose tissue and 3T3–L1 adipocytes.** *Am J Physiol Endocrinol Metab* 2008, **295**:E1502–E1509.

124. Ranjit S, Boutet E, Gandhi P, Prot M, Tamori Y, Chawla A, Greenberg AS, Puri V, Czech MP: **Regulation of fat specific protein 27 by isoproterenol and TNF- alpha to control lipolysis in murine adipocytes.** *J Lipid Res* 2011, **52**:221–236.

125. Price SR, Mizel SB, Pekala PH: **Regulation of lipoprotein lipase synthesis and 3T3-L1 adipocyte metabolism by recombinant interleukin 1.** *Biochim BiophysActa* 1986, **889**:374–381.

126. Feingold KR, Doerrler W, Dinarello CA, Fiers W, Grunfeld C: **Stimulation of lipolysis in cultured fat cells by tumor necrosis factor, interleukin-1, and the interferons is blocked by inhibition of prostaglandin synthesis.** *Endocrinology* 1992, **130**:10–16.

127. Bruun JM, Pedersen SB, Kristensen K, Richelsen B: **Effects of pro-inflammatory cytokines and chemokines on leptin production in human adipose tissue in vitro.** *Mol Cell Endocrinol* 2002, **190**:91–99.

128. Gonzalez RR, Leavis P: **Leptin upregulates beta3-integrin expression and interleukin-1beta, upregulates leptin and leptin receptor expression in human endometrial epithelial cell cultures.** *Endocrine* 2001, **16**:21–28.

129. Muller G, Ertl J, Gerl M, Preibisch G: **Leptin impairs metabolic actions of insulin in isolated rat adipocytes.** *J Biol Chem* 1997, **272**:10585–10593.

130. Trayhurn P, Hoggard N, Mercer JG, Rayner DV: **Leptin: fundamental aspects.** *Int J Obes Relat Metab Disord* 1999, **23**(Suppl 1):22–28.

131. Friedberg M, Zoumakis E, Hiroi N, Bader T, Chrousos GP, Hochberg Z: **Modulation of 11 beta-hydroxysteroid dehydrogenase type 1 in mature human subcutaneous adipocytes by hypothalamic messengers.** *J Clin Endocrinol Metab* 2003, **88**:385–393.

132. Tomlinson JW, Moore J, Cooper MS, Bujalska I, Shahmanesh M, Burt C, Strain A, Hewison M, Stewart PM: **Regulation of expression of 11beta-hydroxysteroid dehydrogenase type 1 in adipose tissue: tissue-specific induction by cytokines.** *Endocrinology* 2001, **142**:1982–1989.

133. Pedersen SB, Jonler M, Richelsen B: **Characterization of regional and gender differences in glucocorticoid receptors and lipoprotein lipase activity in human adipose tissue.** *J Clin Endocrinol Metab* 1994, **78**:1354–1359.

134. Ottosson M, Lonnroth P, Bjorntorp P, Eden S: **Effects of cortisol and growthhormone on lipolysis in human adipose tissue.** *J Clin Endocrinol Metab* 2000, **85**:799–803.

135. Warne JP, Akana SF, Ginsberg AB, Horneman HF, Pecoraro NC, Dallman MF: **Disengaging insulin from corticosterone: roles of each on energy intake and disposition.** *Am J Physiol Regul Integr Comp Physiol* 2009, **296**:R1366–R1375.

136. Fernandez-Real JM, Ricart W: **Insulin resistance and inflammation in an evolutionary perspective: the contribution of cytokine genotype/phenotype to thriftiness.** *Diabetologia* 1999, **42**:1367–1374.

137. Muehlenbein MP, Hirschtick JL, Bonner JZ, Swartz AM: **Toward quantifying the usage costs of human immunity: Altered metabolic rates and hormone levels during acute immune activation in men.** *Am J Hum Biol* 2010, **22**:546–556.

138. Im SS, Yousef L, Blaschitz C, Liu JZ, Edwards RA, Young SG, Raffatellu M, Osborne TF: **Linking lipid metabolism to the innate immune response in macrophages through sterol regulatory element binding protein-1a.** *Cell metabolism* 2011, **13**:540–549.

139. Mathieu P, Lemieux I, Despres JP: **Obesity, inflammation, and cardiovascular risk.** *Clin Pharmacol Ther* 2010, **87**:407–416.

140. Jensen MD: **Role of body fat distribution and the metabolic complications of obesity.** *J Clin Endocrinol Metab* 2008, **93**:S57–S63.

141. Johnson JA, Fried SK, Pi-Sunyer FX, Albu JB: **Impaired insulin action in subcutaneous adipocytes from women with visceral obesity.** *Am J Physiol Endocrinol Metab* 2001, **280**:E4049.

142. Isakson P, Hammarstedt A, Gustafson B, Smith U: **Impaired preadipocyte differentiation in human abdominal obesity: role of Wnt, tumor necrosisfactor-alpha, and inflammation.** *Diabetes* 2009, **58**:1550–1557.

143. Bell ME, Bhargava A, Soriano L, Laugero K, Akana SF, Dallman MF: **Sucrose intake and corticosterone interact with cold to modulate ingestive behaviour, energy balance, autonomic outflow and neuroendocrine responses during chronic stress.** *J Neuroendocrinol* 2002, **14**:330–342.

144. Eckel RH: **Lipoprotein lipase. A multifunctional enzyme relevant to common metabolic diseases.** *N Engl J Med* 1989, **320**:1060–1068.

145. Beutler BA, Cerami A: **Recombinant interleukin 1 suppresses lipoprotein lipase activity in 3 T3-L1 cells.** *J Immunol* 1985, **135**:3969–3971.

146. Hube F, Hauner H: **The role of TNF-alpha in human adipose tissue: prevention of weight gain at the expense of insulin resistance?** *Horm Metab Res* 1999, **31**:626–631.

147. Jager J, Gremeaux T, Cormont M, Le Marchand-Brustel Y, Tanti JF: **Interleukin-1beta-induced insulin resistance in adipocytes through downregulation of insulin receptor substrate-1 expression.** *Endocrinology* 2007, **148**:241–251.

148. Sadur CN, Eckel RH: **Insulin stimulation of adipose tissue lipoprotein lipase. Use of the euglycemic clamp technique.** *J Clin Invest* 1982, **69**:1119–1125.

149. Matsuki T, Horai R, Sudo K, Iwakura Y: **IL-1 plays an important role in lipid metabolism by regulating insulin levels under physiological conditions.** *J Exp Med* 2003, **198**:877–888.

150. Suzuki M, Shinohara Y, Ohsaki Y, Fujimoto T: **Lipid droplets: size matters.** *J Electron Microsc (Tokyo)* 2011, **60**(Suppl 1):S101–S116.

151. Boivin A, Brochu G, Marceau S, Marceau P, Hould FS, Tchernof A: **Regional differences in adipose tissue metabolism in obese men.** *Metabolism* 2007, **56**:533–540.

152. Tchkonia T, Lenburg M, Thomou T, Giorgadze N, Frampton G, Pirtskhalava T, Cartwright A, Cartwright M, Flanagan J, Karagiannides I, et al: **Identification ofdepot-specific human fat cell progenitors through distinct expression profilesand developmental gene patterns.** *Am J Physiol Endocrinol Metab* 2007, **292**:E298–E307.

153. DiGirolamo M, Fine JB, Tagra K, Rossmanith R: **Qualitative regional differences in adipose tissue growth and cellularity in male Wistar rats fed ad libitum.** *Am J Physiol Regul Integr Comp Physiol* 1998, **274**:R1460–R1467.

154. Lu C, Kumar PA, Fan Y, Sperling MA, Menon RK: **A novel effect of growth hormone on macrophage modulates macrophage-dependent adipocyte differentiation.** *Endocrinology* 2010, **151**:2189–2199.

155. Nunn AV, Bell J, Barter P: **The integration of lipid-sensing and anti-inflammatory effects: how the PPARs play a role in metabolic balance.** *Nucl Recept* 2007, **5**:1.

156. Suzawa M, Takada I, Yanagisawa J, Ohtake F, Ogawa S, Yamauchi T, Kadowaki T, Takeuchi Y, Shibuya H, Gotoh Y, et al: **Cytokines suppress adipogenesis and PPAR-gamma function through the TAK1/TAB1/NIK cascade.** *Nat Cell Biol* 2003, **5**:224–230.

157. Alexander CM, Selvarajan S, Mudgett J, Werb Z: **Stromelysin-1 regulates adipogenesis during mammary gland involution.** *J Cell Biol* 2001, **152**:693–703.

158. Kralisch S, Bluher M, Tonjes A, Lossner U, Paschke R, Stumvoll M, Fasshauer M: **Tissue inhibitor of metalloproteinase-1 predicts adiposity in humans.** *Eur J Endocrinol* 2007, **156**:257–261.

7

CaMKII content affects contractile, but not mitochondrial, characteristics in regenerating skeletal muscle

Wouter Eilers[1], Richard T Jaspers[2], Arnold de Haan[1,2], Cline Ferri [3], Paola Valdivieso[3] and Martin Flck [1,3*]

Abstract

Background: The multi-meric calcium/calmodulin-dependent protein kinase II (CaMKII) is the main CaMK in skeletal muscle and its expression increases with endurance training. CaMK family members are implicated in contraction-induced regulation of calcium handling, fast myosin type IIA expression and mitochondrial biogenesis. The objective of this study was to investigate the role of an increased CaMKII content for the expression of the contractile and mitochondrial phenotype *in vivo*. Towards this end we attempted to co-express alpha- and beta-CaMKII isoforms in skeletal muscle and characterised the effect on the contractile and mitochondrial phenotype.

Results: Fast-twitch muscle *m. gastrocnemius* (GM) and slow-twitch muscle *m. soleus* (SOL) of the right leg of 3-month old rats were transfected via electro-transfer of injected expression plasmids for native α/β CaMKII. Effects were identified from the comparison to control-transfected muscles of the contralateral leg and non-transfected muscles. α/β CaMKII content in muscle fibres was 4-5-fold increased 7 days after transfection. The transfection rate was more pronounced in SOL than GM muscle (i.e. 12.6 vs. 3.5%). The overexpressed α/β CaMKII was functional as shown through increased threonine 287 phosphorylation of β-CaMKII after isometric exercise and down-regulated transcripts COXI, COXIV, SDHB after high-intensity exercise *in situ*. α/β CaMKII overexpression under normal cage activity accelerated excitation-contraction coupling and relaxation in SOL muscle in association with increased SERCA2, ANXV and fast myosin type IIA/X content but did not affect mitochondrial protein content. These effects were observed on a background of regenerating muscle fibres.

Conclusion: Elevated CaMKII content promotes a slow-to-fast type fibre shift in regenerating muscle but is not sufficient to stimulate mitochondrial biogenesis in the absence of an endurance stimulus.

Keywords: CaMKII, Skeletal muscle, Plasticity, Excitation, Contraction, Mitochondria

Background

Repeated muscle contractions rely on motoneuron-driven variations in sarcoplasmic calcium though ryanodine receptor-mediated release of calcium from the sarcoplasmic reticulum (SR) and the subsequent re-uptake of calcium via SERCA channels [1]. The observed magnitude of the rise in sarcoplasmic calcium varies between slow and fast muscle types, which suggests it may control the contractile characteristics of muscle fibres [2]. However, this relationship is not fixed and muscle fibre makeup in SR and contractile proteins demonstrates a certain degree of plasticity in response to contractile stimuli [3]. An important feature of repeated muscle work (i.e. endurance training) is the specific increase in mitochondrial content; reflecting a compensatory strategy to meet the energy demand of fibres undergoing frequent rounds of actin and myosin cross-bridge cycling [4]. In the rat, the mitochondrial adaptations of exercised skeletal muscle are associated with a transition of myosin isoform expression towards a slow-twitch phenotype [5,6]. The observed transformation of muscle fibre types is associated with a chronic rise in sarcoplasmic calcium [7-9], which implicates

* Correspondence: mflueck@research.balgrist.ch
[1]Institute for Biomedical Research into Human Movement and Health, Manchester Metropolitan University, John Dalton Building, Oxford Road, M1 5GD Manchester, United Kingdom
[3]Laboratory for Muscle Plasticity, Department of Orthopaedics, University of Zurich, Balgrist University Hospital, Forchstrasse 340, 8008 Zurich, Switzerland
Full list of author information is available at the end of the article

calcium-dependent biochemical pathways in the regulation of muscle plasticity.

The calcium/calmodulin-dependent phosphatase calcineurin and calcium/calmodulin-dependent kinases (CaMK) are important transducers of calcium signals towards gene expression [2,10]. The calcineurin-mediated pathway has been shown to regulate expression of slow fibre type-related myofibrillar proteins [11-13] and affects mitochondrial gene expression although calcineurin does not appear required for exercise-induced mitochondrial biogenesis [14-16]. By contrast, CaMK activation has been implied to regulate mitochondrial biogenesis [9,17,18], type IIA myosin heavy chain (MHCIIA) expression [19,20] and calcium re-uptake into the SR in slow type muscle fibres [21].

However, the current understanding of the physiological role of CaMK holoenzymes in whole muscle is incomplete, as previous studies rely on short-term inhibition studies with pharmacological agents in single muscle fibres [22] or the overexpression of a CaMKIV mutant which is not expressed in skeletal muscle [23] and has lost its calcium-dependent regulation [18]. CaMKII is the main CaMK isoform in skeletal muscle. Importantly, however, the effects of CaMKII on the expression of genes that underlie muscle plasticity have - apart from the study of the glucose transporter GLUT4 [24] - not been addressed.

CaMKII operates as a hetero-meric phospho-transferase which can decode calcium transients through auto-phosphorylation at threonine-287 ([2,25,26]). Threonine-287 phosphorylation of CaMKII is increased after acute exercise in rats and humans [27,28], indicating that CaMKII is part of the signalling pathways integrating the effects of exercise on muscle structure and function (reviewed by [2,29]). These findings emphasize that CaMKII activation is firmly associated with the regulation of the oxidative muscle phenotype with contractile paradigms [2,30]. This is corroborated by the concomitant increase in CaMKII and mitochondrial ATP synthase expression with endurance exercise training [31,32]. However, the question remains to which extent contractile features, as shown by CaMK inhibition in vitro [19,20], depend on CaMKII in vivo, and to which extent down-stream effects of CaMKII-mediated calcium sensing would be differently affected between contractile muscle phenotypes [33,34].

We hypothesized that the content of hetero-multimeric CaMKII controls the mitochondrial and contractile phenotype of skeletal muscle and that this would take place in both slow-twitch *m. soleus* (SOL) and fast-twitch *m. gastrocnemius* (GM). We tested this assumption by assessing the effects of the co-overexpression of native alpha- and beta-CaMKII isoforms, with similar substrate specificity and structure as the skeletal muscle CaMKII isoforms [35,36] on selected protein markers of the contractile and mitochondrial phenotype. Additionally, the corresponding transcript response to high-intensity exercise *in situ* was measured along with functional characteristics of the targeted SOL and GM muscles. Because the muscles under investigation show fibre recruitment during self-initiated locomotion [37] we assumed that the effect of CaMKII overexpression would manifest under normal cage activity without an imposed contraction protocol. Control experiments were carried out to quantify the extent of muscle regeneration being associated with the selected electro-transfer method to produce overexpression from injected expression plasmids [38-40].

Results

CaMKII overexpression and phosphorylation in skeletal muscle

α/β-CaMKII-transfection increased protein levels of α- and β-CaMKII isoforms at 50 and 60 kDa, respectively, compared to control-transfected SOL muscle (Figure 1A). *In vitro* experiments demonstrated Ca^{2+}/CaM-dependent phosphorylation of the introduced β CaMKII (Figure 1C). Overexpression of α/β CaMKII could be detected in 12.6% of fibres in SOL muscle and at a lower level, i.e. 3.5%, in GM muscle (p = 0.002). α- and β-CaMKII content was increased at the level of total protein in SOL muscle (Figure 1D/E). Fibres in SOL and GM muscle which demonstrated elevated CaMKII expression after the transfection of α/β CaMKII plasmid had 5.3 0.8 and 4.0 0.5 fold increased CaMKII levels, respectively. Mean cross sectional area (MCSA) of the transfected muscle fibres was lower than the non-transfected fibres in the α/β CaMKII-transfected SOL muscle (transfected vs. non-transfected muscle fibre: 2675 132 vs. 3706 86 μm2; p = 0.001).

α-and β-CaMKII co-overexpression shifts gene expression towards a fast phenotype with enhanced calcium handling

Factorial analysis of the paired data revealed a main effect (p < 0.05) of the co-overexpression of the native α- and β-CaMKII isoforms on the contractile parameters time-to-peak-twitch force (-16%) and half-relaxation-time (-15%) for the combined data from SOL and GM muscle (Figure 2). In SOL muscle alone, a trend for a shortened half-relaxation-time was identified. Maximum twitch force and maximum tetanic force, and fatigability of tetanic force, did not differ between control- and α/β CaMKII-transfected GM and SOL.

We assessed the effect of α/β CaMKII overexpression on the levels of proteins associated with the acceleration of muscle contraction (i.e. MHCIIA/IIX and IIB) and relaxation (SERCA2, ANXV; [4, 67]). This analysis was limited to SOL, because of the higher transfection efficiency

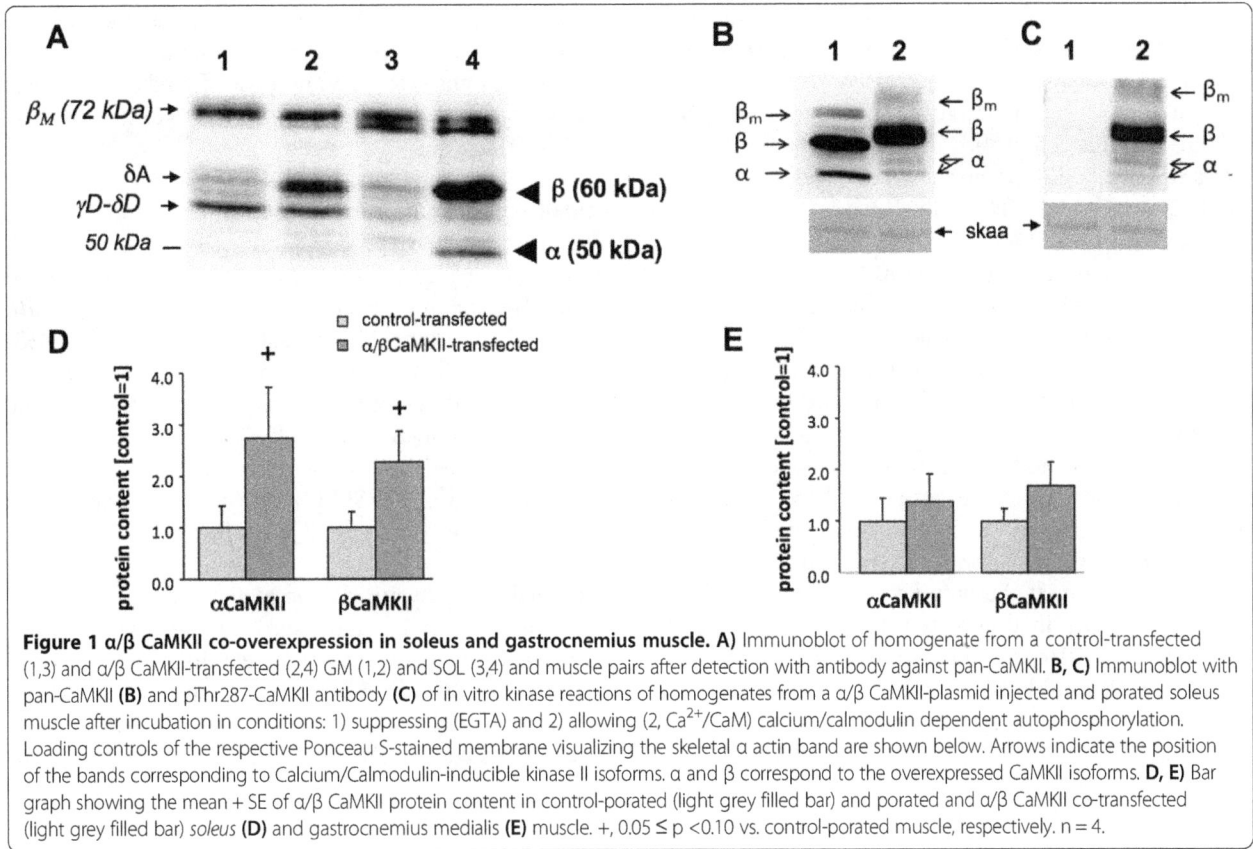

Figure 1 α/β CaMKII co-overexpression in soleus and gastrocnemius muscle. A) Immunoblot of homogenate from a control-transfected (1,3) and α/β CaMKII-transfected (2,4) GM (1,2) and SOL (3,4) and muscle pairs after detection with antibody against pan-CaMKII. **B, C)** Immunoblot with pan-CaMKII **(B)** and pThr287-CaMKII antibody **(C)** of in vitro kinase reactions of homogenates from a α/β CaMKII-plasmid injected and porated soleus muscle after incubation in conditions: 1) suppressing (EGTA) and 2) allowing (2, Ca^{2+}/CaM) calcium/calmodulin dependent autophosphorylation. Loading controls of the respective Ponceau S-stained membrane visualizing the skeletal α actin band are shown below. Arrows indicate the position of the bands corresponding to Calcium/Calmodulin-inducible kinase II isoforms. α and β correspond to the overexpressed CaMKII isoforms. **D, E)** Bar graph showing the mean + SE of α/β CaMKII protein content in control-porated (light grey filled bar) and porated and α/β CaMKII co-transfected (light grey filled bar) *soleus* **(D)** and gastrocnemius medialis **(E)** muscle. +, $0.05 \leq p < 0.10$ vs. control-porated muscle, respectively. n = 4.

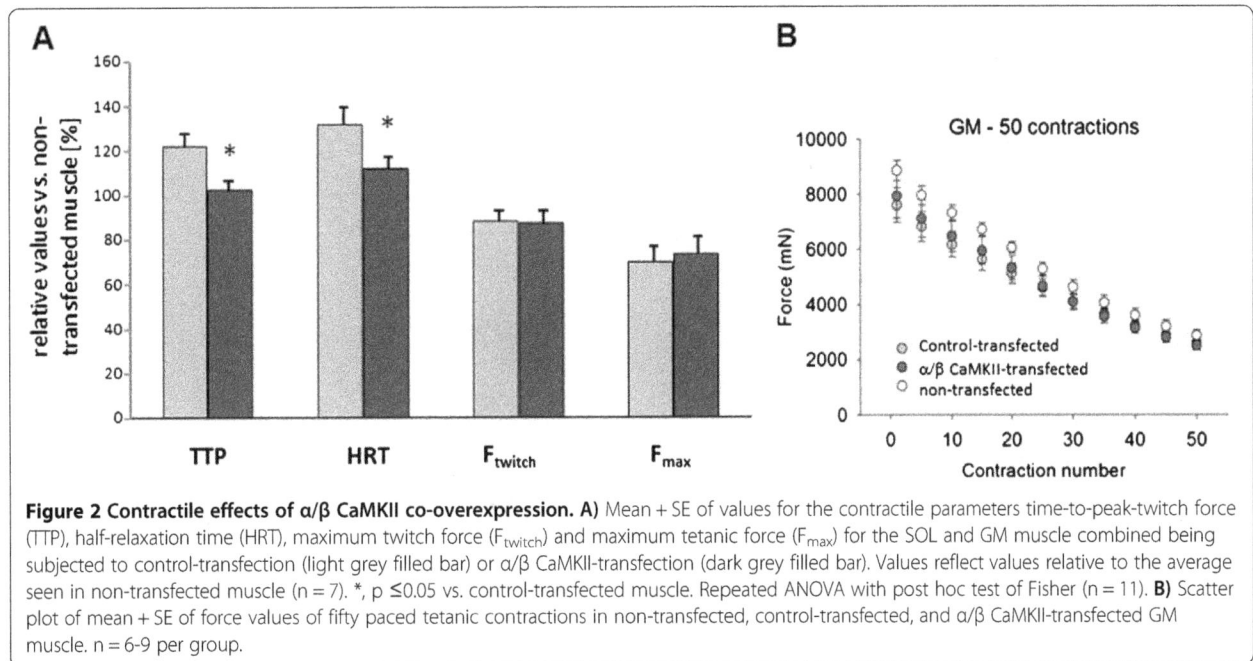

Figure 2 Contractile effects of α/β CaMKII co-overexpression. A) Mean + SE of values for the contractile parameters time-to-peak-twitch force (TTP), half-relaxation time (HRT), maximum twitch force (F_{twitch}) and maximum tetanic force (F_{max}) for the SOL and GM muscle combined being subjected to control-transfection (light grey filled bar) or α/β CaMKII-transfection (dark grey filled bar). Values reflect values relative to the average seen in non-transfected muscle (n = 7). *, p $\leq$0.05 vs. control-transfected muscle. Repeated ANOVA with post hoc test of Fisher (n = 11). **B)** Scatter plot of mean + SE of force values of fifty paced tetanic contractions in non-transfected, control-transfected, and α/β CaMKII-transfected GM muscle. n = 6-9 per group.

achieved in this muscle. We found that the expression of all three proteins, myosin heavy chain isoforms IIA/IIX, SERCA2 and ANXV, was increased in SOL muscle compared to contra-lateral control-transfected SOL muscle (Figures 3 and 4).

Examples of the immunofluorescence detection of CaMKII, MHCI and MHCII are shown in Figure 4A-C. A larger fraction of CaMKII-transfected fibres expressed MHCII than non-transfected fibres (0.36 vs. 0.18; p = 0.0008, Chi2-Test). Quantification of the co-staining of CaMKII and SERCA2 (Figure 4D/E) revealed a significantly higher staining intensity of SERCA2 in CaMKII-overexpressing SOL fibres compared to that in non-transfected fibres of the same muscle (Figure 4F).

Protein levels for constituents of the oxidative phosphorylation chain were not affected by α/β CaMKII overexpression (Figure 5A). We assessed whether overexpression of α/β CaMKII was sufficient to increase COXIV protein expression at the fibre level (Figure 5C). COXIV staining intensity in transfected muscles did not differ between CaMKII-overexpressing and non-transfected fibres in SOL muscle (Figure 5D).

Immunofluorescent signals in muscle fibres were also quantified in GM muscle. In this muscle, COXIV signal intensities did not differ as a function of α/β CaMKII overexpression (Figure 5D), but a larger fraction of CaMKII-transfected than non-transfected muscle fibres demonstrated MHCII staining (0.77 vs. 0.12, p = 0.048; Chi2-Test).

CaMKII signalling after paced contractions in situ

We investigated whether α/β CaMKII-transfected SOL muscle retains responsiveness for contraction-induced CaMKII signalling. Paced isometric exercise *in situ* increased threonine-287 phosphorylation of β CaMKII (Figure 6A). Concomitantly, muscle fibres with elevated CaMKII content demonstrated increased signal for pThr287-CaMKII (Figure 6B-E). RT-PCR experiments demonstrated reduced transcript levels of mitochondrial factors (COXI, COXIV, SDHB) and SERCA2A immediately after high-intensity exercise (Figure 5B).

Transfection affects muscle contractility

Compared to non-transfected muscle, twitch force (-12%) and maximal tetanic force (-30%) were reduced and time-to-peak-twitch force (+22%) and half-relaxation-time (+32%) were prolonged in control-transfected muscle (Table 1). When values were assessed separately for the

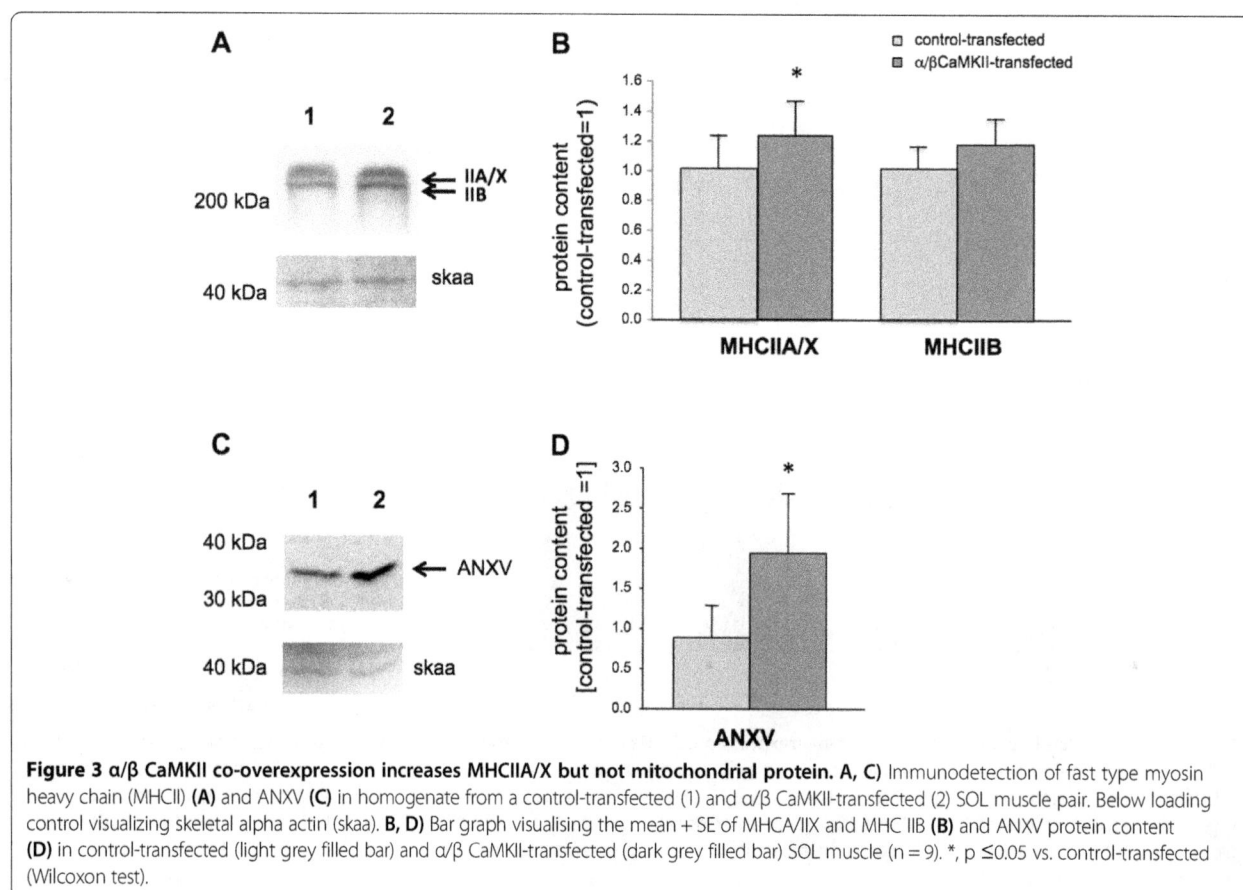

Figure 3 α/β CaMKII co-overexpression increases MHCIIA/X but not mitochondrial protein. A, C) Immunodetection of fast type myosin heavy chain (MHCII) **(A)** and ANXV **(C)** in homogenate from a control-transfected (1) and α/β CaMKII-transfected (2) SOL muscle pair. Below loading control visualizing skeletal alpha actin (skaa). **B, D)** Bar graph visualising the mean + SE of MHCA/IIX and MHC IIB **(B)** and ANXV protein content **(D)** in control-transfected (light grey filled bar) and α/β CaMKII-transfected (dark grey filled bar) SOL muscle (n = 9). *, p $\leq$0.05 vs. control-transfected (Wilcoxon test).

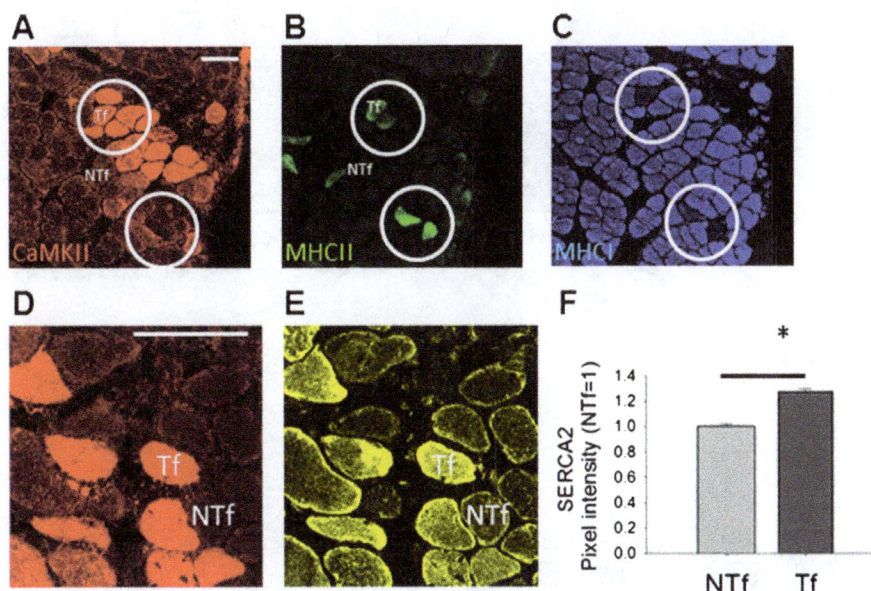

Figure 4 α/β CaMKII co-overexpression in relation to MHC and SERCA2 expression. A-C) Microscopic field of α/β CaMKII-transfected SOL muscle stained for CaMKII **(A, red)**, fast MyHCII **(B, green)** and slow MHCI **(C, blue)**. Corresponding areas are circled. **D, E)** Microscopic field of an α/β CaMKII-transfected SOL muscle after staining for CaMKII **(red, D)** and SERCA2 **(yellow, E). F)** Bar graph visualizing the mean + SE of SERCA2 levels in transfected (Tf, n = 276) and non-transfected (NTf, n = 221) muscle fibers. *, p ≤0.001.

two muscles, twitch force and maximum tetanic force were reduced in SOL muscle with control-transfection. Concomitantly, markers of damage (caveolin 3 mRNA) and regeneration (myogenin protein, fibres with internal nuclei) were elevated in SOL muscle 7 days after transfection (Figure 7).

Discussion

This is the first study that investigates whether increased CaMKII protein expression affects the skeletal muscle phenotype *in vivo*. Transcript measures indicate that α/β CaMKII signalling down-regulates mitochondrial gene expression after high-intensity exercise (Figure 5B). In contrast to our hypothesis, we did not observe altered expression of mitochondrial protein(s) in α/β CaMKII-transfected muscle fibres of rats housed under normal cage activity (Figure 5A/D). By contrast, twitch contraction and relaxation times were reduced in α/β CaMKII-transfected muscles (Figure 2) when major proteins of muscle contraction and relaxation, i.e. MHC IIA/IIX and SERCA2, were increased (Figures 3A/B and 4). Regarding contractile features and MHCII expression in transfected muscle (fibres) the effects of α/β CaMKII overexpression were comparable in the slow-twitch and fast-twitch muscle under investigation. Our results suggest that, in the context of muscle transfection, α/β CaMKII content regulates the expression of proteins involved in muscle contraction and relaxation, but not of proteins involved in mitochondrial biogenesis.

Technical considerations

In order to assess the effect of an increase in CaMKII holoenzymes, we deployed gene electro-transfer with expression constructs for native α- and β-CaMKII isoforms with similar substrate specificity and structure as the skeletal muscle CaMKII isoforms [35,36]. CaMKII overexpression was confined to muscle fibres (Figures 4A, 5C and 6B/D), in which CaMKII content was increased 4.0-5.3 fold compared to CaMKII content in non-transfected fibres. The latter possibly reflects the abundant β M isoform (Figure 1A; [36,41]). Immunodetection of the validated protein band for threonine 287-phosphorylated CaMKII (Figure 1C) demonstrated that the introduced β CaMKII retained responsiveness for contraction-induced CaMKII signalling (Figure 6A). The findings imply that the increased content of native CaMKII resulted in potentially higher CaMKII activity which is amenable to physiological regulation during muscle recruitment *in vivo*. It has been estimated that motor units in SOL muscles of caged, but freely moving rats are active for 25-30% during a 24-hour period [34]. Furthermore, rat SOL is recruited during postural and slow running activity [37]. Therefore, we expected transfected fibres in this muscle to be frequently recruited. We acknowledge, however, that muscle regeneration is inherent to the selected mode of transfection (Figure 7). This is of relevance for our finding that mitochondrial protein levels in α/β CaMKII-transfected SOL muscles were unaffected because muscle regeneration decreases mitochondrial enzyme expression and activity [42,43].

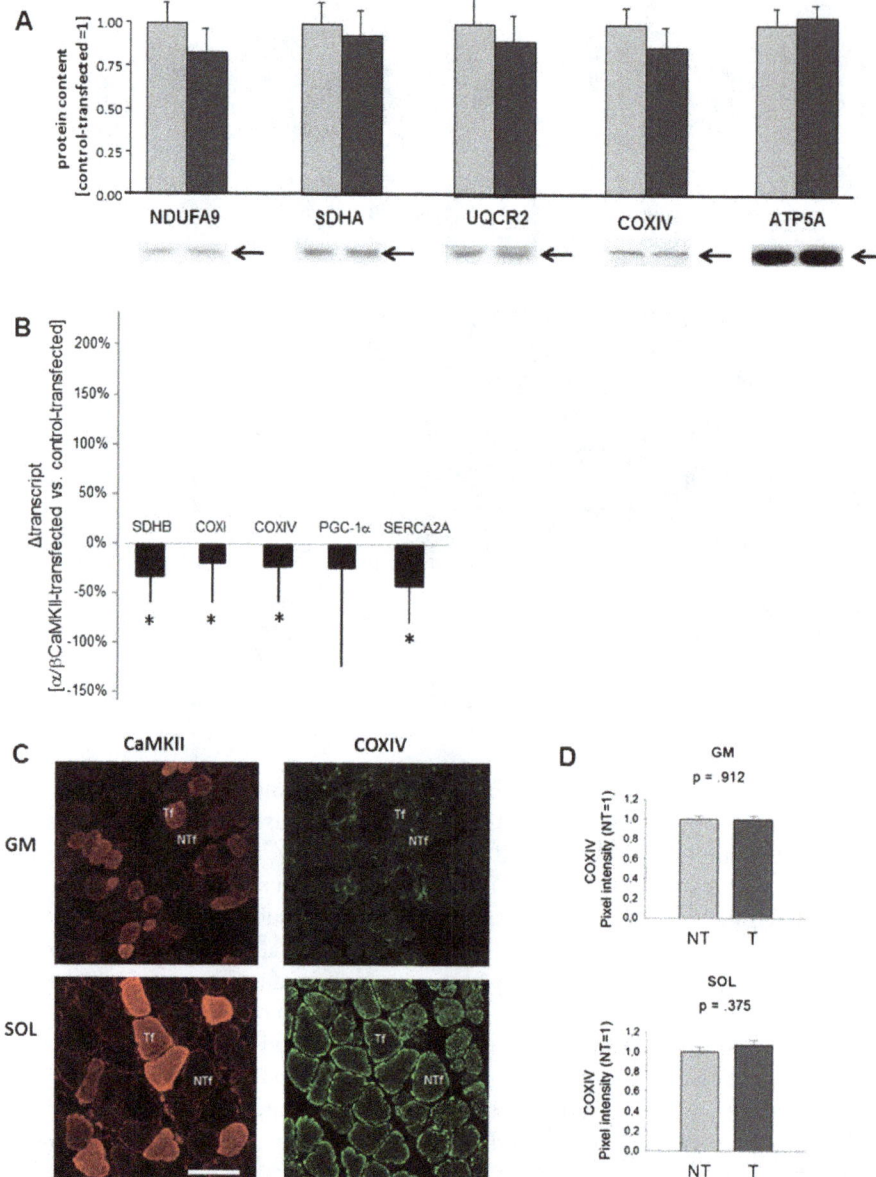

Figure 5 Effect of α/β CaMKII co-overexpression on mitochondrial gene expression. A) Bar graph visualising the mean + SE of assessed mitochondrial proteins in control-transfected (light grey filled bar) and α/β CaMKII-transfected (dark grey filled bar) SOL muscle (n = 6). Representative examples of detected mitochondrial protein are shown below. *, p ≤0.05 vs. control-transfected (Wilcoxon Test). **B)** Bar graph of mean + SE of the differences in expression of selected gene transcripts between α/β CaMKII-transfected and control-transfected SOL muscle (n = 6). * denotes p ≤0.05 vs. control-transfected muscle (T-test). **C)** Microscopic images visualising the association of the mitochondrial marker, COXIV, with transfected (Tf) and non-transfected (NTf) fibres in α/β CaMKII-transfected GM and SOL muscle. **D)** Bar graph showing the mean + SE of COXIV levels in transfected (n = 54 for GM and n = 38 for SOL) and non-transfected (n = 51 for GM and n = 35 for SOL) muscle fibres. The corresponding p-values are indicated.

The identified reduction in time-to-peak-twitch force and half-relaxation time in α/β CaMKII-transfected muscles (Figure 2) support a role of CaMKII content in the regulation of excitation-contraction coupling in skeletal muscle. The comparison to non-transfected muscle reveals that this contractile effect occurred on the background of reduced contractility with transfection-induced muscle damage and regeneration (Table 1; Figure 7). Considering the broad influence of muscle damage on myogenic processes and the expression of factors involved in excitation-contraction coupling [44,45]; a number of factors are likely involved in correcting the detriment in contractility by the overexpression of α/β CaMKII. This potentially includes the calcium channels, SERCA2 and RyR, which control excitation-contraction coupling via calcium release and re-uptake in the sarcoplasmic

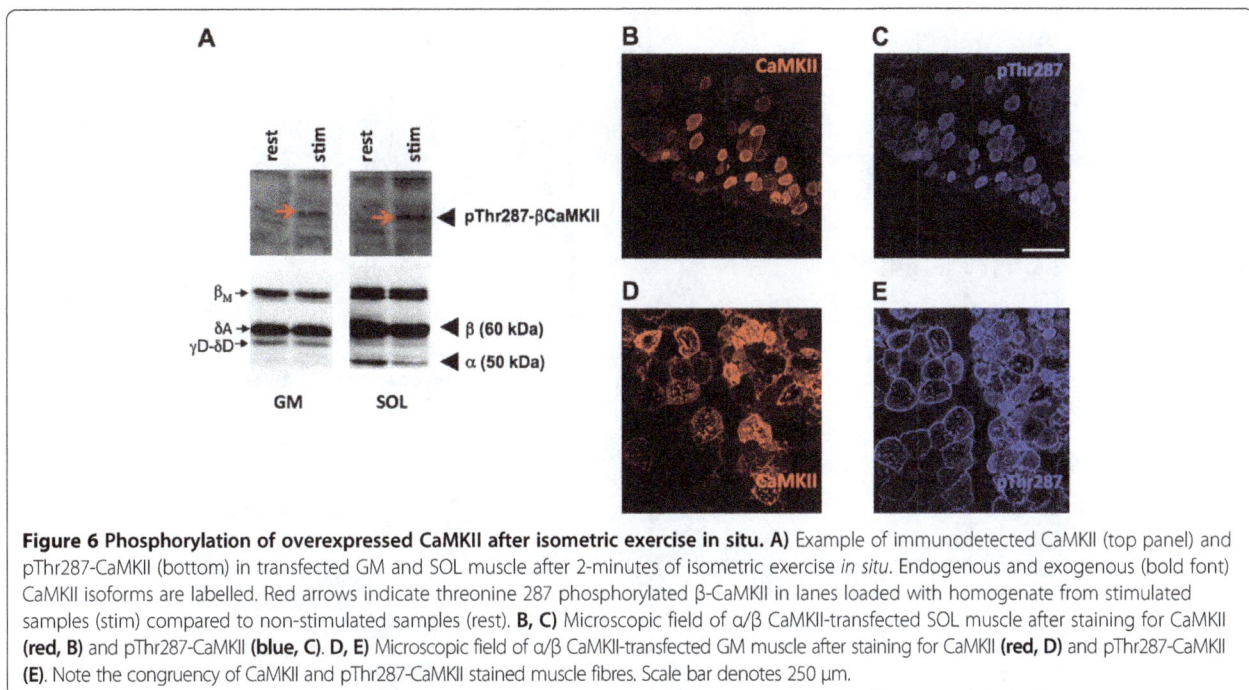

Figure 6 Phosphorylation of overexpressed CaMKII after isometric exercise in situ. A) Example of immunodetected CaMKII (top panel) and pThr287-CaMKII (bottom) in transfected GM and SOL muscle after 2-minutes of isometric exercise *in situ*. Endogenous and exogenous (bold font) CaMKII isoforms are labelled. Red arrows indicate threonine 287 phosphorylated β-CaMKII in lanes loaded with homogenate from stimulated samples (stim) compared to non-stimulated samples (rest). **B, C)** Microscopic field of α/β CaMKII-transfected SOL muscle after staining for CaMKII **(red, B)** and pThr287-CaMKII **(blue, C). D, E)** Microscopic field of α/β CaMKII-transfected GM muscle after staining for CaMKII **(red, D)** and pThr287-CaMKII **(E)**. Note the congruency of CaMKII and pThr287-CaMKII stained muscle fibres. Scale bar denotes 250 μm.

reticulum. *In vitro* and in isolated muscle fibres both channels are regulated by CaMKII-dependent phosphorylation ([22,46], Hawkins et al., [47,48]). The characterisation of CaMKII-mediated phosphorylation was not the focus of this investigation. At present it is therefore unclear if CaMKII-dependent phosphorylation of SERCA and RyR played a role in decreasing twitch contraction and relaxation times in our experiments. Rather we identify that correction of the detriment in time-to-peak contraction and half-relaxation time by α/β CaMKII overexpression was associated with altered expression of SERCA2 and selected factors involved in excitation-contraction coupling (i.e. MHCIIA/X, ANXV). The increased SERCA2 protein levels in SOL were localised to muscle fibres that overexpress α/β CaMKII (Figure 4D-E). The localisation of SERCA2 and ANXV to the sarcoplasmic reticulum [49,50] suggests that the decrease in half-relaxation time with α/β CaMKII overexpression

involves adjustments within the sarcoplasmic reticulum of transfected muscle fibres.

By contrast we observed no effect of α/β CaMKII-transfection on maximal force production (Figure 2). Regeneration has been shown to decrease specific force and increase the ratio of twitch force to tetanic force [44]. This detriment has been shown to last up to seven days after injury [43]. Therefore, it may be that any increase in maximal force was masked by negative effects of transfection on characteristics that limit force production with contraction.

Transfection of SOL muscle is associated with the expression of myosin heavy chain IIA (MHCIIA) in type I muscle fibres [39]. In this regard it is of interest that α/β CaMKII overexpression in slow-twitch SOL muscle further increased MHCIIA/X levels compared to control-transfected muscle (Figure 3A) and that the CaMKII-transfected muscle fibres demonstrated

Table 1 Effect of α/βCaMKII-transfection vs. controls on contractile parameters

	SOL			GM		
	Non-transfected	*Control-transfected*	*α/βCaMKII-transfected*	*Non-transfected*	*Control-transfected*	*α/βCaMKII-transfected*
F_{twitch} (mN)	2169.3	178 15 [a]	174 20	2548 86	2377 175 [a]	2380 178
F_{max} (mN)	108357	555 57 [a]	568 80	8864 395	7594 638 [a]	8078 723
Fatigue (%)	10.5 3.6	18.8 5.3	22.7 5.4	67.5 2.1	65.3 2.9	67.6 2.2
TTP (ms)	105 14	133 7.9 [a]	108 7.3 [b]	43.0 3.3	50.9 4.0 [a]	44.2 2.4 [b]
HRT (ms)	121 18	168 4.6 [a]	142 6.9 [b]	42.9 5.9	54.0 6.0 [a]	46.2 3.9 [b]

Data are shown as mean ? SE. For abbreviations see Figure 2. Fatigue: % decrease in force after the 50 maximal tetanic contractions of the high-intensity exercise, relative to first contraction; [a]: Main effect of electro-transfer procedure (p<0.05); [b]: Main effect of α/βCaMKII overexpression (p<0.05).

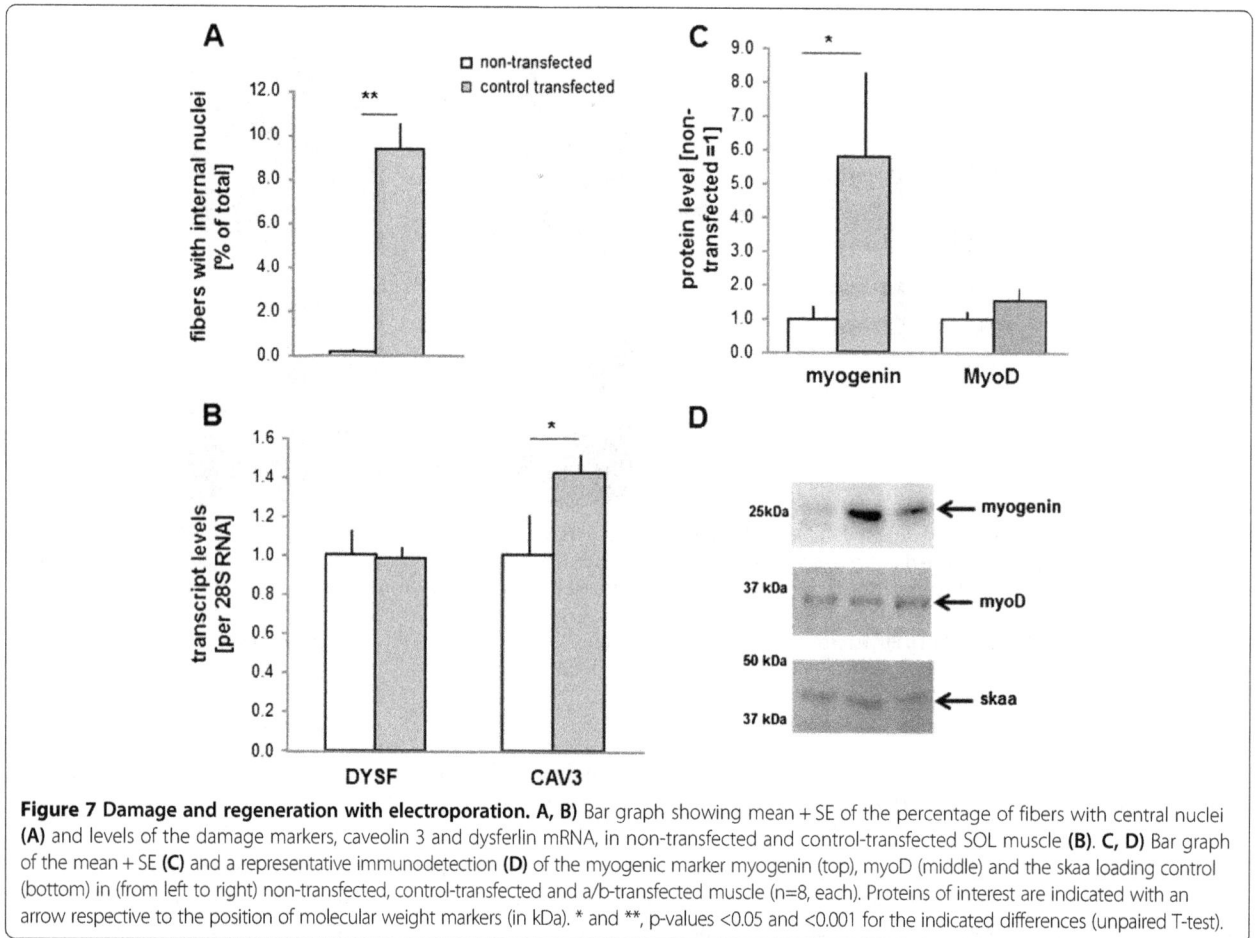

Figure 7 Damage and regeneration with electroporation. A, B) Bar graph showing mean + SE of the percentage of fibers with central nuclei **(A)** and levels of the damage markers, caveolin 3 and dysferlin mRNA, in non-transfected and control-transfected SOL muscle **(B)**. **C, D)** Bar graph of the mean + SE **(C)** and a representative immunodetection **(D)** of the myogenic marker myogenin (top), myoD (middle) and the skaa loading control (bottom) in (from left to right) non-transfected, control-transfected and a/b-transfected muscle (n=8, each). Proteins of interest are indicated with an arrow respective to the position of molecular weight markers (in kDa). * and **, p-values <0.05 and <0.001 for the indicated differences (unpaired T-test).

an increased fraction of MHCII expression in SOL (0.36 vs. 0.18) and GM muscle (0.77 vs. 0.12). The identified increase in SERCA2 and ANXV content with α/β CaMKII-overexpression compare to the demonstrated influence of overexpressed native CaMKII on gene expression being associated with excitation-contraction coupling and hypertrophy in cardiac myocytes [51,52]. Our findings are also in accordance with the results of Allen & Leinwand [19], who demonstrated that the calcium-ionophore A23187 increased MHCIIA promoter activity in C2C12 cells, which was attenuated by the CaMK inhibitor KN62. This raises the hypothesis that an increase in sarcoplasmic calcium levels in injured muscle fibres enhances expression of the fast fibre type program, through a CaMKII-dependent mechanism.

In contrast to our expectations, we observed no increase in mitochondrial protein (Figure 5A) and fatigue resistance (Figure 2B) in α/β CaMKII-overexpressing muscles compared to control-transfected muscles. To the best of our knowledge, this is the first study investigating whether increased content of native CaMKII increases the expression of a mitochondrial protein in any tissue type. Constitutively active CaMKIV increases mitochondrial

biogenesis when overexpressed from an embryonic stage onward [18], but this CaMK is not endogenously expressed in skeletal muscle [23,32] and CaMKIV knock-out mice do not display altered muscle adaptation in response to training [23]. Whether CaMKIV would have a similar function in skeletal muscle compared to CaMKII is questionable, since the two proteins have different substrate specificity and intracellular localisation [53-55].

The results demonstrate that increased α/β CaMKII content is not sufficient to increase mitochondrial gene expression. We can therefore not rule out the possibility that CaMKII is required in conjunction with other signalling pathways for the response to exercise as shown before for the activity of a GLUT4-enhancer in mouse *m. tibialis anterior* [56]. In this regard, we identify that the reduced mitochondrial and SERCA2 transcript levels after high-intensity exercise in α/β CaMKII-transfected SOL muscle (Figure 5B) reproduce the reduced transcript expression within hour after high-load type of bicycle exercise [57] which contrasts to the up-regulation of gene transcripts with low-load endurance type exercise [58]. This suggests that effects of regeneration on mitochondrial transcript expression possibly interact with insufficient endurance type stimuli in the α/β CaMKII-transfected muscle of the rats housed under normal cage activity.

Conclusion

Our results support a role for elevated sarcoplasmic CaMKII content for accelerating muscle contraction and relaxation in regenerating muscle via effects that include the enhanced expression of fast myosin heavy chain and sarcoplasmic reticulum associated SERCA2 and ANXV protein, but not in mitochondrial biogenesis. These observations *in vivo* are the first to point out a role for quantitative changes in this multi-functional calcium-dependent enzyme in control of the contractile muscle phenotype.

Methods

Experimental design

Three experimental groups from two phenotypically distinct muscles (i.e. the fast GM and slow SOL muscle) were compared in this experiment: group 1: α/β *CaMKII-transfection*, group 2: *control-transfection*, and group 3: *non-transfected controls*. The comparison of group 1 vs. 2 allows identifying the feasibility and effect of CaMKII overexpression, while the comparison of groups 2 vs. 3. allows conclusions on the effects of transfection alone.

Transfection of muscle fibres was achieved via intramuscular injection of plasmid prior to the application of defined electric pulses (electro-transfer). Thereby a paired design was adopted where α/β CaMKII-transfected right SOL and GM muscles of animals were compared to the respective contralateral (i.e. left) muscles that were subjected to a control-transfection.

Effects were assessed seven days after the intervention through measurements of selected molecular, cellular and functional parameters. Functional effects were assessed *in situ* in intact muscle-tendon preparations (for abbreviations see Figure 2). The molecular measures included the quantification of the content in selected proteins using western blotting/immunodetection and the content of selected gene transcripts after high-intensity exercise *in situ*. The specificity of detecting CaMKII and threonine 287 phosphorylated CaMKII (pThr287-CaMKII) was assessed based on western blotting and immunodetection of homogenates from control-transfected and α/β CaMKII-transfected muscle, and homogenates which were incubated *in vitro* to assess calcium/calmodulin-dependent threonine 287 phosphorylation with commercial antibodies. The cellular specificity of CaMKII overexpression and downstream effects were assessed by quantifying immunofluorescent signals as recorded using confocal microscopy or by quantifying conventional colorimetric staining as documented with light microscopy.

Animals

Female Wistar rats were used for the experiments described here. *In situ* contraction protocols and the majority of the electroporation experiments were carried out at the MOVE Research Institute Amsterdam, VU University Amsterdam, The Netherlands, and approved by the local committee on ethics of animal experimentation. Rat handling and experiments conformed with the Dutch Research Councils guide for the care and use of laboratory animals. Two series of electroporation experiments were carried out at the Department of Cardiovascular Surgery, University Hospital Bern, Switzerland. These experiments were carried out according to the permission of the Animal Care Committee of the Canton of Berne (Switzerland) and following the recommendations provided by the European Convention for the protection of Vertebrate Animals used for Experimental and Scientific purposes (Strasbourg, 18.III.1986).

Transfection

Plasmid injection followed by electropulsing was essentially carried out with modifications as described [39]. Three-month-old female Wistar rats (Harlan Laboratories/ Charles River; 191-230 grams, n = 13) were used to transfect GM and SOL muscle. Both, left and right muscles were injected with a reporter plasmid prior to electropulsing; the right muscles only were also injected with plasmid for native α and β CaMKII. pCDNA3 plasmids vectors encoding full-length cDNA for α CaMKII (pCDNA3-CaMKIIα) and β CaMKII (pCDNA3-CaMKIIβ) were a gift from Dr. M Neal Waxham (University of Texas, Houston, USA). The reporter plasmid encoding full-length luciferase under control of 424 basepairs upstream of the transcription start site of the chicken skeletal α-actin gene [59] was a gift from Dr. Frank W. Booth (University of Missouri, Columbia, USA). Animals were anaesthetized with 2-4% isoflurane through inhalation. Hindlimbs were shaved, and skin was disinfected with 70% ethanol. An incision was made into the skin and fascia between GM and *m. tibialis anterior*. SOL muscle was subsequently exposed and liberated, after which four injections of a plasmid mixture with a total volume of 90 μl were administered intramuscularly with a 29-gauge insulin syringe. Subsequently four injections of a total volume of 180 μl were administered to the GM along the length of the muscle. 5 minutes after DNA injection, the muscles were subjected to electroporation as established. 6-mm long needle electrodes (BD microlance TM3, 27G 1⁄2″; distance 4 mm) were inserted perpendicular to the fibre orientation of the injected muscle and subjected to discrete pulse protocols as established in previous experiments. For SOL the protocol involved the delivery of

3 trains of 80 100 microsecond pulses at 100 mA, with 992 milliseconds of interrupt on 2 locations using needle electrodes with a GET42EV generator (E.I.P. Electronique et Informatique du Pilat, Jonzieux, France) [39]. For the GM, this included the delivery of 8 trains of 60 100 microsecond duration at 50 mA, with 994 milliseconds interrupt on 3 locations. A mix of expression plasmid pCDNA3-CaMKIIα(0.22 μg μl^{-1}) and pCDNA3-CaMKIIβ(0.22 μg μl^{-1}) in TBE buffer was injected into muscles of the right leg together with the reporter plasmid (0.55 μg μl^{-1}). Data obtained from this reporter construct are beyond the scope of this paper, and are therefore not reported. Muscles of the left leg were injected with the reporter plasmid only (1 μg μl^{-1}). Right and left muscles of this experiment will henceforth be referred to as α/β CaMKII-transfected and control-transfected, respectively. For the study of CaMKII activation by isometric exercise *in situ*, both left and right muscles were transfected with α/β CaMKII plasmid.

After electropulsing, the skin wound was closed with sutures, and the animal was allowed to recover from anaesthesia. Animals were kept in cages afterwards, where they resumed normal activity within hours after surgery. After seven days, animals were anaesthetized for further measurement of contraction parameters (see below) and euthanized by intra-cardiac injection of Euthasol (VU University Amsterdam) or anaesthetized with 3% isoflurane and euthanized by dislocation of the cervical vertebrae and rapid exsanguination (University Hospital Bern). Treated muscles were harvested from both legs and snap-frozen in liquid nitrogen.

In situ measures of muscle contraction

For measurement of isometric muscle contraction parameters, rats were anaesthetized by intra-peritoneal injections of 1.2 ml/100 gram body weight of 12.5% urethane [60]. Ear and foot reflexes were tested to check whether the animal was sufficiently anesthetized. Subsequent injections of 0.3-0.5 ml, up to a maximum of 1.5 ml, were given every 10 min afterwards until reflexes had disappeared. Experiments were carried out at room temperature (24C). Rats were kept on a heated pad to prevent hypothermia. Hindlimbs were shaved and skin was removed, after which GM and SOL muscles were exposed and mechanically isolated by removing as much as possible the myofascial connections to surrounding muscles. Blood supply to, and nerve innervations of, both muscles were kept intact and tendons of GM and SOL muscles were attached to a force transducer via Kevlar wires. The sciatic nerve was severed proximally and connected to an external electrode that was controlled by a computer to receive pulse wave stimulation.

Optimum length of the muscle-tendon complex (the length of the muscle-tendon complex at which maximum tetanic force was produced) for isometric contractions was first estimated using twitches, then determined using a protocol consisting of two twitches and one tetanic contraction (pulse duration 100 μsec, tetanic stimulation frequency: 100 Hz, train duration: 400 ms [61]. Muscles were kept below slack length between contractions and rest duration between maximal contractions was approximately one minute. After determination of optimum length, muscles rested for five minutes. Subsequently, while muscles were set to optimum length, *a protocol of high-intensity exercise* (stimulation frequency: 100 Hz; train duration: 300 ms, one train every 800 ms, 50 trains/contractions) was applied to induce muscle fatigue. GM and SOL muscles were dissected after the end of stimulation and snap-frozen in liquid nitrogen. Animals were killed by intra-cardiac injection of Euthasol, while still fully anaesthetized. Frozen muscles were stored at -80C until use for western blotting/immunodetection and microscopic analysis as described below.

Force data during muscle stimulation were sampled at a frequency of 1000 Hz and collected using custom written software based on Matlab (v 7.5.0, The Mathworks Inc., MA, USA). Time-to-peak-twitch force, half-relaxation time, maximum twitch force and maximum tetanic force were determined. The same contraction parameters were determined for a group of non-transfected muscles (NT; SOL/GM, n = 8). Values obtained for the two twitch values in each trace were averaged.

Isometric exercise in situ

A two-minute stimulation protocol consisting of intermittent isometric tetanic contractions of GM muscle at 100 Hz stimulation frequency [27] was applied via the sciatic nerve to α/β-CaMKII-transfected SOL muscle *in situ*. The stimulated muscles (n = 6) were freeze-clamped between liquid nitrogen-cooled aluminium grips during stimulation after two minutes. Non-stimulated, α/β-CaMKII-transfected contra-lateral muscles were subsequently dissected and frozen in liquid nitrogen. Proteins were extracted from the muscle and subjected to SDS-PAGE followed by western blotting and immunodetection as described below.

Protein biochemistry
Western blotting/immunodetection

To analyse protein expression, frozen 25 μm thick cross-sections taken from the centre portion of the muscle were homogenized in ice-cold RIPA buffer (50 mM TRIS-HCl (pH 7.5), 150 mM NaCl, 1 mM EDTA, 1% v/v Nonidet P40 substitute, 0.25% w/v sodium deoxycholate) plus freshly added protease/phosphatase inhibitors: 1 mM NaF, 1 mM Na$_3$VO$_4$, 0.1 mM PMSF, 1 μg ml^{-1} leupeptin, 0.2 μg ml^{-1} pepstatin, 0.1 μg ml^{-1} aprotinin, using a Polytron homogenizer (Kinematica,

Luzern, Switzerland). Chemicals were obtained from Sigma-Aldrich (Dorset, United Kingdom). Crude homogenates were aspirated 5-10 times through a 0.8 mm syringe needle, and stored at -80C until use for analysis. An aliquot of the aspirated homogenate was taken for determination of protein concentration with the bicinchoninic acid protein assay (Pierce, Rockford IL, USA).

Protein levels of total CaMKII and pThr287-CaMKII were analysed by western blotting followed by immunodetection. Homogenates were denatured by addition of SDS-PAGE buffer (final concentration: 50 mM TRIS-HCl (pH 6.8), 2% w/v bromophenol blue, 10% v/v glycerol, 2% β-mercaptoethanol) and five minutes heating at 95C. 20-40 μg of protein was separated by SDS-PAGE and transferred overnight onto a nitrocellulose membrane (GE Healthcare, Little Chalfont, UK). Membranes were stained with Ponceau S solution to confirm equal protein loading and transfer. The membrane was blocked in 5% skimmed milk in TRIS-buffered saline (pH 7.4) with 0.05% Tween-20 (TBS-T), followed by incubation with a primary antibody for pan-CaMKII (BD Bioscience #611292, dilution: 1/2500), pThr287-CaMKII (Cell Signalling Technology #3361, dilution: 1/1000), fast myosin heavy chain (Sigma-Aldrich #M4276, dilution 1/1000), myogenin (Santa Cruz Biotechnology, sc-12732 (F5D); 1:200) or myoD (Santa Cruz Biotechnology, sc-304; 1:200) or OxPhos proteins (succinate dehydrogenase Fp subunit (SDHA), ATP synthase subunit α (ATP5A), ubiquinol cytochrome c oxioreductase subunit 2 (UQCRC2) and NADH ubiquinone oxidoreductase subunit 9 (NDUFA9); #458199, Invitrogen, dilution 1/1000, and COXIV (#4850, Cell Signalling Technology, 1/2000)) for 2 hours. Antibody incubation solutions were 5% milk or 5% bovine serum albumin (BSA) in TBS-T. Finally, membranes were incubated with species-specific horseradish peroxidase-conjugated secondary antibodies (Millipore, Watford, UK). Membranes were washed in TBS-T for 4 5 minutes after both antibody incubations. Antibodies were detected with an enhanced chemiluminescence kit (Pierce, Rockford IL, USA). Light signals were captured with a ChemiDoc XRS system (Biorad, Hemel Hempstead, UK).

Transfected muscle pairs from the same animal were run on the same blot. Measures were limited to animals whose CaMKII injected & porated muscles showed increased expression in either of the exogenous CaMKII isoforms on a western blot. Protein bands were quantified with Quantity One version 4.6.8 (Biorad). These values were subsequently expressed as relative to the mean of the control-transfected muscles for the respective immunoblot.

Establishing CaMKII detection

To identify CaMKII isoforms in skeletal muscle [41] buffer components were added to muscle homogenate

to promote, or suppress, calcium/calmodulin dependent protein phosphorylation *in vitro* as described [62]. The reaction products were subjected to SDS-PAGE and immunoblotted for CaMKII as described in the section on western blotting and immunodetection below. CaMKII isoforms were labelled in reference to a previous report [41]. The phosphorylated form of exogenous β CaMKII was identified based on its molecular weight (60.4 kDa), which is very similar to that of δa (60.1 kDa), the second largest CaMKII isoform in skeletal muscle [29].

Microscopic analysis

To investigate differences in protein expression at the single fibre level, immunofluorescent staining was performed on cryosections of transfected muscles. Sections (12 μm thickness) were cut on a cryostat (CM3050, Leica, Germany) and dried for 30 minutes on glass slides. Sections were then fixed with ice-cold acetone and blocked with 5% normal goat serum in phosphate buffered saline, pH 7.5 (PBS). CaMKII and SERCA2, COXIV, MHCI or MHCII, were detected simultaneously using commercially available primary antibodies (anti-CaMKII; anti-SERCA2 (Abcam #Ab3625 or Abcam #2A7-A1, dilution 1/200); anti-COXIV (#4850, Cell Signalling Technology); anti-MHCI (#MAB1628, Millipore, dilution 1/100); anti-MHCII (#M4277, Sigma Chemicals, dilution 1/100) and species-specific Alexa 488/555 secondary antibodies (Invitrogen). Sections were washed with PBS for 4 5 minutes after both antibody incubations. To detect nuclei, sections were incubated for 10 minutes with TO-PRO-3 iodide (Invitrogen, Paisley, UK). Immuno-labelled sections were embedded in fluorescence compatible mounting medium (DAKO, Ely, UK).

Protein expression in electroporated fibres was analysed on a TCS SP5 confocal microscope (Leica, Milton Keynes, UK). A 10 objective was used in combination with 4 optical zoom. The fluorescent labels were excited with an Argon laser at 488 nm and HeNe lasers at 543 nm and 633 nm. The pinhole was set to match the thickness of the stained section and the focus plane was adjusted to maximize signal detection. Dyes were excited separately using a sequential scanning mode. Detected light spectra were set to maximize signal detection, but care was taken to prevent cross-excitation of dyes. Laser intensity was set to produce images with few under- or overexposed pixels, and low levels of non-specific staining, as indicated by light emission from sections that had been labelled with the secondary antibodies only. 8-Bit images were captured at 2048 2048 pixels, using 100 Hz scanning speed and 5-times line averaging.

The efficiency of overexpression was estimated by taking a tile scan of one cryosections of the belly portion of each α/β CaMKII-transfected muscle, which was stained for CaMKII using immunofluorescence or colorimetric staining. Subsequently individual microscopic fields were assessed for the number of fibres with prominent staining for CaMKII and the total fiber number. On average 234 and 386 fibres were counted for SOL and GM muscle, respectively. MCSA of transfected and non-transfected fibres was estimated in colorimetrically stained cross sections using Adobe Photoshop CC (Adobe Systems Incorporated) in regions of α/β CaMKII-transfected SOL muscle as described [63]. Only fibres which met the criteria of a circularity factor >0.5 were included. On average 30 transfected and 60 non-transfected fibres from the same transfected region were assessed per cross section.

SERCA2, COXIV and CaMKII staining intensity in muscle fibres overexpressing CaMKII (identified based on CaMKII staining intensity by visual inspection) was quantified with ImageJ (*rsbweb.nih.gov/ij/*). Fibres were circumscribed manually and the average pixel intensity within the fibre was measured. An approximately equal number of fibres in the same image which did not demonstrate elevated CaMKII content (designated non-transfected fibers) was measured as well, and acted as the control group of fibres to which the CaMKII-overexpressing fibres (designated transfected fibers) were compared. MHCII expression in transfected and non-transfected fibers was assessed in the transfected region based on the presence or absence of MHC-staining as this staining was rather discrete than continuous.

Fibres with internal nuclei were assessed on 12-μm cryosections being stained with and counterstained with hematoxylin (MERCK, Germany). Microscopic files were taken at a 10-fold magnification (Axioskop 2, Carl Zeiss Ltd, Welwyn Garden City, UK) and assembled with AxioVision software (Carl Zeiss Ltd). Subsequently a grid with 250-μm unit length was superimposed and microscopic fields corresponding to 0.0625 μm2 were assessed in a random initiation, systematic manner counting fibre profiles and fibre profiles with internal (blue) nuclei. On average 475 + 50 fibre were counted per muscle.

RT-PCR

RNA extraction from muscle tissue and RT-PCR analysis were carried out as described elsewhere [64]. Total RNA was extracted from frozen 25 μm-sections of transfected SOL muscles using the RiboPure kit (Applied Biosystems). RNA concentration and purity (260/280 nm ratio; mean: 2.06, range: 1.92-2.09) were determined using a spectrophotometer (Nanodrop Technologies, Wilmington, DE). Total RNA concentration in muscle tissue was expressed as RNA (ng) per weight of the analysed sample (mg). Five hundred nanogram of total RNA per muscle was reverse-transcribed using the high capacity RNA-to-cDNA kit (Applied Biosystems) containing random primers in a 20 μl total reaction volume. Tubes were heated at 25C for

5 min, followed by 42C for 30 min. Finally; the tubes were heated to 85C for 5 min to stop the reaction and stored at -80C until used in the PCR reaction.

For each PCR target, 5 μl of the RT reaction product was amplified in duplicate using Fast Sybr Green mastermix (Applied Biosystems). The following transcripts were targeted: 18S ribosomal RNA (18S rRNA), caveolin 3 (CAV3), dysferlin (DYSF), cytochrome-c oxidase subunit 1 (COXI), cytochrome-c oxidase 4 (COXIV), succinate dehydrogenase subunit b (SDHB), peroxisome proliferator-activated receptor γ-co-activator 1 α (PGC-1α), Annexin V (ANXV), and SERCA2A. PCR primers were designed using Primer-BLAST (http://www.ncbi.nlm.nih.gov/tools/primer-blast/). Primer sequences and Genbank accession numbers for the transcripts are shown in Table 2. Amplification efficiency of the primers used was 92.7-102.0%, and melting curve analysis demonstrated specific amplification. The range of cycle threshold values was 13-25. For all transcripts, the 18S rRNA cycle threshold was subtracted from the mean cycle threshold value of the specific target to obtain ΔC_t and converted into relative concentrations by $2^{-\Delta Ct}$.

Statistics

Statistical analyses were carried out with STATISTICA for windows (V10.0, StatSoft, Inc. (2011), www.statsoft.com) or SPSS16 (SPSS Inc, IL, USA). One sample was identified as an outlier in the RT-PCR experiments based on the Grubbs test and excluded from the further analysis. Immunofluorescence data from fibres demonstrating

Table 2 Primers sequences used for RT-PCR analysis of mRNA targets

mRNA target mRNA	PCR primer sequence 5 → 3	Genbank
18S RNA	Forward: CGAACGTCTGCCCTATCAACTT	EU 139318.1
	Reverse: ACCCGTGGTCACCATGGTA	
COXI	Forward: TGCCAGTATTAGCAGCAGGT	X14848.1
	Reverse: GAATTGGGTCTCCACCTCCA	
COXIV	Forward: AGTCCAATTGTACCGCATCC	NM 017202.1
	Reverse: ACTCATTGGTGCCCTTGTTC	
SDHB	Forward: CAGAGAAGGGATCTGTGGCT	NM 001100539.1
	Reverse: TGTTGCCTCCGTTGATGTTC	
PGC-1α	Forward: ATGAGAAGCGGGAGTCTGAA	NM 031347.1
	Reverse: GCGCTCTTCAATTGCTTTCT	
SERCA2A	Forward: GGCCCGAAACTACCTGGAGCC	NM 001110139
	Reverse: CAACGCACATGCACGCACCC	
CAV3	Forward: CCCAAGAACATCAATGAGGAC	U31968
	Reverse: GGAGACGGTGAAAGTGGTGT	
DYSF	Forward: TGGGAACCGCTACCATCTAC	NM001107869
	Reverse: CTCTGGTGCAGGAAGGAGAC	

elevated or normal CaMKII levels in the same α/β CaMKII-transfected muscle were analysed with two-tailed t-tests (unpaired). The fractions of MHCII-positive muscle fibres in the α/β CaMKII-transfected and non-transfected fibre pool, respectively, were analysed with Chi-squared tests because they represent categorical values. Western blot/immunodetection data from control-transfected and α/β CaMKII-transfected muscles were analysed with two-tailed Wilcoxon signed ranks tests. The effect of transfection on twitch and tetanic force parameters from α/β CaMKII-transfected and control-transfected muscles was tested by relating force values to the respective mean of measures from the respective non-transfected muscles (i.e. GM and SOL) and running an ANOVA for the factors muscle (SOL, GM) x transfection (CaMKII-transfected, control-transfected). Non-parametric tests were run with exact significance. Significance level was set at $p < 0.05$. Values are provided as mean standard error (SE).

Abbreviations

18S rRNA: 18S ribosomal RNA; ANXV: Annexin V; ATP5A: ATP synthase H + transporting mitochondrial F1 complex; CaMKII: Calcium/calmodulin-dependent protein kinase II; CAV3: Caveolin 3; COXI: Cytochrome-c oxidase subunit 1; COXIV: Cytochrome-c oxidase subunit 4; CaM: Calmodulin; DYSF: Dysferlin; EGTA: Ethylene glycol-bis(2-aminoethylether) -tetraacetic acid ; Ftwitch: Maximum twitch force; Fmax: Maximum tetanic force; GM: Musculus gastrocnemius; HRT: Half-relaxation time; MHCIIA: Type IIA myosin heavy chain; MHCIIB: Type IIB myosin heavy chain; MHCIIX: Type IIX myosin heavy chain; myoD: Myogenic factor 3; NDUFA9: NADH dehydrogenase (ubiquinone) 1 alpha subcomplex 9; NTf: Non-transfected; PGC-1α: Peroxisome proliferator-activated receptor γ-co-activator 1 α; PCR: Polymerase chain reaction; pThr287-CaMKII: Threonine 287 phosphorylated CaMKII; SERCA2: Sarco/endoplasmic reticulum Ca2 + -ATPase; SDHA: Succinate dehydrogenase subunit b; SDHB: Succinate dehydrogenase subunit b; SE: Standard error; skaa: Skeletal alpha actin; SOL: Musculus soleus; SR: Sarcoplasmic reticulum; Tf: Transfected; TTP: Time-to-peak-twitch force; UQCRC2: Ubiquinol-cytochrome c reductase core II protein.

Competing interests

The authors declare that no academic, financial or non-financial competing interest exists.

Authors contributions

Conception and design of research: WE, RTJ, ADH, MF; Performed experiments: WE, CF, PV, MF; Analyzed data: WE, MF, RTJ; Interpreted results of experiments: WE, RTJ, MF; Funding: ADH, MF; Prepared figures: WE, MF; Drafted manuscript: WE, MF; Edited and revised manuscript: WE, RTJ, ADH, MF. All authors read and approved the final version of manuscript.

Authors information

WE carried out his work during the course of his PhD project under supervision of MF, RJ and AdH. He is currently a postdoctoral fellow involved in developing gene therapies for muscular dystrophies and type 2 diabetes. RJ is assistant professor and head of the Laboratory for Myology of the MOVE Research Institute Amsterdam. His research interest is in molecular physiology with a focus on mechano-transduction and adaptation of muscle size and oxidative capacity. Basic insights are translated into research on improvement of muscle function in sports, neuromuscular disorders and aging. AdH is Professor in Exercise Physiology at the Faculty of Human Movement Sciences, VU University Amsterdam, the Netherlands and Director of MOVE Research Institute Amsterdam, the Netherlands. His main professional interests concern short-term changes in metabolic and functional muscle characteristics (fatigue, potentiation) and adaptations to increased and decreased muscle activity as a result of training, disease, bedrest, spinal

cord injury and aging. With integrative and translational research, he tries to bridge the gap between research at the genetic/molecular level and research performed at the whole human body level.
CF is a research assistant who contributed to critical experimentation during the revision of the manuscript.
PV is a postdoctoral fellow assessing molecular pathways of muscle plasticity who provided substantial input on the control experiments.
MF is Professor of Muscle Plasticity at the Orthopedics Clinics of the University of Zurich at Balgrist. His research centers on the signaling pathways that integrate muscle plasticity in response to use-related and clinical forms of stimuli. Towards this end he deploys an integrative approach combining the use of modern omics platforms, gene technology and classical physiological measures in rodent and human models. He is in the editorial board of The European Journal of Applied Physiology, Physiological Genomics and BMC Physiology.

Acknowledgements

We thank Carla Offringa for carrying out the RT-PCR experiments and Guus C. Baan for assistance with the muscle contraction measures, Dr. M. Neal Waxham (The University of Texas Medical School, Houston, USA) for donating the α/β-CaMKII plasmids, Dr. Frank W. Booth (University of Missouri, Columbia, USA) for donating the skeletal alpha-actin reporter plasmid and Dr. Marie-Nolle Giraud (University of Bern, Bern, Switzerland) for donating the SERCA2 antibodies.
The study was supported through start-up grants from Manchester Metropolitan University (Manchester, United Kingdom), and VU University Amsterdam (Amsterdam, the Netherlands Kingdom), and grant 310000-112139 from the Swiss National Science Foundation.

Author details

[1]Institute for Biomedical Research into Human Movement and Health, Manchester Metropolitan University, John Dalton Building, Oxford Road, M1 5GD Manchester, United Kingdom. [2]Laboratory for Myology, MOVE Research Institute Amsterdam, Faculty of Human Movement Sciences, VU University Amsterdam, Van der Boechorststraat 7, 1081 BT Amsterdam, The Netherlands. [3]Laboratory for Muscle Plasticity, Department of Orthopaedics, University of Zurich, Balgrist University Hospital, Forchstrasse 340, 8008 Zurich, Switzerland.

References

1. Berchtold MW, Brinkmeier H, Muntener M: **Calcium ion in skeletal muscle: its crucial role for muscle function, plasticity, and disease.** *Physiol Rev* 2000, **80**:1215 1265.
2. Chin ER: **Role of Ca2+/calmodulin-dependent kinases in skeletal muscle plasticity.** *J Appl Physiol* 2005, **99**:414 423.
3. Fluck M, Hoppeler H: **Molecular basis of skeletal muscle plasticity from gene to form and function.** *Rev Physiol Biochem Pharmacol* 2003, **146**:159 216.
4. Darveau CA, Suarez RK, Andrews RD, Hochachka PW: **Allometric cascade as a unifying principle of body mass effects on metabolism.** *Nature* 2002, **417**:166 170.
5. Daz-Herrera P, Torres A, Morcuende JA, Garca-Castellano JM, Calbet JA, Sarrat R: **Effect of endurance running on cardiac and skeletal muscle in rats.** *Histol Histopathol* 2001, **16**:29 35.
6. Wada M, Inashima S, Yamada T, Matsunaga S: **Endurance training-induced changes in alkali light chain patterns in type IIB fibers of the rat.** *J Appl Physiol* 2003, **4**:923 9.
7. Kubis HP, Haller EA, Wetzel P, Gros G: **Adult fast myosin pattern and Ca2 + -induced slow myosin pattern in primary skeletal muscle culture.** *Proc Natl Acad Sci U S A* 1997, **94**:4205 4210.
8. Sreter FA, Lopez JR, Alamo L, Mabuchi K, Gergely J: **Changes in intracellular ionized Ca concentration associated with muscle fiber type transformation.** *Am J Physiol* 1987, **253**:C296 C300.
9. Wright DC, Geiger PC, Han DH, Jones TE, Holloszy JO: **Calcium induces increases in peroxisome proliferator-activated receptor gamma coactivator-1alpha and mitochondrial biogenesis by a pathway leading to p38 mitogen-activated protein kinase activation.** *J Biol Chem* 2007, **282**:18793 18799.

10. Tavi P, Westerblad H: The role of in vivo Ca(2)(+) signals acting on Ca(2)(+)-calmodulin-dependent proteins for skeletal muscle plasticity. *J Physiol* 2011, **589**:5021 5031.

11. Chin ER, Olson EN, Richardson JA, Yang Q, Humphries C, Shelton JM, Wu H, Zhu W, Bassel-Duby R, Williams RS: A calcineurin-dependent transcriptional pathway controls skeletal muscle fiber type. *Genes Dev* 1998, **12**:2499 2509.

12. Parsons SA, Millay DP, Wilkins BJ, Bueno OF, Tsika GL, Neilson JR, Liberatore CM, Yutzey KE, Crabtree GR, Tsika RW, Molkentin JD: Genetic loss of calcineurin blocks mechanical overload-induced skeletal muscle fiber type switching but not hypertrophy. *J Biol Chem* 2004, **279**:26192 26200.

13. Serrano AL, Murgia M, Pallafacchina G, Calabria E, Coniglio P, Lomo T, Schiaffino S: Calcineurin controls nerve activity-dependent specification of slow skeletal muscle fibers but not muscle growth. *Proc Natl Acad Sci U S A* 2001, **98**:13108 13113.

14. Garcia-Roves PM, Huss J, Holloszy JO: Role of calcineurin in exercise-induced mitochondrial biogenesis. *Am J Physiol Endocrinol Metabol* 2006, **290**:E1172 E1179.

15. Jiang LQ, Garcia-Roves PM, De Castro BT, Zierath JR: Constitutively active calcineurin in skeletal muscle increases endurance performance and mitochondrial respiratory capacity. *Am J Physiol Endocrinol Metabol* 2010, **298**:E8 E16.

16. Long YC, Glund S, Garcia-Roves PM, ZIERATH JR: Calcineurin regulates skeletal muscle metabolism via coordinated changes in gene expression. *J Biol Chem* 2007, **282**:1607 1614.

17. Ojuka EO, Jones TE, Han DH, Chen M, Holloszy JO: Raising Ca2+ in L6 myotubes mimics effects of exercise on mitochondrial biogenesis in muscle. *FASEB J* 2003, **17**:675 681.

18. Wu H, Kanatous SB, Thurmond FA, Gallardo T, Isotani E, Bassel-Duby R, Williams RS: Regulation of mitochondrial biogenesis in skeletal muscle by CaMK. *Science* 2002, **296**:349 352.

19. Allen DL, Leinwand LA: Intracellular calcium and myosin isoform transitions. Calcineurin and calcium-calmodulin kinase pathways regulate preferential activation of the IIa myosin heavy chain promoter. *J Biol Chem* 2002, **277**:45323 45330.

20. Mu X, Brown LD, Liu Y, Schneider MF: Roles of the calcineurin and CaMK signaling pathways in fast-to-slow fiber type transformation of cultured adult mouse skeletal muscle fibers. *Physiol Genomics* 2007, **30**:300 312.

21. Hawkins C, Xu A, Narayanan N: Sarcoplasmic reticulum calcium pump in cardiac and slow twitch skeletal muscle but not fast twitch skeletal muscle undergoes phosphorylation by endogenous and exogenous Ca2+/calmodulin-dependent protein kinase. Characterization of optimal conditions for calcium pump phosphorylation. *J Biol Chem* 1994, **269**:31198 31206.

22. Tavi P, Allen DG, Niemela P, Vuolteenaho O, Weckstrom M, Westerblad H: Calmodulin kinase modulates Ca2+ release in mouse skeletal muscle. *J Physiol* 2003, **551**:5 12.

23. Akimoto T, Ribar TJ, Williams RS, Yan Z: Skeletal muscle adaptation in response to voluntary running in Ca2+/calmodulin-dependent protein kinase IV-deficient mice. *Am J Physiol Cell Physiol* 2004, **287**:C1311 C1319.

24. Witczak CA, Jessen N, Warro DM, Toyoda T, Fujii N, Anderson ME, Hirshman MF, Goodyear LJ: CaMKII regulates contraction- but not insulin-induced glucose uptake in mouse skeletal muscle. *Am J Physiol Endocrinol Metabol* 2010, **298**:E1150 E1160.

25. Anderson ME, Brown JH, Bers DM: CaMKII in myocardial hypertrophy and heart failure. *J Mol Cell Cardiol* 2011, **51**:468 473.

26. De Koninck P, Schulman H: Sensitivity of CaM kinase II to the frequency of Ca2+ oscillations. *Science* 1998, **279**:227 230.

27. Rose AJ, Alsted TJ, Kobbero JB, Richter EA: Regulation and function of Ca2+-calmodulin-dependent protein kinase II of fast-twitch rat skeletal muscle. *J Physiol* 2007, **580**:993 1005.

28. Rose AJ, Kiens B, Richter EA: Ca2+-calmodulin-dependent protein kinase expression and signalling in skeletal muscle during exercise. *J Physiol* 2006, **574**:889 903.

29. Eilers W, Gevers W, Van Overbeek D, De Haan A, Jaspers RT, Hilbers PA, Van Riel N, Fluck M: Muscle-Type Specific Autophosphorylation of CaMKII Isoforms after Paced Contractions. *BioMed Res Internat* 2014, 943806. doi:10.1155/2014/943806. Epub 2014 Jun 26.

30. Jain SS, Paglialunga S, Vigna C, Ludzki A, Herbst EA, Lally JS, Schrauwen P, Hoeks J, Tupling AR, Bonen A, Holloway GP: High-fat diet-induced mitochondrial biogenesis is regulated by mitochondrial derived reactive oxygen species activation of CaMKII. *Diabetes* 2014, **63**(6):1907 1913.

31. Benziane B, Burton TJ, Scanlan B, Galuska D, Canny BJ, Chibalin AV, Zierath JR, Stepto NK: Divergent cell signaling after short-term intensified endurance training in human skeletal muscle. *Am J Physiol Endocrinol Metab* 2008, **295**:E1427 E1438.

32. Rose AJ, Frosig C, Kiens B, Wojtaszewski JF, Richter EA: Effect of endurance exercise training on Ca2+ calmodulin-dependent protein kinase II expression and signalling in skeletal muscle of humans. *J Physiol* 2007, **583**:785 795.

33. Baylor SM, Hollingworth S: Sarcoplasmic reticulum calcium release compared in slow-twitch and fast-twitch fibres of mouse muscle. *J Physiol* 2003, **551**:125 138.

34. Hennig R, Lomo T: Firing patterns of motor units in normal rats. *Nature* 1985, **314**:164 166.

35. Gaertner TR, Kolodziej SJ, Wang D, Kobayashi R, Koomen JM, Stoops JK, Waxham MN: Comparative analyses of the three-dimensional structures and enzymatic properties of alpha, beta, gamma and delta isoforms of Ca2+-calmodulin-dependent protein kinase II. *J Biol Chem* 2004, **279**:12484 12494.

36. Woodgett JR, Cohen P, Yamauchi T, Fujisawa H: Comparison of calmodulin-dependent glycogen synthase kinase from skeletal muscle and calmodulin-dependent protein kinase-II from brain. *FEBS Lett* 1984, **170**:49 54.

37. Gorassini M, Eken T, Bennett DJ, Kiehn O, Hultborn H: Activity of hindlimb motor units during locomotion in the conscious rat. *J Neurophysiol* 2000, **83**:2002 2011.

38. Durieux AC, Bonnefoy R, Manissolle C, Freyssenet D: High-efficiency gene electrotransfer into skeletal muscle: description and physiological applicability of a new pulse generator. *Biochem Biophys Res Commun* 2002, **296**:443 450.

39. Durieux AC, D'antona G, Desplanches D, Freyssenet D, Klossner S, Bottinelli R, Fluck M: Focal adhesion kinase is a load-dependent governor of the slow contractile and oxidative muscle phenotype. *J Physiol* 2009, **587**:3703 3717.

40. Rizzuto G, Cappelletti M, Maione D, Savino R, Lazzaro D, Costa P, Mathiesen I, Cortese R, Ciliberto G, Laufer R, La Monica N, Fattori E: Efficient and regulated erythropoietin production by naked DNA injection and muscle electroporation. *Proc Natl Acad Sci U S A* 1999, **96**:6417 6422.

41. Bayer K, Harbers K, Schulman H: alphaKAP is an anchoring protein for a novel CaM kinase II isoform in skeletal muscle. *EMBO J* 1998, **17**:5598 5605.

42. Duguez S, Feasson L, Denis C, Freyssenet D: Mitochondrial biogenesis during skeletal muscle regeneration. *Am J Physiol Endocrinol Metabol* 2002, **282**:E802 E809.

43. Shu B, Shen Y, Wang AM, Fang XQ, Li X, Deng HY, Yu ZQ: Histological, enzymohistochemical and biomechanical observation of skeletal muscle injury in rabbits. *Chin J Traumatol* 2007, **10**:150 153.

44. Esposito A, Germinario E, Zanin M, Palade PT, Betto R, Danieli-Betto D: Isoform switching in myofibrillar and excitation-contraction coupling proteins contributes to diminished contractile function in regenerating rat soleus muscle. *J Appl Physiol* 2007, **102**:1640 1648.

45. Fluck M, Schmutz S, Wittwer M, Hoppeler H, Desplanches D: Transcriptional reprogramming during reloading of atrophied rat soleus muscle. *Am J Physiology Regul Integ Comp Physiol* 2005, **289**:R4 R14.

46. Wang J, Best PM: Inactivation of the sarcoplasmic reticulum calcium channel by protein kinase. *Nature* 1992, **359**:739 741.

47. Dulhunty AF, Laver D, Curtis SM, Pace S, Haarmann C, Gallant EM: Characteristics of irreversible ATP activation suggest that native skeletal ryanodine receptors can be phosphorylated via an endogenous CaMKII. *Biophysical J* 2001, **81**:3240 3252.

48. Xu A, Narayanan N: Ca2+/calmodulin-dependent phosphorylation of the Ca2+-ATPase, uncoupled from phospholamban, stimulates Ca2+-pumping in native cardiac sarcoplasmic reticulum. *Biochem Biophys Res Commun* 1999, **258**:66 72.

49. Arcuri C, Giambanco I, Bianchi R, Donato R: Annexin V, annexin VI, S100A1 and S100B in developing and adult avian skeletal muscles. *Neuroscience* 2002, **109**:371 388.

50. Zador E, Mendler L, Ver Heyen M, Dux L, Wuytack F: Changes in mRNA levels of the sarcoplasmic/endoplasmic-reticulum Ca(2+)-ATPase isoforms in the rat soleus muscle regenerating from notexin-induced necrosis. *Biochem J* 1996, **320**(Pt 1):107 113.

51. Ramirez MT, Zhao XL, Schulman H, Brown JH: The nuclear deltaB isoform of Ca2+/calmodulin-dependent protein kinase II regulates atrial

natriuretic factor gene expression in ventricular myocytes. *J Biol Chem* 1997, **272**:31203 31208.

52. Ronkainen JJ, Hanninen SL, Korhonen T, Koivumaki JT, Skoumal R, Rautio S, Ronkainen VP, Tavi P: **Ca2 + -calmodulin-dependent protein kinase II represses cardiac transcription of the L-type calcium channel alpha(1C)-subunit gene (Cacna1c) by DREAM translocation.** *J Physiol* 2011, **589**:2669 2686.

53. Srinivasan M, Edman CF, Schulman H: **Alternative splicing introduces a nuclear localization signal that targets multifunctional CaM kinase to the nucleus.** *J Cell Biol* 1994, **126**:839 852.

54. Sun P, Enslen H, Myung PS, Maurer RA: **Differential activation of CREB by Ca2+/calmodulin-dependent protein kinases type II and type IV involves phosphorylation of a site that negatively regulates activity.** *Genes Dev* 1994, **8**:2527 2539.

55. Sun P, Lou L, Maurer RA: **Regulation of activating transcription factor-1 and the cAMP response element-binding protein by Ca2+/calmodulin-dependent protein kinases type I, II, and IV.** *J Biol Chem* 1996, **271**:3066 3073.

56. Murgia M, Elbenhardt Jensen T, Cusinato M, Garcia M, Richter EA, Schiaffino S: **Multiple signalling pathways redundantly control GLUT4 gene transcription in skeletal muscle.** *J Physiol* 2009, **587**(Pt 17):4319 4327.

57. Klossner S, Dapp C, Schmutz S, Vogt M, Hoppeler H, Fluck M: **Muscle transcriptome adaptations with mild eccentric ergometer exercise.** *Pflugers Arch* 2007, **455**:555 562.

58. Schmutz S, Dapp C, Wittwer M, Vogt M, Hoppeler H, Fluck M: **Endurance training modulates the muscular transcriptome response to acute exercise.** *Pflugers Arch* 2006, **451**:678 687.

59. Marsh DR, Carson JA, Stewart LN, Booth FW: **Activation of the skeletal alpha-actin promoter during muscle regeneration.** *J Muscle Res Cell Motil* 1998, **19**:897 907.

60. Haan A, Huijing PA, Vliet MR: **Rat medial gastrocnemius muscles produce maximal power at a length lower than the isometric optimum length.** *Pflugers Archiv Europ J Physiol* 2003, **445**:728 733.

61. De Haan A, De Ruiter CJ, Lind A, Sargeant AJ: **Age-related changes in force and efficiency in rat skeletal muscle.** *Acta Physiol Scand* 1993, **147**:347 355.

62. Fluck M, Waxham MN, Hamilton MT, Booth FW: **Skeletal muscle Ca(2+)-independent kinase activity increases during either hypertrophy or running.** *J Appl Physiol* 2000, **88**:352 358.

63. Desplanches D, Amami M, Dupr-Aucouturier S, Valdivieso P, Schmutz S, Mueller M, Hoppeler H, Kreis R, Flck M: **Hypoxia refines plasticity of mitochondrial respiration to repeated muscle work.** *Eur J Appl Physiol* 2014, **114**(2):405 417.

64. Van Wessel T, De Haan A, van der Laarse WJ, Jaspers RT: **The muscle fiber type-fiber size paradox: hypertrophy or oxidative metabolism?** *Eur J Appl Physiol* 2010, **110**:665 694.

Liver-derived endocrine IGF-I is not critical for activation of skeletal muscle protein synthesis following oral feeding

Britt-Marie Iresjö[1*], Johan Svensson[2], Claes Ohlsson[2] and Kent Lundholm[1]

Abstract

Background: Insulin-like growth factor-1 (IGF-1) is produced in various tissues to stimulate protein synthesis under different conditions. It is however, difficult to distinguish effects by locally produced IGF-1 compared to liver-derived IGF-1 appearing in the circulation. In the present study the role of liver-derived endocrine IGF-I for activation of skeletal muscle protein synthesis following feeding was evaluated.

Results: Transgenic female mice with selective knockout of the IGF-I gene in hepatocytes were freely fed, starved overnight and subsequently refed for 3 hours and compared to wild types (wt). Liver IGF-I knockout mice had 70% reduced plasma IGF-I. Starvation decreased and refeeding increased muscle protein synthesis ($p < 0.01$), similarly in both IGF-I knockouts and wt mice. Phosphorylation of p70s6k and mTOR increased and 4EBP1 bound to eIF4E decreased in both IGF-I knockouts and wt mice after refeeding ($p < 0.05$). Muscle transcripts of IGF-I decreased and IGF-I receptor increased ($p < 0.01$) in wild types during starvation but similar alterations did not reach significance in knockouts ($p > 0.05$). mTOR mRNA increased in knockouts only during starvation. Plasma glucose decreased during starvation in all groups in parallel to insulin, while plasma IGF-I and GH did not change significantly among the groups during starvation-refeeding. Plasma amino acids declined and increased during starvation-refeeding in wild type mice ($p < 0.05$), but less so in IGF-I $^{(-/-)}$ knockouts ($p < 0.08$).

Conclusion: This study demonstrates that re-synthesis of muscle proteins following starvation is not critically dependent on endocrine liver-derived IGF-I.

Keywords: IGF-I, Muscle protein synthesis, Cell signaling, Amino acid

Background

Protein synthesis is rapidly increased in skeletal muscles after oral feeding due to intracellular signaling for activation of initiation or protein translation [1], which is quantitatively the most important alteration in the control of short term protein balance in skeletal muscles [2,3]. Meal feeding is a complex stimuli where nutrients are provided and appear simultaneously with changes in circulating levels of hormones and substrates as well as hormone binding proteins. Our earlier studies have suggested that amino acids are important substrate factor(s) behind post-feeding activation of muscle protein synthesis, whereas insulin seems rather permissive [4,5]. On the other hand, it can be expected that insulin-like growth factor I (IGF-I) should be involved since provision of anti IGF-I antibodies before meal feeding attenuated a subsequent rise in protein synthesis [5], besides its well-recognized effects on muscle cell proliferation and regeneration [6-8]. Furthermore, blood levels and muscle expression of IGF-I are significantly changed during starvation and feeding [5,9]. The role of endocrine liver-derived and locally tissue produced IGF-I to promote protein synthesis in response to feeding is however unclear, in part due to complex conditions with different IGF-binding proteins, which may also have independent control functions of net protein metabolism at tissue levels [10-12]. This complexity makes it uncertain to define roles of locally produced versus endocrine liver-derived IGF-I for activation of protein translation and synthesis in skeletal muscle tissue following feeding [13,14]. The aim of the present study was therefore to evaluate the

* Correspondence: britt-marie.iresjo@surgery.gu.se
[1]Department of Surgery Sahlgrenska University Hospital Kir., Metabol lab
Bruna Stråket 20-413 45, Gothenburg, Sweden
Full list of author information is available at the end of the article

Liver-derived endocrine IGF-I is not critical for activation of skeletal muscle protein synthesis...

99

role of endocrine liver-derived IGF-I for activation of translation initiation of muscle proteins at refeeding in a transgenic mouse model with selectively and conditionally deleted liver IGF-I [15]. This deletion caused levels of circulating IGF-I to be reduced by 70% compared to wild type controls in combination with normal muscle expression of IGF-I [15].

Methods

Animals

Transgenic female mice (C57BL/6) with inducible inactivation of the Insulin-like growth factor-1 gene constructed with the Cre/LoxP system were used. Animals were bred as described earlier [15]. Recombination was induced by polyinosinic-polycytidylic acid (PiPc) treatment at 10–12 weeks of age in mice homozygous for loxP and heterozygous for Mx-Cre, [15,16]. These mice are referred to as liver IGF-I knockouts, Li-IGF-I $^{(-/-)}$. PiPc treated siblings, homozygous for LoxP but lacking Mx-Cre, were used as controls and referred to as wild type animals, WT $^{(+/+)}$. Adult weight stable Li-IGF-I $^{(-/-)}$ mice housed with 5 animals per cage, matured normally with normal body composition as compared to our previous experiments on partially IGF-I knockouts $^{(+/-)}$ [9]. Body weight was 22.2 ±0.1 g in knockouts and 23.8±0.10 g in wild types at the start of experiments, in 5 months old mice; which is before any alterations in body composition in knockouts [17]. Male animals were not used since they must be housed individually in this kind of experiment; a condition which is associated with stress reactions and adaptations. However, females are subjected to hormone alterations during the estrous cycle, which could theoretically induce alterations in muscle protein metabolism. However, comparisons of rates of muscle protein synthesis between phases of the menstrual cycle are limited. Miller *et.al.* found no effect of the menstrual cycle phases in human females [18], while Toth *et.al.* reported minor changes in the gastrocnemius fractional synthesis rate related to estradiol or progesterone replacement therapy in ovariectomized rats [19]. Therefore, all our experiments were carried out with mice randomly divided across cages housed simultaneously and close together, in order to promote estrous synchronization within and across cages.

Liver IGF-I knockouts and wild type mice were used across the groups; freely fed, starved and refed animals. Freely fed animals had continuous access to water ad lib. and standard rodent chow (2016 Global Tekland®, Netherlands). Starved mice had no access to food overnight for 12 hours before experiments, while refed animals were similarly starved overnight for 12 hours and had then free access to food during 3 hours before termination according to previous findings [4,9,20]. Animals were killed by cervical dislocation and blood samples were drawn by cardiac puncture. Mixed hind limb muscles from both legs were excised. Muscles from one leg were used for measurements of fractional protein synthesis and protein measurements. Muscle tissue from the other leg was used for RNA extraction and RNA expression analyses.

All animal procedures were performed in accordance to Swedish law (Animal welfare act, 1988:538) and national guidelines for care and use of research animals (DFS 2004:4) and approved by the regional ethics committee for animal research in Gothenburg (450–2008).

RNA expression

Hind limb mixed muscle tissue were snap-frozen in liquid nitrogen and kept in –70°C until analysis. RNA was extracted using RNeasy fibrous tissue kit (Qiagen) with DNAse step included. Total RNA concentrations were measured by spectrophotometer (Nanodrop ND-100) and RNA quality was checked by calculating the 18S/28S ratio using an Agilent 2100 bioanalyser. One µg of total RNA was reverse transcribed using oligo d(T)-primer according to kit instructions (Advantage RT for PCR kit,) for cDNA synthesis. Positive and negative controls were included in each run of cDNA synthesis. Realtime PCR was performed with a LightCycler 1.5 instrument (Roche) using the LightCycler FastStart DNA Master^{PLUS}SYBR Green 1 kit. For analysis of Igf-1, 2 µl cDNA and 10 pmol of forward (GCT CTT CAG TTC GTG TGT GGA C) and reverse (CAT CTC CAG TCT CCT CAG ATC) primers were used to each reaction of 20 µl. PCR were performed with the following settings; denaturation 95°C for 10 sec., annealing 64°C, 4 sec. and extension 72°C, 6 sec. For analysis of Igf-1r (Quantitect Primer assay Nr QT00155351, Qiagen), 2 µl cDNA and 2 µl of premixed Quantitect primers were used for each reaction of 20 µl. PCR were performed with the following settings; denaturation 95°C for 10 sec., annealing 60°C, 6 sec. and extension 72°C, 5 sec. For analysis of Akt (QT00114401), mTOR (QT01532916) and PI3-kinase (QT00149709), 2 µl cDNA and 2 µl of premixed Quantitect primers were used for each reaction of 20 µl. Real time PCR were performed using QuantiFast™SYBR Green PCR kit (Qiagen). Quantitative results were produced by the relative standard curve method. All samples were analyzed in duplicates and negative controls were included in each run. All results are related to the expression of Gapdh as housekeeping gene according to separate evaluations among 12 gene alternatives, where Gapdh showed minimal alterations in response to starvation/refeeding with 8% variation among all the groups at extreme conditions as starvation/refeeding ($0.15 < p > 0.80$).

Protein synthesis

Fractional liver and skeletal muscle protein synthesis were measured by the flooding dose technique as described [21,22]. A single dose injection of L-[U-^{14}C] phenylalanine

(0.4 µCi/g) in 150 mM phenylalanine was provided ip. 30 minutes before killing. Liver tissue and mixed hind limb muscles were rapidly excised and frozen in liquid nitrogen until analysis. Blood samples were heparinized and immediately centrifuged at +4°C and plasma was frozen until analysis. Fractional synthesis rate ($\% \times hr^{-1}$) was calculated as described [9].

Western blotting

Mixed hind limb muscles were rapidly excised and frozen in liquid nitrogen until next day when biopsies were thawed and homogenized in seven volumes of ice-cold buffer A (20 mM Hepes, pH 7.4, 100 mM KCl, 0.2 mM EDTA, 2 mM EGTA, 1 mM DTT, 50 mM NaF, 50 mM β–glycerophosphate, 0.1 mM AEBSF, 1 mM bensamidine, 0.5 mM sodium vanadate). The homogenate was centrifuged at 10 000 × g for 10 min at 4°C. Aliquots of the supernatant were used for western blot analysis of phosphorylation state of 4EBP1 and p70s6 kinase or immunoprecipitated for analysis of 4EBP1 · eIF4E complexes as previously described [23]. Anti-eIF4E antibodies used were a kind gift from Dr Scot Kimball, Pennsylvania State University, USA. All blot membranes were exposed to Hyperfilm ECL (Amersham Biosciences, UK) and quantification was carried out with Quantity One software (Bio-Rad Laboratories AB, Sundbyberg, Sweden). For quantification of 4EBP1 · eIF4E complex the total optical density was measured and the results were corrected for eIF4E content. Optical density is expressed in arbitrary units. The phosphorylation state of 4EBP1 is expressed as percentage of the most phosphorylated γ-form compared to the total and calculated as optical density of the γ-band/optical density of all bands [(α+β+γ)*100]. Phosphorylation state of p70s6 kinase was measured by gel mobility shift and is expressed as percentage of the least phosphorylated α form compared to the total and calculated as optical density of the α-band/optical density of all bands [(α+β+γ)*100]. For measurement of mTOR and phosphorylated mTOR[2448], aliquots of the homogenate supernatant were mixed with equal volumes of 2x SDS electrophoresis sample buffer and separated in a 3-8% NuPage Tris-acetate mini gel (Invitrogen). Proteins were transferred to PVDF membranes, which were incubated over night at +4°C with a rabbit anti mouse mTOR[2448] antibody (#2971, Cell Signaling Technology) after blocking in 10% nonfat dry milk in Tris-buffered Saline-Tween 20. The blots were then washed, incubated with secondary antibodies and developed using an ECL Western Blotting Kit according to the manufacturers description (Amersham Biosciences, UK) and exposed against Hyperfilm ECL (Amersham Biosciences, UK). After detection of signals, antibodies were removed by 45 minutes incubation at +50°C in stripping buffer (100 mM 2-mercaptoethanol, 2% sodium dodecyl sulfat (SDS), 62.5 mM Tris–HCl pH 7.6) and membranes were thereafter reprobed for measurement of total mTOR by incubating membranes 75 min at room temperature with a rabbit anti human mTOR antibody (sc-8319, Santa Cruz biotechnology, Santa Cruz, USA) Quantification of signals was carried out with GS-710 imaging densitometer and Quantity One software (Bio-Rad Laboratories AB, Sundbyberg, Sweden). Measured optical density was expressed as arbitrary units. On each gel, 2 lanes were loaded with MagicMark XP Western Protein Standards (Invitrogen). The average optical density for the standard band with most similar molecular size as the measured protein was used to normalize signal intensity between blots.

Western ligand blotting

IGF-I ligand blotting was performed under conditions described by Hosssenlopp et.al. [24]. Equal volumes from each supernatant with similar amount of proteins of the prepared muscle homogenates in one group were pooled and mixed with an equal volume of Laemmli sample buffer and heated to 95°C. 15 µl of the samples were separated by electrophoresis on 12% Tris-Glycine gels using non-reduced conditions and transferred to PVDF membranes. Membranes were blocked and incubated overnight with ^{125}I-labelled IGF-I (PerkinElmer). After washing, blots were exposed to Hyperfilm MP at –70°C. Films were scanned and band intensity was measured (Quantity One software, GS-710 densitometer, BioRad). The molecular weight of IGFBPs was estimated from prestained standards.

Plasma concentrations

Plasma IGF-I was measured by an IGF-I binding protein blocked RIA (Mediagnost). Glucose was measured with the glucose oxidase method according to the manufacturers' instructions (Roche). Plasma amino acids were analyzed by HPLC as described elsewhere [25,26], in order to relate alterations in Igf-I/Igf-Ir transcript expression to changes in plasma amino acids, which may be stimulators of muscle protein synthesis [20,27]. Growth hormone (GH) and insulin were measured with ELISA methods (Linco research). Plasma IGFBPs were not measured since IGFBPs were estimated in the muscle tissue compartment.

Statistics

Results are presented as mean ± SEM based on 8 animals in each group except for 7 mice in starved wild type and 9 in Li-IGF-I $^{(-/-)}$. Factorial ANOVA was used to test within groups and among groups followed by Fisher PLSD test for multiple comparisons. P<0.05 was considered statistically significant and p < 0.10 a trend to significance in two tailed tests.

Results

Plasma concentrations

Plasma levels of IGF-I were reduced by 70% in liver IGF-I knockout mice (Li-IGF-I $^{(-/-)}$) compared to wild type mice at all nutritional conditions (<0.001), while glucose and insulin levels were comparable among Li-IGF-I $^{(-/-)}$ and wild type mice. Overnight starvation caused a significant decrease in plasma glucose compared to freely fed mice in both knockout and wt mice (p<0.05) (Table 1). Growth hormone did not change significantly within groups during freely feeding, starvation and refeeding and it was not significantly altered when comparing between groups. Branched chain and essential amino acids were significantly altered during starvation-refeeding in wild type mice, but not in liver IGF-I knockouts. These alterations were also reflected in concentrations of the sum of all amino acids (Table 2).

Protein synthesis

The magnitude of basal fractional synthesis rate in liver and muscle tissue was comparable in freely fed wild type and liver IGF-I knockout mice. Refeeding increased similarly liver (p < 0.10) and muscle protein synthesis (p < 0.01) compared to starvation in both wild type and liver IGF-I knockout animals (Figure 1A,B).

RNA transcripts in skeletal muscles

mRNA transcript levels were comparable in freely fed wild type and knockout mice (Igf-I, Igf-Ireceptor, PI3-kinase, Akt and mTOR). However, Igf-I transcripts decreased significantly in muscles from wild type mice during starvation but with a different time course in knockouts. Igf-Ir increased similarly during starvation in both wild type and knockout mice and remained increased during refeeding (Figure 2A-B). Significant changes in transcript levels of PI3k and Akt were not observed (PI3-kinase: WT, FF 1.40±0.15, ST 1.12±0.16, RF 1.54±0.21; Li-IGF$^{(-/-)}$, FF 1.13±0.18, ST 1.62±0.17, RF 1.50±0.26) (Akt: WT, FF 1.09±0.15, ST 1.14±0.08,

RF 1.41±0.16; Li-IGF$^{(-/-)}$, FF 1.12±0.13, ST 1.54±.24, RF 1.49±0.17). By contrast, mTOR expression was significantly increased in starved knockout animals compared to refed mice without any similar change in wild type mice (Figure 2C). However, this increased transcript level did not correspond to altered mTOR protein levels among animal groups (not shown).

Translational and cell signaling proteins in skeletal muscle tissue

The 4EBP1·eIF4E complex, 4EBP1 phosphorylation state (% γ of total), p70s6k phosphorylation (% α of total) and mTOR posporylation (p-mTOR^{ser2448}/mTOR^{total}) were comparable among wild type and liver IGF-I knockout mice. Starvation significantly increased muscle content of 4EBP1·eIF4E complexes with corresponding normalization in refed animals (Figure 3A). The 4EBP1 phosphorylation state was significantly and similarly decreased in starved mice compared to freely fed mice with significant increase in refed wild type and liver IGF-I knockout mice (Figure 3B). p70s6k and mTOR^{2448} was less phosphorylated in starved wild type and liver IGF-I knockout mice with complete reversal in both groups during refeeding (Figure 3C,D,E). IGFBP content was similar among all groups (Figure 4) indicating comparable extracellular conditions of binding proteins among the groups.

Discussion

Anabolic effects by IGF-I are well recognized, particularly such as stimulation of protein synthesis related to cell proliferation, tissue growth and cell differentiation [6,28]. Parts of these effects are probably mediated by muscle tissue specific IGF-I isoforms such as the mechano growth factor [29]. We have earlier assumed that circulating IGF-I is involved in promotion of diurnal alterations of muscle protein synthesis in response to meal feeding [14]; where a similar role may be assumed for insulin [5]. Our earlier studies have, however, not confirmed an important and primary role of insulin in physiologic resynthesis of skeletal

Table 1 Plasma concentrations in study (starved, refed) and control mice (freely fed) from wild type and liver IGF-I knockout mice

		Freely fed	Starved	Refed	Within groups p<	Among groups p<
Glucose (mmol/l)	wt	10.4 ± 0.5	8.0 ± 0.6	11.3 ± 0.4	0.05	
	IGF-	12.3 ± 1.2	8.1 ± 0.6	10.0 ± 0.8	0.05	ns
Insulin (µg/l)	wt	0.58±0.09	0.35±0.05	0.93±0.16	0.01	
	IGF-	1.11±0.26	0.43±0.07	0.98±0.20	0.05	ns
IGF-I (µg/l)	wt	172 ± 13	138 ± 13	159 ± 8	ns	
	IGF-	58 ± 7	40 ± 7	46 ± 7	ns	0.01
GH (µg/l)[a]	wt	2.0±0.8	5.1±2.1	12.6±7.3	ns	
	IGF-	11.5±8.5	15±6.1	17.6±11.3	ns	ns

Mean±SEM.
A measured at 9 a.m.

Table 2 Plasma amino acids in freely fed, starved and refed mice as described in material and methods

		Freely fed	Starved	Refed	Within groups p<0.05	Among groups p<0.05
			μmol/liter			
Essential AA						
Isoleucine	wt	61 ± 6	56 ± 4	67 ± 9	ns	
	IGF-	59 ± 6	72 ± 7	50 ± 6	ns	ns
Leucine	wt	124 ± 17	84 ± 6	179 ± 29	0.05	
	IGF-	111 ± 12	114 ± 11	131 ± 20	ns	ns
Valine	wt	161 ± 16	120 ± 6	176 ± 20	ns	
	IGF-	152 ± 12	156 ± 13	143 ± 17	ns	ns
BCAA	**wt**	**346 ± 38**	**260 ± 16**	**422 ± 58**	**0.05**	
	IGF-	**321 ± 28**	**342 ± 31**	**325 ± 43**	**ns**	ns
Lysine	wt	258 ± 16	246 ± 16	277 ± 14	ns	
	IGF-	281 ± 21	282 ± 26	273 ± 21	ns	ns
Methionine	wt	55 ± 7	41 ± 5	97 ± 10	0.001	
	IGF-	48 ± 5	38 ± 3	77 ± 13	0.01	ns
Phenylalanine	wt	287 ± 37	389 ± 107	386 ± 93	ns	
	IGF-	402 ± 86	277 ± 36	311 ± 72	ns	ns
Threonine	wt	147 ± 14	119 ± 10	207 ± 13	0.05	
	IGF-	125 ± 7	114 ± 8	162 ± 20	0.05	0.05
Tryptophan	wt	34 ± 4	30 ± 3	42 ± 4	ns	
	IGF-	36 ± 3	35 ± 4	33 ± 3	ns	ns
Essential AA	**wt**	**1127 ± 80**	**1086 ± 119**	**1433 ± 89**	**0.05**	
	IGF-	**1213 ± 112**	**1089 ± 70**	**1181 ± 91**	**ns**	ns
Non-essential AA						
Alanine	wt	337 ± 33	262 ± 37	547 ± 47	0.001	
	IGF-	283 ± 26	194 ± 13	459 ± 44	0.001	0,01
Arginine	wt	77 ± 12	20 ± 7	43 ± 10	0.01	
	IGF-	56 ± 14	41 ± 9	30 ± 10	ns	ns
Aspartic acid	wt	37 ± 6	34 ± 3	25 ± 3	ns	
	IGF-	22 ± 2	40 ± 6	33 ± 4	ns	ns
Asparagine	wt	31 ± 2	27 ± 2	41 ± 2	0.01	
	IGF-	25 ± 2	25 ± 1	32 ± 3	ns	0.01
Citrulline	wt	30 ± 3	20 ± 2	34 ± 2	0.01	
	IGF-	29 ± 2	20 ± 1	30 ± 3	0.01	ns
Glutamic acid	wt	166 ± 18	152 ± 16	129 ± 15	ns	
	IGF-	166 ± 11	138 ± 13	158 ± 23	ns	ns
Glutamine	wt	538 ± 36	520 ± 30	578 ± 31	ns	
	IGF-	553 ± 27	516 ± 42	560 ± 35	ns	ns
Glycine	wt	174 ± 18	170 ± 17	178 ± 10	ns	
	IGF-	150 ± 9	140 ± 15	175 ± 24	ns	ns
Histidine	wt	53 ± 4	50 ± 3	70 ± 4	0.01	
	IGF-	57 ± 4	52 ± 4	64 ± 4	ns	ns
Serine	wt	108 ± 12	85 ± 5	136 ± 5	0.01	
	IGF-	93 ± 16	75 ± 5	118 ± 9	0.01	ns
Tyrosine	wt	330 ± 23	395 ± 65	339 ± 82	ns	

Table 2 Plasma amino acids in freely fed, starved and refed mice as described in material and methods *(Continued)*

	IGF-	323 ± 39	239 ± 40	285 ± 59	ns	ns
Ornitine	wt	88 ± 22	90 ± 12	109 ± 16	ns	
	IGF-	109 ± 16	83 ± 15	115 ± 10	ns	ns
α-Aba	wt	7 ± 1	8 ± 1	9 ± 1	ns	
	IGF-	6 ± 1	6 ± 1	8 ± 1	ns	ns
Non-ess. AA	**wt**	**1977 ± 142**	**1835 ± 149**	**2237 ± 89**	**ns**	
	IGF-	1872 ± 71	1570 ± 112	2065 ± 125	0.05	ns
Total AA	**wt**	**3103 ± 219**	**2921 ± 264**	**3669 ± 143**	**0.05**	
	IGF-	3085 ± 171	2659 ± 180	3246 ± 205	0.08	ns

Mean±SEM.
wt = wild type mice.
IGF- = hepatic deficient IGF-I $^{(-/-)}$ mice.

muscles during animal starvation-refeeding experiments [4], as well as in human skeletal muscles, where insulin only attenuated break down of non-myofibrillar proteins [2]. Therefore, we assumed that endocrine IGF-I may have a role in stimulation of diurnal variations of protein synthesis in skeletal muscles related to feeding with increased flux of substrates and amino acids across cell membranes [30]. A role of IGF-1 was also tempting, when we observed that locally expressed IGF-I decreased in muscle tissue following overnight starvation and increased in response to meal feeding [5]. However, the complex situation, with protein bound circulating IGF-I and locally produced IGF-I, makes

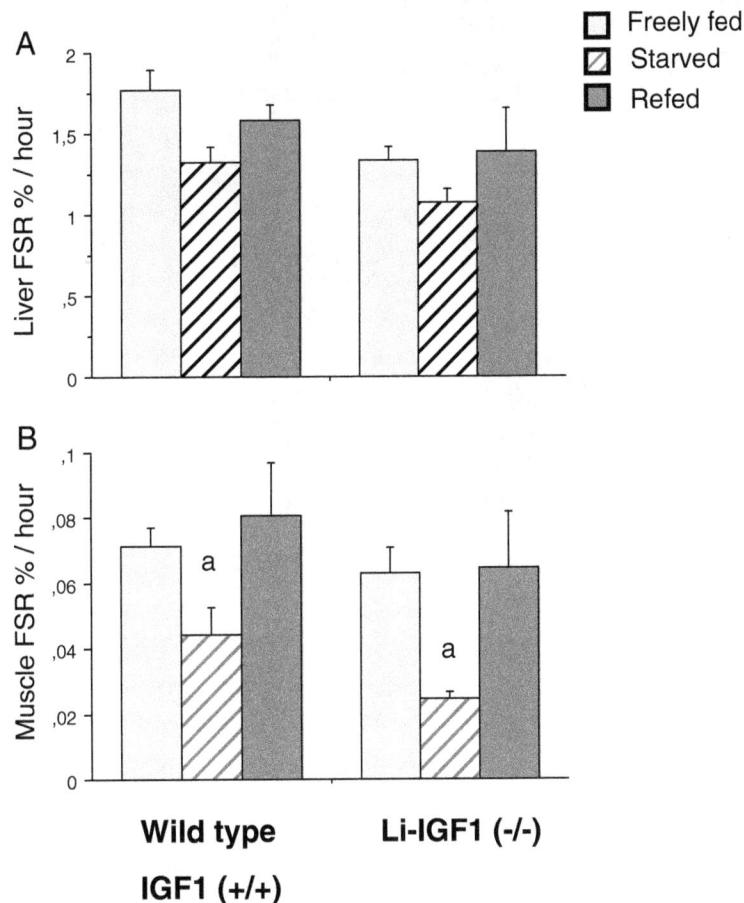

Figure 1 A,B Effects of starvation-refeeding on synthesis rate of proteins in mixed skeletal muscle and liver tissue. FSR% was measured with the "flooding dose" technique ($[^{14}C]$-Phe) as described. Animals were freely fed, starved for 12 hours or refed during 3 hours after starvation period as described in Methods. Results are mean ± SEM for 7–9 animals per group. a-p<0.05 vs. freely fed and refed mice.

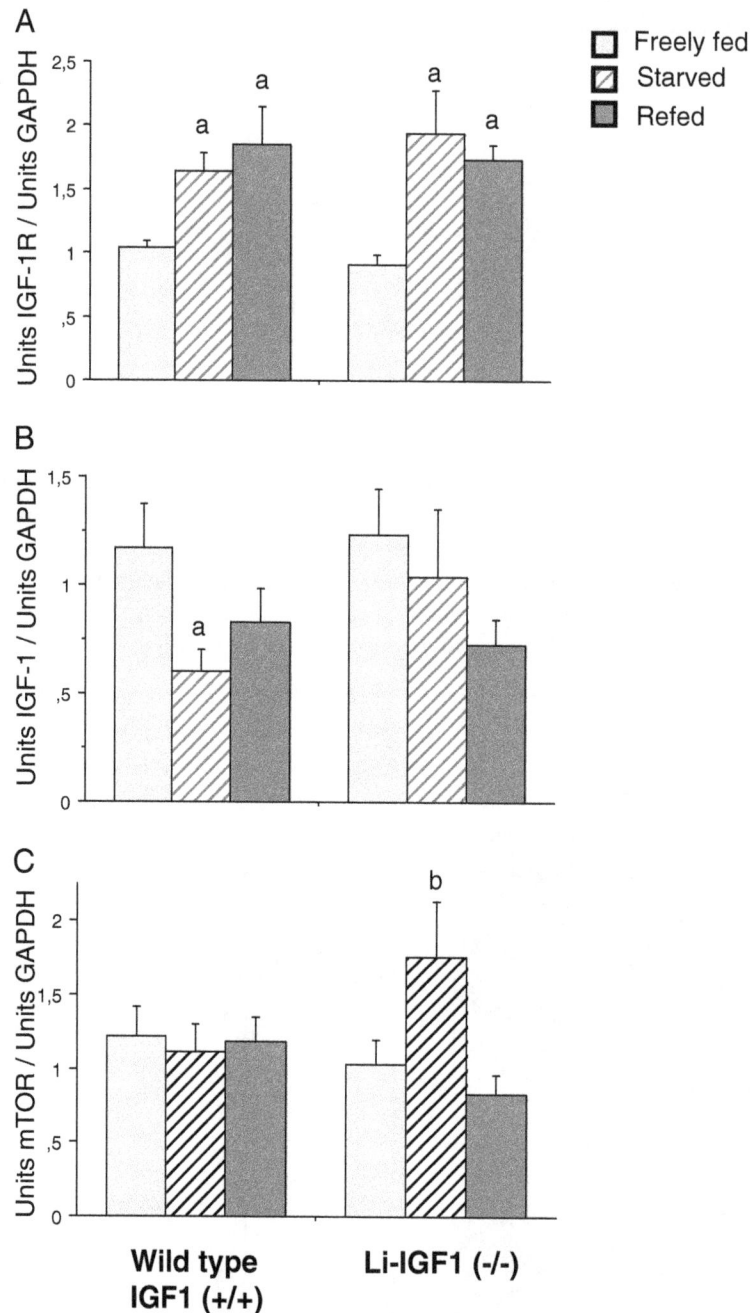

Figure 2 A-C Effects of starvation-refeeding on Igf-I, Igf-Ir and mTOR mRNA content in skeletal muscle tissue. Analyzed by quantitative PCR using SYBRgreen detection. Results are mean ± SEM for 7–9 animals per group. a-p<0.05 vs. freely fed animals. b-<0.05 vs. freely fed and refed animals.

it difficult to demonstrate defined roles for the various IGF-I compartments, particularly when binding proteins themselves may have independent regulatory functions across muscle membranes [11,12]. Therefore, it seemed interesting to apply investigations in liver IGF-I knockout mice, where IGF-I in the circulation is low due to a lack in production of IGF-I in the liver and spleen, in order to re-examine the role of circulating level versus local tissue

expression of IGF-I/IGF-IR for alterations in skeletal muscle protein synthesis during starvation-refeeding [5,9].

Earlier attempts to study nutritional effects by IGF-I have not provided unanimous and conclusive results [5,9,31]. We found that injection of anti IGF-I antibodies before feeding of mice attenuated a subsequent rise in protein synthesis by 25%, while ip. injections of IGF-I to overnight starved mice only increased protein synthesis

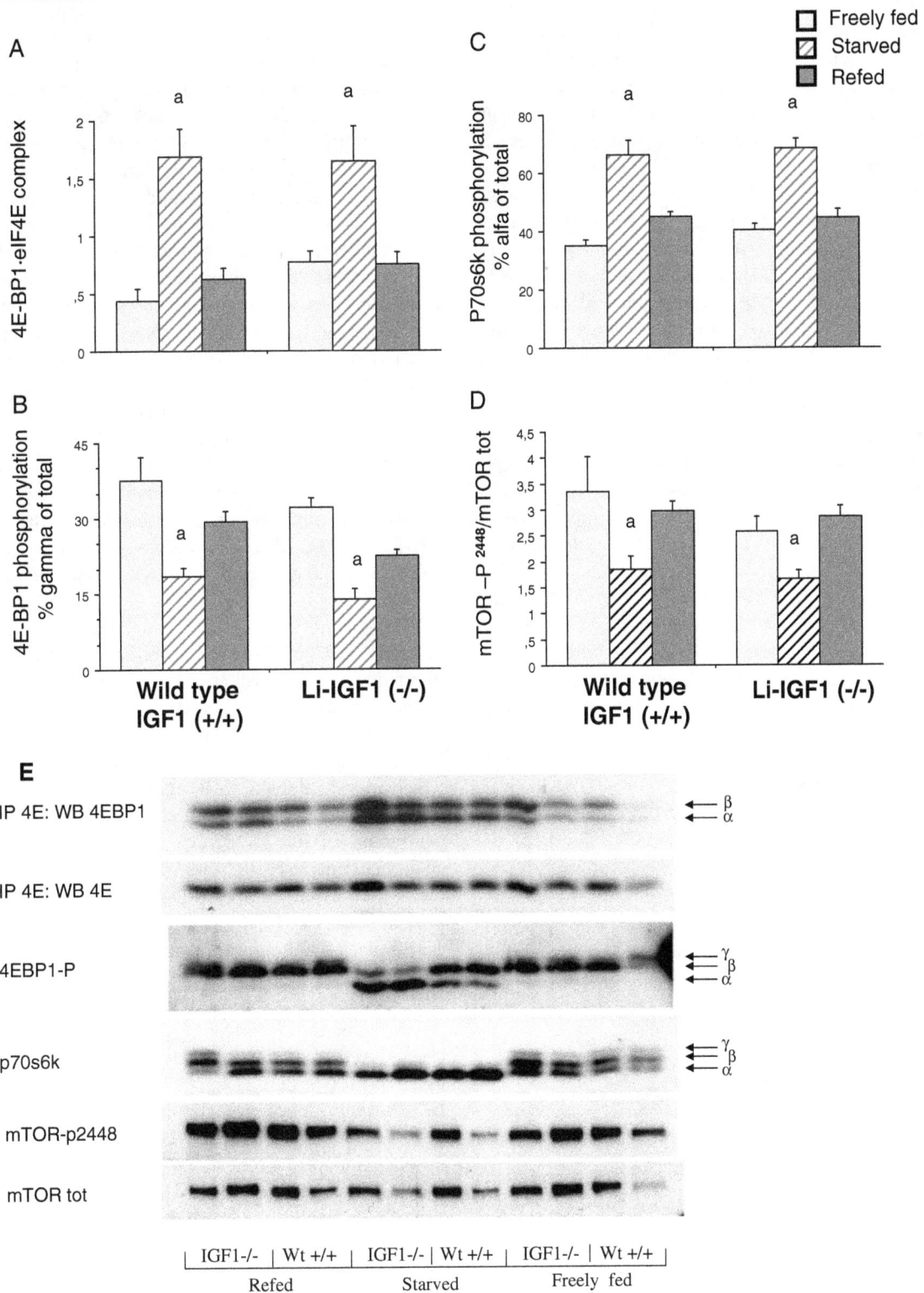

Figure 3 A-E Effects of starvation-refeeding on total 4E-BP1 · eIF4E complex (A), 4E-BP1 · phosphorylation (B) p70s6kinase phosphorylation (C) and mTOR phosphorylation in skeletal muscle tissue. Figure 3E is a representative blot, one of four, of each analysis. Proteins were immunoprecipitated with a monoclonal anti-eIF4E antibody and thereafter analyzed by Western blot with an antibody against 4E-BP1 in analysis of 4E-BP1 · eIF4E complex. Results are mean ± SEM with 7–9 animals per group. a-p<0.01 vs. freely fed and refed mice. All blot analyses were perfomed on the same protein extracts with the same amount of total protein applied among the groups (not shown).

marginally [5], and studies on genetically altered mice implied that fractional resynthesis of muscle protein was not clear-cut related to circulating GH, blood IGF-I and locally produced IGF-I mRNA [9]. Others have however reported that a one hour iv. infusion of IGF-I to over-night starved mice increased muscle protein synthesis to levels comparable to fed mice [32]. Furthermore, re-duced free plasma IGF-I by 50% of normal levels, by in-fusion of IGF binding protein 1, decreased muscle protein synthesis by 25% with decreased phosphorylation of p70s6 kinase [33], while provision of IGF-I/IGFBP-3 complex improved sepsis induced muscle catabolism [34]. However, plasma IGF-I did not diverge from basal levels in humans who received a drink of essential amino acids at a time when muscle protein synthesis was stim-ulated by more than 100% [35]. Another study in humans evaluated effects by IGF-I when infused directly into arm muscle bed compared to systemically raised IGF-I [36], where protein synthesis was only increased subsequently to locally infused IGF-I. A study, based on microdialysis, revealed that concentrations of free IGF-I in muscle interstitial fluid were 20 fold higher than sim-ultaneous plasma levels, supporting that circulating IGF-I is not directly determining rates of protein synthesis during feeding [37]; observations in line with our own findings that infused amino acids improved protein bal-ance across human muscles independently of plasma in-sulin, IGF-I and IGF-I-binding proteins-1 and −3 [3].

A compensatory factor in the present study may be that increased levels of growth hormone (GH) in liver-IGF-I knockouts, observed in the present and a previous study, would counteract subnormal IGF-I levels in the circulation [15] since cell experiments indicate that GH phosphorylates similar or the same downstream targets for protein synthesis as amino acids and IGF-I through PI3-kinase dependent transduction [38]. Also, GH treat-ment increased fractional muscle protein synthesis in fed but not in starved pigs [39]. However, in a previous study we used mice where circulating levels of both GH and IGF-I were low and found that fractional muscle protein synthesis increased normally to expected levels after food intake [9]. Re-synthesis of muscle protein fol-lowing starvation-refeeding did not relate to plasma GH concentrations in either knockouts or wild type mice. Therefore, we find it unlikely that GH explains rapid al-terations in the feeding related muscle protein synthesis evaluated in the present model.

We found no difference between liver IGF-I deficient and wild type mice regarding translational control of muscle protein synthesis. Both liver IGF-I knockouts and wild type mice showed increased phosphorylation of 4EBP1 protein and decreased association of the 4E-BP1 · eIF4E complex. Also, p70s6 kinase phosphorylation was increased similarly in both groups including upstream phosphorylation of $mTOR^{ser2448}$. Thus, effects by circulat-ing IGF-I were less critical for the control of translation initiation compared to other possible factors such as plasma or extracellular amino acids, although consistent changes in plasma amino acids were not observed among IGF-I deficient and wild type mice at starvation-refeeding. However, we did not measure eIF4G · eIF4E complexes, which may be influenced by IGF-I as reported by others using a hindlimb perfusion model, where physiologic con-centrations of IGF-I (10 nM) in the presence of amino acids were unable to dissociate 4E-BP1 from eIF4E, but in-creased the assembly of eIF4G-4E complex and stimulated protein synthesis [40].

Both liver IGF-I knockouts and wild type mice showed increased muscle expression of the IGF-IR during starva-tion, which usually reflects cellular processes related to regeneration and hypertrophy of muscle cells [6]. This in-creased receptor expression may reflect a positive feed-back control of IGF-I signaling secondary to decreased IGF-I protein close to membranes; a conclusion supported by observations in cultured cells on increased IGF-IR number and promoted amino acid transport related to decreased extracellular concentration of amino acids, par-ticularly glutamine [30,41]. Increased transcript and IGF-IR protein levels have also been reported in response to exercise [42-44], but information of similar changes in re-lation to feeding are sparse, although equivalent observa-tions have been reported [45,46]. Thus, IGF-IR expression appears more tightly controlled than tissue IGF-I expres-sion in skeletal muscle metabolism in response to starva-tion – refeeding. By contrast to feeding, a recent report in mice with non-functional IGF-IR showed that load-

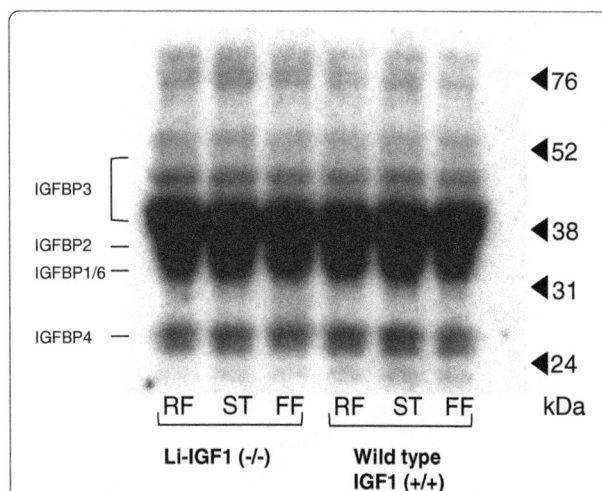

Figure 4 Radioligand blot which demonstrates similar levels of IGF binding proteins in skeletal muscle tissue among groups in relationship to molecular weights (24–76 kD). Approximate mobility of IGF-I binding proteins 1–6 is indicated to the left. The same amount of proteins (±3%) was loaded in all tracks determined by spectrophotometry.

induced hypertrophy occurred [47], which suggested that increased protein synthesis following exercise was not entirely dependent on IGF-IR signaling.

There were no changes in either PI3K or AKT expression during starvation-refeeding, while mTOR transcript expression was up-regulated in liver-IGF-I knockouts during starvation, but without apparent change in protein phosphorylation. This up-regulation in starved knockouts may therefore reflect compensatory effects unrelated to phosphorylation of mTOR, secondary to consistently decreased circulating IGF-I. If so, it remains to be explored which factor(s) that up-regulates mTOR expression in muscle tissue when endocrine IGF-I is declined, particularly during starvation of knockout mice (Figure 2C).

Conclusion

In conclusion, our present results confirm previous reports that alteration in muscle protein synthesis during starvation–refeeding relates to alteration in muscle mTOR signaling, but not to Akt and PI3-kinase. Present findings also support our previous conclusions that muscle produced IGF-I/IGF-IR are related to translation initiation of muscle proteins at oral feeding. [5]. New information is that endocrine IGF-I is not, critical for this effect. It remains to determine to what extent local muscle IGF-I signaling is critical, since systemically IGF-I $^{(+/-)}$ knockout mice had normal fractional synthesis rate (%/hrs) in skeletal muscles at refeeding [9]. Whether a lack of effects by liver derived IGF-I may be overcome by alternative signals upstream to mTOR remains also to be determined, but insulin and GH are probably not such candidates.

Abbreviations
AEBSF: 4-(2-aminoethyl)benzenesulfonyl fluoride; EGTA: Ethylene-bis [oxyethylenenitrilo]tetraacetic acid; KCl: Potassium chloride; NaF: Sodium fluoride; eIF4E: Eukaryotic initiation factor 4E; eIF4G: Eukaryotic initiation factor 4G; 4E-BP1: Eukaryotic initiation factor 4E binding protein 1; p70s6k: Ribosomal protein S6 Kinase, 70-kDa; Li-IGF-I: Liver derived IGF-I; IGF-IR: IGF-I receptor; PiPc: Polyinosinic- polycytidylic acid; mTOR: mammalian target of Rapamycin; PI3K: Phosphatidylinositol 3-kinase; Akt: Proteinkinase B-alpha; DTT: Ditiotreitiol; EDTA: Ethylenediaminetetraacetic acid.

Competing interests
The authors' declare that they have no competing interests.

Authors' contributions
B.I carried out the analyses, calculated statistics, and drafted manuscript, JS CO generated the transgenic mice KL. Conceived of the study and drafted manuscript. All authors participated in study design and critical revision of manuscript. All authors have read and approved the manuscript.

Acknowledgements
Supported in parts by grants from the Swedish Cancer Society (2014), the Swedish Research Council (08712), Assar Gabrielsson Foundation (AB Volvo), Jubileumskliniken Foundation, IngaBritt & Arne Lundberg Research Foundation, Swedish and Gothenburg Medical Societies and the Medical Faculty, University of Gothenburg, Sahlgrenska University Hospital Foundation, Swedish Nutrition Foundation Wilhelm and Martina Lundgren Research foundation.

Author details
[1]Department of Surgery Sahlgrenska University Hospital Kir., Metabol lab Bruna Stråket 20-413 45, Gothenburg, Sweden. [2]Department of Internal Medicine, Sahlgrenska Academy, University of Gothenburg, Gothenburg, Sweden.

References
1. Vary TC, Lynch CJ: Meal feeding enhances formation of eIF4F in skeletal muscle: role of increased eIF4E availability and eIF4G phosphorylation. *Am J Physiol Endocrinol Metab* 2006, **290**(4):E631–642.
2. Moller-Loswick AC, Zachrisson H, Hyltander A, Korner U, Matthews DE, Lundholm K: Insulin selectively attenuates breakdown of nonmyofibrillar proteins in peripheral tissues of normal men. *Am J Physiol* 1994, **266**(4 Pt 1):E645–652.
3. Svanberg E, Moller-Loswick AC, Matthews DE, Korner U, Andersson M, Lundholm K: Effects of amino acids on synthesis and degradation of skeletal muscle proteins in humans. *Am J Physiol* 1996, **271**(4 Pt 1):E718–724.
4. Svanberg E, Jefferson LS, Lundholm K, Kimball SR: Postprandial stimulation of muscle protein synthesis is independent of changes in insulin. *Am J Physiol* 1997, **272**(5 Pt 1):E841–847.
5. Svanberg E, Zachrisson H, Ohlsson C, Iresjo BM, Lundholm KG: Role of insulin and IGF-I in activation of muscle protein synthesis after oral feeding. *Am J Physiol* 1996, **270**(4 Pt 1):E614–620.
6. Philippou A, Halapas A, Maridaki M, Koutsilieris M: Type I insulin-like growth factor receptor signaling in skeletal muscle regeneration and hypertrophy. *J Musculoskelet Neuronal Interact* 2007, **7**(3):208–218.
7. Stewart CE, Pell JM: Point: Counterpoint: IGF is/is not the major physiological regulator of muscle mass. Point: IGF is the major physiological regulator of muscle mass. *J Appl Physiol* 2010, **108**(6):1820–1821. discussion 1823–1824; author reply 1832.
8. Flueck M, Goldspink G: Point: Counterpoint: IGF is/is not the major physiological regulator of muscle mass. Counterpoint: IGF is not the major physiological regulator of muscle mass. *J Appl Physiol* 2010, **108**(6):1821–1823. discussion 1823–1824; author reply 1833.
9. Svanberg E, Powell-Braxton L, Ohlsson C, Zachrisson H, Lundholm K: The role of the growth hormone/insulin-like growth factor I axis in stimulation of protein synthesis in skeletal muscles following oral refeeding. *Endocrinology* 1998, **139**(12):4906–4910.
10. Awede B, Thissen J, Gailly P, Lebacq J: Regulation of IGF-I, IGFBP-4 and IGFBP-5 gene expression by loading in mouse skeletal muscle. *FEBS Lett* 1999, **461**(3):263–267.
11. Frost RA, Lang CH: Differential effects of insulin-like growth factor I (IGF-I) and IGF-binding protein-1 on protein metabolism in human skeletal muscle cells. *Endocrinology* 1999, **140**(9):3962–3970.
12. Spangenburg EE, Abraha T, Childs TE, Pattison JS, Booth FW: Skeletal muscle IGF-binding protein-3 and −5 expressions are age, muscle, and load dependent. *Am J Physiol Endocrinol Metab* 2003, **284**(2):E340–350.
13. Wang W, Iresjo BM, Karlsson L, Svanberg E: Provision of rhIGF-I/IGFBP-3 complex attenuated development of cancer cachexia in an experimental tumor model. *Clin Nutr* 2000, **19**(2):127–132.
14. Svanberg E, Ohlsson C, Kimball SR: Lundholm K: rhIGF-I/IGFBP-3 complex, but not free rhIGF-I, supports muscle protein biosynthesis in rats during semistarvation. *Eur J Clin Invest* 2000, **30**(5):438–446.
15. Sjogren K, Liu JL, Blad K, Skrtic S, Vidal O, Wallenius V, LeRoith D, Tornell J, Isaksson OG, Jansson JO, et al: Liver-derived insulin-like growth factor I (IGF-I) is the principal source of IGF-I in blood but is not required for postnatal body growth in mice. *Proc Natl Acad Sci U S A* 1999, **96**(12):7088–7092.
16. Sjogren K, Wallenius K, Liu JL, Bohlooly YM, Pacini G, Svensson L, Tornell J, Isaksson OG, Ahren B, Jansson JO, et al: Liver-derived IGF-I is of importance for normal carbohydrate and lipid metabolism. *Diabetes* 2001, **50**(7):1539–1545.
17. Svensson J, Sjogren K, Faldt J, Andersson N, Isaksson O, Jansson JO, Ohlsson C: Liver-derived IGF-I regulates mean life span in mice. *PloS one* 2011, **6**(7):e22640.
18. Miller BF, Hansen M, Olesen JL, Flyvbjerg A, Schwarz P, Babraj JA, Smith K, Rennie MJ, Kjaer M: No effect of menstrual cycle on myofibrillar and connective tissue protein synthesis in contracting skeletal muscle. *Am J Physiol Endocrinol Metab* 2006, **290**(1):E163–E168.

19. Toth MJ, Poehlman ET, Matthews DE, Tchernof A, MacCoss MJ: **Effects of estradiol and progesterone on body composition, protein synthesis, and lipoprotein lipase in rats.** *Am J Physiol Endocrinol Metab* 2001, **280**(3):E496–501.

20. Svanberg E, Ohlsson C, Hyltander A, Lundholm KG: **The role of diet components, gastrointestinal factors, and muscle innervation on activation of protein synthesis in skeletal muscles following oral refeeding.** *Nutrition* 1999, **15**(4):257–266.

21. Garlick PJ, McNurlan MA, Preedy VR: **A rapid and convenient technique for measuring the rate of protein synthesis in tissues by injection of [3H] phenylalanine.** *Biochem J* 1980, **192**(2):719–723.

22. Lundholm K, Ternell M, Zachrisson H, Moldawer L, Lindstrom L: **Measurement of hepatic protein synthesis in unrestrained mice- evaluation of the 'flooding technique'.** *Acta Physiol Scand* 1991, **141**(2):207–219.

23. Iresjo BM, Svanberg E, Lundholm K: **Reevaluation of amino acid stimulation of protein synthesis in murine- and human-derived skeletal muscle cells assessed by independent techniques.** *Am J Physiol Endocrinol Metab* 2005, **288**(5):E1028–1037.

24. Hossenlopp P, Seurin D, Segovia-Quinson B, Hardouin S, Binoux M: **Analysis of serum insulin-like growth factor binding proteins using western blotting: use of the method for titration of the binding proteins and competitive binding studies.** *Analytical biochemistry* 1986, **154**(1):138–143.

25. Georgi G, Pietsch C, Sawatzki G: **High-performance liquid chromatographic determination of amino acids in protein hydrolysates and in plasma using automated pre-column derivatization with o-phthaldialdehyde/2-mercaptoethanol.** *J Chromatogr* 1993, **613**(1):35–42.

26. Iresjo BM, Korner U, Larsson B, Henriksson BA, Lundholm K: **Appearance of individual amino acid concentrations in arterial blood during steady-state infusions of different amino acid formulations to ICU patients in support of whole-body protein metabolism.** *JPEN J Parenter Enteral Nutr* 2006, **30**(4):277–285.

27. Svanberg E, Moller-Loswick AC, Matthews DE, Korner U, Andersson M, Lundholm K: **The role of glucose, long-chain triglycerides and amino acids for promotion of amino acid balance across peripheral tissues in man.** *Clin Physiol* 1999, **19**(4):311–320.

28. Sievers C, Schneider HJ, Stalla GK: **Insulin-like growth factor-1 in plasma and brain: regulation in health and disease.** *Front Biosci* 2008, **13**:85–99.

29. Goldspink G: **Loss of muscle strength during aging studied at the gene level.** *Rejuvenation Res* 2007, **10**(3):397–405.

30. Wang HS, Wasa M, Okada A: **Amino acid transport in a human neuroblastoma cell line is regulated by the type I insulin-like growth factor receptor.** *Life Sci* 2002, **71**(2):127–137.

31. Sandstrom R, Svanberg E, Hyltander A, Haglind E, Ohlsson C, Zachrisson H, Berglund B, Lindholm E, Brevinge H, Lundholm K: **The effect of recombinant human IGF-I on protein metabolism in post- operative patients without nutrition compared to effects in experimental animals.** *Eur J Clin Invest* 1995, **25**(10):784–792.

32. Bark TH, McNurlan MA, Lang CH, Garlick PJ: **Increased protein synthesis after acute IGF-I or insulin infusion is localized to muscle in mice.** *Am J Physiol* 1998, **275**(1 Pt 1):E118–123.

33. Lang CH, Vary TC, Frost RA: **Acute in vivo elevation of insulin-like growth factor (IGF) binding protein-1 decreases plasma free IGF-I and muscle protein synthesis.** *Endocrinology* 2003, **144**(9):3922–3933.

34. Svanberg E, Frost RA, Lang CH, Isgaard J, Jefferson LS, Kimball SR, Vary TC: **IGF-I/IGFBP-3 binary complex modulates sepsis-induced inhibition of protein synthesis in skeletal muscle.** *Am J Physiol Endocrinol Metab* 2000, **279**(5):E1145–1158.

35. Cuthbertson D, Smith K, Babraj J, Leese G, Waddell T, Atherton P, Wackerhage H, Taylor PM, Rennie MJ: **Anabolic signaling deficits underlie amino acid resistance of wasting, aging muscle.** *Faseb J* 2005, **19**(3):422–424.

36. Fryburg DA, Jahn LA, Hill SA, Oliveras DM, Barrett EJ: **Insulin and insulin-like growth factor-I enhance human skeletal muscle protein anabolism during hyperaminoacidemia by different mechanisms.** *J Clin Invest* 1995, **96**(4):1722–1729.

37. Desvigne N, Barthelemy JC, Frere D, Gay-Montchamp JP, Costes F: **Microdialysis of insulin-like growth factor-I in human muscle.** *Eur J Appl Physiol* 2005, **94**(1–2):216–219.

38. Hayashi AA, Proud CG: **The rapid activation of protein synthesis by growth hormone requires signaling through mTOR.** *Am J Physiol Endocrinol Metab* 2007, **292**(6):E1647–1655.

39. Bush JA, Kimball SR, O'Connor PM, Suryawan A, Orellana RA, Nguyen HV, Jefferson LS, Davis TA: **Translational control of protein synthesis in muscle and liver of growth hormone-treated pigs.** *Endocrinology* 2003, **144**(4):1273–1283.

40. Vary TC, Jefferson LS, Kimball SR: **Role of eIF4E in stimulation of protein synthesis by IGF-I in perfused rat skeletal muscle.** *Am J Physiol Endocrinol Metab* 2000, **278**(1):E58–64.

41. Lundholm K, Bennegard K, Zachrisson H, Lundgren F, Eden E, Moller-Loswick AC: **Transport kinetics of amino acids across the resting human leg.** *J Clin Invest* 1987, **80**(3):763–771.

42. Willis PE, Chadan SG, Baracos V, Parkhouse WS: **Restoration of insulin-like growth factor I action in skeletal muscle of old mice.** *Am J Physiol* 1998, **275**(3 Pt 1):E525–530.

43. Owino V, Yang SY, Goldspink G: **Age-related loss of skeletal muscle function and the inability to express the autocrine form of insulin-like growth factor-1 (MGF) in response to mechanical overload.** *FEBS Lett* 2001, **505**(2):259–263.

44. Willis PE, Chadan S, Baracos V, Parkhouse WS: **Acute exercise attenuates age-associated resistance to insulin-like growth factor I.** *Am J Physiol* 1997, **272**(3 Pt 1):E397–404.

45. Oldham JM, Hodges AK, Schaare PN, Molan PC, Bass JJ: **Nutritional dependence of insulin-like growth factor (IGF) receptors in skeletal muscle: measurement by light microscopic autoradiography.** *J Histochem Cytochem* 1993, **41**(3):415–421.

46. Lowe WL Jr, Adamo M, Werner H, Roberts CT Jr, LeRoith D: **Regulation by fasting of rat insulin-like growth factor I and its receptor.** *Effects on gene expression and binding. J Clin Invest* 1989, **84**(2):619–626.

47. Spangenburg EE, Le Roith D, Ward CW, Bodine SC: **A functional insulin-like growth factor receptor is not necessary for load-induced skeletal muscle hypertrophy.** *J Physiol* 2008, **586**(1):283–291.

9

Differential role of STIM1 and STIM2 during transient inward (T_{in}) current generation and the maturation process in the *Xenopus* oocyte

Barbara Serrano-Flores, Edith Garay, Francisco G Vázquez-Cuevas and Rogelio O Arellano[*]

Abstract

Background: The *Xenopus* oocyte is a useful cell model to study Ca^{2+} homeostasis and cell cycle regulation, two highly interrelated processes. Here, we used antisense oligonucleotides to investigate the role in the oocyte of stromal interaction molecule (STIM) proteins that are fundamental elements of the store-operated calcium-entry (SOCE) phenomenon, as they are both sensors for Ca^{2+} concentration in the intracellular reservoirs as well as activators of the membrane channels that allow Ca^{2+} influx.

Results: Endogenous STIM1 and STIM2 expression was demonstrated, and their synthesis was knocked down 48–72 h after injecting oocytes with specific antisense sequences. Selective elimination of their mRNA and protein expression was confirmed by PCR and Western blot analysis, and we then evaluated the effect of their absence on two endogenous responses: the opening of SOC channels elicited by G protein-coupled receptor (GPCR)-activated Ca^{2+} release, and the process of maturation stimulated by progesterone. Activation of SOC channels was monitored electrically by measuring the T_{in} response, a Ca^{2+}-influx-dependent Cl^- current, while maturation was assessed by germinal vesicle breakdown (GVBD) scoring and electrophysiology.

Conclusions: It was found that STIM2, but not STIM1, was essential in both responses, and T_{in} currents and GVBD were strongly reduced or eliminated in cells devoid of STIM2; STIM1 knockdown had no effect on the maturation process, but it reduced the T_{in} response by 15 to 70%. Thus, the endogenous SOCE response in *Xenopus* oocytes depended mainly on STIM2, and its expression was necessary for entry into meiosis induced by progesterone.

Keywords: SOCE, STIM1, STIM2, *Xenopus* oocyte, Ca^{2+}-entry, Maturation

Background

For approximately three decades, the *Xenopus* oocyte has been a useful cell model to determine the underlying mechanisms responsible for the increase of the cytoplasmic Ca^{2+} concentration through its release from intracellular reservoirs [1,2] and by calcium influx either through Ca^{2+}-dependent voltage-dependent channels or via store-operated Ca^{2+} (SOC) channels [3-5]. The latter results from the activation of the phenomenon known as store-operated Ca^{2+} entry (SOCE), which allows the replenishment of emptied reservoirs [5] after the stimulation of Ca^{2+} release through IP_3/diacylglycerol synthesis by

phospholipase C (PLC). Release of Ca^{2+} from intracellular reservoirs and SOCE activation are common responses in the *Xenopus* oocytes since they endogenously express the machinery that activates PLC by stimulating endogenous G protein-coupled receptors (GPCR); cytoplasmic Ca^{2+}-increase, through either release or influx, opens Ca^{2+}-dependent Cl^- channels in the oocyte membrane generating conspicuous current responses [6]. SOCE activation in the membrane of the *Xenopus* oocyte was first detected by measuring the transient inward (T_{in}) current response [6] after Ca^{2+} release in the oocyte. The T_{in} response is generated by hyperpolarizing steps, and is mainly due to the Ca^{2+}-influx that subsequently opens Ca^{2+}-dependent Cl^- channels; this membrane response has been used as a reliable monitor of SOC channel activation [3,7].

* Correspondence: arellano.ostoa@comunidad.unam.mx
Departamento de Neurobiología Celular y Molecular, Instituto de Neurobiología, Universidad Nacional Autónoma de México, Boulevard Juriquilla 3001, Juriquilla Querétaro, Querétaro, C.P. 76230, Mexico

The SOCE current is most likely driven through Ca^{2+}-permeable channels formed by Orai, a channel activated by association with the stromal interaction molecule (STIM) [8], a protein that is localized mainly in the endoplasmic reticulum (ER) membrane and that senses the Ca^{2+} concentration in its lumen [9]. Although transcripts for endogenous Orai and STIM molecules have been reported in the oocyte [10], the role for the different types and isoforms of these proteins and their relation with endogenous responses in the oocyte have not been thoroughly studied; these issues are of interest given that the roles for the different SOC molecular elements are also incompletely understood, and their study in a well-known model such as the *Xenopus* oocyte might reveal important information.

Two STIM proteins, STIM1 and STIM2, are expressed in eukaryotic cells [11]. A different role for each of them has been proposed; for example, the ER Ca^{2+} content must be greatly reduced in order to activate STIM1 protein, while the more Ca^{2+}-sensitive STIM2 seems to require only a slight reduction in ER Ca^{2+} concentration [12-14]. It has been proposed that STIM2 participates in maintaining the cytoplasmic Ca^{2+} concentration [12-15]. Although the fundamental role of STIM1 in activating SOCE has been demonstrated in several cell types [16-18], other information indicates that STIM2 is the main protein involved in SOCE generation in neurons, dendritic cells, and mammary epithelial cells [19-21]. Thus, it is plausible that the specific functions of STIM1 and STIM2 depend on the cell type, their relative rates of expression, and other factors such as interactions among them or with regulatory proteins.

It has also been shown that during maturation, the Ca^{2+}-signaling pathway in the oocyte is significantly reconfigured, probably as part of the mechanism that prepares the gamete for fertilization and subsequent embryonic development. This reconfiguration includes Orai1 channels and STIM1, which are regulated during maturation thus eliminating the SOCE response [22-25]. Due to the importance of this phenomenon for cell cycle control in general, it is also of interest to explore the effects on oocyte maturation of altered STIM expression [26,27].

In the present study, we specifically knocked down STIM1 or STIM2 in the *Xenopus* oocyte to analyze the effect on two endogenous phenomena, the generation of the T_{in} current response (i.e., SOC channel activation) and the maturation process. We found that STIM2 expression was essential in both phenomena, while STIM1 expression was not.

Methods
Cell preparation
Xenopus laevis frogs were obtained from Xenopus I (Ann Arbor, MI, USA). Ovary lobules [28] were surgically removed under sterile conditions from frogs that had been anaesthetized using 0.1% aminobenzoic acid ethyl ester and rendered hypothermic. After surgery, frogs were sutured and allowed to recover from anesthesia. Frogs were maintained for 3–7 days in individual tanks until healing was complete; they were then housed in larger groups, and no further oocytes were taken from them for at least 2 months. Procedures were approved by the institutional animal committees (INB-UNAM). The lobules were placed in sterile Barth's solution containing (in mM): 88 NaCl, 1 KCl, 2.4 $NaHCO_3$, 0.33 $Ca(NO_3)_2$, 0.41 $CaCl_2$, 0.82 $MgSO_4$, and 5 HEPES, with 75 µg/ml gentamicin and adjusted to pH 7.4. Studies were carried out using oocytes at stage VI [29] dissected from the ovaries and defolliculated by collagenase (1 mg/ml) treatment at room temperature for 30 min in normal frog Ringer's solution (NR, containing in mM: 115 NaCl, 2 KCl, 1.8 $CaCl_2$, 5 Hepes, pH 7.0). After washing, the oocytes were stored at 18°C in sterile Barth's solution, and electrical recordings were performed over a period of 2–4 days in either uninjected oocytes or in those injected with cRNA for specific receptors and/or with antisense oligonucleotide to knock down specific proteins.

Reverse transcription polymerase chain reactions
Total RNA from the oocytes was purified using Trizol Reagent (Life Technologies). First-strand cDNA was synthesized using 2 µg of DNase-treated RNA as template and 1 µg of oligo (dT), 0.25 µg random hexamers, and reverse transcriptase. The cDNA was used as template in a polymerase chain reaction to amplify cDNA fragments for *stim1* and *stim2*, and the ribosomal protein S2 (*rps2*) was used as a control. All the PCR programs started at 95°C for 2 min. The amplification in the 35 cycles consisted in 45 s at 95°C, 40 s at 55°C, and 35 s at 72°C, and a final extension at 72°C for 5 min. The sequences of oligonucleotides used were: *stim1*, forward, 5'-CGACGAGTTTCTCAGGGAAG-3' and reverse, 5'-CTTCATGTGGTCCTCGGAGT-3'; *stim2*, forward, 5'-CCAGCCTTGAGGCAATATGT-3' and reverse, 5'-GCAACCTCCAACTCCGATTA-3'; *rps2*, forward, 5'-TGGTAACAGGGGAGGTTTCCGC-3' and reverse, 5'-ATACCAGCCATCATGAGCAGC-3'.

The amplified products were isolated, purified (QIAEX II, QIAGEN, Hilden, Germany), and subcloned into the pJET 1.2 vector (Thermo Fisher Scientific Inc., Waltham, MA). Finally, their nucleotide sequences were confirmed by Sanger sequencing (ABI PRISM 310 Genetic Analyzer, Applied Biosystems).

Western blot
Protein expression was assessed by Western blot in either control oocytes or in those injected with as-STIM1 or as-STIM2. For each group, 10 oocytes were homogenized 72 h post-injection in a buffer containing (in mM): 20

Tris–HCl pH 7.6, 1 EDTA pH 8, 80 sucrose, and 1X complete mini protease inhibitor (Hoffmann-La Roche, Switzerland). Then samples were centrifuged at 4°C and 500 rpm for 5 min, at 3500 rpm for 10 min, and at 14,000 rpm for 20 min. Subsequently, the final pellets were resuspended in 50 μl of buffer containing (in mM): 50 Tris–HCl pH 7.6, 1 EDTA pH 8, 100 NaCl, 100 $MgCl_2$, and 1X complete mini protease inhibitor. Total membrane protein concentration was quantified with a Bradford assay. For electrophoresis, samples (1.5 μg per lane) were fractionated in a 10% SDS-polyacrylamide gel and transferred to a nitrocellulose membrane (BioRad, Hercules, CA, USA). Membranes were blocked for 1 h at room temperature in TBS-T solution (in mM): 150 NaCl, 20 Tris, pH 7.4, and 0.1% Tween 20, containing 5% nonfat dry milk and then incubated overnight at 4°C with a 1:1000 dilution of rabbit primary antibody. The antibody denoted NH-STIM1 (Alomone, Jerusalem, Israel) was directed against a region of the amino-terminus of the STIM1 protein, and the antibodies denoted NH-STIM2 (Alomone, Jerusalem, Israel) and COOH-STIM2 (ProSci Inc., Poway CA, USA) were against the amino and carboxy termini, respectively, of STIM2. Western blot analysis was also used to detect SERCA2 expression, used as a loading control (antibody from Cell Signaling Technology Inc. Danvers, MA, USA). After incubation, the membranes were washed with TBS-T and incubated for 45 min at room temperature with HRP-conjugated goat anti-rabbit antibody (Life Technologies) in TBS-T. The immunoreactive proteins were detected by chemiluminescence, and analyzed with ImageJ Software (NIH, USA); the results were normalized against the control condition and expressed in optical density units. To analyze loading controls such as SERCA2, the same membranes used to detect STIM proteins were incubated for 30 min in striping solution (in mM): 50 Tris pH 6.8, 100 β-mercaptoethanol, and 2% SDS at 55°C and then washed twice with TBS-T. Then the membranes were treated with a primary antibody against the SERCA2 protein and finally with an HRP-conjugated goat anti-rabbit antibody (Life Technologies) in TBS-T and quantified as above.

Expression of purinergic and muscarinic receptors and transcript knockdown using antisense oligonucleotides in *Xenopus laevis* oocytes

In order to express the desired membrane receptors, cDNA coding for P2Y2, P2Y8, or M1 receptors were cloned into the plasmid pEXENEX1 and linearized with SalI or HindIII, then purified and transcribed to capped RNA with T7 polymerase using the mMESSAGE mMACHINE kit (Life Technologies CA, USA). Oocytes were injected with 25–50 ng of the respective cRNA (1 ng/nl). For purinergic receptors the P2Y8 *Xenopus laevis* [cDNA clone

MGC: 52559, Source BioScience Nottingham, UK], and the P2Y2 *Xenopus tropicalis* [cDNA clone IMAGE 5383884, ATCC Manassas, USA] subtypes were used, and for muscarinic receptors, the M1 subtype [human cDNA Clone ID IOH56940 (Life Technologies CA, USA)]. Another group was injected with 25–50 nl of H_2O for control experiments.

The antisense sequences were designed to target the initiation translation region, a strategy that has been successfully used in several experimental protocols; antisense oligonucleotide strongly inhibits mRNA expression via an RNAse-H-dependent mechanism [30].

Expression of endogenous STIM1 or STIM2 was knocked down by the injection of 25–50 ng of antisense oligonucleotides with the following sequences: for antisense oligonucleotide STIM1 (as-STIM1), 5′-ATAGCAGAGTCCGACACCAAAGCATTCCGC-3′, and for antisense oligonucleotide STIM2 (as-STIM2), 5′-TCCTCTTCTTCTTTCTCCCGTTCATGGCTG-3′. Control experiments for antisense oligonucleotides were performed injecting (50 ng per oocyte) scrambled sequences for both as-STIM, and a second control for antisense oligonuleotide injection (as-Cx38) was made knocking down the expression of connexin 38 (Cx38) which was monitored measuring the I_c current in Ca^{2+}-free Ringer solution [28], the sequence for as-Cx38 was: 5′-GCTTTAGTAATTCCCATCCTGCCATGTTTC-3′. In general, after injection, oocytes were incubated at 18°C in Barth's solution, and the effects of these procedures on protein expression and current responses were examined by biochemical and electrophysiological methods. Unless otherwise stated, groups of injected oocytes that were induced to express purinergic receptors were incubated in Barth's solution containing 5 U/ml apyrase to hydrolyze the ATP that is released from the oocyte into the medium, thus avoiding stimulation of purinergic receptors during the incubation period [31].

Electrophysiology

Oocyte membrane currents were monitored using the two-electrode voltage-clamp technique. The cells were continuously superfused (10 ml/min) with NR solution and held at −10 mV. Voltage steps to −100 mV with a duration of 4 s were applied every 40 s to activate the T_{in} current response, and the oocytes were stimulated for 120 s (acute protocol stimulation) with one of the agonists (100 μM ATP or ACh, or a 1:1000 dilution of FBS) added to the bath solution. For long-lasting stimulation, GPCR-expressing oocytes were incubated for 1–4 h with 1 μM agonist, and P2Y8- or P2Y2-expressing oocytes were incubated in medium devoid of apyrase; in this condition, endogenously released ATP activated the receptors in most cases.

Intra-oocyte injection of antibodies during electro-physiological recording was achieved by pneumatic pressure ejection from a third micropipette [32]. The injection micropipette was loaded with antibody dissolved in 5 mM HEPES, adjusted to pH 7.0 with KOH.

Oocyte maturation assays

Maturation studies were carried out on batches of 15–25 defolliculated oocytes, stage VI, incubated in 2 ml of Barth's solution plus 10 μM progesterone. GVBD was scored by white-spot formation and confirmed by cutting the oocytes through the equator after incubating them in hot NR for 1 min [32]. Maturation was analyzed in groups of oocytes that had been injected 72 h earlier with as-STIM1 or as-STIM2, and they were compared with uninjected oocytes or those injected with H_2O. Electrical properties of oocytes from the different groups were analyzed after 9–12 h in the presence of progesterone.

Reagents

ATP, ACh, apyrase, collagenase type I, progesterone, FBS, and all salts were from Sigma Chemical Co. (St Louis, MO, USA).

Statistical analysis

All data are expressed as mean ± SEM of at least 10–15 oocytes from three different frogs for each condition. Statistical analysis was performed using the Igor Pro Wavemetrics, Inc. software through analysis of variance (ANOVA). The means of two different experimental groups were compared using a Student's t-test. Differences were considered to be significant at $p < 0.01$.

Results

Expression of endogenous STIM1 and STIM2 in *Xenopus* oocytes

Expression of RNA transcripts *stim1* and *stim2* was determined in oocytes using RT-PCR. In RNA samples from control (non-injected) oocytes (Figure 1A) the use of oligonucleotide primers for *stim1* resulted in an amplicon of 463 bp, while *stim2* primers amplified a fragment of 494 bp. Both had the expected size for the corresponding transcript, and the amplified fragments were then cloned into the pJET 1.2 vector, sequenced, and analyzed using BLAST. The sequences obtained were highly homologous to those reported for *stim1* (99%) from *Xenopus laevis* [GenBank: NM_001097037.1] and for *stim2* (90%) from *Xenopus tropicalis* [GenBank: XM_004916759.1] (Additional file 1). Control amplifications without RT or without a cDNA template did not produce any PCR products (Figure 1A). Groups of oocytes that had been injected 48–72 h earlier with either the as-STIM1 or the as-STIM2 oligonucleotide sequences showed a dramatic decrease in the corresponding transcripts.

To determine whether the injection of antisense oligonucleotides induced a parallel reduction in level of STIM1 and STIM2 proteins, these were evaluated using Western blot analysis with specific antibodies (Figures 1 and 2). As expected, NH-STIM1 detected a band above 75 KDa in total membrane fractions from control oocytes, and from the mouse brain (Figure 1B) [33,34]. Then, a group of oocytes injected with as-STIM1 was tested; as illustrated in Figure 1C, antisense-injected oocytes showed a significant STIM1 decrease compared to the control group.

Similarly, STIM2 was detected using two distinct antibodies, COOH-STIM2 (Figures 1B-C) and NH-STIM2, which revealed STIM2 as a band about 100 KDa, in both the total membrane preparation of control oocytes and in total protein from mouse brain, in agreement with previous reports [12,21]. Western blot analysis in oocytes injected with as-STIM2 indicated that antisense produced a large decrease in the amount of STIM2 as compared to control oocytes (Figure 1C).

These results showed that the antisense sequences used specifically decreased the endogenous transcripts for

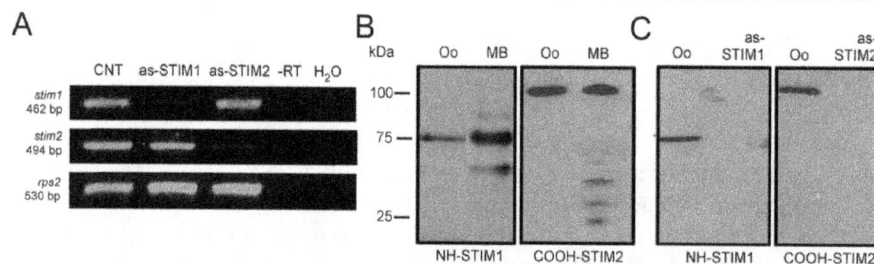

Figure 1 STIM expression in the *Xenopus* oocyte and its downregulation by as-STIM injection. A) shows the RT-PCR amplification of products that corresponded to the size expected for either *stim1* or *stim2* in native oocytes (CNT); the corresponding amplicons were absent in oocytes from the same batch that had been injected with either as-STIM1 or as-STIM2 48 h before the assay. The *rps2* amplicon indicates the reaction efficiency, and -RT and H_2O lanes correspond to negative controls, either RNA without RT, or to the reaction mix without a cDNA template, respectively. **B)** STIM1 and STIM2 were identified by Western blot analysis in protein extracts from oocytes (Oo) or mouse brain (MB, positive control) using either NH-STIM1 (left panel) or COOH-STIM2 (right panel) as antibody. **C)** A similar analysis as in **B** was made for batches of oocytes injected with H_2O as control (CNT), or with as-STIM1 or as-STIM2 48 h before the protein extraction, in which cases proteins were eliminated. (in all cases 10 oocytes per condition).

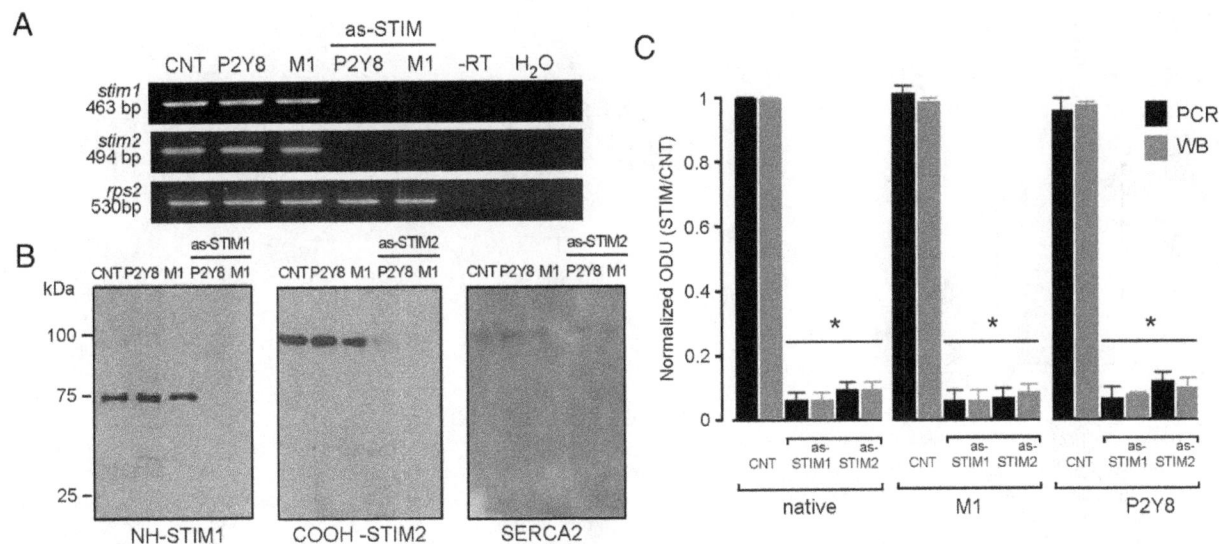

Figure 2 Knockdown of STIM expression in oocytes co-injected with GPCR mRNA. A) RT-PCR amplification of *stim1*, *stim2*, or *rps2* in batches of oocytes injected with H_2O (CNT) or with cRNA (50 ng per oocyte) coding for either P2Y8 or M1 GPCR. In oocytes co-injected with as-STIM1 or as-STIM2 (50 ng per oocyte) together with P2Y8 or M1 cRNA, the corresponding STIM amplicon was downregulated. Control reactions illustrate specificity; *rps2* amplicons are positive controls, and -RT and H_2O lanes show negative controls. **B)** Similar groups of oocytes as in **A)** were assayed using the Western blot technique; in this case oocytes from the same donor injected with one GPCR mRNA (P2Y8 or M1) alone, or co-injected with as-STIM1, were tested with NH-STIM1, while as-STIM2-injected oocytes were probed with COOH-STIM2. In both as-STIM groups SERCA was used as gel-loading control. **C)** The graph shows the densitometric analysis of bands, summarizing the results obtained in different preparations of 10 oocytes per group and repeated in 3–5 frogs. Both PCR products and bands detected by Western blot (WB) were analyzed for batches of oocytes injected with H_2O (CNT) or with either 50 ng as-STIM1 or as-STIM2 alone (native group). Similar analysis was made for batches of control oocytes injected with P2Y8 or M1 cRNA alone, and oocytes from the same frogs co-injected with either as-STIM or as-STIM together with the GPCR cRNA. Optical density units (ODU) for each band were normalized against the value obtained in the corresponding CNT conditions (*p < 0.01).

stim1 or *stim2*, with a concomitant depletion of STIM1 and STIM2 proteins.

STIM1 and STIM2 levels were decreased by injection of antisense-STIM sequences in oocytes co-expressing GPCR

Most of the following experiments were made using oocytes exogenously expressing muscarinic or purinergic receptors due to injection of the respective cRNA in order to get a robust and consistent response; therefore, it was determined if GPCR expression affected either the endogenous expression of STIM or its decrease due to as-STIM injection. Seventy-two hours after injection with cRNA coding for GPCR, oocytes exhibited strong current responses in the presence of their respective agonists (see below); this GPCR expression did not affect the level of *stim1* or *stim2* transcripts, as illustrated in Figure 2A. Moreover, the decrease of *stim1* or *stim2* expression due to antisense injection was also not affected in oocytes that were co-injected with either P2Y8 or M1 receptor cRNA (Figure 2A). Consistent with this result, knockdown of neither STIM1 nor STIM2 protein was altered by co-injecting oocytes with cRNA to express GPCR, as shown in Figure 2B. In all cases, SERCA2 (114 KDa, used as the loading control) did not show significant changes in response to the various experimental conditions (Figure 2B).

The results obtained for all conditions described above are summarized in Figure 2C. Taken together, they confirm that antisense knockdown of endogenous STIM proteins in the oocyte was specific and effective and that this was not affected by simultaneous exogenous GPCR expression.

STIM protein knockdown did not affect the generation of the oscillatory Cl⁻ current induced by agonist

To evaluate the role of STIM1 and STIM2 in SOC current activation, we monitored the T_{in} response generation. Prior to this analysis we tested whether or not as-STIM injection affected the Ca^{2+}-dependent Cl⁻ oscillatory current (I_{osc}) generated by the first application of one of the agonists (Figure 3A). For this, groups of oocytes were exposed to either FBS (stimulation of the endogenous LPA receptor (LPAR)) [35], ACh, or ATP in order to monitor the I_{osc} amplitude, as a measure of the oocyte capacity to release Ca^{2+} from intracellular reservoirs [2,36-39]. I_{osc} elicited by FBS were recorded from native oocytes, and those generated by ACh or ATP were recorded from oocytes expressing M1 or P2Y receptors. The I_{osc} amplitude was then compared among control oocytes and oocytes co-injected with as-STIM1 or as-STIM2. The results showed no significant difference among the various groups

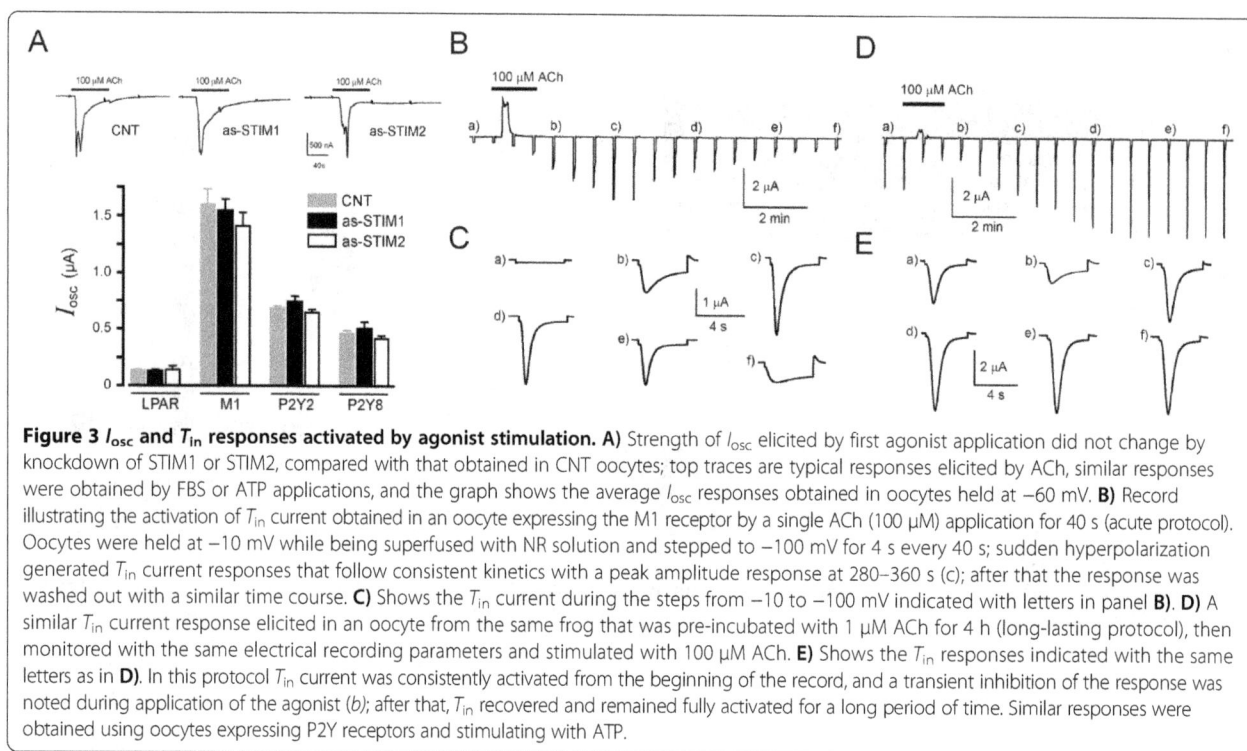

Figure 3 I_{osc} and T_{in} responses activated by agonist stimulation. **A)** Strength of I_{osc} elicited by first agonist application did not change by knockdown of STIM1 or STIM2, compared with that obtained in CNT oocytes; top traces are typical responses elicited by ACh, similar responses were obtained by FBS or ATP applications, and the graph shows the average I_{osc} responses obtained in oocytes held at −60 mV. **B)** Record illustrating the activation of T_{in} current obtained in an oocyte expressing the M1 receptor by a single ACh (100 μM) application for 40 s (acute protocol). Oocytes were held at −10 mV while being superfused with NR solution and stepped to −100 mV for 4 s every 40 s; sudden hyperpolarization generated T_{in} current responses that follow consistent kinetics with a peak amplitude response at 280–360 s (c); after that the response was washed out with a similar time course. **C)** Shows the T_{in} current during the steps from −10 to −100 mV indicated with letters in panel **B)**. **D)** A similar T_{in} current response elicited in an oocyte from the same frog that was pre-incubated with 1 μM ACh for 4 h (long-lasting protocol), then monitored with the same electrical recording parameters and stimulated with 100 μM ACh. **E)** Shows the T_{in} responses indicated with the same letters as in **D)**. In this protocol T_{in} current was consistently activated from the beginning of the record, and a transient inhibition of the response was noted during application of the agonist (b); after that, T_{in} recovered and remained fully activated for a long period of time. Similar responses were obtained using oocytes expressing P2Y receptors and stimulating with ATP.

of oocytes tested for a particular agonist (Figure 3A), although average current amplitude was consistently smaller for LPAR stimulation, and larger for M1-stimulated responses. Together, these results showed that the injection of antisense oligonucleotides did not affect I_{osc} activation, strongly suggesting that the Ca^{2+}-release mechanism remained intact and showing that its strength was dependent on the receptor type stimulated.

Participation of STIM1 in T_{in} generation

To analyze the role of STIM1 and STIM2, T_{in} current was monitored by applying hyperpolarizing voltage steps of −90 mV every 40–60 s, from a holding potential of −10 mV (Figure 3B-E). As illustrated in Figure 3B, the T_{in} current amplitude generally increased after acute agonist application (either ATP, ACh, or FBS for 120 s), reached a peak after 400–480 s, and then slowly returned to basal levels after 680–800 s (65 oocytes, 12 frogs). Consistent with previous studies [6], T_{in} was a Cl$^-$ current that was dependent on extracellular Ca^{2+}, and it was blocked by lanthanides with an IC$_{50}$ for La^{3+} of 41 ± 0.21 nM and for Gd^{3+} of 7 ± 0.23 μM, potencies similar to those shown to block SOC channels in other studies [3,6,40].

Then the effect of as-STIM1 injection on T_{in} current generation (121 oocytes, 9 frogs) was assessed. In control oocytes, application of FBS (1:1000) elicited T_{in} current responses of 2.5 ± 0.28 μA (Figure 4A-B). However, in as-STIM1-injected oocytes, the average T_{in} generated was 0.92 ± 0.38 μA, which represented a decrease of 60 ± 5.2%.

Similarly, oocytes exposed to 100 μM ACh (expressing M1 receptor) showed a 70 ± 9.7% decrease in T_{in} in the as-STIM1-injected group. However, oocytes expressing P2Y8 and exposed to 100 μM ATP exhibited a 20 ± 1.4% decrease in T_{in} and oocytes expressing P2Y2 exhibited a reduction of only 15 ± 1.5% (Figure 4B). The results clearly indicated that elimination of STIM1 did not cause a complete loss of the T_{in} response elicited by any of the agonists used.

STIM2 knockdown potently inhibited T_{in} generation regardless of the receptor stimulated

We next tested whether STIM2 knockdown affected T_{in} currents activated either by P2Y or M1 receptors with experiments similar to those described above. In contrast to what happened with STIM1 knockdown, as-STIM2 injection drastically reduced the T_{in} response elicited by the acute stimulation of any of the receptors tested (Figure 4C-D). T_{in} current amplitude was reduced by 96 ± 6.6% in oocytes stimulated with FBS, by 96 ± 3.6% with ACh, by 93 ± 7.1% with ATP for oocytes expressing P2Y8 receptors, and by 94 ± 8% for those expressing P2Y2. In this case, the amount of decrease observed did not differ among the receptors studied (Figure 4D). As shown above, it was evident that the decrease in the T_{in} response was not due to uncoupling of the IP$_3$/Ca^{2+}-release system since the oscillatory responses in all the oocyte groups remained unchanged.

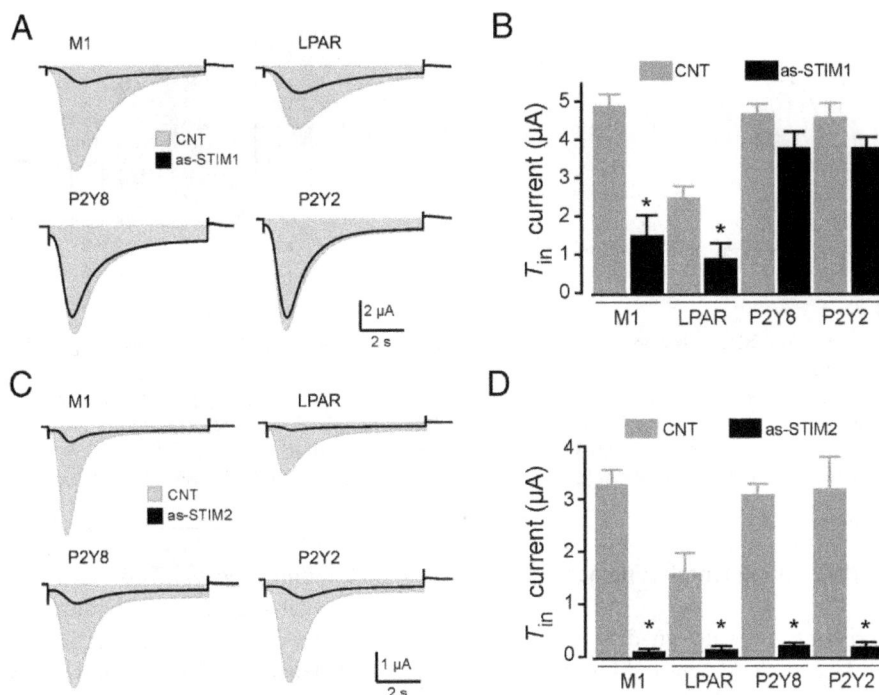

Figure 4 Specific STIM knockdown by oocyte injection of as-STIM differentially decreased the T_{in} current. A) Oocytes induced to express M1, P2Y8, or P2Y2 receptors were stimulated with either ACh or ATP (100 μM), and LPAR in native oocytes were stimulated by FBS (1:1000 dilution); the resulting T_{in} currents (CNT, gray areas) were compared with the T_{in} obtained in oocytes from the corresponding group that were also injected with 50 ng as-STIM1 (superimposed black traces); all responses were monitored 48–72 h after oocyte injection. **B)** The graph shows the results obtained using the different experimental conditions illustrated in **A)**. **C)** In a set of experiments similar to those shown in **A)**, T_{in} currents were monitored, and the peak amplitudes of non-injected CNT oocytes were compared with those of oocytes injected (48–72 h before recording) with 50 ng as-STIM2 and stimulated with the agonists. **D)** The graph shows the results obtained using the different experimental conditions illustrated in **C)**. Bars correspond to the mean (± SEM) of the T_{in} peak amplitude of 10–15 oocytes from 5–6 frogs (*p < 0.01, as-STIM vs. CNT).

Control experiments were also made using scrambled oligonucleotide sequences as well as as-Cx38 a different antisense oligonucleotide sequence to rule out the possibility that injection *per se* yielded nonspecific results, in these cases no effects were observed on T_{in} current amplitude. For example, as-Cx38 was used to knockdown connexons formed by Cx38, whose opening by superfusion of Ca^{2+}-free Ringer's solution [28,32] results in a fast and reliable test for Cx38 expression. Thus, in control oocytes the I_c current response was elicited by superfusion of Ca^{2+}-free Ringer's solution (3.06 ± 0.16 μA; 9 oocytes, 3 frogs) while in as-Cx38 injected oocytes the current response was eliminated. However, in the same oocytes from both groups, the Tin current amplitude was similar, regardless the membrane receptor stimulated, either M1 (2.98 ± 0.17 μA vs. 2.95 ± 0.18 μA) or P2Y8 (3.14 ± 0.14 μA vs. 3.15 ± 0.15 μA) (16 oocytes, 4 frogs).

All together, these results indicate that T_{in} generation in the *Xenopus* oocyte requires STIM2 protein.

COOH-STIM2 antibody enhances the T_{in} current response

Envisioning that specific binding of antibody to STIM1 or STIM2 might affect the function of these proteins and then serve as a specific tool to evaluate the involvement of STIM in a particular response, we tested the same antibodies used in the Western blot for their effect on T_{in} generation. For this purpose, antibodies were microinjected into the oocyte cytoplasm to reach a final dilution of 1:1000. Figure 5 shows that ACh application onto oocytes pre-loaded with COOH-STIM2 resulted in a robust potentiation of the T_{in} response, increasing the amplitude by 158 ± 25% (15 oocytes, 5 frogs). COOH-STIM2 injection also potentiated by 168 ± 30% the T_{in} responses elicited by FBS, and a similar effect was observed in oocytes stimulated through the P2Y8 (126 ± 37%) or the P2Y2 receptor (129 ± 23%) (Figure 5). However, in oocytes (n = 22) from the same frogs that were injected with denatured COOH-STIM2 (incubated for 10 min at 70°C), T_{in} potentiation was completely abolished (Figure 5B). Also, injection of NH-STIM1 or NH-STIM2 antibody did not produce any changes in the T_{in} response, nor did the injection of a P2Y2 antibody.

All these results clearly indicated that the COOH-STIM2 antibody specifically potentiated the T_{in} current, regardless of the receptor stimulated.

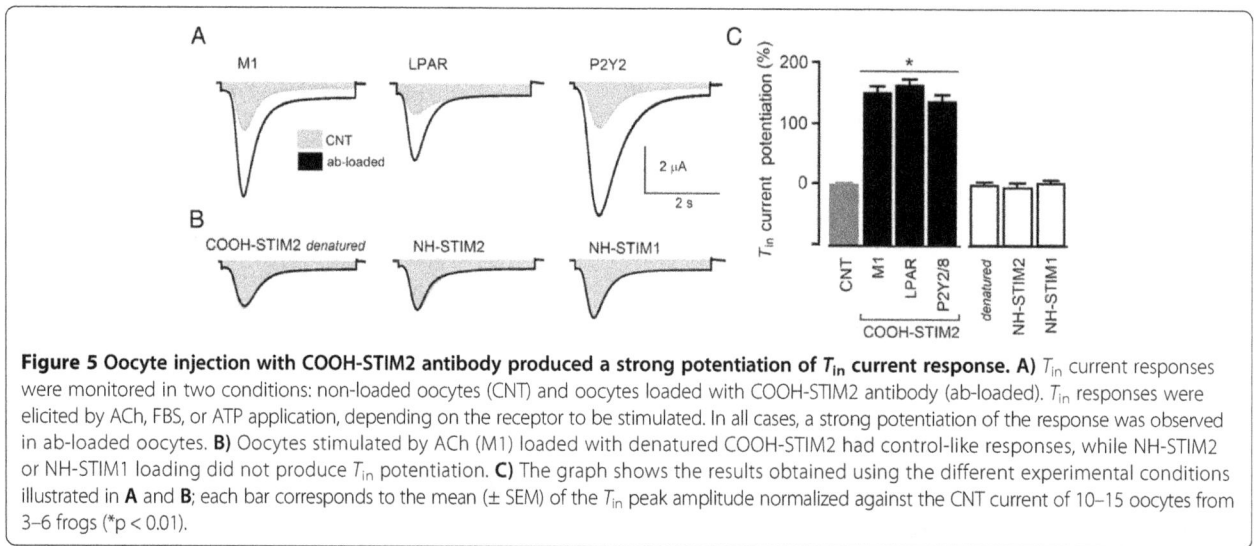

Figure 5 Oocyte injection with COOH-STIM2 antibody produced a strong potentiation of T_{in} current response. A) T_{in} current responses were monitored in two conditions: non-loaded oocytes (CNT) and oocytes loaded with COOH-STIM2 antibody (ab-loaded). T_{in} responses were elicited by ACh, FBS, or ATP application, depending on the receptor to be stimulated. In all cases, a strong potentiation of the response was observed in ab-loaded oocytes. **B)** Oocytes stimulated by ACh (M1) loaded with denatured COOH-STIM2 had control-like responses, while NH-STIM2 or NH-STIM1 loading did not produce T_{in} potentiation. **C)** The graph shows the results obtained using the different experimental conditions illustrated in **A** and **B**; each bar corresponds to the mean (± SEM) of the T_{in} peak amplitude normalized against the CNT current of 10–15 oocytes from 3–6 frogs (*p < 0.01).

Role of STIM1 and STIM2 during long-lasting agonist stimulation

The following experiments were designed to explore the possibility that STIM1 and STIM2 have different effects, depending on the duration of the stimulus. Thus, oocytes injected with as-STIM1 or with as-STIM2 and expressing M1, P2Y8, or P2Y2 receptors were incubated for 1–4 h in the presence of their respective agonists at 1 μM (Figure 3D-E). Extended agonist incubation generated strong T_{in} currents that remained stable for more than the 60-min recording time, even under constant superfusion of the oocytes with NR solution, and it began to decrease after 120–180 min of wash; we assumed that in this condition the SOC machinery was over-stimulated, and that the time spent in the activated state reflected the time necessary to refill the reservoirs.

In the oocytes knocked down for STIM1, T_{in} currents activated by long-lasting stimulation with any of the agonists analyzed were no different from those observed in control oocytes. In contrast, in oocytes injected with as-STIM2 and expressing P2Y or M1 receptors that had been stimulated for long intervals with their respective agonists, the T_{in} current was no longer generated (10–15 oocytes in each group, 5 frogs), strongly suggesting that STIM2 in the oocyte was essential for responses generated through both the acute and long-lasting stimulation protocols.

STIM proteins and the maturation process

During the maturation process, molecular elements that control the Ca^{2+} dynamics in the *Xenopus* oocyte undergo an important reconfiguration; this observation has been extended to different species, and similar changes are known to occur during mitosis [23,31,41]. Given the importance of these events for cell cycle control, we asked whether or not the knockdown of STIM proteins affected

the maturation process. Thus, batches of control oocytes, and those that were injected with as-STIM1 or as-STIM2 were assayed 48–72 h after injection with 10 μM progesterone in Barth's solution to induce maturation. Oocyte maturation entry was scored by the appearance of GVBD after 8–12 h in the presence of progesterone. The GVBD score obtained was compared against progesterone-treated control oocytes. The results are illustrated in Figure 6A; as-STIM1-injected oocytes did not show any effect on the efficiency of maturation, while STIM2 knockdown produced a strong inhibition of the process (the experiment was repeated in oocytes from 3 different donors). Lack of GVBD in as-STIM2-injected oocytes seemed to indicate a failure to enter meiosis and a consequent incomplete maturation process; this interpretation was also supported by monitoring electrophysiological parameters in all of the groups tested. As illustrated in Figure 6B-C, electrical parameters of as-STIM2-injected oocytes (progesterone-treated) were different from those displayed by as-STIM1-injected oocytes and control oocytes maintained in progesterone for the same period of time.

Taken together, these results clearly showed that in oocytes where STIM2 was knocked down, the process of maturation was inhibited at some early point. The first manifestation of this was the complete blockage of GVBD, i.e., of the signal for meiosis entry; this result was clearly different from that observed in STIM1-deprived oocytes.

Discussion

Here, using biochemical strategies and electrophysiology, we studied what effects the knockdown of endogenous STIM proteins had on two important *Xenopus* oocyte responses: the activation of SOCE monitored by measuring T_{in} current generation, and the maturation process induced by progesterone. We found that: *i)* Both STIM1

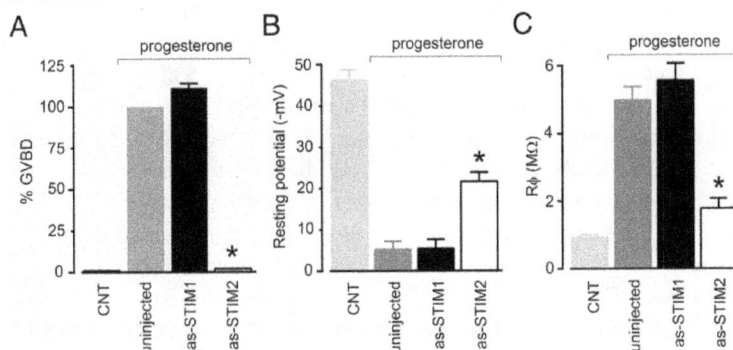

Figure 6 Effect of as-STIM2 on GVBD and oocyte membrane characteristics during maturation induced by progesterone. A) The maturation process promoted by progesterone (10 µM) was analyzed in uninjected oocytes, or in oocytes injected 72 h prior to the assay with either as-STIM1 or as-STIM2, and compared with control oocytes in the absence of progesterone. GVBD was quantified after 8–12 h in presence of progesterone (10 oocytes per group, repeated using 3 different frogs) and is normalized against the value observed in uninjected oocytes. **B)** Resting membrane potential was monitored 8–12 h after addition of progesterone in the same groups of oocytes (n = 3-5, repeated in 3 frogs) as in **A**). **C)** The input membrane resistance (Rφ) was estimated over the range from −80 to −20 mV in the different oocyte groups treated in the same conditions. Control groups, without progesterone, included both uninjected and antisense-injected oocytes. In all cases, values for as-STIM2-injected groups were different from as-STIM1-injected or uninjected groups (*p < 0.01).

and STIM2 proteins were endogenously expressed in the *Xenopus* oocyte; *ii)* Injection of antisense oligonucleotide sequences of STIM1 or STIM2 potently knocked down the expression of both the corresponding mRNA and the protein; *iii)* STIM1 or STIM2 knockdown did not seem to affect the Ca^{2+}-signaling machinery responsible for generating oscillatory Ca^{2+}-signals in the oocyte; *iv)* STIM2, but not STIM1, proved to be fundamental for T_{in} current generation; this was observed both in acute stimulation protocols or after long-lasting stimulation periods, and it did not depend on the receptor type stimulated; *v)* STIM2 protein knockdown blocked entry into the process of maturation induced by progesterone, while STIM1 elimination did not affect this process; and *vi)* an antibody against the COOH terminus of STIM2 potentiated T_{in} current generation.

Calcium release and influx are two phenomena well studied in the *Xenopus* oocyte. The main subject addressed here is the identity and role of STIM proteins during calcium influx stimulated through endogenous responses. It is known that after GPCR stimulation, both endogenous as well as exogenously expressed GPCR generate in the oocyte mainly two Ca^{2+}-dependent Cl^- ion currents, one due to intracellular Ca^{2+} release that is normally followed by another current dependent on Ca^{2+} influx; this pattern is generated through an enzymatic cascade involving IP_3 synthesis, a common mechanism in most cell systems [1]. Following the original nomenclature, in the oocyte the first response is named I_{osc}, while the second generates the T_{in} current response [6]. The Ca^{2+}-influx magnitude is directly related to the amplitude of Ca^{2+}-release; the main molecular element responsible for this linkage is the STIM protein, since it is the Ca^{2+}-sensor within the Ca^{2+} reservoir. As in previous

studies [8,42,43], to monitor the $[Ca^{2+}]_i$ increase produced by both mechanisms in the oocyte, here we used the Ca^{2+}-dependent Cl^- current as an endogenous sensor whose amplitude accurately reflects the concentration of Ca^{2+} beneath the plasmatic membrane. This is especially true for Ca^{2+} influx, since this occurs in the plasma membrane where the Ca^{2+}-dependent Cl^- channels are co-expressed with the SOC channels responsible for the influx. Thus, monitoring an endogenous Ca^{2+} sensor such as the Cl^- channel offers not only spatial and temporal advantages, but also amplifies the normally small Ca^{2+} current through SOC channels and avoids altering the Ca^{2+} dynamics with further pharmacological manipulations. STIM protein expression and function was then studied in the *Xenopus* oocyte using this tool.

It is well known that when Ca^{2+} is released from the ER, STIM proteins are activated, rapidly translocated, and oligomerized into junctions formed between the ER and the plasma membrane, where they bind to and activate highly selective Ca^{2+} channels formed by Orai proteins that allow Ca^{2+} influx [44,45]. The main trigger for this phenomenon is a decrease in ER Ca^{2+} content; however, evidence indicates that isoforms of STIM2 protein might maintain a basal activation of Orai channels without prior Ca^{2+} release, thereby controlling the cytoplasmic Ca^{2+} concentration [12,46]. The ratio of STIM1 to STIM2 expression seems to depend on the cell type, and perhaps on the pathophysiological state; as shown here for the *Xenopus* oocyte, other cells such as T cells, myoblasts, skeletal muscle, and liver cells also co-express both STIM proteins [20,47-49]. Studies to distinguish the roles of STIM1 and STIM2 in various cells have employed diverse silencing strategies and overexpression. The injection of an antisense oligonucleotide sequence for each STIM protein was chosen here for its simplicity and because it excludes potential non-specific effects caused by protein over-expression. The effect of antisense injection on STIM expression was demonstrated by analyzing both its mRNA and protein expression by RT-PCR and Western blot, respectively. This analysis demonstrated that expression of STIM1 or STIM2 was strongly down-regulated in oocytes injected with the corresponding antisense oligonucleotide sequence. This antisense effect was not affected by co-expression of GPCR proteins, used experimentally to stimulate Ca^{2+}-release. Also, it was shown that STIM protein knockdown did not affect the IP_3 increase and subsequent Ca^{2+} release, as indicated by the I_{osc} amplitude responses evoked at the beginning of each experiment by acute application of one of the agonists studied. In addition, preliminary results using RT-PCR showed amplification of transcripts for Orai1 and Orai2 in the oocyte (not shown).

Oocytes injected with either antisense STIM1 or STIM2 were then monitored to analyze their ability to generate T_{in} current using two stimulation protocols. In the first, acute application of the agonist produced the typical I_{osc} response; in control conditions it was followed by T_{in} generation that declined after 680–800 s. In the second protocol, long-lasting (1–4 h) stimulation of control oocytes with a low concentration of agonist (1 μM) gave strong T_{in} current responses that remained active for 60–180 min, even in constant superfusion with NR solution. A possible explanation for this difference in response kinetics is that prolonged stimulation produced a stronger activation of the SOCE mechanism, probably due to a more marked decrease in ER Ca^{2+} concentration. Both protocols were applied in oocytes in which STIM1 or STIM2 expression had been eliminated. The STIM2 knockdown produced a severe decrease in T_{in} current generation (93 - 100%) in both stimulation protocols, indicating that STIM2 was indispensable to induce the T_{in} current response. Using acute receptor stimulation, elimination of STIM1 caused a smaller but significant decrease in T_{in} current generation thus, STIM2 alone was unable to support full T_{in} activation during acute stimulation, suggesting that an association of STIM2 with STIM1 was necessary in order to activate the endogenous response. Also it was observed that STIM1 requirement seemed to be minor during P2Y purinergic stimulation, this difference cannot be explained by the amplitudes of I_{osc} generated by the agonists, given that ACh and LPA were the more and less effective, respectively, in generating the response, and both agonists showed similar patterns of T_{in} decrease by STIM1 knockdown. Thus, this result might indicate some type of molecular specificity, perhaps intrinsic to the molecules involved or as a consequence of their differential expression and localization in the oocyte membrane. Differential insertion

of several proteins expressed in the oocyte membrane has been demonstrated; thus, membrane domains with greater expression of STIM2 together with P2Y receptors are plausible.

A central role for STIM2 protein in SOCE generation has been shown before in some cell types such as neurons [20,50] and dendritic cells [19]; however, there is no information indicating whether or not the expression of STIM1 might affect the full endogenous response in these cases. For example, it has been shown the essential role of STIM2 in SOCE activation in dendritic spines [50], which was not substituted by overexpression of STIM1. The authors concluded that this is due to differences in STIM-Ca^{2+} sensitivity and subcellular localization of the proteins. In many other cell systems, co-participation or complementary roles for the two STIM proteins have been postulated [15,48]. Finally, when the oocytes were stimulated using the long-lasting protocol, elimination of STIM1 had no effect indicating that, in this case, the T_{in} current was activated by STIM2 alone. The central role for STIM2 is supported by the latter result as well as by the finding that injecting the antibody (COOH-STIM2) against STIM2 specifically increased the current amplitude by more than 100%, regardless of the agonist used to generate the T_{in} response. It is known that the COOH region, in both STIM1 and STIM2, contains the domain necessary to interact and activate the SOC channel formed by Orai [44]. Thus, a potentiating effect of the COOH-STIM2 antibody indicates that the strength of the STIM2-Orai interaction might be regulated, either positively or negatively, through a site that is affected by the antibody, indirectly confirming the central role of STIM2 during T_{in} generation. As expected given the STIM structure proposed, the two antibodies that recognized domains close to the amino-terminus had no effect on the T_{in} response.

Significant inhibition of the maturation process was observed in oocytes devoid of STIM2 protein. Here, we provided clear-cut evidence of STIM2 involvement during or in preparation for maturation, since its absence eliminated the process of GVBD. Once again, this result contrasted with the lack of effect in STIM1-knockdown oocytes, whose maturation was similar to that of control oocytes. Indeed, it has been shown that the function of STIM1 is downregulated during the maturation process, which contributes to elimination of the SOC response in *Xenopus* oocytes [22-24]; a similar condition has been shown in the mammalian oocyte [25], although in the latter this phenomenon remains controversial [51]. There is no previous information regarding the effect produced by lack (or overexpression) of STIM2 during maturation either in frog or mammalian oocytes, as most previous studies focused on the role of STIM1. However, mouse oocyte is known to express STIM2 protein in the ER; during maturation, STIM2 re-localizes from a homogeneous distribution to one closer to the meiotic spindles, suggesting a role during this process [52]. In frog, is possible that the inhibitory effect of STIM2 knockdown was unrelated to its role in SOCE activation, since meiosis entry in *Xenopus* does not require Ca^{2+}-influx [42]. Further studies will be necessary to characterize the level at which the lack of STIM2 had such a dramatic effect on the maturation process, and to determine if it might have more general implications. One possibility is that as-STIM2 might cause downregulation of a STIM2 isoform different from that involved in SOCE activation. Another possibility relates to its role regulating cytoplasmic $[Ca^{2+}]$, in which case as-STIM2 might affect the activation of Ca^{2+}-dependent processes required prior to meiosis entry.

Conclusion

In this study, STIM2 is fundamental for the endogenous SOC response in the oocyte, although an association with STIM1 seemed to be necessary for its full generation. The mechanism responsible for the clear dependence of meiosis entry on STIM2 expression is a fundamental question that remains open, and its elucidation might help to understand the function of STIM proteins in the *Xenopus* oocyte and in other cell types as well.

Competing interests
The authors declare that they have no competing interests.

Author's contributions
B.S.-F. performed experiments, collected data, provided input in data analysis and was involved in drafting the manuscript. F.G.V.-C. and E. G. performed experiments and provided substantial input in design and interpretation of data. R.O.A. designed research, performed experiments and drafted the manuscript. All authors gave final approval to the version to be published.

Acknowledgments
The author's thank to Dr. Dorothy D. Pless for editing the manuscript. We also thank Mr. Horacio Ramírez Leyva, M. en C. Leonor Casanova, Ing. Ramón Martínez Olvera, and ISC Omar González Hernández, for their expert technical assistance. B.S.-F. as a doctoral student from Programa de Doctorado en Ciencias Biomédicas at Universidad Nacional Autónoma de México (UNAM) is grateful that she received fellowship 215719 from CONACyT-México. R.O. A. received grants by CONACyT-México 82340 and PAPIIT-UNAM-México IN205312, lastly, F.G.V.-C. is grateful for the grants received by CONACyT-México No. 166725 and PAPIIT-UNAM-México No. IN205114.

References

1. Berridge MJ, Lipp P, Bootman MD: The versatility and universality of calcium signalling. *Nat Rev Mol Cell Biol* 2000, 1:11–21.
2. Parker I, Miledi R: Changes in intracellular calcium and in membrane currents evoked by injection of inositol trisphosphate into *Xenopus* oocytes. *Proc R Soc Lond B Biol Sci* 1986, 228:307–315.
3. Yao Y, Tsien R: Calcium current activated by depletion of calcium stores in *Xenopus* oocytes. *J Gen Physiol* 1997, 109:703–715.
4. Hartzell HC: Activation of different Cl⁻ currents in Xenopus oocytes by Ca²⁺ liberated from stores and by capacitative Ca²⁺ influx. *J Gen Physiol* 1996, 108:157–175.
5. Parekh AB, Penner R: Store depletion and calcium influx. *Physiol Rev* 1997, 77:901–930.
6. Parker I, Gundersen C, Miledi R: A transient inward current elicited by hyperpolarization during serotonin activation in *Xenopus* oocytes. *Proc R Soc Lond B Biol Sci* 1985, 223:279–292.
7. Sun L, Machaca K: Ca²⁺(cyt) negatively regulates the initiation of oocyte maturation. *J Cell Biol* 2004, 165:63–75.
8. Williams RT, Manji SS, Parker NJ, Hancock MS, Van Stekelenburg L, Eid JP, Senior PV, Kanzenwadel JS, Shandala T, Saint R, Smith PJ, Dziadek MA: Identification and characterization of the STIM (stromal interaction molecule) gene family: coding for a novel class of transmembrane proteins. *Biochem J* 2001, 357:673–685.
9. Roos J, DiGregorio PJ, Yeromin AV, Ohlsen K, Lioudyno M, Zhang S, Safrina O, Kozak JA, Wagner SL, Cahalan MD, Veliçelebi G, Stauderman KA: STIM1, an essential and conserved component of store-operated Ca²⁺ channel function. *J Cell Biol* 2005, 169:435–445.
10. Klein SL, Strausberg RL, Wagner L, Pontius J, Cllifton SW, Richardson P: Genetic and genomic tools for *Xenopus* research: The NIH *Xenopus* initiative. *Dev Dyn* 2002, 225:384–391.
11. Soboloff J, Rothberg BS, Madesh M, Gill DL: STIM proteins: dynamic calcium signal transducers. *Nat Rev Mol Cell Biol* 2012, 13:549–565.
12. Brandman O, Liou J, Park WS, Meyer T: STIM2 is a feedback regulator that stabilizes basal cytosolic and endoplasmic reticulum Ca²⁺ levels. *Cell* 2007, 131:1327–1339.
13. Frischauf I, Schindl R, Derler I, Bergsmann J, Fahrner M, Romanin C: The STIM/Orai coupling machinery. *Channels (Austin)* 2008, 2:261–268.
14. López E, Salido GM, Rosado JA, Berna-Erro A: Unraveling STIM2 function. *J Physiol Biochem* 2012, 68:619–633.
15. Gruszczynska-Biegala J, Pomorski P, Wisniewska MB, Kuznicki J: Differential roles for STIM1 and STIM2 in store-operated calcium entry in rat neurons. *PLoS One* 2011, 6:e19285.
16. Stiber J, Hawkins A, Zhang ZS, Wang S, Burch J, Graham V, Ward CC, Seth M, Finch E, Malouf N, Williams RS, Eu JP, Rosenberg P: STIM1 signalling controls store-operated calcium entry required for development and contractile function in skeletal muscle. *Nat Cell Biol* 2008, 10:688–697.
17. Varga-Szabo D, Authi KS, Braun A, Bender M, Ambily A, Hassock SR, Gudermann T, Dietrich A, Nieswandt B: Store-operated Ca²⁺ entry in platelets occurs independently of transient receptor potential (TRP) C1. *Pflugers Arch* 2008, 457:377–387.
18. Zhang SL, Yu Y, Roos J, Kozak JA, Deerinck TJ, Ellisman MH, Stauderman KA, Cahalan MD: STIM1 is a Ca²⁺ sensor that activates CRAC channels and migrates from the Ca²⁺ store to the plasma membrane. *Nature* 2005, 437:902–905.
19. Bandyopadhyay BC, Pingle SC, Ahern GP: Store-operated Ca²⁺ signaling in dendritic cells occurs independently of STIM1. *J Leukoc Biol* 2010, 89:57–62.
20. Berna-Erro A, Braun A, Kraft R, Kleinschnitz C, Schuhmann MK, Stegner D, Wultsch T, Eilers J, Meuth SG, Stoll G, Nieswandt B: STIM2 regulates capacitive Ca²⁺ entry in neurons and plays a key role in hypoxic neuronal cell death. *Sci Signal* 2009, 2:ra67.
21. Song MY, Makino A, Yuan JX-J: STIM2 Contributes to enhanced store-operated Ca²⁺ entry in pulmonary artery smooth muscle cells from patients with idiopathic pulmonary arterial hypertension. *Pulm Circ* 2011, 1:84–94.
22. El-Jouni W, Jang B, Haun S, Machaca K: Calcium signaling differentiation during *Xenopus* oocyte maturation. *Dev Biol* 2005, 288:514–525.
23. Machaca K, Haun S: Induction of maturation-promoting factor during *Xenopus* oocyte maturation uncouples Ca²⁺ store depletion from store-operated Ca²⁺ entry. *J Cell Biol* 2002, 156:75–85.
24. Yu F, Sun L, Machaca K: Orai1 internalization and STIM1 clustering inhibition modulate SOCE inactivation during meiosis. *Proc Natl Acad Sci U S A* 2009, 106:17401–17406.
25. Cheon B, Lee H-C, Wakai T, Fissore RA: Ca²⁺ influx and the store-operated Ca²⁺ entry pathway undergo regulation during mouse oocyte maturation. *Mol Biol Cell* 2013, 24:1396–1410.
26. Abdullaev IF, Bisaillon JM, Potier M, Gonzalez JC, Motiani RK, Trebak M: Stim1 and Orai1 mediate CRAC currents and store-operated calcium entry important for endothelial cell proliferation. *Circ Res* 2008, 103:1289–1299.
27. El Boustany C, Katsogiannou M, Delcourt P, Dewailly E, Prevarskaya N, Bprpwiec AS, Capiod T: Differential roles of STIM1, STIM2 and Orai1 in the

control of cell proliferation and SOCE amplitude in HEK293 cells. *Cell Calcium* 2010, **47**:350–359.

28. Arellano RO, Robles-Martínez L, Serrano-Flores B, Vázquez-Cuevas F, Garay E: Agonist-activated Ca^{2+} influx and Ca^{2+} -dependent Cl$^-$ channels in *Xenopus* ovarian follicular cells: functional heterogeneity within the cell monolayer. *J Cell Physiol* 2012, **227**:3457–3470.

29. Dumont JN: Oogenesis in *Xenopus laevis* (Daudin). I. Stages of oocyte development in laboratory maintained animals. *J Morphol* 1972, **136**:153–179.

30. Hulstrand AM, Schneider PN, Houston DW: The use of antisense oligonucleotides in *Xenopus* oocytes. *Methods* 2010, **51**:75–81.

31. Saldaña C, Garay E, Rangel GE, Reyes LM, Arellano RO: Native ion current coupled to purinergic activation via basal and mechanically induced ATP release in *Xenopus* follicles. *J Cell Physiol* 2009, **218**:355–365.

32. Arellano RO, Woodward RM, Miledi R: A monovalent cationic conductance that is blocked by extracellular divalent cations in Xenopus oocytes. *J Physiol* 1995, **484**:593–604.

33. Galán C, Zbidi H, Bartegi A, Salido GM, Rosado JA: STIM1, Orai1 and hTRPC1 are important for thrombin- and ADP-induced aggregation in human platelets. *Arch Biochem Biophys* 2009, **490**:137–144.

34. López JJ, Salido GM, Pariente JA, Rosado JA: Interaction of STIM1 with endogenously expressed human canonical TRP1 upon depletion of intracellular Ca^{2+} stores. *J Biol Chem* 2006, **281**:28254–28264.

35. Tigyi G, Dyer D, Matute C, Miledi R: A serum factor that activates the phosphatidylinositol phosphate signaling system in *Xenopus* oocytes. *Proc Natl Acad Sci U S A* 1990, **87**:1521–1525.

36. Miledi R, Parker I: Chloride current induced by injection of calcium into *Xenopus* oocytes. *J Physiol* 1984, **357**:173–183.

37. Nomura Y, Kaneko S, Kato K, Yamagishi S, Sugiyama H: Inositol phosphate formation and chloride current responses induced by acetylcholine and serotonin through GTP-binding proteins in *Xenopus* oocyte after injection of rat brain messenger RNA. *Brain Res* 1987, **388**:113–123.

38. Oron Y, Dascal N, Nadler E, Lupu M: Inositol 1,4,5-trisphosphate mimics muscarinic response in *Xenopus* oocytes. *Nature* 1985, **313**:141–143.

39. Takahashi T, Neher E, Sakmann B: Rat brain serotonin receptors in Xenopus oocytes are coupled by intracellular calcium to endogenous channels. *Proc Natl Acad Sci U S A* 1987, **84**:5063–5067.

40. Putney JW: Pharmacology of store-operated calcium channels. *Mol Interv* 2010, **10**:209–218.

41. Preston SF, Sha'afi RI, Berlin RD: Regulation of Ca^{2+} influx during mitosis: Ca^{2+} influx and depletion of intracellular Ca2+ stores are coupled in interphase but not mitosis. *Cell Regul* 1991, **2**:915–925.

42. Petersen CC, Berridge MJ: The regulation of capacitative calcium entry by calcium and protein kinase C in *Xenopus* oocytes. *J Biol Chem* 1994, **269**:32246–32253.

43. Parker I, Ivorra I: Characteristics of membrane currents evoked by photoreleased inositol trisphosphate in *Xenopus* oocytes. *Am J Physiol* 1992, **263**:C154–C165.

44. Cahalan MD: STIMulating store-operated Ca^{2+} entry. *Nat Cell Biol* 2009, **11**:669–677.

45. Rothberg BS, Wang Y, Gill DL: Orai channel pore properties and gating by STIM: implications from the Orai crystal structure. *Sci Signal* 2013, **6**:pe9.

46. Hoth M, Niemeyer BA: The neglected CRAC proteins: Orai2, Orai3, and STIM2. *Curr Top Membr* 2013, **71**:237–271.

47. Oh-Hora M, Yamashita M, Hogan PG, Sharma S, Lamperti E, Chung W, Prakriya M, Feske S, Rao A: Dual functions for the endoplasmic reticulum calcium sensors STIM1 and STIM2 in T cell activation and tolerance. *Nat Immunol* 2008, **9**:432–443.

48. Kar P, Bakowski D, Di Capite J, Nelson C, Parekh AB: Different agonists recruit different stromal interaction molecule proteins to support cytoplasmic Ca^{2+} oscillations and gene expression. *Proc Natl Acad Sci U S A* 2012, **109**:6969–6974.

49. Darbellay B, Arnaudeau S, Ceroni D, Bader C, Koning S, Bernheim L: Human muscle economy myoblast differentiation and excitation-contraction coupling use the same molecular partners, STIM1 and STIM2. *J Biol Chem* 2010, **285**:22437–22447.

50. Sun S, Zhang H, Liu J, Popugaeva E, Xu NJ, Feske S, White CL, Bezprozvanny I: Reduced synaptic STIM2 expression and impaired store-operated calcium entry cause destabilization of mature spines in mutant presenilin mice. *Neuron.* 2014, **82**:79–93.

51. Gomez-Fernandez C, Lopez-Guerrero AM, Pozo-Guisado E, Álvarez IS, Matín-Romero FJ: Calcium signaling in mouse oocyte maturation: the roles of STIM1, ORAI1 and SOCE. *Mol Hum Reprod* 2012, **18**:194–203. Miao Y-L, Williams CJ: Calcium signaling in mammalian egg activation and embryo development: the influence of subcellular localization. *Mol Reprod Dev* 2012, **79**:742–756.

52. Miao Y-L, Williams CJ: Calcium signaling in mammalian egg activation and embryo development: the influence of subcellular localization. *Mol Reprod Dev* 2012, **79**:742–756.

10

Genomic homeostasis is dysregulated in favour of apoptosis in the colonic epithelium of the azoxymethane treated rat

Caroline A Kerr[1,2,6*], Barney M Hines[1,3], Janet M Shaw[1,2], Robert Dunne[1,4], Lauren M Bragg[1,4], Julie Clarke[1,5], Trevor Lockett[1,2] and Richard Head[1]

Abstract

Background: The acute response to genotoxic carcinogens in rats is an important model for researching cancer initiation events. In this report we define the normal rat colonic epithelium by describing transcriptional events along the anterior-posterior axis and then investigate the acute effects of azoxymethane (AOM) on gene expression, with a particular emphasis on pathways associated with the maintenance of genomic integrity in the proximal and distal compartments using whole genome expression microarrays.

Results: There are large transcriptional changes that occur in epithelial gene expression along the anterior-posterior axis of the normal healthy rat colon. AOM administration superimposes substantial changes on these basal gene expression patterns in both the distal and proximal rat colonic epithelium. In particular, the pathways associated with cell cycle and DNA damage and repair processes appear to be disrupted in favour of apoptosis.

Conclusions: The healthy rats' colon exhibits extensive gene expression changes between its proximal and distal ends. The most common changes are associated with metabolism, but more subtle expression changes in genes involved in genomic homeostasis are also evident. These latter changes presumably protect and maintain a healthy colonic epithelium against incidental dietary and environmental insults. AOM induces substantial changes in gene expression, resulting in an early switch in the cell cycle process, involving p53 signalling, towards cell cycle arrest leading to the more effective process of apoptosis to counteract this genotoxic insult.

Keywords: Colorectal cancer, Azoxymethane, Rats, Gene expression

Background

Colorectal cancer (CRC) is the third most common cancer in males and second most common in females world-wide [1]. The majority of these cancers are considered preventable by appropriate diet and associated lifestyle factors [2]. Dietary patterns consisting of micronutrient dense, low-fat, high-fibre food patterns protect against colorectal cancer [3,4]. Conversely, specific sources of dietary protein have been linked to increased CRC risk [5] and animal studies have indicated that different dietary proteins can induce DNA damage in the rats' colon [6]. Consequently, the challenge is to translate this information into strategies that prevent CRC. One of the first steps to doing this is to understand the early molecular events involved in oncogenesis and develop hypotheses on the role played by environmental factors such as diet in this process.

The azoxymethane (AOM)-treated rodent provides an important tool in the study of sporadic CRC development and progression [7]. It has been used extensively to study colon carcinogenesis and its prevention, in at least two formats that model different aspects of CRC [8,9]. One version of this model studies tumour development (at least 14 weeks post-treatment) to find the underlying signalling pathways of colon carcinogenesis. For instance, it has been used to investigate mouse models of colorectal carcinogenesis using gene expression profiling and has provided significant insights into the role of reactivated

* Correspondence: Caroline_Kerr@uow.edu.au
[1]CSIRO Preventative Health Flagship, CSIRO, North Ryde, NSW 2113, Australia
[2]CSIRO, Food and Nutritional Sciences, North Ryde, NSW 2113, Australia
Full list of author information is available at the end of the article

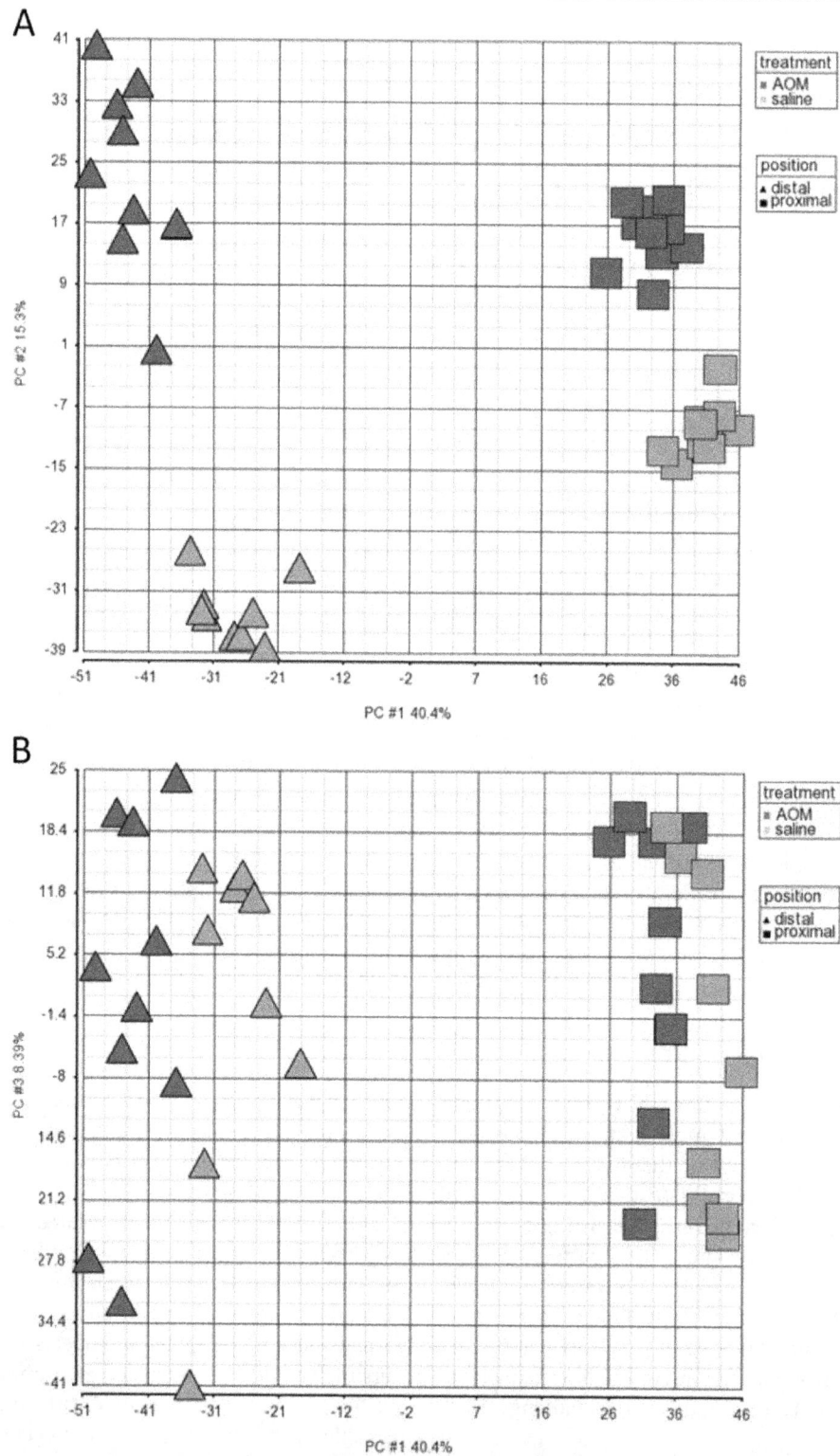

Figure 1 Global gene expression depicted as a principal component analyses (PCA, covariate) showing the A) PC1 and PC2 and B) PC1 and PC3, illustrating the effect of six hours post-AOM on proximal and distal sections of the rat colon (AOM distal ▲, AOM proximal ■, saline distal "light gray triangle symbol" and saline proximal "light gray square symbol").

embryonic signatures in colon tumours [10]. The other main version of the AOM model is the 'cancer initiation' model, which is used to study the early response to the carcinogen, where tissues are harvested shortly after treatment (around 0–48 hours) [11]. Using this latter acute AOM model, we report here some of the early transcriptional events induced by this carcinogen in mucosal tissue along the length of the colon in rats.

Results and discussion

The colonic epithelium is one of the largest epithelial barriers in the body and is in a constant state of self-renewal. In order to understand the effects of a carcinogenic insult to this tissue, it is important to develop an understanding of the natural morphologic and molecular features of the normal rat colon. It has been demonstrated that rat colonic stem cells are located in different positions and behave differently in crypts sampled from different points along the anterior-posterior length of the colon [12]. In distal sections, stem cells are located in the crypt base from whence progeny differentiating cells then migrate up towards the lumen, ultimately undergoing anoikis and sloughing off into the digesta [12]. In proximal sections, stem cells are located in the middle one-third of the crypt. Differentiating cells migrate bi-directionally from this source with some differentiating colonocytes migrating towards the lumen, while others migrate into the crypt base [12]. Our own data confirm the observations of others that the crypt height in the normal rat distal colon is greater than that for the proximal colon (34.4 ± 0.26 and 27.4 ± 0.27 cells respectively, $P<0.0001$, n=10). Despite these morphological differences, no significant differences in rates of baseline apoptosis between the proximal and distal normal (saline treated) colon (0.018 ± 0.012 and 0.057 ± 0.028 cells per crypt, respectively) were observed.

It has been shown in mice that significant numbers of genes are differentially expressed along functionally distinct regions of the gastrointestinal tract [13,14] and this is also true for the normal human colon [15,16]. When gene expression in the normal colon of the rat was examined at the level of individual genes, the proximal expression profile differed markedly from that of the distal colonic epithelium with 4527 genes differentially expressed (False Discovery Rate (FDR) 0.05) (Figure 1). These genes are listed in Additional file 1: Table S1. This microarray dataset was also validated by demonstrating that the top 8 genes most differentially expressed between the proximal and distal colon were also 100% consistently differentially expressed using real time RTPCR (as shown in Additional file 1: Table S3).

When the functional groupings of these genes were considered through pathway analysis, most of the top 20 pathways identified were broadly associated with intestinal metabolism functions (see Figure 2 for the top 20

pathways). The magnitude of these changes in expression can be very large (changes up to 104 fold). We consider this association with metabolism most likely reflects the changing profile of digestive functions naturally occurring along the length of the colon. Consequently, these position-associated profiles provide the background against which changes in gene expression induced by colonic carcinogens need to be assessed.

The carcinogens AOM and 1,2-Dimethylhydrazine are metabolised by cytochrome P450 (CYP2E1) into methylazoxymethanol. In turn this breaks down to form highly reactive alkylating species which can lead to the addition of methyl adducts at the O^6 position of Guanine residues in the DNA to form the promutagenic modified base O^6 methyl guanine (O6-mdGua). If this modified base is not repaired, it can lead to G:C to A:T transition mutations during replication Tan [17,18]. These DNA adduct-induced mutations are found commonly in colorectal cancers [18]. So not surprisingly, AOM induces substantial transcriptional changes in the mucosa of the rat colon six hours after subcutaneous administration (Figure 1). The genes differentially expressed in response to AOM are listed in Additional file 1: Table S1. There were 1960 and 9441 genes differently expressed (FDR 0.05) in the proximal and distal colons respectively of AOM-treated rats when compared with the same tissues from normal (saline treated) animals. The fold changes were up to 6.6 in the proximal and 10.7 in the distal colon.

At a whole genome level, principal component analysis (PCA) revealed that the magnitude of the site effect on gene expression (proximal versus distal colon) was equal to or greater than that of AOM for the two highest principal components (PCs) (Figure 1A). Further examination of the PCA revealed that PC1 and PC3 best explained the effect of AOM (Figure 1B), and PC1 and PC4 best explained the effect of 'site' (not shown). As it has been previously shown that the greatest effects of AOM in the rat, in terms of tumours numbers are exhibited in the distal colon [10] and human tumours predominately occur in the most distal colonic region, i.e. sigmoid colon and the rectum [16], it is not surprising that there almost 10-fold more genes expressed in the distal rat colon at 6 hours post treatment. As a consequence, this report will concentrate predominantly on the effects this carcinogen in this colonic region with a particular focus on DNA damage and repair.

In a previous study using the "cancer initiation" AOM model in Sprague Dawley rats, Tan et al. measured levels of O6-mdGua accumulating in the DNA from a number of tissues harvested 6 hours and 48 hours after subcutaneous injection of this carcinogen. They observed that 6 hours after AOM exposure, the highest levels O6-mdGua occurred in the following tissues (in order of highest to lowest): liver, distal colon, proximal colon, proximal small intestine (SI), and kidney. The stomach, distal SI, bladder,

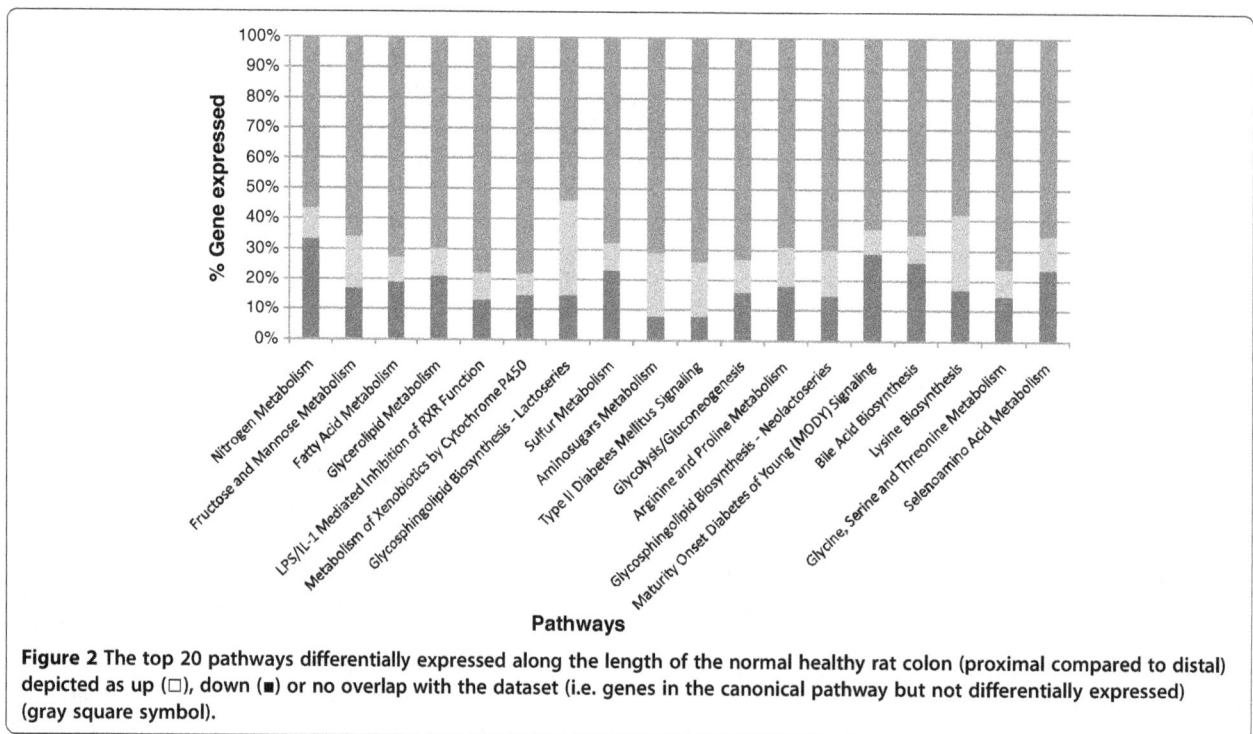

Figure 2 The top 20 pathways differentially expressed along the length of the normal healthy rat colon (proximal compared to distal) depicted as up (□), down (■) or no overlap with the dataset (i.e. genes in the canonical pathway but not differentially expressed) (gray square symbol).

spleen, blood and lung had relatively low levels O6-mdGua. While levels of this highly mutagenic alkylation product had dropped in most tissues tested by 48 h post AOM administration, O6-mdGua levels remained high at this time point in the proximal and distal colon, kidney and bladder. This is a significant finding as the distal colon is more prone to AOM induced tumours than any other tissue [17] and tumours in the bladder and kidney have been observed in animals treated with high levels of dimethyl hydrazine, a precursor of AOM [19].

A key enzyme involved in the repair of O6-mdGua is O-6-methylguanine DNA methyltransferase (MGMT). In a 'suicide' reaction the methyl adduct from one modified guanine base is transferred to a cysteine residue in the active site of one molecule of enzyme resulting in the inactivation of that molecule of enzyme and earmarking it for ubiquitination and degradation [20]. Interestingly, in the current study, in the normal colon, the level of expression of MGMT was greater in the distal section compared to the proximal section (Figure 3). This would be consistent with an adaptation to a higher basal metabolic demand for DNA adduct repair in the distal colonic mucosa relative to the proximal. This could arise in response to dietary mutagens in the colonic digesta becoming more concentrated as more and more water is removed during its transit from proximal to distal colon. Whatever the drivers may be, however, this change in MGMT levels from proximal to distal colon is likely to form a part of an innate homeostatic

process to maintain genomic integrity in a healthy colonic mucosa.

Six hours after the administration of AOM, MGMT expression was down-regulated in both the proximal and distal colonic epithelium (fold changes −1.39 and −1.79 respectively). As there are high levels of O6-mdGua present in the DNA of the distal colon at this time [17] and with MGMT being the primary enzyme for repair of DNA methyl adducts, it appears that MGMT is rapidly depleted instead of being up-regulated in response to AOM. As the animals survive AOM challenge well with no apparent significant loss of colonic function, this observation suggests that other repair mechanisms are brought into play to ensure the rapid return to normal colonic function.

Further analysis revealed that the expression of a number of other DNA repair and damage genes was also altered in response to AOM, particularly in the distal colon (see Figure 3 and Additional file 1: Table S2). Expression of the damaged DNA binding and sensing H2A histone family member X (H2AFX) gene was significantly up-regulated in response to AOM (p=3.08E-08, fold change 1.5) (Figure 3), confirming that repair mechanisms other than MGMT are deployed in response to the AOM perturbation. In terms of single strand break repair, there are a number of nucleotide-excision repair (NER) (n=16) genes differentially expressed in the distal colon in response to AOM treatment and 80% of them were up-regulated. This is

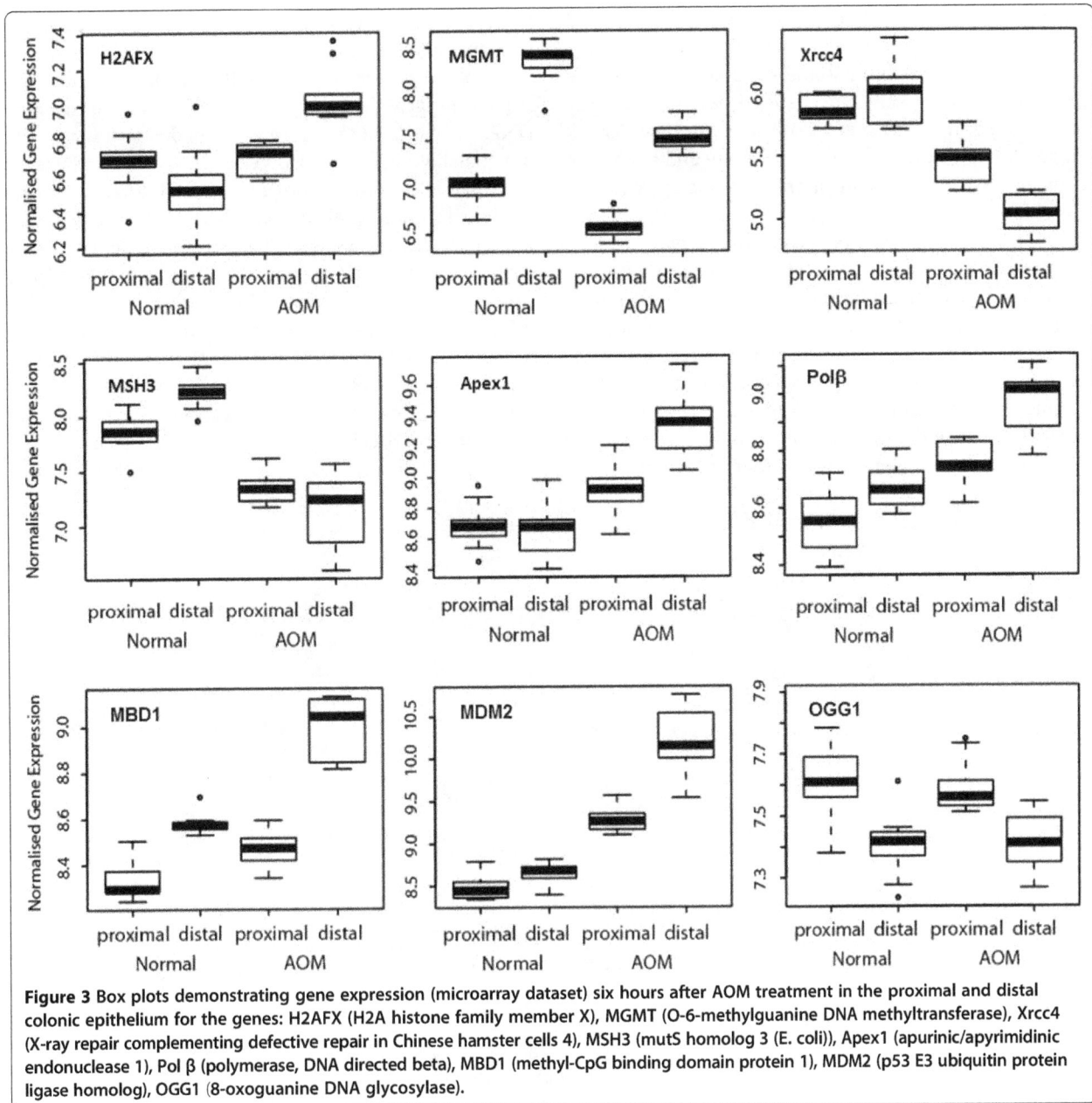

Figure 3 Box plots demonstrating gene expression (microarray dataset) six hours after AOM treatment in the proximal and distal colonic epithelium for the genes: H2AFX (H2A histone family member X), MGMT (O-6-methylguanine DNA methyltransferase), Xrcc4 (X-ray repair complementing defective repair in Chinese hamster cells 4), MSH3 (mutS homolog 3 (E. coli)), Apex1 (apurinic/apyrimidinic endonuclease 1), Pol β (polymerase, DNA directed beta), MBD1 (methyl-CpG binding domain protein 1), MDM2 (p53 E3 ubiquitin protein ligase homolog), OGG1 (8-oxoguanine DNA glycosylase).

important as NER is the most flexible of the DNA repair pathways as it repairs bulky DNA lesions [21]. Other base-excision repair associated genes also showing increased expression in response to treatment with AOM include Apex1 (apurinic/apyrimidinic endonuclease 1) had a 1.6 fold change and Polβ, (polymerase, DNA directed beta) a 1.4 fold change (see Figures 3). The mismatch repair (MMR) pathway is an important pathway involved in the DNA damage response to carcinogen induced lesions resulting in cell cycle arrest and, at high lesion load, apoptosis [22]. However, AOM treatment led to the down-regulated response of MMR genes (n=4). For instance, MSH3 (mutS homolog 3 (E. coli)), which recognises insertion/deletion mismatches containing two or more extra bases [23] showed decreased expression (–2.1 fold change) with AOM (Figure 3). These observations suggest that the MMR pathway in general may be down-regulated in response to AOM and are consistent with AOM's major mode of action involving DNA adduct formation and induction of point mutations rather than the formation of multi-base mismatches.

Double-strand breaks (DSB), in which both strands in the DNA double helix are severed, are particularly hazardous to the cell because they can lead to genome rearrangements [24]. DSB repair via homologous recombination (HR) is an important process as it takes place late in the S- and G2-

phases of the cell cycle to prevent unrepaired double strand breaks from causing down-stream problems in transcription, replication and chromosome segregation [25]. In the distal colon there were nine genes from this pathway up-regulated in response to AOM. For instance, Xrcc2, which plays a central role in this pathway and encodes a member of the Rad51 family of proteins, was up-regulated 1.5-fold. Conversely, the DSB repair via non-homologous end-joining (NHEJ) pathway was down-regulated with AOM, demonstrated by the decreased expression of Xrcc4 (X-ray repair complementing defective repair in Chinese hamster cells 4, -1.94 fold change) (Figure 3). Consequently, there is some evidence that single and double strand break repair functions may be compromised in response to AOM treatment. These data coupled with the accumulation of unrepaired O6-mdGua lesions in colonic epithelium in response to carcinogen, indicates that at six hours post

treatment other cellular processes such as cell cycle arrest and apoptosis becomes more important in maintaining mucosal integrity in response to this genomic insult.

To investigate the biological consequences of unrepaired DNA damage, such as the O6-mdGua lesions, the functionality of the top 800 genes differentially expressed in response to AOM in the proximal and distal colon, was examined through pathways analysis. The top 12 pathways in which the highest percentage of component genes displayed AOM-associated differential expression relative to the saline treated control in the distal and proximal colonic mucosa are shown in Figure 4. There was a number of cell cycle regulation pathways differentially expressed in the distal colon 6 hours after the treatment with AOM. These included, "p53 signalling" and "Cell cycle regulation by B cell translocation (BTG)" (see Figure 4 for more cell cycle pathways). This is noteworthy as

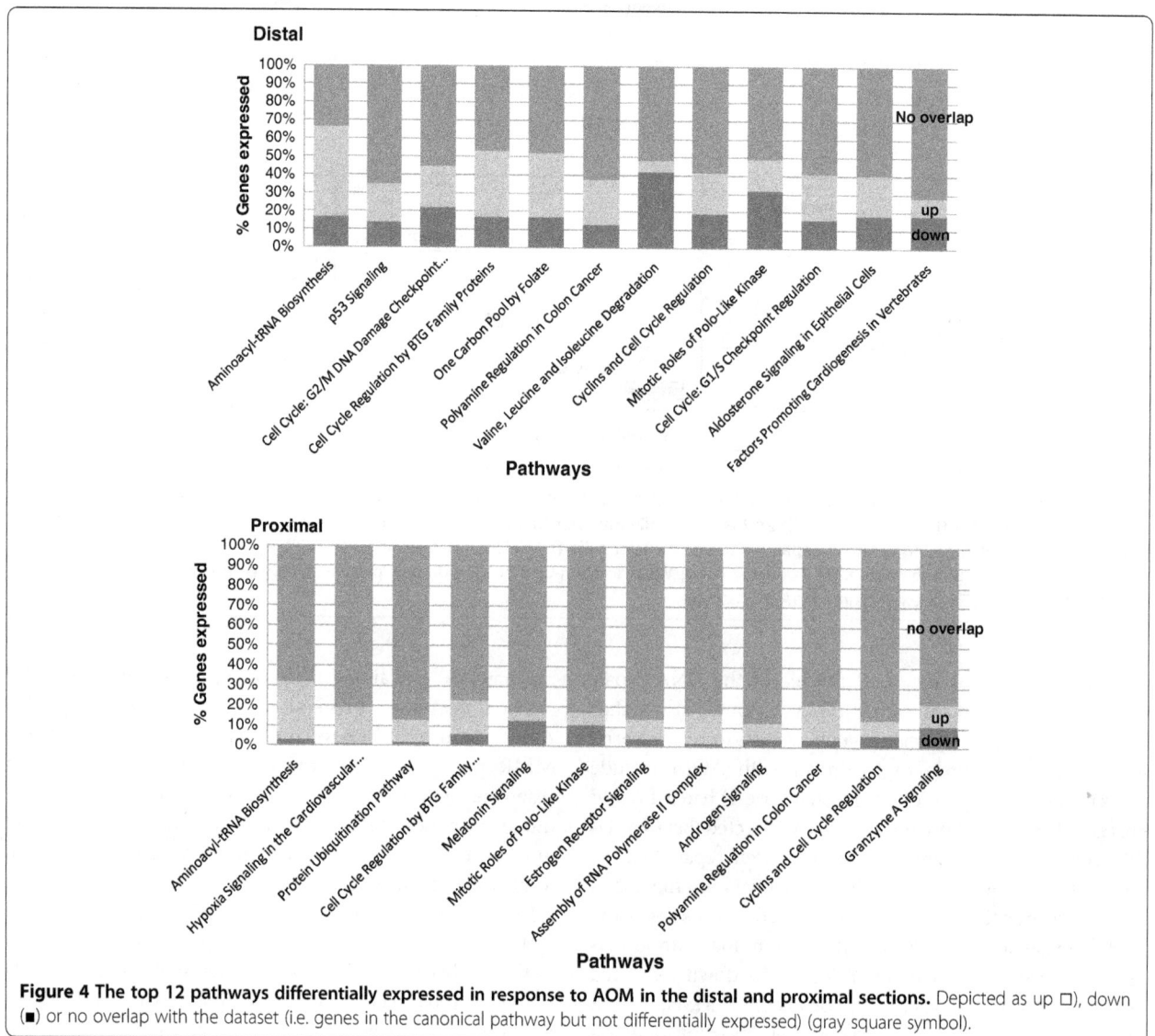

Figure 4 The top 12 pathways differentially expressed in response to AOM in the distal and proximal sections. Depicted as up □), down (■) or no overlap with the dataset (i.e. genes in the canonical pathway but not differentially expressed) (gray square symbol).

deregulated cell cycle processes are a prominent feature of oncogenesis [25]. Overall, the response suggests a trend towards cell cycle arrest in response to AOM.

DNA damage checkpoint control mechanisms tightly regulate progression through the cell cycle, ensuring the fidelity of cell division which is an important self-defence mechanism for the maintenance of genome stability [26]. A number of observations support the involvement of the p53 signalling (see Figure 5) and BTG pathways in AOM-induced cell cycle arrest in the distal colon: Cyclin G1, a protein involved in G2/M phase arrest and regulates p53 [27] expression increased 4.34 fold; cyclin dependent kinase inhibitor 1 (p21Cip1), which inhibits the activity of cyclin-CDK2 or -CDK4 complexes [28], is marginally up-regulated, and as a result Retinoblastoma 1 (Rb1) is down-regulated (1.5 fold); BTG family member 2 (BTG2), an important transcriptional regulator that impairs G1-S cell cycle progression [29] increased 2.34 fold and MDM2 (p53 binding protein homolog, 2.81 fold change increase) (Figure 3) which is also a member of another expressed

pathway, "Cell Cycle: G2/M DNA Damage Checkpoint Regulation" (p= 0.002). This latter cell cycle pathway has other genes differentially expressed. For example, Chek1, which is a checkpoint regulator of cell cycle arrest and putative tumour suppressor in response to DNA damage [30], is up-regulated (1.6 fold change). Most cancer cells harbour mutations in tumour suppressors and/or onco-genes which would normally control cell cycle checkpoints [26]. Therefore, cell cycle regulation is important in the maintenance of genomic stability and to prevent cells that have undergone malignant transformation progressing through the cell cycle phases.

The p53 signaling pathway (pvalue 1.66×10^{-4}) is significantly expressed (the second most highly expressed pathway in the distal colon) in response to AOM. Loss of p53 function is thought to be a contributing factor in colorectal cancer, because the p53-dependent pathway shuts down damaged cells, either through apoptosis, cell-cycle arrest or cellular senescence [31]. Apoptosis was observed histologically to have significantly increased

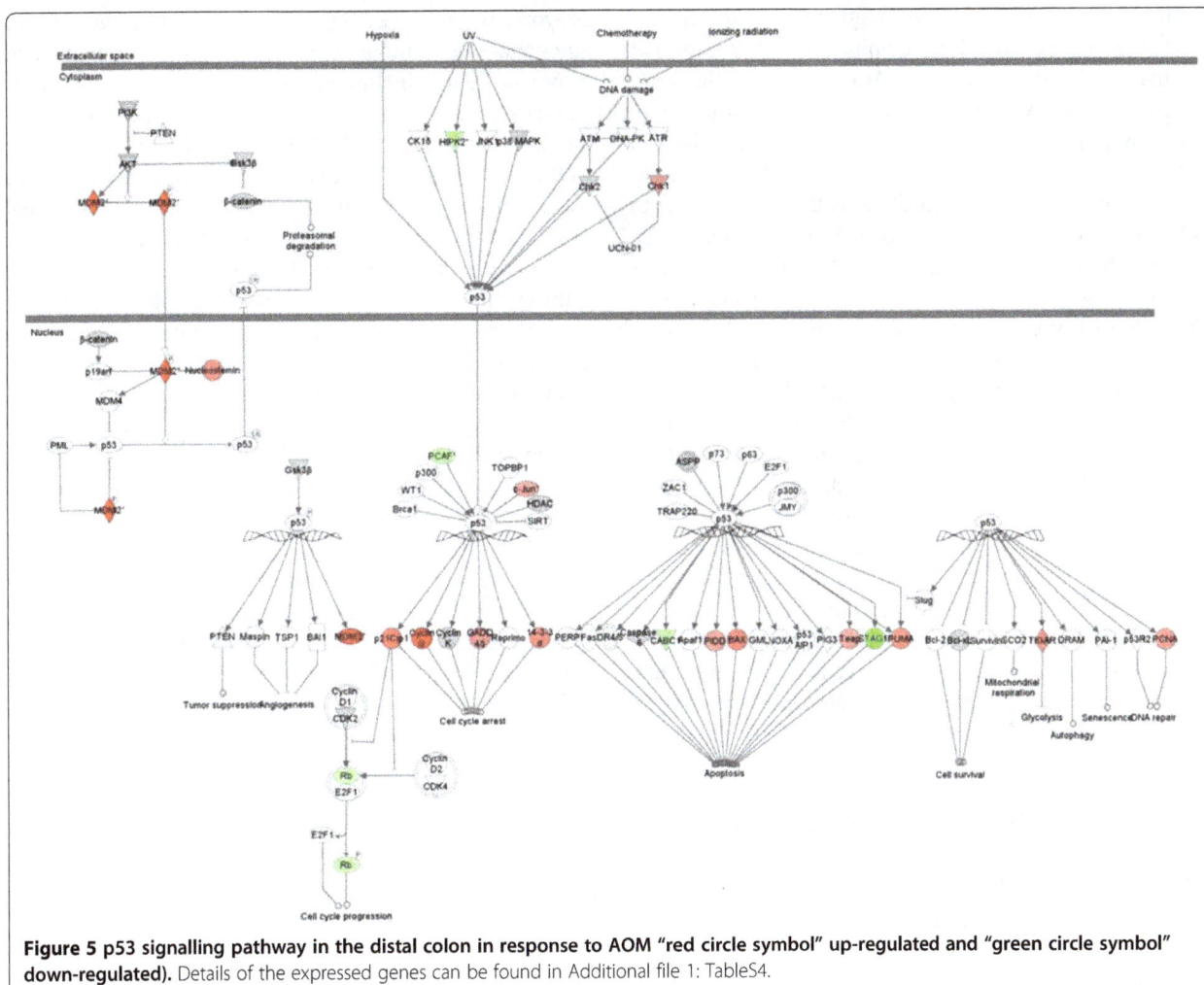

Figure 5 p53 signalling pathway in the distal colon in response to AOM "red circle symbol" up-regulated and "green circle symbol" down-regulated). Details of the expressed genes can be found in Additional file 1: TableS4.

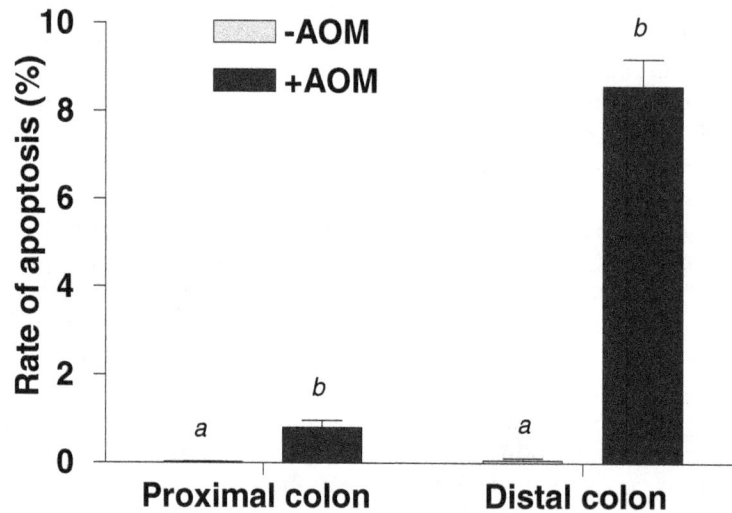

Figure 6 Apoptotic indices (% apoptotic cells per crypt height) of the proximal and distal colonic epithelium of rats 6 h after injection with saline (–AOM) and AOM (+AOM) as determined by morphological assessment of the colonic mucosa. Data are mean±SEM (n=20). Means within the same colonic section with different superscripts are significantly different (P<0.0001).

at six hours after the AOM treatment (Figure 6). As MGMT is depleted at this time point, we hypothesise that the main cellular response to AOM involves the early depletion of MGMT then a switch to the induction of apoptosis and this most likely first occurs through the p53 signalling pathway. This is demonstrated through closer examination of the p53 signalling pathway response to AOM in the distal colon (see Figure 5). Firstly, genes such as TP53INP1 (tumour protein p53 inducible nuclear protein 1), which is a key transcriptional regulator that responds to a variety of cellular stresses, including DNA damage, oxidative stress and activated oncogenes, to regulate key cellular processes including the induction of apoptosis [32], is up-regulated 1.5 fold. Furthermore, Caspases 1 (Casp1) and Casp3 are up-regulated in response to AOM in the distal colon (1.2 fold change for both). The activation of Casp3 triggers an execution arm of the apoptosis response initiating DNA fragmentation [33]. The apoptotic function of caspases is regulated by the Bcl-2 family of proteins [34]. Accordingly, in response to AOM, Bcl-associated X protein (Bax) which is critically important in the up-regulation of apoptosis, is increased two fold. Furthermore, there is also decreased expression of the caspase-activated inhibitor Avon by 1.2-fold. Therefore, these results indicate that at 6 hours after being treated with AOM, one of the major effects of this carcinogen occurs through the p53 signalling pathway and the result is cell cycle arrest and a cellular switch towards apoptosis.

Gene network analysis was used to further understand the function of genes expressed in response to AOM in each colonic segment, in particular the early induction of apoptosis. When the top three AOM/proximal networks were merged (Figure 7) there were 13 genes with functional annotations (p= 7.16×10^{-4}) associated with colorectal cancer including the up-regulation (1.6-fold) of transcriptional regulator c-JUN (jun proto-oncogene) and the down-regulation of MGMT (1.4-fold). In terms of the AOM/distal network there were eight genes associated with colon cancer (p= 5.04×10^{-4}), including the transcriptional regulator MYC (up-regulated 1.6 -fold) and the previously mentioned c-JUN (Figure 8). When the p53 signalling pathway and apoptosis genes were cross-referenced in this network, c-Jun Kinase (JNK), which regulates cJUN and is an important regulator of cell death [35], was a gene common to both and is linked through the gene network to the down-regulated p53 signalling transcriptional regulator, Retinoblastoma 1 (Rb1). Taken together these results suggest that the early genomic damage effects of AOM on the colonic mucosa may be mediated through the p53 pathway, favouring apoptosis through c-JUN/ JNK signalling and preventing cell cycle progression through reduced Rb1 expression. Whilst this mechanism is hypothetical, it provides a framework for the further elucidation of the key mechanisms underpinning the cellular switch towards apoptosis in the gut mucosa in response to alkylating carcinogen challenge.

Conclusion

The healthy rat colonic mucosa exhibits extensive gene expression changes from its proximal to distal end reflecting regional changes in metabolic function. The normal rat colon also has naturally occurring protective and genomic repair mechanisms expressed dynamically, albeit subtly, along the proximal/distal axis. Six hours

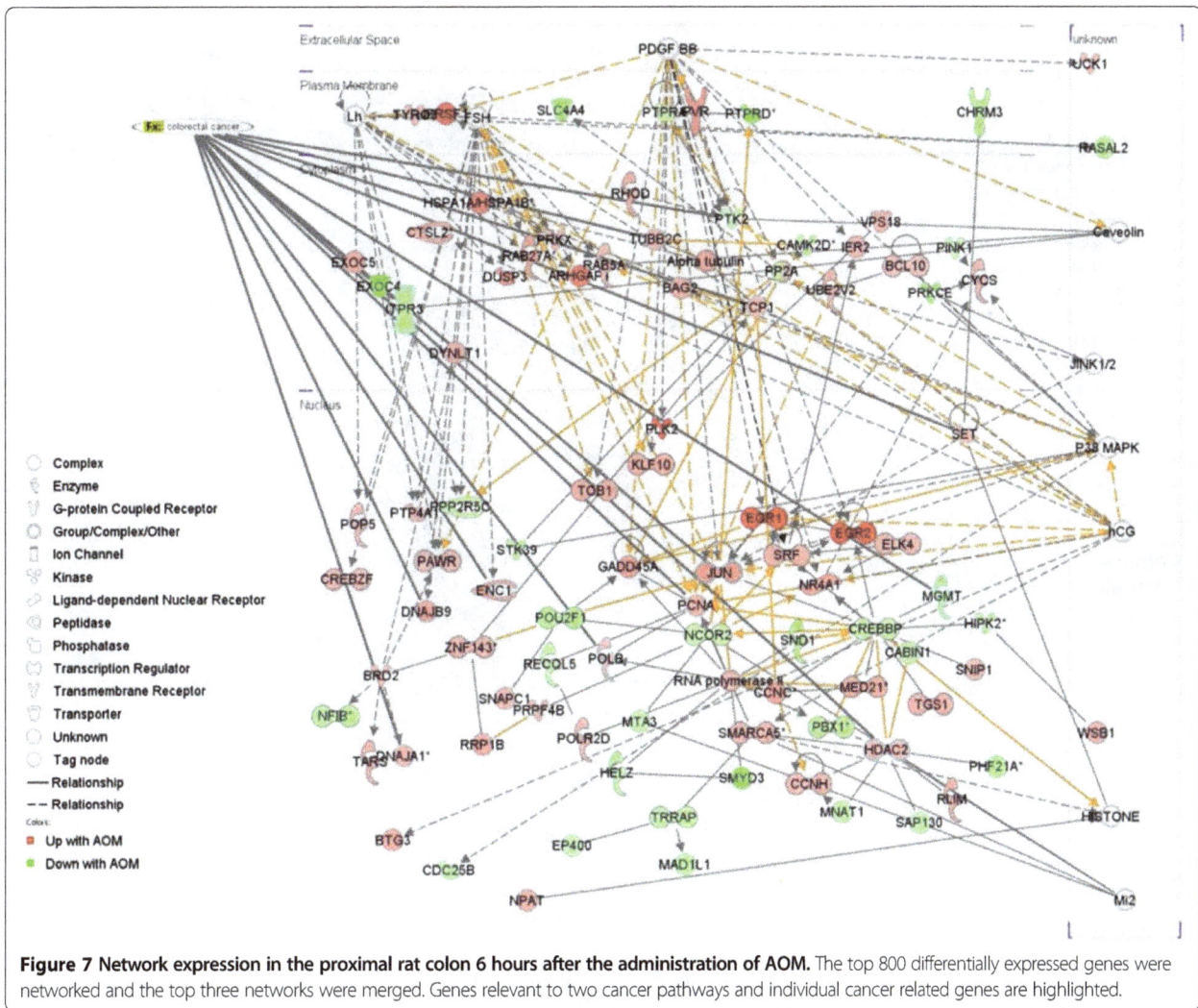

Figure 7 Network expression in the proximal rat colon 6 hours after the administration of AOM. The top 800 differentially expressed genes were networked and the top three networks were merged. Genes relevant to two cancer pathways and individual cancer related genes are highlighted.

after administration of AOM, substantial changes in gene expression have occurred in the colonic mucosa and these also differ along the length of the colon. The changes are greater in the distal colon and appear particularly associated with the sensing of genomic damage, associated cell cycle arrest and a cellular switch towards the induction of apoptosis. Consequently, the genomic homeostasis mechanisms that naturally exist to combat dietary and environmental insults in the colon of the normal rat appear to be dysregulated by AOM resulting in a cellular switch through p53 signaling to more efficient genes associated with the apoptotic response, a genetic response that is also reflected histologically.

Methods

Animals and diets

Forty male Sprague Dawley rats weighing approximately 176 ± 2.4 g were purchased from the Animal Resource Centre, Western Australia. They were housed in wire-bottomed caging in a temperature controlled room

(22-24°C) with a 12 h light/dark cycle. They were randomly allocated into two groups (n=20) with approximately equal body weights. They were given free access to water and a modified AIN-93G diet [36]. Both groups were fed this diet for 28 days. One group was then injected subcutaneously with azoxymethane (AOM; 15 mg/kg; Sigma Chemical Co., St. Louis, MO, USA) the other with saline. Six hours after injection the rats were anaesthetised with isoflurane and killed by exsanguination. The large bowel (excluding the rectum) was removed, opened longitudinally along the mesenteric border and digesta removed. The colon was rinsed clean with PBS and transferred to a chilled ceramic plate for dissection. The colons were on average 15 ± 0.5 cm long. The last 0.5 cm distal and first 0.5 cm proximal sections of the colon were discarded and the next 2 cm from both ends placed into 10% buffered formalin (Sigma) for morphological assessment of apoptosis. Mucosal samples for gene expression and protein analyses were collected by scraping the next 4 cm of proximal and distal colon with new microscope slides. The mucosal

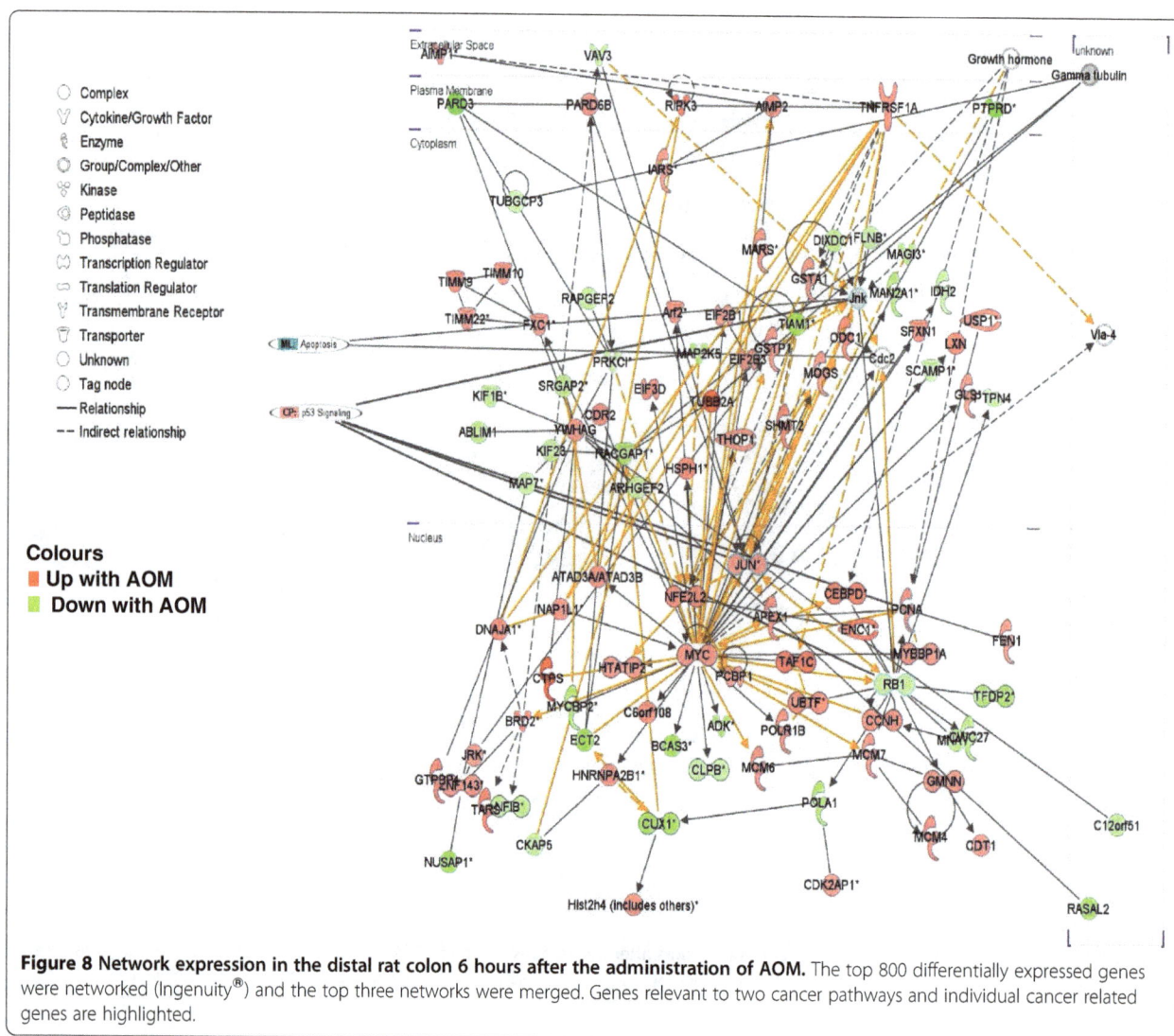

Figure 8 Network expression in the distal rat colon 6 hours after the administration of AOM. The top 800 differentially expressed genes were networked (Ingenuity®) and the top three networks were merged. Genes relevant to two cancer pathways and individual cancer related genes are highlighted.

samples were placed in RNA*later* (Sigma Chemical Co., St. Louis, MO, USA) and then stored at −80°C for later processing. All instruments were replaced or cleaned thoroughly between animals.

All procedures involving animals were approved by the Commonwealth Scientific and Industrial Research Organisation (CSIRO) Human Nutrition Animal Ethics Committee and complied with the *Australian code of practice (2004).* [http://www.nhmrc.gov.au/publications/synopses/ea16syn.htm].

Measurement of crypt height and colonocyte apoptosis

The rate of apoptosis was determined on paraffin-embedded sections (4 μm) stained with haematoxylin (Harris, BDH Laboratory Supplies, England). An Olympus BX-41 light microscope (Olympus Corp., Japan) was used to identify 20 randomly chosen intact crypts and to determine the crypt height by counting the total number of cells from the base to the lumen using a previously

validated technique [37]. The number of apoptotic cells was identified by cell shrinkage, presence of condensed chromatin, and sharply delineated cell borders surrounded by a clear halo as described by [38]. All histological analyses were performed in a blinded fashion by a single operator. The rates of apoptosis for each section of colon (±AOM) were analysed with Mann Whitney t-tests using GraphPad Prism Version 4.00 (GraphPad Software Inc. San Diego, CA, USA). Data are expressed as mean ± standard error of the mean (SEM).

Acquisition and data analysis

Proximal and distal sections from ten rats were used from each group. It was ascertained in a preliminary study that investigated baseline variation in this model and tissue type, that n=10 was a sufficient sample (see Gene Expression Omnibus (GEO) accession number GSE13802 for the complete dataset of this pilot study). The distal and proximal colonic mucosal samples from the AOM and saline treated rats were removed from the RNAlater stabilisation reagent (Sigma, Australia) and placed in 1ml of TRIzol® Reagent (Invitrogen, Sydney, N.S.W., Australia). Samples were then homogenised using beads (mix of 2.5 mm glass and 0.1 - 1.0 mm diameter silicon-zirconian beads) in a MiniBeadbeater-8™ (BioSpec Products Inc. Oklahoma, US). Total RNA was extracted according to the TRIzol® Reagent manufacturer's instruction after which samples were further purified using RNAeasy mini spin columns (QIAGEN, Doncaster, Victoria, Australia) with a DNase on-column digestion as per the manufacturer's instructions. The integrity of the RNA was checked using a Bioanalyzer 2100 (Agilent Technologies) and quantified using a NanoDrop® ND-1000 Spectrophotometer. Ten AOM rat and nine saline rat proximal and distal colonic epithelia (one saline set was dropped due to substandard RNA quality), i.e. 38 RNA (4.5 µg) samples, were processed for microarray expression analysis using high-density oligonucleotide arrays (Affymetrix® GeneChip array, Affymetrix®, Santa Clara, CA, USA) commensurate with the manufacturer's instructions. The complete microarray dataset from this study can be sourced at NCBI's Gene Expression Omnibus (GEO accession GSE15184).

Affymetrix® Gene Chip Rat Expression 230® results were analysed using the Partek® genomics suite software for differential expression, using an RMA normalization method. This software was used to Principal Component Analysis (PCA) which is a mathematical algorithm that reduces the dimensionality of the data by identifying directions, called principal components (e.g. PC1, PC2, etc.), along which the variation in the data is maximal [39]. The results were then plotted so that it is possible to visually assess similarities and differences between samples and determine whether samples can be grouped. The Partek software was also used to generate lists of differentially expressed genes by obtaining estimates of variance components for mixed models, using the method of moments estimation [40], restricted maximum likelihood estimation (REML) [41], and minimum variance quadratic unbiased estimation (MIVQUE) [42] using Analysis of Variance model that included rat number, colonic position (proximal or distal) and treatment (AOM or saline). As there is multiplicity of genes in microarray datasets, particularly for genes with small standard errors that can generate false discoveries, we used the False Discovery Rate (FDR) [43] to restrict our gene lists beyond p-values. The Gene Ontology Biological Processing and Molecular function terms [44] were added to the lists of differentially expressed. Individual gene data is presented using Box and Whisker plots which describes the dataset on an interval scale, i.e. as explanatory data analysis, to demonstrate the shape of the distribution, its central value, and its variability. The ends of the box are the upper and lower quartiles, so the box spans the interquartile range, the median is marked by a vertical line inside the box and the whiskers are the two lines outside the box that extend to the highest and lowest observations.

Pathway and network expression

While the characterization of each gene that is differentially expressed in response to AOM as outlined above provides useful data, the identification of specific pathways that are changed in response to the AOM treatment is important for understanding the early changes that occur at a transcriptome level. To further understand the biology of gene expression comparisons, beyond the lists of expressed gene, pathway and network analysis was also performed using Ingenuity Pathway Analysis (Ingenuity® Systems, Inc., Redwood City, CA, USA, http://www.ingenuity.com), a curated knowledge base with over 1·5 million entries to determine the pathways that are perturbed by AOM. IPA identifies differentially expressed pathways based on the probability of having the observed number of differentially expressed genes associated with the dataset for that pathway in Ingenuity's propriety database, by random chance and the p-value is calculated with the right-tailed Fisher's Exact Test (Ingenuity® Systems, www.ingenuity.com). This analysis was applied to lists of the top 800 differentially expressed genes from comparisons of normal proximal rat colon to normal distal rat colon and the AOM-induced changes in both the proximal and distal colon. The gene network analysis was performed as described by [45] and Ingenuity® Systems, www.ingenuity.com.

Real-time PCR validation

As there is a risk of false discovery associated with microarray experiments (see above) it is important to verify data using an independent technology platform such as RTPCR. As a result the top eight differentially expressed genes between proximal and distal rat colon that were identified by microarray data analysis were chosen to be a representative subset and were measured by qRTPCR using TaqMan® Universal PCR Master Mix commensurate with the manufacturer's instructions). Reactions were performed in 20 ul reaction volumes using an ABI PRISM® 7700 Sequence Detection System. Data were normalised using the Relative Quantitation of Gene Expression method as outlined in the ABI 7700 manual. An aliquot of any given RNA sample used for microarray gene expression analysis was reverse-transcribed to provide the substrate for qRTPCR quantification.

Competing interests

The authors declare that they have no competing interests.

Authors' contributions

CK co-designed the study with JC, co-authored the manuscript with RD, LMB, JC, TL and RH, lead the molecular work, guided the study concept and helped with data interpretation. BMH and JMS performed the molecular work, JC carried out the animal study and the tissue results, RD, JMS and LMB carried out the data analysis, TL and RH developed the concept of the study and sought funding. All authors read and approved the final manuscript.

Acknowledgements

We thank Glenn Brown for running the GeneChip slides and Ben Scherer and Jessica Southwood for their help with the animal samples. We would also like to thank Kim Fung and Konsta Duesing for their valuable manuscript critique.

Author details

[1]CSIRO Preventative Health Flagship, CSIRO, North Ryde, NSW 2113, Australia. [2]CSIRO, Food and Nutritional Sciences, North Ryde, NSW 2113, Australia. [3]CSIRO Division of Livestock Industries, Queensland Biosciences Precinct, St Lucia, Queensland 4067, Australia. [4]CSIRO, Mathematical and Information Sciences, North Ryde, New South Wales 1670, Australia. [5]CSIRO Food and Nutritional Sciences, Adelaide 5000, South Australia. [6]Graduate School of Medicine, University of Wollongong, Wollongong, NSW, Australia.

References

1. Parkin DM, Bray F, Ferlay J, Pisani P: Global cancer statistics, 2002. *CA Cancer J Clin* 2005, **55**(2):74–108.
2. Platz EA, Willett WC, Colditz GA, Rimm EB, Spiegelman D, Giovannucci E: Proportion of colon cancer risk that might be preventable in a cohort of middle-aged US men. *Cancer Cause Control* 2000, **11**(7):579–588.
3. Park Y, Hunter DJ, Spiegelman D, Bergkvist L, Berrino F, van den Brandt PA, Buring JE, Colditz GA, Freudenheim JL, Fuchs CS, et al: Dietary fiber intake and risk of colorectal cancer - A pooled analysis of prospective cohort studies. *Jama-J Am Med Assoc* 2005, **294**(22):2849–2857.
4. Wirfalt E, Midthune D, Reedy J, Mitrou P, Flood A, Subar AF, Leitzmann M, Mouw T, Hollenbeck AR, Schatzkin A, et al: Associations between food patterns defined by cluster analysis and colorectal cancer incidence in the NIH-AARP diet and health study. *Eur J Clin Nutr* 2009, **63**(6):707–717.
5. Norat T, Bingham S, Riboli E: Re: Meat, fish, and colorectal cancer risk: The European prospective investigation into cancer and nutrition - Reply. *J Natl Cancer I* 2005, **97**(23):1788–1789.
6. Toden S, Bird AR, Topping DL, Conlon MA: Differential effects of dietary whey, casein and soya on colonic DNA damage and large bowel SCFA in rats fed diets low and high in resistant starch. *Brit J Nutr* 2007, **97**(3):535–543.
7. Boivin GP, Washington K, Yang K, Ward JM, Pretlow TP, Russell R, Besselsen DG, Godfrey VL, Doetschman T, Dove WF, et al: Pathology of mouse models of intestinal cancer: Consensus report and recommendations. *Gastroenterology* 2003, **124**(3):762–777.
8. Perse M, Cerar A: Morphological and Molecular Alterations in 1,2 Dimethylhydrazine and Azoxymethane Induced Colon Carcinogenesis in Rats. *J Biomed Biotechnol* 2011, **2011**:473964.
9. Chen JZ, Huang XF: The signal pathways in azoxymethane-induced colon cancer and preventive implications. *Cancer Biol Ther* 2009, **8**(14):1313–1317.
10. Kaiser S, Park YK, Franklin JL, Halberg RB, Yu M, Jessen WJ, Freudenberg J, Chen XD, Haigis K, Jegga AG, et al: Transcriptional recapitulation and subversion of embryonic colon development by mouse colon tumor models and human colon cancer. *Genome Biol* 2007, **8**(7):R131.
11. Hu Y, Martin J, Le Leu R, Young GP: The colonic response to genotoxic carcinogens in the rat: regulation by dietary fibre. *Carcinogenesis* 2002, **23**(7):1131–1137.
12. Sato M, Ahnen DJ: Regional Variability of Colonocyte Growth and Differentiation in the Rat. *Anat Rec* 1992, **233**(3):409–414.

13. Mutch DM, Simmering R, Donnicola D, Fotopoulos G, Holzwarth JA, Williamson G, C-T I: Impact of commensal microbiota on murine gastrointestinal tract gene ontologies. *Physiol Genomics* 2004, **19**(1):22–31.
14. Anderle P, Sengstag T, Mutch DM, Rumbo M, Praz V, Mansourian R, Delorenzi M, Williamson G, Roberts MA: Changes in the transcriptional profile of transporters in the intestine along the anterior-posterior and crypt-villus axes. *BMC Genomics* 2005, **6**.
15. Glebov OK, Rodriguez LM, Nakahara K, Jenkins J, Cliatt J, Humbyrd CJ, DeNobile J, Soballe P, Simon R, Wright G, et al: Distinguishing right from left colon by the pattern of gene expression. *Cancer Epidem Biomar* 2003, **12**(8):755–762.
16. LaPointe LC, Dunne R, Brown GS, Worthley DL, Molloy PL, Wattchow D, Young GP: Map of differential transcript expression in the normal human large intestine. *Physiol Genomics* 2008, **33**(1):50–64.
17. Tan SL, Gerber JP, Cosgrove LJ, Lockett TJ, Clarke JM, Williams DB, Head RJ: Is the tissue persistence of O-6-methyl-2′-deoxyguanosine an indicator of tumour formation in the gastrointestinal tract? *Mutat Res-Gen Tox En* 2011, **721**(2):119–126.
18. Al-Saleh I, Arif J, El-Doush I, Al-Sanea N, Jabbar AA, Billedo G, Shinwari N, Mashhour A, Mohamed G: Carcinogen DNA adducts and the risk of colon cancer: case–control study. *Biomarkers* 2008, **13**(2):201–216.
19. Toth B, Malick L, Shimizu H: Production of Intestinal and Other Tumors by 1,2-Dimethylhydrazine Dihydrochloride in Mice .1. Light and Transmission Electron-Microscopic Study of Colonic Neoplasms. *Am J Pathol* 1976, **84**(1):69–86.
20. Nilsen H, Lindahl T, Verreault A: DNA base excision repair of uracil residues in reconstituted nucleosome core particles. *EMBO J* 2002, **21**(21):5943–5952.
21. de Boer J, Hoeijmakers JHJ: Nucleotide excision repair and human syndromes. *Carcinogenesis* 2000, **21**(3):453–460.
22. Iyer RR, Pluciennik A, V B, Modrich PL: DNA mismatch repair: Functions and mechanisms. *Chem Rev* 2006, **106**(2):302–323.
23. Larrea AA, Lujan SA, Kunkel TA: SnapShot: DNA Mismatch Repair. *Cell* 2010, **141**(4):730–730.el.
24. Michailidi C, Papavassiliou AG, Troungos C: DNA Repair Mechanisms in Colorectal Carcinogenesis. *Curr Mol Med* 2012, **12**(3):237–246.
25. Yuan J, Strebhardt K: Targeting the G2/M transition for antitumor therapy. *Lett Drug Des Discov* 2005, **2**(4):274–281.
26. Bucher N, Britten CD: G2 checkpoint abrogation and checkpoint kinase-1 targeting in the treatment of cancer. *Brit J Cancer* 2008, **98**(3):523–528.
27. Kimura SH, Ikawa M, Ito A, Okabe M, Nojima H: Cyclin G1 is involved in G2/M arrest in response to DNA damage and in growth control after damage recovery. *Oncogene* 2001, **20**(25):3290–3300.
28. Gartel AL, Tyner AL: The role of the cyclin-dependent kinase inhibitor p21 in apoptosis. *Mol Cancer Ther* 2002, **1**(8):639–649.
29. Cortes U, Moyret-Lalle C, Falette N, Duriez C, El Ghissassi F, Barnas C, Morel AP, Hainaut P, Magaud JP, Puisieux A: BTG gene expression in the p53-dependent and -independent cellular response to DNA damage. *Mol Carcinogen* 2000, **27**(2):57–64.
30. Golan A, Pick E, Tsvetkov L, Nadler Y, Kluger H, Stern DF: Centrosomal Chk2 in DNA damage responses and cell cycle progression. *Cell Cycle* 2010, **9**(13):2647–2656.
31. Fearon ER: Molecular Genetics of Colorectal Cancer. *Annu Rev Pathol-Mech* 2011, **6**:479–507.
32. Tomasini R, Samir AA, Carrier A, Isnardon D, Cecchinelli B, Soddu S, Malissen B, Dagorn JC, Iovanna JL, Dusetti NJ: TP53INP1s and homeodomain-interacting protein kinase-2 (HIPK2) are partners in regulating p53 activity. *J Biol Chem* 2003, **278**(39):37722–37729.
33. Shanmugathasan M, Jothy S: Apoptosis, anoikis and their relevance to the pathobiology of colon cancer. *Pathol Int* 2000, **50**(4):273–279.
34. Adams JM, Cory S: Life-or-death decisions by the Bcl-2 protein family. *Trends Biochem Sci* 2001, **26**(1):61–66.
35. Donauer J, Schreck I, Liebel U, Weiss C: Role and interaction of p53, BAX and the stress-activated protein kinases p38 and JNK in benzo(a)pyrene-diolepoxide induced apoptosis in human colon carcinoma cells. *Arch Toxicol* 2012, **86**(2):329–337.
36. Bajka BH, Topping DL, Cobiac L, Clarke JM: Butyrylated starch is less susceptible to enzymic hydrolysis and increases large-bowel butyrate

more than high-amylose maize starch in the rat. *Brit J Nutr* 2006, **96**(2):276–282.

37. Le Leu RK, Hu Y, Brown IL, Young GP: **Effect of high amylose maize starches on colonic fermentation and apoptotic response to DNA-damage in the colon of rats.** *Nutr Metab (Lond)* 2009, **6**:11.

38. Potten CS, Li YQ, Oconnor PJ, Winton DJ: **A Possible Explanation for the Differential Cancer Incidence in the Intestine, Based on Distribution of the Cytotoxic Effects of Carcinogens in the Murine Large-Bowel.** *Carcinogenesis* 1992, **13**(12):2305–2312.

39. Ringner M: **What is principal component analysis?** *Nat Biotechnol* 2008, **26**(3):303–304.

40. Eisenhart C: **The assumptions underlying the analysis of variance.** *Biometrics* 1947, **3**(1):1–21.

41. Thompson W: **The problem of negative estimates of variance components.** *Ann Math Stat* 1962, **26**:721–733.

42. Rao CR: **Minque Estimation of Variance and Covariance Components.** *Ann Math Stat* 1971, **42**(4):1477.

43. Pawitan Y, Michiels S, Koscielny S, Gusnanto A, Ploner A: **False discovery rate, sensitivity and sample size for microarray studies.** *Bioinformatics* 2005, **21**(13):3017–3024.

44. Laulederkind SJF, Shimoyama M, Hayman GT, Lowry TF, Nigam R, Petri V, Smith JR, Wang SJ, de Pons J, Kowalski G, *et al*: **The Rat Genome Database curation tool suite: a set of optimized software tools enabling efficient acquisition, organization, and presentation of biological data.** *Database-Oxford* 2011:Bar002.

45. van Baarlen P, Troost F, van der Meer C, Hooiveld G, Boekschoten M, Brummer RJM, Kleerebezem M: **Human mucosal in vivo transcriptome responses to three lactobacilli indicate how probiotics may modulate human cellular pathways.** *P Natl Acad Sci USA* 2011, **108**:4562–4569.

11

Contractile properties and movement behaviour in neonatal rats with axotomy, treated with the NMDA antagonist DAP5

Konstantinos Petsanis[1†], Athanasios Chatzisotiriou[1*†], Dorothea Kapoukranidou[1], Constantina Simeonidou[2], Dimitrios Kouvelas[3] and Maria Albani[1]

Abstract

Background: It is well known that axotomy in the neonatal period causes massive loss of motoneurons, which is reflected in the reduction of the number of motor units and the alteration in muscle properties. This type of neuronal death is attributed to the excessive activation of the ionotropic glutamate receptors (glutamate excitotoxicity). In the present study we investigated the effect of the NMDA antagonist DAP5 [D-2-amino-5-phosphonopentanoic acid] in systemic administration, on muscle properties and on behavioural aspects following peripheral nerve injury.

Methods: Wistar rats were subjected to sciatic nerve crush on the second postnatal day. Four experimental groups were included in this study: a) controls (injection of 0.9% NaCl solution) b) crush c) DAP5 treated and d) crush and DAP5 treated. Animals were examined with isometric tension recordings of the fast extensor digitorum longus and the slow soleus muscles, as well as with locomotor tests at four time points, at P14, P21, P28 and adulthood (2 months).

Results: 1. Administration of DAP5 alone provoked no apparent adverse effects. 2. In all age groups, animals with crush developed significantly less tension than the controls in both muscles and had a worse performance in locomotor tests ($p < 0.01$). Crush animals injected with DAP5 were definitely improved as their tension recordings and their locomotor behaviour were significantly improved compared to axotomized ones ($p < 0.01$). 3. The time course of soleus contraction was not altered by axotomy and the muscle remained slow-contracting in all developmental stages in all experimental groups. EDL, on the other hand, became slower after the crush ($p < 0.05$). DAP5 administration restored the contraction velocity, even up to the level of control animals 4. Following crush, EDL becomes fatigue resistant after P21 ($p < 0.01$). Soleus, on the other hand, becomes less fatigue resistant. DAP5 restored the profile in both muscles.

Conclusions: Our results confirm that contractile properties and locomotor behaviour of animals are severely affected by axotomy, with a differential impact on fast contracting muscles. Administration of DAP5 reverses these devastating effects, without any observable side-effects. This agent could possibly show a therapeutic potential in other models of excitotoxic injury as well.

* Correspondence: achatzisot@med.auth.gr
†Equal contributors
[1]Department of Physiology, Faculty of Medicine, Aristotle University of Thessaloniki, Thessaloniki, Greece
Full list of author information is available at the end of the article

Background

Peripheral nerve injury during the critical period of development imparts severe structural and functional consequences on the muscles of the growing animal. It has been well documented that axotomy in the early postnatal period reduces the number of surviving motoneurons in the ventral horn of the lumbar segments and induces changes in the contractile properties of limb muscles [1,2]. These consequences have been ascribed to the critical dependency of the developing motoneurons on their interaction with their target muscle [3,4], as well as to their increased susceptibility to the excitotoxic effects of glutamate [5,6].

Glutamate is the major excitatory neurotransmitter in the CNS. Ionotropic receptors of glutamate (NMDA and AMPA/kainate) have been identified throughout the brain and the spinal cord. In case of overactivation of these receptors, the excessive Ca^{2+} influx into the cell induces a cell death cascade, which comprises the activation of proteases, lipases and other enzymes leading to cell lysis [7]. As it has been shown by previous studies [8-10], this is a time-dependent process, as motoneurons are particularly vulnerable to excitotoxic cell death, only during the first five days of postnatal life.

In the present study we performed sciatic nerve crush in neonatal rats and we investigated the effect of the NMDA antagonist DAP5 [D-2-amino-5-phosphonopentanoic acid] in systemic administration, on muscle properties and on behavioural aspects following injury. This agent has been largely implemented for its antinociceptive action [11-13], as well as for its effects on memory consolidation and hippocampal rhythm [14,15]. In all these studies, the above agent was either delivered intrathecally, or in ex vivo experiments. Systemic application of NMDA

Table 1 EDL tension recordings-comparisons

	AGE	PROCEDURE			
		CRUSH	DAP5	CRUSH-DAP5	P-VALUE
BODY WEIGHT	P14	-	-	-	0.617
	P21	-	-	-	0.205
	P28	-	-	-	0.771
	ADULT	-	-	-	0.523
MUSCLE WEIGHT	P14	*	-	-	0.005
	P21	*	-	#	0.001
	P28	*	-	#	0.001
	ADULT	*	-	#	0.001
TIME TO PEAK	P14	*	-	-	0.011
	P21	*	-	-	0.003
	P28	*	-	-	0.018
	ADULT	*	-	-	0.003
HALF RELAXATION TIME	P14	*	-	-	0.025
	P21	*	-	-	0.003
	P28	*	-	-	0.007
	ADULT	*	-	-	0.005
SINGLE TWITCH	P14	*	-	-	0.011
	P21	*	-	-	0.003
	P28	*	-	#	0.001
	ADULT	*	-	#	0.001
TETANIC-100	P14	*	-	#	0.002
	P21	*	-	-	0.003
	P28	*	-	#	0.001
	ADULT	*	-	#	0.001
FATIGUE INDEX	P14	-	-	*	0.007
	P21	*	-	#	0.003
	P28	*	-	-	0.003
	ADULT	*	-	-	0.009

Post-hoc multiple comparisons. The actual parameters are presented in the graphs. *: different from control. #: different from crush. Level of significance was a = 0.05.

Table 2 EDL tension recordings

EDL

	AGE	PROCEDURE				ANOVA ON THE RANKS
		CONTROL	CRUSH	DAP5	CRUSH-DAP5	P-VALUE
WEIGHT-INDEX	P14	0.04 ± 0.01	$0.02 \pm 0.^{*}$	0.04 ± 0.01	0.03 ± 0.01	0.017
	P21	0.05 ± 0.01	$0.02 \pm 0.^{*}$	0.04 ± 0.01	$0.03 \pm 0.^{\#}$	0.002
	P28	0.06 ± 0.01	$0.02 \pm 0.^{*}$	0.06 ± 0.01	$0.04 \pm 0.^{\#}$	0.001
	ADULT	0.08 ± 0.01	$0.01 \pm 0.^{*}$	0.09 ± 0.01	0.08 ± 0.01	0.003
TETANIC-10 (g)	P14	6.59 ± 0.89	$1.94 \pm 0.16^{*}$	7.21 ± 1.21	6.79 ± 0.29	0.011
	P21	9.96 ± 0.63	$4.68 \pm 0.79^{*}$	10.66 ± 1.37	9.39 ± 1.71	0.010
	P28	17.4 ± 1.39	$4.94 \pm 0.26^{*}$	18.24 ± 0.53	$15.05 \pm 1.95^{\#}$	0.002
	ADULT	86.72 ± 3.55	$6.05 \pm 0.63^{*}$	87.42 ± 4.1	$72.59 \pm 2.85^{\#}$	0.001
TETANIC-20 (g)	P14	8.13 ± 1.3	$2.5 \pm 0.34^{*}$	8.06 ± 1.02	7.62 ± 0.46	0.012
	P21	13.27 ± 1.52	$6.04 \pm 0.64^{*}$	12.51 ± 0.86	10.65 ± 1.54	0.003
	P28	24.51 ± 1.19	$5.6 \pm 0.41^{*}$	24.45 ± 0.98	$20.88 \pm 1.68^{\#}$	0.001
	ADULT	117.45 ± 5.37	$7.71 \pm 0.96^{*}$	119.52 ± 4.78	105.08 ± 13.66	0.004
TETANIC-40 (g)	P14	9.46 ± 1.64	$3.3 \pm 0.48^{*}$	9.79 ± 1.65	8.87 ± 0.46	0.011
	P21	18.46 ± 1.06	$8.15 \pm 0.37^{*}$	17.53 ± 0.91	$14.61 \pm 1.44^{\#}$	0.001
	P28	37.92 ± 1.44	$8.9 \pm 0.58^{*}$	38.75 ± 1.66	$31.48 \pm 2.91^{\#}$	0.001
	ADULT	177.78 ± 14.95	$13.22 \pm 1.15^{*}$	179.26 ± 8.94	$140.83 \pm 10.29^{\#}$	0.001
TETANIC-80 (g)	P14	10.35 ± 1.78	$3.91 \pm 0.52^{*}$	10.63 ± 1.82	9.57 ± 0.32	0.012
	P21	22.42 ± 1.22	$10.87 \pm 1.29^{*}$	21.36 ± 0.96	$17.49 \pm 1.94^{\#}$	0.001
	P28	49.95 ± 1.34	$10.79 \pm 0.97^{*}$	52.9 ± 1.06	$41.66 \pm 1.97^{\#}$	0.001
	ADULT	208.5 ± 8.55	$14.43 \pm 0.88^{*}$	205.65 ± 6.95	$164.84 \pm 11.33^{\#}$	0.001
FORCE/WEIGHT (g/g)	P14	1559.86 ± 292.25	$834.2 \pm 150.66^{*}$	1379.97 ± 404.56	1565.73 ± 367.12	0.018
	P21	1021.27 ± 308.81	$1474.97 \pm 340.35^{*}$	1081.54 ± 86.26	$1390.81 \pm 306.78^{*}$	0.034
	P28	1124.87 ± 156.98	$571.16 \pm 89.02^{*}$	1099.9 ± 152.2	1247.61 ± 53.81	0.006
	ADULT	1460.03 ± 89.47	$792.95 \pm 138.6^{*}$	1407.11 ± 44.59	1341.69 ± 81.63	0.005

Values are expressed as Mean ± Standard deviation. Post-hoc multiple comparisons. *: different from control. #: different from crush. Level of significance was a = 0.05.

receptor antagonists is usually restricted, due to serious side-effects [16,17]. This is the first time, to our best knowledge, that DAP5 has been administered systemically. Our goal was to evaluate both the drug effective dose and its effect on locomotor behaviour and muscular properties.

Methods

All procedures were performed in accordance with institutional guidelines for the use and care of animals (86/609/EEC) and the 'Principles of Laboratory animal care' (NIH publication No 85–23, revised 1985) and were approved by the Ethical Committee for animal experimentation of the Medical School of Thessaloniki (2-3-2006). One hundred seven Wistar rats of both sexes were used in this study. The animals were provided with ad libitum access to food and water and housed in standard cages in a 22°C environment with a 12:12-h light–dark cycle. All efforts were made to minimize the number of animals and their suffering in the experiments.

The pups (N = 80) were divided into four different groups. Unoperated littermates either received DAP5 (N = 20) or remained as untreated controls (injected with normal saline, N = 20). The third experimental group (N = 20) comprised animals subjected to nerve crush and treated with vehicle, whereas in the fourth group (N = 20) were those animals with nerve crush, which underwent treatment with DAP5. The study was performed in four stages of postnatal development (5 animals per age group), on postnatal days, 14, 21, 28 and during adulthood (2 months). The twenty seven remaining rats participated in the titration study.

Surgical procedures
Nerve crush

Adequate anesthesia was initiated and maintained by ether inhalation. Surgery was performed under an operating stereoscope. On the second postnatal day, a small incision was performed in the posterior surface of the left mid-

Table 3 Soleus recordings-comparisons

	AGE	PROCEDURE			
		CRUSH	DAP5	CRUSH-DAP5	P-VALUE
BODY WEIGHT	P14	-	-	-	0.891
	P21	-	-	-	0.064
	P28	-	-	-	0.918
	ADULT	-	-	-	0.944
MUSCLE WEIGHT	P14	-	-	-	0.257
	P21	*	-	-	0.006
	P28	*	-	#	0.001
	ADULT	*	-	#	0.001
TIME TO PEAK	P14	-	-	-	0.630
	P21	-	*	-	0.007
	P28	*	-	-	0.048
	ADULT	-	-	-	0.744
HALF RELAXATION TIME	P14	-	-	-	0.447
	P21	-	*	-	0.009
	P28	-	-	-	0.219
	ADULT	-	-	*	0.009
SINGLE TWITCH	P14	*	-	-	0.005
	P21	*	-	-	0.036
	P28	*	-	#	0.002
	ADULT	*	-	#	0.002
TETANIC-100	P14	*	-	-	0.003
	P21	*	-	-	0.023
	P28	*	#	#	0.001
	ADULT	*	-	#	0.001
FATIGUE INDEX	P14	*	-	-	0.009
	P21	*	-	-	0.031
	P28	-	-	-	0.063
	ADULT	*	-	-	0.010

Post-hoc multiple comparisons. The actual parameters are presented in the graphs. *: different from control. #: different from crush. Level of significance was $a = 0.05$.

thigh and the sciatic nerve was identified. The crush was performed just proximal to its division to the peroneal and tibial nerve. Attention was paid to avoid damage in the nerve muscular surroundings. Crush was performed by means of a fine pair of forceps which was tightly applied for 30 seconds. Afterwards, the nerve was examined to ensure that the epineural sheath was intact, though translucent. Bleeding was controlled with haemostatic cellulose and the wounds were sutured with 6–0 silk threads. All procedures were carried out by the same researcher. Three hours after recovery from anaesthesia, peanut oil was applied to the wound (to avoid autophagia) and the pups were returned to their mother.

In order to confirm the efficacy of the procedure, the plantar and dorsiflexion reflexes, as well as the inability of normal movement of the left hind limb, with animals suspended from their tail, were assessed daily, for the first 7 days, as described elsewhere [1]. Only animals with verified successful axotomy were included in our study.

Drug titration-administration

9 groups, each consisting of 3 animals were tested for each dose. Under ether anesthesia, the animals were injected subcutaneously at the interscapular region. The injection was performed daily from P2 to P13. The dose of 50 mg/kg was lethal 24 hours after treatment for all animals. Escalating doses of 10, 20, 30, 40 mg/kg resulted in no changes in rat growth, eating, water drinking, and weight gaining. Doses of 45 mg/kg resulted lethal after 3 days. Doses ranging from 42-45 mg/kg resulted in weight loss or were lethal. At the end, 40 mg/kg was chosen as the treatment dose.

Table 4 Soleus tension recordings

SOLEUS

	AGE	PROCEDURE				ANOVA ON THE RANKS
		CONTROL	CRUSH	DAP5	CRUSH-DAP5	P-VALUE
WEIGHT-INDEX	P14	$0.03 \pm 0.$	$0.03 \pm 0.$	0.03 ± 0.01	0.03 ± 0.01	0.364
	P21	$0.03 \pm 0.$	$0.03 \pm 0.^*$	0.03 ± 0.01	$0.03 \pm 0.$	0.039
	P28	$0.04 \pm 0.$	$0.02 \pm 0.^*$	$0.04 \pm 0.$	$0.03 \pm 0.^\#$	0.001
	ADULT	$0.06 \pm 0.$	$0.01 \pm 0.^*$	$0.06 \pm 0.$	$0.04 \pm 0.^\#$	0.001
TETANIC-10 (g)	P14	5.85 ± 1.35	$1.65 \pm 0.18^*$	5.06 ± 0.59	4.64 ± 0.67	0.005
	P21	11.99 ± 0.68	$9.88 \pm 1.02^*$	$13.84 \pm 1.26^\#$	$13.3 \pm 0.69^\#$	0.005
	P28	21.43 ± 2.06	$10.92 \pm 1.04^*$	20.1 ± 1.83	18.39 ± 2.03	0.004
	ADULT	44.65 ± 0.81	$9.15 \pm 0.59^*$	$41.72 \pm 2.27^\#$	$40.77 \pm 2.31^\#$	0.002
TETANIC-20 (g)	P14	6.78 ± 1.29	$2.47 \pm 0.44^*$	6.59 ± 0.75	5.45 ± 0.74	0.003
	P21	16.94 ± 0.97	$14.49 \pm 0.74^*$	$14.73 \pm 1.51^*$	$14.25 \pm 0.9^*$	0.020
	P28	35.76 ± 2.16	$15.44 \pm 0.6^*$	$27.75 \pm 2.08^\#$	$26.39 \pm 2.57^\#$	0.001
	ADULT	54.1 ± 0.92	$10.62 \pm 0.89^*$	53.01 ± 1.65	$49.61 \pm 2.56^\#$	0.002
TETANIC-40 (g)	P14	8.46 ± 1.65	$2.84 \pm 0.3^*$	9.98 ± 0.73	8.05 ± 0.83	0.003
	P21	24.27 ± 0.98	$19.96 \pm 2.02^*$	23.76 ± 1.39	$21.71 \pm 1.34^\#$	0.007
	P28	52.11 ± 2.51	$17.63 \pm 2.33^*$	$32.62 \pm 2.99^\#$	$29.19 \pm 1.82^\#$	0.001
	ADULT	89.15 ± 7.15	$14.16 \pm 1.22^*$	91.78 ± 6.08	$80.85 \pm 3.04^\#$	0.002
TETANIC-80 (g)	P14	10.65 ± 1.32	$3.48 \pm 0.37^*$	11.91 ± 0.96	$9.54 \pm 0.65^\#$	0.002
	P21	33.56 ± 1.09	$29.96 \pm 1.7^*$	34.41 ± 2.25	32.47 ± 1.66	0.013
	P28	69.89 ± 1.69	$20.71 \pm 2.92^*$	$40.38 \pm 2.1^\#$	$37.79 \pm 1.83^\#$	0.001
	ADULT	130.03 ± 1.92	$16.89 \pm 0.98^*$	129.45 ± 2.36	$121.16 \pm 5.06^\#$	0.002
FORCE/WEIGHT (g/g)	P14	2037.05 ± 529.05	$787.3 \pm 156.^*$	2534.11 ± 461.66	1648.11 ± 392.76	0.003
	P21	2046.25 ± 187.04	$2370.38 \pm 252.19^*$	1980.12 ± 357.46	2225.41 ± 213.59	0.131
	P28	2710.54 ± 134.72	1272.12 ± 108.09	$1421.89 \pm 223.69^\#$	$1687.99 \pm 175.58^\#$	0.001
	ADULT	1111.12 ± 25.62	$787.93 \pm 195.12^*$	1104.13 ± 20.91	$1591.63 \pm 127.07^\#$	0.001

Values are expressed as Mean ± Standard deviation. Post-hoc multiple comparisons. *: different from control. #: different from crush. Level of significance was $a = 0.05$.

Tension recordings

All animals were examined for the contractile properties of two hind limb muscles, the extensor digitorum longus (EDL) and soleus, which represent a fast contracting, easily fatigable and a slow, fatigue resistant muscle, respectively. Animals were anaesthetized with chloral hydrate (4.5%, 10 µl/g body weight, i.p.). The sciatic nerve was identified and prepared proximal to its division. Indifferent to the examined muscle branches of the sciatic nerve were cut. The distal tendons were dissected from the surrounding tissues, cut at their insertion at the bone and attached to a strain gauge transducer (Dynamometer UFI, Devices) by a short silk suture and the exposed parts of the muscles were kept moist with warm (37°C) Krebs-Henseleit solution. (NaCl 118.08 mM, $NaHCO_3$ 25 mM, glucose 5.55 mM and $CaCl_2$ 1.89 mM). Two pins were inserted in the femoral and calcaneus condyles, thereby adjusting the leg in a position of 90° flexion of the knee and the ankle joints. Muscle length was appropriately adjusted in order to produce maximal single twitch tension (optimal length),

through a micromanipulator allowing motion on the 3 axes (Prior, England). The tension elicited by sciatic nerve stimulation (Digitimer DS9A stimulator) was displayed on the monitor using a specific Micro 1501 CED (Cambridge Instruments, UK), after amplification by a DC transducer amplifier (Neurolog NL 107).

Stimulus intensity was adjusted in order to elicit maximal tension, using supramaximal (3–9 volts) square pulses each of 0.5 msec duration. Time to peak (TTP) was calculated by measuring the time taken to reach maximum twitch tension. Time to half relaxation (1/2 RT) was calculated as the time taken for peak twitch tension to decrease to half its original value.

Tetanic contractions were then elicited by stimulating the nerve at 10, 20, 40, 80 and 100 Hz. All devices during the tension recording procedure were controlled by a pulse programmer (Digitimer D4030). The fatigability of the muscles was tested by stimulating the nerve at 40 Hz for 250 ms per second for 180 seconds. During this process, the recorded muscle tension

Table 5 Locomotor tests

	AGE	PROCEDURE				ANOVA ON THE RANKS
		CONTROL	CRUSH	DAP5	CRUSH-DAP5	P-VALUE
Rotarod (sec)	P14	264.20 ± 12.28	$8.40 \pm 2.70^*$	256.00 ± 12.02	19.00 ± 3.39 [#]	0.001
	P21	289.80 ± 14.94	$20.40 \pm 6.50^*$	276.40 ± 16.02	$51.40 \pm 7.86^{\#}$	0.001
	P28	289.20 ± 11.80	$37.20 \pm 9.15^*$	290.60 ± 12.92	$104.20 \pm 9.98^{\#}$	0.001
	ADULT	285.80 ± 13.57	$45.80 \pm 7.98^*$	289.40 ± 15.03	$229.80 \pm 12.34^{\#}$	0.001
Bridge 1 cm	P14	1.20 ± 0.45	$8.60 \pm 0.55^*$	1.00 ± 0.71	$4.20 \pm 0.84^{\#}$	0.001
	P21	0.80 ± 0.84	$7.40 \pm 0.89^*$	0.60 ± 0.55	2.60 ± 1.52	0.003
	P28	0.80 ± 0.84	$7.20 \pm 0.84^*$	1.00 ± 0.71	$2.80 \pm 0.45^{\#}$	0.001
	ADULT	0.80 ± 0.45	$6.20 \pm 1.10^*$	0.80 ± 0.45	$3.00 \pm 0.71^{\#}$	0.001
Bridge 3 cm	P14	0.80 ± 0.84	$7.60 \pm 0.89^*$	0.60 ± 0.55	$2.80 \pm 0.84^{\#}$	0.001
	P21	0.40 ± 0.89	$7.00 \pm 0.71^*$	0.40 ± 0.55	$2.80 \pm 0.84^{\#}$	0.001
	P28	0.60 ± 0.55	$5.80 \pm 1.30^*$	0.60 ± 0.89	$2.20 \pm 0.84^{\#}$	0.002
	ADULT	0.20 ± 0.45	$5.00 \pm 1.58^*$	0.60 ± 0.55	$2.20 \pm 0.84^{\#}$	0.001
Bridge 5 cm	P14	0.60 ± 0.55	$6.20 \pm 0.45^*$	0.00 ± 0.00	$2.40 \pm 0.55^{\#}$	0.001
	P21	0.40 ± 0.55	$4.40 \pm 1.14^*$	0.40 ± 0.55	1.60 ± 1.14	0.004
	P28	0.40 ± 0.55	$4.40 \pm 1.14^*$	0.20 ± 0.45	$2.00 \pm 1.00^{\#}$	0.001
	ADULT	0.00 ± 0.00	$2.80 \pm 0.84^*$	0.20 ± 0.45	$1.80 \pm 0.84^*$	0.001
Gait 1 cm	P14	2.80 ± 0.84	$4.60 \pm 0.89^*$	2.60 ± 1.14	3.40 ± 0.89	0.037
(errors)	P21	2.40 ± 1.14	$4.60 \pm 0.55^*$	2.20 ± 1.48	3.00 ± 0.71	0.016
	P28	2.80 ± 0.84	3.80 ± 0.84	2.40 ± 1.14	2.60 ± 0.89	0.149
	ADULT	2.40 ± 1.14	4.00 ± 1.00	2.00 ± 1.58	2.00 ± 1.22	0.091
Gait 3 cm	P14	2.40 ± 0.89	$4.00 \pm 0.71^*$	2.20 ± 0.84	2.80 ± 1.10	0.025
(errors)	P21	1.80 ± 0.84	$3.80 \pm 0.84^*$	1.80 ± 1.30	1.80 ± 1.30	0.036
	P28	1.80 ± 1.48	$4.20 \pm 0.84^*$	1.60 ± 0.89	2.00 ± 0.00	0.014
	ADULT	1.80 ± 1.30	3.80 ± 1.30	1.60 ± 1.14	1.80 ± 1.30	0.094
Gait 5 cm	P14	2.40 ± 1.52	3.40 ± 0.55	1.60 ± 1.14	3.00 ± 1.00	0.098
(errors)	P21	1.40 ± 1.14	$3.00 \pm 0.71^*$	0.80 ± 0.84	1.40 ± 0.55	0.019
	P28	1.80 ± 1.48	$3.60 \pm 0.89^*$	1.80 ± 0.45	1.20 ± 1.30	0.029
	ADULT	1.20 ± 1.30	3.40 ± 1.52	1.20 ± 0.84	1.20 ± 0.84	0.089
Limb Rotation	P14	13.40 ± 0.98	0.00 ± 0.00	13.18 ± 0.76	14.42 ± 0.89	0.194
	P21	17.88 ± 0.44	$21.24 \pm 0.86^*$	17.90 ± 0.53	$20.00 \pm 0.83^*$	0.002
	P28	18.62 ± 1.21	$22.56 \pm 0.79^*$	18.50 ± 0.86	$22.12 \pm 0.79^*$	0.002
	ADULT	20.76 ± 1.87	$27.28 \pm 0.56^*$	20.62 ± 1.64	$24.60 \pm 0.72^{\#}$	0.001
Stride Length (cm)	P14	3.78 ± 0.53	0.00 ± 0.00	3.70 ± 0.29	$2.30 \pm 0.51^*$	0.010
	P21	11.86 ± 0.56	$9.94 \pm 0.44^*$	12.02 ± 0.57	$10.10 \pm 0.70^*$	0.003
	P28	15.78 ± 1.18	$13.56 \pm 0.41^*$	15.42 ± 1.19	$13.76 \pm 0.60^*$	0.006
	ADULT	17.82 ± 0.68	$13.14 \pm 0.95^*$	18.02 ± 0.51	$16.44 \pm 0.54^{\#}$	0.001
DBF(cm)	P14	0.98 ± 0.18	0.00 ± 0.00	0.98 ± 0.22	$0.64 \pm 0.13^*$	0.027
	P21	1.86 ± 0.18	$1.30 \pm 0.19^*$	2.02 ± 0.20	$1.36 \pm 0.13^*$	0.002
	P28	2.70 ± 0.19	2.96 ± 0.11	2.78 ± 0.16	$2.20 \pm 0.14^*$	0.003
	ADULT	3.34 ± 0.23	$3.80 \pm 0.19^*$	3.43 ± 0.19	$2.92 \pm 0.16^{\#}$	0.003

Values are expressed as Mean ± Standard deviation. Post-hoc multiple comparisons. *: different from control. #: different from crush. Level of significance was a = 0.05.

gradually declined as the muscle fibers one by one were losing their contraction ability. Then the fatigue index was calculated as FI = (Initial tension-tension after 180 min)/Initial tension. After tension recordings were completed, the animals were sacrificed and muscles were excised and weighed.

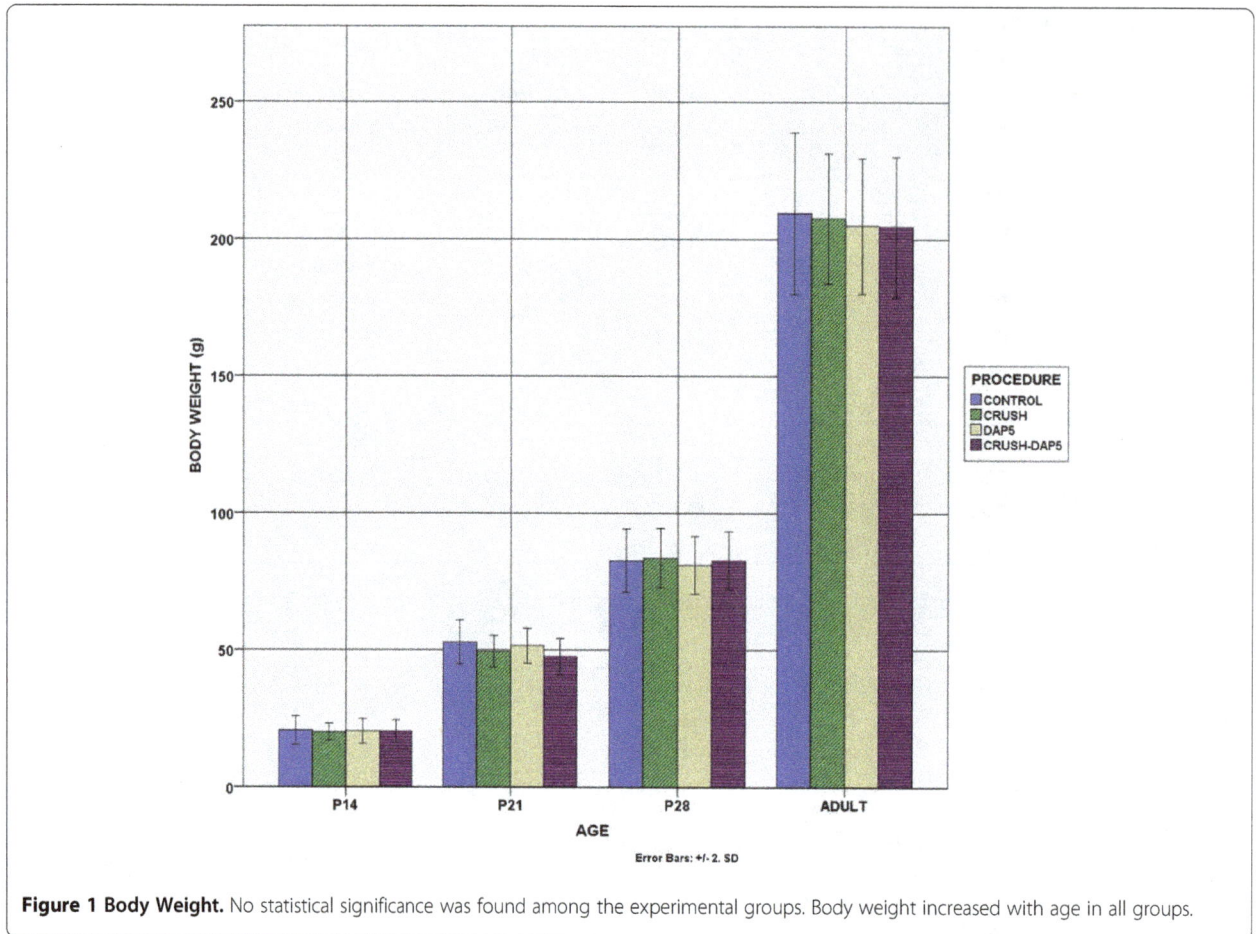

Figure 1 Body Weight. No statistical significance was found among the experimental groups. Body weight increased with age in all groups.

Movement behaviour

Movement behaviour was examined by performing 3 kinds of tests. All tests were performed at the same day (P14, P21, P28, 2 months).

1. The Rotarod test in which a rodent was placed on a rotating treadmill. The speed of rotation was gradually increased at an accelerated speed of 4-40 rpm/min. The animals were placed at the treadmill at which time the individual timers started and the rodent's ability to remain on the rotating rod was recorded. The test lasted for a maximum of 10 minutes. When the animals fell off the treadmill the timer stopped. The purpose of the Rotarod test is to assess the rodent's sensorimotor coordination [18,19].

2. Bridging: rats are placed in three different (1, 3 and 5 cm wide) narrow wooden lanes of one meter long. Two parameters were examined; the number of errors in passing the bridge and the gait type measured using a particular scale, ranging from 0 to 5 (corresponding to fluent gait with 2 stops, fluent gait with many stops, fearful but with no stops, fearful with stops, particularly difficult).

3. Footprint analysis: The footprint analysis was performed according to Jeroen et al and Alexander Klein et al [20,21] to evaluate hindlimb walking patterns. Briefly, the rats had to walk on strips of paper through a walk away (1 m long, 6 cm wide). Their hindpaws were dipped in blue fountain pen ink. Three series of at least one stepping cycle per side (four sequential steps) were performed per experimental day. The parameters examined were: stride length (distance between left and right footprints), limb rotation (angle between a virtual line through the third digit and the centre of the palm and a virtual line parallel to the walking direction) and distance between feet (distance between feet of the left and right stepping cycle) were analyzed.

Statistical analysis

Analysis was performed using SPSS 19.0 software for Windows. Animals of the same age group were compared among the different interventions and animals subjected to the same procedure were compared among the different developmental stages. Nonparametric tests were applied.

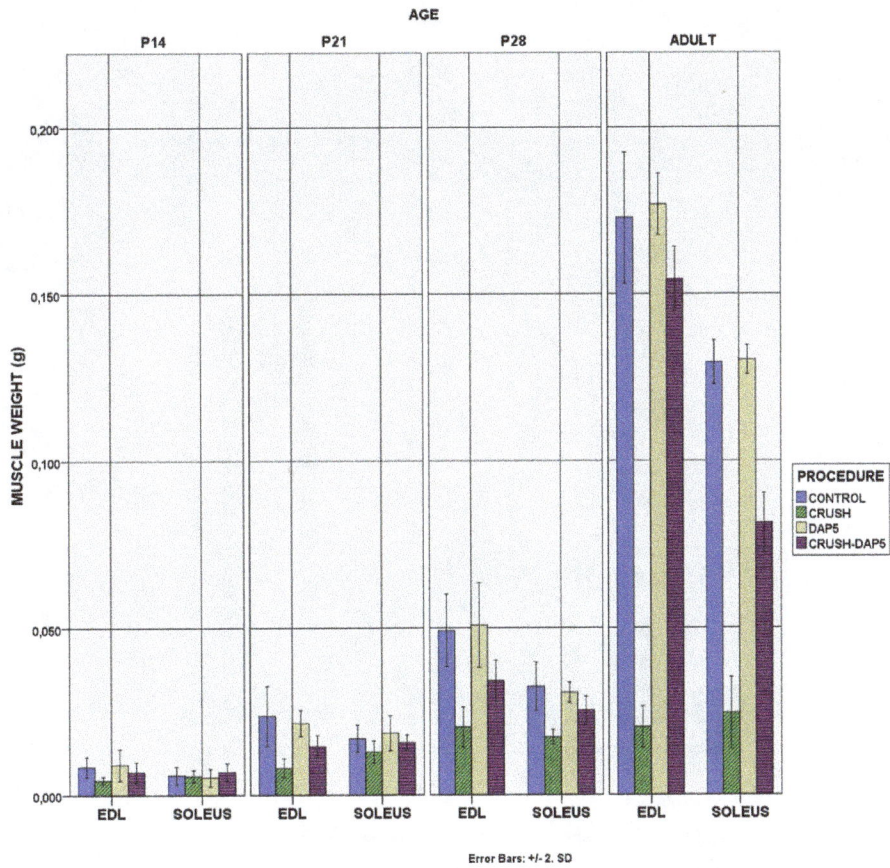

Figure 2 Muscle Weight. Muscle weight was reduced by crush, after P14 in EDL and after P21 in soleus (p < 0.01). DAP-5 increased muscle weight, but not to the level of control animals.

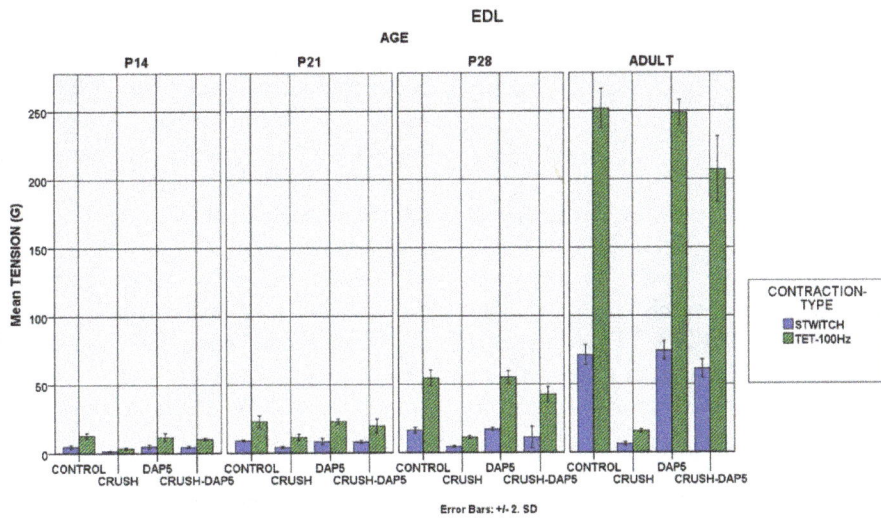

Figure 3 EDL Force Generation. Bar chart showing the contractile force of the EDL muscle. Single twitch and maximum tetanic contraction at 100 Hz is depicted for all experimental groups in all ages. It is evident that crush animals developed significantly less tension than the controls and DAP5 administration clearly improved muscle performance.

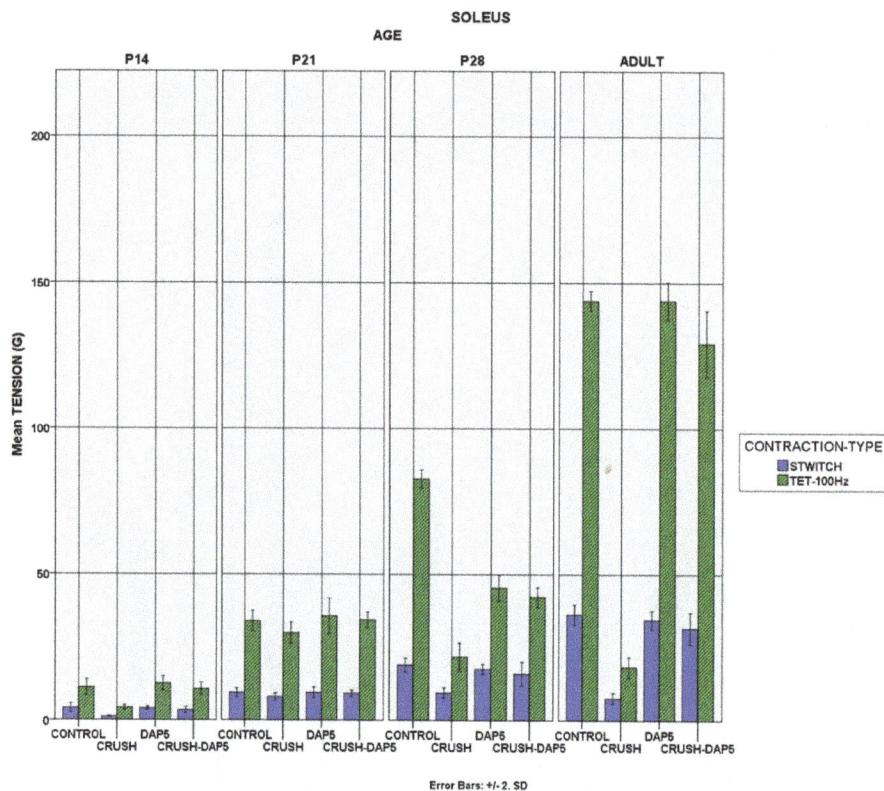

Figure 4 Soleus Force Generation. Similar to Figure 1, showing the contractile force of soleus muscle.

Kruskal – Wallis procedure was initially used in order to detect differences between groups, following which post-hoc pairwise comparisons were performed, by means of a stepwise, step-down method. Criterion of statistical significance was set at p < 0.05.

Results

The results are presented in detail in Tables 1, 2, 3, 4, 5.

A. Body-weight-muscle weight

Body weight did not differ between the experimental groups (Figure 1). Muscle weight (Figure 2) and weight index (muscle/body weight) in crush animals was definitely reduced compared to controls (p < 0.01). This reduction was already apparent by P14 in EDL, whereas in soleus was evident after P21. Similarly, in crush animals which received DAP5, the difference compared to controls was evident after P14 in EDL and after P21 in soleus. These animals also differed from animals with crush, with differences becoming evident earlier, already at P14 in EDL and at P21 in soleus. We have to note that during normal development weight index changed (increased in adulthood compared to P14, p < 0.01). Axotomy progressively reduced the index, presumably due to muscle weight decrease. DAP-5 reversed this situation for both muscles.

B. Isometric tension recordings

Tension development: Treatment with DAP5 did not alter the normal muscle properties, the only exception being the soleus muscle in P21 and P28 animals, in which the tetanic tensions were unexpectedly lower (p < 0.01). The absence of muscle "side effects" was consistent for both muscles in all age groups. In adult rats, EDL single twitch in controls, DAP5–treated, crush and crush + DAP5 treatment was 71.37 ± 3.64, 74.43 ± 3.30, 6.27 ± 0.67 and 61.24 ± 3.32gr, respectively (values expressed as mean ± SD).When soleus was considered, the respective values were 36.41 ± 1.71, 34.62 ± 1.56, 7.72 ± 0.93 and 31.76 ± 2.71gr. In all age groups, animals with crush exhibited significantly less tension than the controls in both muscles (p < 0.01). Crush animals injected with DAP5 were definitely improved as their tension recordings were significantly higher than the crush ones without DAP5 in both muscles (p < 0.01). This improvement however, did not generally reach the level of control animals, nor those with DAP5 injection (Figure 3–4).

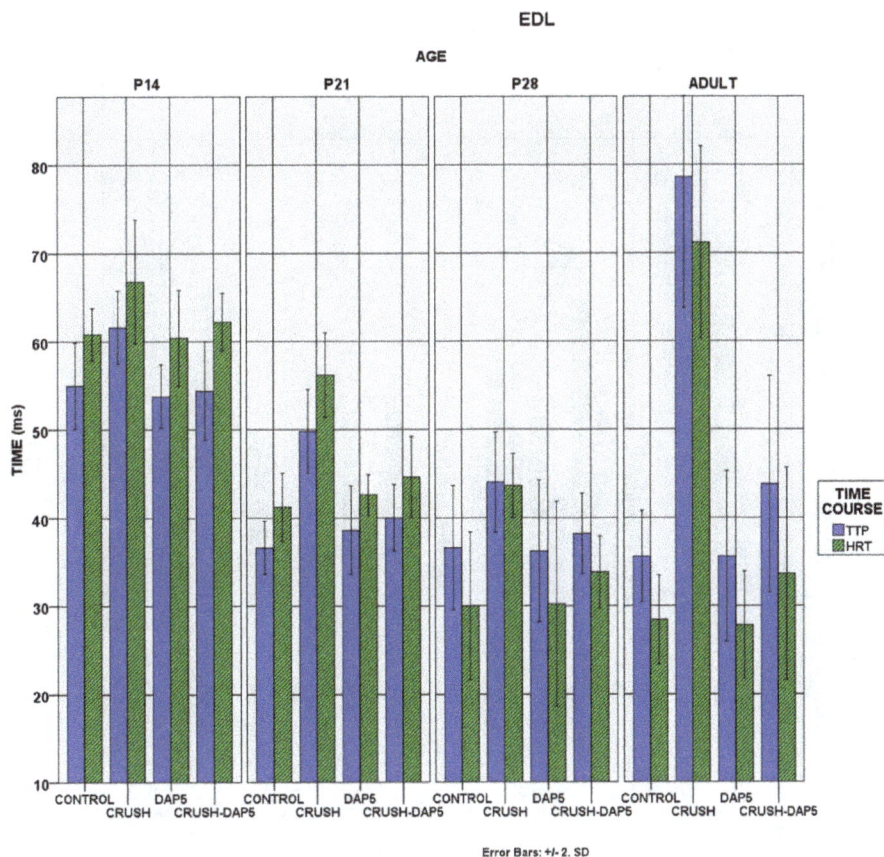

Figure 5 EDL Time course of Contraction. Bar chart showing the evolution of the two parameters of the time course of contraction, among the different experimental groups. TTP:time-to-peak and HRT:Half-relaxation-time. Immature EDL is a slow muscle, but progressively its contraction is shortened in order to attain the fast profile of the adult animal. Crush disrupts this process and the muscle remains slow in all developmental stages.

Time course of contraction: The time course of soleus contraction was not altered by axotomy and the muscle remained slow-contracting in all developmental stages, in all experimental groups. EDL, on the other hand, became slower after the crush ($p < 0.05$). DAP5 administration restored the contraction velocity, up to the level of control animals (Figure 5–6).

Fatigue index: Following crush, EDL becomes fatigue resistant after P21. In adult animals with crush the index was 0.18 ± 0.03 vs 0.48 ± 0.03 in controls ($p < 0.01$). Soleus, on the other hand, becomes less fatigue resistant (0.2 ± 0.06 in controls vs 0.34 ± 0.09 in axotomized adults, $p < 0.01$). DAP5 administration restored the profile in both muscles (EDL: $0,48 \pm 0.02$, soleus: 0.24 ± 0.03, $p < 0.01$ compared to crush), up to the level of control animals (no difference after P28)(Figure 7).

Specific tension: This parameter (tetanic tension 100 Hz/muscle weight) was reduced in crush animals in both muscles ($p < 0.01$). DAP5 administration reversed this effect.

C. Movement behaviour

The results are presented in Table 5 and the performance in rotarod test is shown in Figure 8. It should be noticed that P14-crush animals were not able to perform the limb rotation, stride length and DBF, presumably due to their young age to participate in these tests.

Injection of DAP5 had no impact in animal locomotion, as there was no significant difference compared to controls, in any age group, in any parameter studied.

Among the various experimental groups, crush animals had definitely lower motor scores than the controls ($p < 0.05$). These differences remained throughout all ages, apart from adults, in which the gaits exhibited no significant changes. DAP5 administration in axotomized animals improved motor behaviour ($p < 0.05$ compared to axotomized). For limb rotation, stride length and DBF, the difference became evident after P28. This improvement, however, reached the level of neither the controls ($p < 0.05$), nor those with intact nerve and DAP5 treatment ($p < 0.05$).

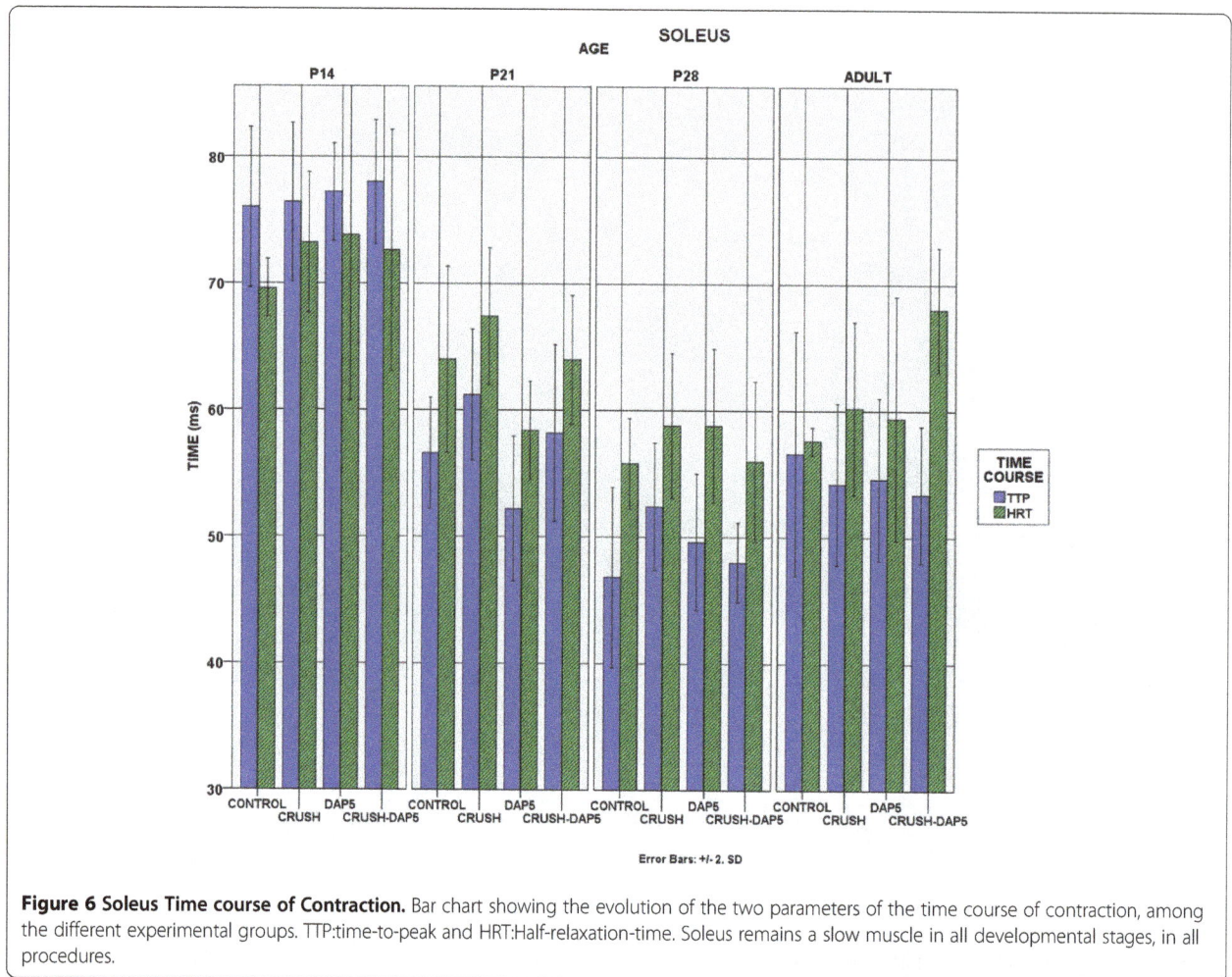

Figure 6 Soleus Time course of Contraction. Bar chart showing the evolution of the two parameters of the time course of contraction, among the different experimental groups. TTP:time-to-peak and HRT:Half-relaxation-time. Soleus remains a slow muscle in all developmental stages, in all procedures.

Concerning the evolution of locomotor behaviour, the animal performance in the gaits and the bridges did not exhibit any discernible difference, as the animals grew older. On the other hand, the rotarod, the limb rotation, the stride length and the DBF provided a more robust index of the differentiation of the animals' locomotion, with significant differences between the age groups ($p < 0.05$).

Discussion

It is well established that peripheral nerve crush injury, during early postnatal development, results in significant loss of motor neurons and extensive muscle atrophy [1,9]. The mechanism of cell death involves, on the one hand, the activation of several apoptotic pathways [22] and on the other hand the necrotic cell death, probably caused by glutamate-mediated excitotoxicity [2,6]. The differential response between mature and immature motoneurons following injury is attributed to the quantity of glutamate receptors on the cell membrane [23,24].

Administration of an NMDA or AMPA/Kainate receptor antagonist within this critical period of development is thought to reverse the neurotoxic effects of axotomy and result in increased survival of motoneurons [2,5,7,25,26]. Unfortunately, the protective effects for many of these factors are only transient, lasting 2–3 weeks [27]. Dizocilpine malate (MK-801), an NMDA antagonist, has been used in animal models in vivo with success, in order to prevent motoneuron death after axotomy. It was badly tolerated by rats, however, due to side effects and high mortality [2,25]. Furthermore, magnesium, which is known to act as a voltage-dependent blocker of the N-methyl-D-aspartate (NMDA) channel, by coupling with the specific Mg^{2+} site within the pore of the ion channel [28,29], was found to inhibit the death of ventral horn motoneurons and to restore the alteration in contractile properties provoked by axotomy [1].

In the present study we assessed the contractile properties and the movement behaviour in rats of different age groups, following neonatal sciatic nerve crush and administration of DAP5. This is a selective

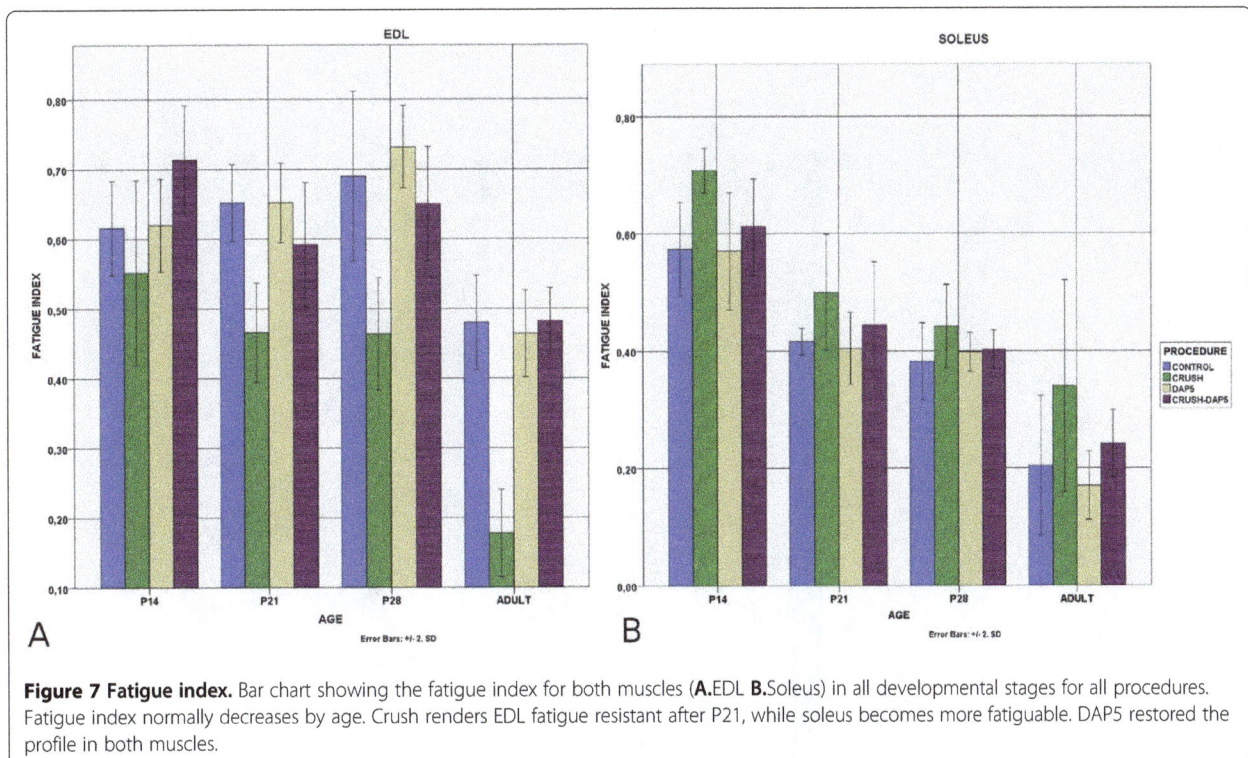

Figure 7 Fatigue index. Bar chart showing the fatigue index for both muscles (**A.**EDL **B.**Soleus) in all developmental stages for all procedures. Fatigue index normally decreases by age. Crush renders EDL fatigue resistant after P21, while soleus becomes more fatiguable. DAP5 restored the profile in both muscles.

NMDA receptor antagonist that competitively inhibits the ligand (glutamate) binding site of NMDA receptors. DAP5 is generally very fast acting as indicated by in vitro preparations, and can block NMDA receptor action at a reasonably small concentration [30]. Our hypothesis was that, by delivering an agent with a direct action on the NMDA receptor, we would be able to achieve a more profound effect, than the one observed with the indirect action of magnesium. A drawback in our study is that axotomized hindlimbs were not compared with the ones of the opposite side (right), but with those of control animals, thus rendering our observations more vulnerable to interanimal differences. We chose that design, however, to achieve a correlation with the behavioural tests, which necessarily had to entail a control group of animals. Moreover, body weight did not differ among the experimental groups and consequently the differences in tension recordings may be directly ascribed to the muscle changes.

According to our knowledge, this is the first time that DAP5was administered in vivo. Systematic administration of DAP5 has been discouraged by other researchers, due to poor cerebrospinal fluid (CSF) absorption and probable toxic features [17]. By initially following titration trials, we did not observe any side effects. In all age groups, no significant difference was found between control animals and those that the agent was administered, in both contractile properties and behavioural tests. These results

allowed us to conclude that a safe and effective therapeutic profile is evident for the aforementioned drug, at least for the parameters studied.

Apart from reducing the number of surviving motoneurons, axotomy in the early postnatal period alters the contractile properties of limb muscles, as well [3]. Our results are in accordance with our previous work [1], as well as other researchers [2], showing that axotomy severely impairs tension development by the muscle. The main feature in this study is that DAP5 resulted in the recovery of the contractile properties of both muscles, up to the level of control animals, thus fully eliminating the debilitating effect of axotomy. We assume that the direct action of the agent on the NMDA receptor accounts for the improved results.

Concerning the time evolution of contraction, we reconfirmed that immature (P14) muscles are not yet differentiated into fast- or slow-contracting ones and that fast contracting muscles are more severely affected by axotomy [1,3,31]. In the early developmental stages, contraction in both muscles is rather prolonged, with a high fatigue index. In control animals, EDL attains its normal features by adulthood, in the case of axotomy, however, the muscle becomes slow and fatigue resistant. At this point, there was a differentiation concerning our previous work, as DAP5 succeeded in recuperating in a greater degree the original features of the muscle. In agreement with the majority of researchers, it was of no

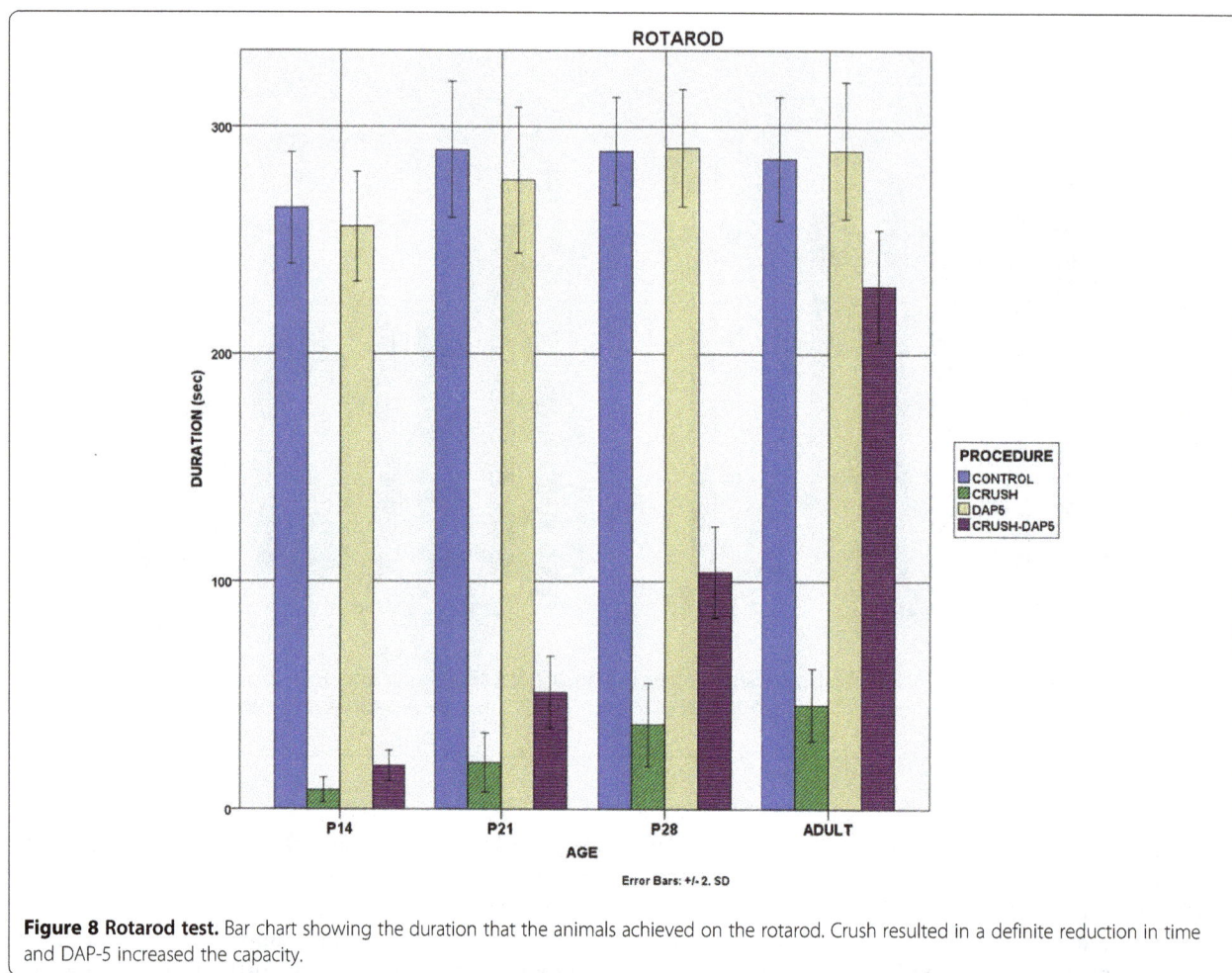

Figure 8 Rotarod test. Bar chart showing the duration that the animals achieved on the rotarod. Crush resulted in a definite reduction in time and DAP-5 increased the capacity.

surprise that soleus did not present any alteration in its time course of contraction, as its contractile properties are not significantly altered throughout early postnatal life. Concerning fatigability, normally soleus is converted progressively into a fatigue resistant muscle. This process is halted, in case of axotomy and is partially reversed by DAP5 administration. We also have to point out that differences were statistically significant in most parameters among the various age groups (within the same experimental group), reflecting the fact that all animals underwent the natural course of contractile properties maturation (force augmentation during development).

In order to evaluate the locomotion, a series of tests was applied, which comprised the rotarod, as well as passing along bridges of different width and footprint analysis. The results were in full correlation with the isometric recordings. Rats with axotomy exhibited overt changes in their locomotor behaviour, compared with controls. Treatment with DAP5 improved movement, although the difference with controls was still discernible. Improvement in locomotor behaviour, following DAP5 administration,

however, was not as impressive as the one observed in tension recordings. Axotomy provokes a serious sensori-motor disruption, early in development, and coordination of the limbs during walking does not entirely rely on the reinforcement of individual muscles. Adaptive mechanisms are activated to compensate for the lack of function; the injured rat exerts a notifying effort to use the crushed leg and eventually succeeds in walking, nevertheless, with uncontestable difference with respect to the non-injured one. In addition, it seems that some tests are more specific in delineating subtle differences between the different groups. The rotarod and the footprint analysis turned out to evaluate locomotor behaviour in a more efficient way, than the observation and the grading of the gait.

The lack of side-effects seems rather unexpected in our study, compared to what has been described in the literature [32]. The NMDA receptor contributes to plasticity, neuronal differentiation and synaptogenesis in the developing nervous system [33]. NMDA antagonists are notorious for causing a multitude of behavioural sequelae. The disfunction of this receptor is frequently considered to contribute to the pathophysiology of schizophrenia, depression, anxiety and, indeed, these agents are usually implemented in the research of several psychotic states [34]. Moreover, MK-801, one of the most extensively studied drugs in this category, is known to induce long term behavioural disturbances, when administered in neonatal rats [35]. One could argue that our locomotor models may not be so sensitive to detect this kind of behavioural defect. Furthermore, despite sharing nominally common mechanisms of action and often presumed biological equivalence, the NMDA antagonists present very diverse effects [36]. Most antagonists used in animal studies, such as MK-801, act via an uncompetitive antagonism, whereas DAP5 utilizes a competitive mode of action. It might be that, this mode of action, in association with the affinity of the receptor, should provide an effective combination which varies among the different substances and explains the magnitude of primary actions as well as the side effects.

Conclusions

Our results show that contractile properties and locomotor behaviour of animals are severely affected by axotomy, with a differential impact on fast contracting muscles. Administration of DAP5 reverses these devastating effects. To our knowledge, this is the first time that the systematic action of DAP5 is studied and the absence of apparent side-effects is very important, although further research is certainly required, in order to detect direct or indirect, local or systemic actions, which were not identified in our study.

The implications of such findings are apparent. By possessing a relatively safe pharmacologic profile and the encouraging results described above, this agent could be explored in a variety of animal models dealing with excitotoxic cell death.

Abbreviations
NMDA: N-methy-D-Aspartate; AMPA: A-amino-isoxazolopropionic acid; DAP5: D-2-Amino-5-phosphonopentanoic acid; EDL: Extensor digitorum longus; DBF: Distance between feet.

Competing interests
The authors declare that they have no competing interests.

Author details
[1]Department of Physiology, Faculty of Medicine, Aristotle University of Thessaloniki, Thessaloniki, Greece. [2]Department of Experimental Physiology, Faculty of Medicine, Aristotle University of Thessaloniki, Thessaloniki, Greece. [3]2nd Department of Pharmacology, Faculty of Medicine, Aristotle University of Thessaloniki, Thessaloniki, Greece.

Authors' contribution
CP was the primary researcher, was involved in the initial design of the study and contributed to the writing of the manuscript. AC carried out the data analysis and drafted the manuscript. CS has contributed to the design of the behavioural part of the study and helped to draft the manuscript. DK conducted a part of the experimental procedures. DK had a substantial involvement in the pharmacologic design of the study and the performance of the titration procedure. MA conceived of the study and participated in its design, coordination and supervision. All authors read and approved the final manuscript.

References
1. Gougoulias N, Chatzisotiriou A, Kapoukranidou D, Albani M: Magnesium administration provokes motor unit survival, after sciatic nerve injury in neonatal rats. BMC Muscoloskeletal Disorders 2004, 5(1):33.
2. Mentis GZ, Greensmith L, Vrbova G: Motoneurons destined to die are rescued by blocking N-methyl-D-aspartate receptors. Neuroscience 1993, 54(2):283–285.
3. Lowrie MB, Vrbová G: Different pattern of recovery of fast and slow muscles following nerve injury in the rat. J Physiol 1984, 349:397–410.
4. Schmalbruch H: Motoneurone death after sciatic nerve section in newborn rats. J Comp Neurol 1984, 224:252–258.
5. Greensmith L, Hasan H, Vrbova G: Nerve injury induces the susceptibility of motoneurons to N-methyl-D-aspartate- induced neurotoxicity in the developing rat. Neuroscience 1994, 58:727–733.
6. Lawson SJ, Lowrie MB: The role of apoptosis and excitotoxicity in the death of spinal motoneurons and interneurons after neonatal nerve injury. Neuroscience 1998, 87(2):337–348.
7. Lodge D, Johnson KM: Noncompetitive excitatory amino acid receptor antagonists. TIPS 1990, 11:81–86.
8. Albani M, Lowrie MB, Vrbova G: Reorganization of motor units in reinervated muscles of the rat. J Neurol Sci 1988, 88:195–206.
9. Lowrie MB, Krishnan S, Vrbová G: Permanent changes in muscle and motoneurons induced by nerve injury during a critical period of development of the rat. Brain Res 1987, 428:91–101.
10. Rothman SM, Olney JW: Excitotoxicity and the NMDA receptor. TINS 1987, 10(7):299–302.
11. Choia BT, Leea JH, Wanb Y, Hanb JS: Involvement of ionotropic glutamate receptors in low frequency electroacupuncture analgesia in rats. Neurosci Lett 2005, 377:185–188.
12. McNally W: Effects of systemic, intracerebral or intrathecal administration of an N-methyl-D-aspartate receptor antagonist on associative morphine analgesic tolerance and hyperalgesia in rats. Behavioural Neuroscience 1998, 112(4):966–978.
13. Cahusac E: The behavioural effects of NMDA receptor following application to the lumbar spinal cord of conscious rats. Neuropharmacology 1984, 23:719–724.
14. Leung LS, Desborough KA: APV, an N-methyl-D-aspartate receptor antagonist, blocks the hippocampal theta rhythm in behaving rats. Brain Res 1988, 463:148–152.
15. Puma V, Monmaur A, Sharif P, Monmaur: Intraseptal infusion of selective and competitive glutamate receptor agonist NMDA and antagonist o-2-amino-5-phosphonopentanoic acid Spectral implications for the physostigmine-induced hippocampal theta rhythm in urethane-anesthetized rats. Exp Brain Res 1996, 109:384–392.
16. Manahan-Vaughan D, von Haebler D, Winter C, Juckel G, Heinemann U: A single application of MK801 causes symptoms of acute psychosis, deficits in spatial memory, and impairment of synaptic plasticity in rats. Hippocampus 2008, 18(2):125–134.
17. Lipton SA: Failures and successes of NMDA receptor antagonists: molecular basis for the use of open-channel blockers like memantine in the treatment of acute and chronic neurologic insults. Neuropharmacology 2004, 1(1):101–110.
18. Atman J, Sudarshan K: Postnatal development on locomotion in the laboratory rat. Anim Behav 1975, 23:896–920.
19. Kaner T, Karadag T, Cirak B, Erken HA, Karabulut A, Kiroglu Y, Akkaya S, Acar F, Coskun E, Genc O, Colakoglu N: The effects of human umbilical cord blood transplantation in rats with experimentally induced spinal cord injury. J Neurosurg Spine 2010, 13(4):543–551.
20. Dijkstra Jeroen R, Meek Marcel F, Robinson Peter H, Albert Gramsbergen: Methods to evaluate functional nerve recovery in adult rats: walking track analysis, video analysis and the withdrawal reflex. J Neurosci Methods 2000, 96:89–96.
21. Klein A, Wessolleck J, Papazoglou A, Metz F, Nikkhah G: Walking pattern analysis after unilateral 6-OHDA lesion and transplantation of foetal dopaminergic progenitor cells in rats. Behav Brain Res 2009, 199(2):317–325.

22. Sun W, Oppenheim RW: **Response of motoneurons to neonatal sciatic nerve axotomy in Bax-knockout mice.** *Mol Cell Neurosci* 2003, **24**:875–886.

23. Harding DI, Greensmith L, Anderson PN, Vrbová G: **Motoneurons innervating partially denervated rat hindlimb muscles remain susceptible to axotomy induced cell death.** *Neuroscience* 1998, **86**:291–299.

24. Virgo L, Dekkers J, Mentis GZ, *et al*: **Changes in expression of NMDA receptor subunits in the rat lumbar spinal cord following neonatal nerve injury.** *Neuropathol Appl Neurobiol* 2000, **26**(3):258–272.

25. Greensmith L, Mentis GZ, Vrbova G: **Blockade of N-methyl-D-aspartate receptors by MK-801 (dizocilpine maleate) rescues motoneurons in developing rats.** *Developmental Brain Research* 1994, **81**:162–170.

26. Gougoulias N, Kouvelas D, Albani M: **Protective effect of PNQX on motor units and muscle property after sciatic nerve crush in neonatal rats.** *Pharmacol Res* 2007, **55**(5):370–377.

27. Greensmith L, Vrbova G: **Motoneurone survival: a functional approach.** *Trends Neurosci* 1996, **19**:450–455.

28. Antonov SM, Johnson JW: **Permeant ion regulation of NMDA receptor channel block by Mg2+.** *Proc Natl Acad Sci* 1999, **96**(25):14571–14576.

29. Kuner T, Schoepfer R: **Multiple structural elements determine subunit specificity of Mg2+ block in NMDA receptor channels.** *J Neurosci* 1996, **16**(11):3549–3558.

30. Lodge D, Davies S, Jones M, Millar J, Manallack D, Ornstein P, Verberne A, Young N, Beart P: **A comparison between the in vivo and in vitro activity of five potent and competitive NMDA antagonists.** *Br J Pharmacol* 1988, **95**:957–965.

31. Navarrete R, Vrbová G: **Differential effect of nerve injury at birth on the activity pattern of reinnervated slow and fast muscles of the rat.** *J Physiol* 1984, **351**:675–685.

32. Milton A, Lee Jonathan L, Butler Victoria J, Gardner R, Everitt B: **Intra-amygdala and systemic antagonism of NMDA receptors prevents the reconsolidation of drug-associated memory and impairs subsequently both novel and previously acquired drug-seeking behaviours.** *J Neurosci* 2008, **28**(33):8230–8237.

33. McDonald JW, Johnston MV: **Physiological and pathophysiological roles of excitatory amino acids during central nervous system development.** *Brain Res Brain Res Rev* 1990, **15**:41–70.

34. Kantrowitz JT, Javitt DC: **N-methyl-d-aspartate (NMDA) receptor dysfunction or dysregulation: the final common pathway on the road to schizophrenia?** *Brain Res Bull* 2010, **83**(3–4):108–121.

35. Uehara T, Sumiyoshi T, Seo T, Itoh H, Matsuoka T, Suzuki M, Kurachi M: **Long-term effects of neonatal MK-801 treatment on prepulse inhibition in young adult rats.** *Psychopharmacology (Berlin)* 2009, **206**(4):623–630.

36. Gilmour G, Pioli EY, Dix SL, Smith JW, Conway MW, Jones WT, Loomis S, Mason R, Shahabi S, Tricklebank MD: **Diverse and often opposite behavioural effects of NMDA receptor antagonists in rats: implications for "NMDA antagonist modelling" of schizophrenia.** *Psychopharmacology (Berlin)* 2009, **205**(2):203–216.

12

White-nose syndrome initiates a cascade of physiologic disturbances in the hibernating bat host

Michelle L Verant[1], Carol U Meteyer[2,5], John R Speakman[3], Paul M Cryan[4], Jeffrey M Lorch[1] and David S Blehert[2*]

Abstract

Background: The physiological effects of white-nose syndrome (WNS) in hibernating bats and ultimate causes of mortality from infection with *Pseudogymnoascus* (formerly *Geomyces*) *destructans* are not fully understood. Increased frequency of arousal from torpor described among hibernating bats with late-stage WNS is thought to accelerate depletion of fat reserves, but the physiological mechanisms that lead to these alterations in hibernation behavior have not been elucidated. We used the doubly labeled water (DLW) method and clinical chemistry to evaluate energy use, body composition changes, and blood chemistry perturbations in hibernating little brown bats (*Myotis lucifugus*) experimentally infected with *P. destructans* to better understand the physiological processes that underlie mortality from WNS.

Results: These data indicated that fat energy utilization, as demonstrated by changes in body composition, was two-fold higher for bats with WNS compared to negative controls. These differences were apparent in early stages of infection when torpor-arousal patterns were equivalent between infected and non-infected animals, suggesting that *P. destructans* has complex physiological impacts on its host prior to onset of clinical signs indicative of late-stage infections. Additionally, bats with mild to moderate skin lesions associated with early-stage WNS demonstrated a chronic respiratory acidosis characterized by significantly elevated dissolved carbon dioxide, acidemia, and elevated bicarbonate. Potassium concentrations were also significantly higher among infected bats, but sodium, chloride, and other hydration parameters were equivalent to controls.

Conclusions: Integrating these novel findings on the physiological changes that occur in early-stage WNS with those previously documented in late-stage infections, we propose a multi-stage disease progression model that mechanistically describes the pathologic and physiologic effects underlying mortality of WNS in hibernating bats. This model identifies testable hypotheses for better understanding this disease, knowledge that will be critical for defining effective disease mitigation strategies aimed at reducing morbidity and mortality that results from WNS.

Keywords: White-nose syndrome, Bats, Doubly labeled water

Background

Since emergence of white-nose syndrome (WNS) in 2007, bat populations of eastern North America have declined precipitously due to disease-related mortality [1-3]. The causative agent of WNS is the fungus *Pseudogymnoascus* (formerly *Geomyces*) *destructans* [4-6], which erodes unfurred skin comprising wing membranes, muzzles, and ears of hibernating bats, inducing

physiological perturbations, altered behavior, and death [7]. Although underlying causes for mortality from this invasive cutaneous mycosis remain unclear, proposed mechanisms include disruptions to vital homeostatic functions such as thermoregulation and water balance [8]. For example, water and electrolyte losses across the ulcerated wing epithelium have been proposed to cause hypotonic dehydration [9] and acid base disturbances [10]. Consequently, alterations in behavior have been observed in infected bats, including increased frequency of arousal from torpor during hibernation [11,12] and unusual day flights during winter [3]. High metabolic

* Correspondence: dblehert@usgs.gov
[2]US Geological Survey National Wildlife Health Center, 6006 Schroeder Rd., Madison, Wisconsin, USA
Full list of author information is available at the end of the article

demands of such activities [13-15] likely also contribute to mortality of bats prior to spring emergence by accelerating depletion of fat reserves. However, physiological data linking altered behavior to increased energy demands in bats with WNS are lacking.

The doubly labeled water (DLW) method is widely applicable to the study of energetics in relation to homeostasis, behavioral adaptations, and resource allocation in both animals and humans [16]. This method is based on dynamic flux of hydrogen and oxygen through the body and ability to measure these flux rates over a period of time using labeled isotopes, ^{2}H and ^{18}O [17]. Following administration of these exogenous isotopes, they equilibrate throughout the body water pool. The total body water volume (TBW) can then be estimated from the dilution spaces of the isotopes when introduced at known concentrations and serves as a valuable indicator of body composition (ratio of lean body mass to fat) [18]. Notably the DLW method has been used in temperate-zone insectivorous bats in the wild (*e.g.*, *Myotis lucifugus* [19] and *Eptesicus fuscus* [20]), but there are no published reports of this method being used in bats hibernating over a protracted time period (*i.e.*, months).

To evaluate proposed causes of mortality from WNS, we used the DLW method to quantify energy expenditure and changes in body composition of hibernating little brown bats (*M. lucifugus*) experimentally infected with *P. destructans* to test the hypothesis that WNS increases metabolic demands during hibernation. We predicted that infected bats would exhibit greater changes in body composition, specifically decreased proportion of fat mass, over the course of the experiment compared to negative control bats as a result of higher daily energy expenditures and fat utilization. To further characterize previously reported physiologic outcomes associated with WNS, we analyzed blood chemistries of all bats at the end of the experiment to assess acid base balance, electrolytes, and hydration status.

Results
Infection status and torpor patterns
Of the 39 bats treated with conidia from *P. destructans*, 32 bats (14 male, 18 female) developed epidermal wing lesions characteristic of WNS by the end of the 98-d experiment. The majority of these bats (n = 30) had mild to moderate WNS (severity scores 1 or 2 with median score of 1), while the remaining two had moderate to severe WNS (severity scores 3 and 4). Sex had no effect on the probability that a bat developed WNS (Fisher s Exact Test, p = 0.4075). All infected bats, including animals that did not develop detectable WNS by histology (n = 7), were PCR-positive for *P. destructans*; all bats in the control (non-infected) group were PCR-negative for

the fungal pathogen. Four infected bats and five control bats died prior to the end of the experiment.

Average torpor bout duration for infected bats following DLW injection was 9.13 (2.31) d with average arousal duration of 54 (10) min. Average torpor bout duration for control bats following DLW injection was 8.52 (2.34) d with average arousal duration of 55 (11) min. Differences in torpor-arousal patterns of bats between treatment groups were not significant (torpor bout duration, p = 0.5337; arousal duration p = 0.6508).

Blood chemistry
Blood chemistry parameters were analyzed for 27 infected bats (10 male, 17 female) and 11 control bats (6 male, 5 female) from which sufficient blood sample volumes were collected. One infected bat did not have skin lesions characteristic of WNS on histopathology, but there were no discernible differences across parameters when compared to infected bats with confirmed WNS. Additionally, we were unable to collect sufficient blood volume for analysis from the two bats with most advanced pathology (WNS severity scores 3 and 4). Thus, blood chemistry values presented herein for infected bats represent bats with mild WNS pathology (median severity score of 1).

Infected bats had significantly lower blood pH than controls (Table 1, Figure 1a). This acidemia was associated with a significant elevation of pCO_2 in infected bats compared to controls (Table 1, Figure 1a), indicating that bats had respiratory acidosis. Bicarbonate levels of infected bats were also significantly higher than those of non-infected controls (Table 1, Figure 1a), evident of a compensatory renal response to a chronic acidosis. The accumulation of bicarbonate in blood of infected bats was also reflected in an elevated base excess compared to controls (Table 1). There were no differences in sodium or chloride concentrations between treatment groups, but potassium concentration was significantly higher in the infected bats than it was in the controls (Table 1, Figure 1b). Glucose concentrations were lower in infected bats but not significantly (Table 1), and anion gap values were not different from controls nor elevated as would be expected if acidemia resulted from metabolic lactic or keto-acidosis. Other measures of hydration status (hematocrit, blood urea nitrogen, and total protein) were equivalent between treatment groups (Table 1, Figure 1c). Overall, there were no effects of sex (two-way MANOVA, Pillais Trace = 0.48, F (9,14) = 1.46, p = 0.25) or the interaction of sex and treatment (two-way MANOVA, Pillais Trace = 0.53, F (9,14) = 1.79 , p = 0.16) on measured blood parameters. See Additional file 1 for a complete table of blood chemistry parameter estimations compared to available reference values.

Table 1 Blood chemistry comparisons

Parameter	k	df	Unadjusted p-value α = 0.05	Holm-Bonferroni corrected p-value (α/k)
pCO_2	12	38	<0.0001*	.0042
K	11	35	<0.0001*	.0045
pH	10	38	<0.0001*	.0050
HCO_3^-	9	36	<0.0001*	.0056
BE	8	37	<0.0001*	.0063
Glucose	7	26	.0144	.0071
AG	6	26	.0483	.0083
Cl^-	5	22	.0646	.01
BUN	4	36	.2093	.0125
TP	3	36	.6085	.0167
Na^+	2	36	.7079	.025
Hct	1	23	.8396	.05

Abbreviations: pCO_2 dissolved carbon dioxide, *K* potassium, HCO_3^- bicarbonate, *BE* base excess, *AG* anion gap, Cl^- chloride, *BUN* blood urea nitrogen, *TP* total protein, Na^+ sodium, *Hct* hematocrit.

Results of *t*-tests used to compare mean blood chemistry parameters for little brown bats (*Myotis lucifugus*) either experimentally infected with *Pseudogymnoascus destructans* or negative (non-infected) controls. Significant differences between treatment groups (*) were determined by p-values < Holm-Bonferroni p-values corrected by the index of comparison (*k*).

Measurements of daily energy expenditure and total body water

Upon collection of final blood samples, 67 d after injection with DLW, labeled isotope concentrations had decreased to levels statistically indistinguishable from background levels. Consequently, isotope turnover rates and daily energy expenditure (DEE) could not be determined for bats euthanized at the end of the experiment. However, one bat in the control group that died 35 d after initial injection of DLW had detectable isotope concentrations at time of death. For this bat, k_d and k_o were 0.004, calculated respiratory CO_2 production (rCO_2) was 0.01 ml/min, and resultant DEE was 0.44 kJ/day.

Measurements of total body water (TBW) were available for 26 bats (19 infected, 7 controls) following initial injection of DLW and for 24 bats (17 infected, 7 controls) after final injection (Table 2). The reduction in sample size is attributed to mortality of bats during the experiment or inability to collect a sufficient amount of blood for isotope analyses. At the time of initial DLW injection, mean TBW as percent of body mass (TBW % BM) was significantly lower for infected bats than controls (Tables 2 and 3), but mean body mass was not different between groups (t = −0.5925, df = 30, p = 0.558). After 67 d hibernation, changes in TBW and body mass were compared for infected and control bats for which paired measurements were available. Body mass decreased significantly in both treatment groups (infected: t = 11.32, df = 13, p <0.0001; control: t = 14.24, df = 3, p = 0.0008), but the loss in body mass was equal between groups. Changes in TBW % BM were marginally significant between infected and control bats, but not when corrected for multiple comparisons (Tables 2 and 3). Within groups,

infected bats, which all developed mild WNS (n = 14; median WNS severity score 1, range 1 2) exhibited a significant increase in TBW % BM (Tables 2 and 3); increase in TBW % BM among control bats (n = 4) was not significant (Tables 2 and 3).

As trends in TBW, namely TBW % BM, reflect changes in body composition, net fat energy utilization was calculated from the change in TBW (in g) and body mass measurements for all bats with paired data assuming constant 73% water content of lean mass (see Additional file 2). Based upon these calculations, mean total fat energy utilization for the 67 d after which bats were administered DLW was significantly higher for bats with WNS compared to negative controls (Tables 2 and 3).

Discussion

Results of this study support the hypothesis that infection with *P. destructans* and subsequent development of WNS increases energy (fat) use in hibernating bats and provide key information for understanding the progression of physiologic disturbances that ultimately lead to mortality from this disease. Specifically, isotope-based estimates of changes in body composition provided evidence that hibernating little brown bats with WNS utilized twice as much energy as non-infected control bats housed under equivalent experimental conditions. However, the greater energy use by infected bats was not associated with an increased rate or duration of arousals from torpor. This implies that bats, even with mild WNS lesions, have an elevated metabolism prior to the onset of altered arousal patterns characteristic of late-stage infections [12]. Additionally, bats with early-stage WNS developed severe, chronic respiratory acidosis and hyperkalemia

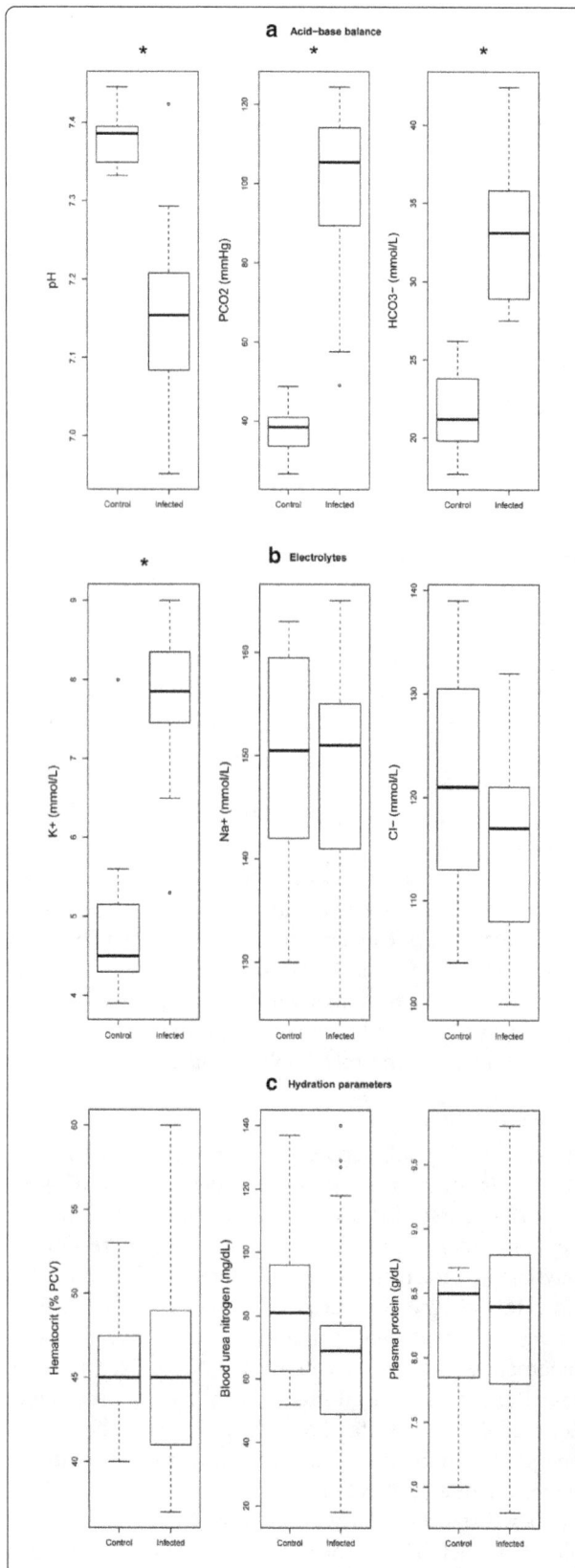

Figure 1 Blood chemistry parameters. Box-and-whisker plots of blood chemistry values for hibernating little brown bats (*Myotis lucifugus*) experimentally infected with *Pseudogymnoascus destructans* and negative (non-infected) controls. Parameters for acid-base balance **(a)**, electrolytes **(b)** and hydration status **(c)** are shown. The median (bold line), upper and lower quartiles (box), and maximum and minimum values (whiskers) are shown. Potential outliers (points) shown were not confirmed by Bonferonni outlier tests. Significant differences (*) were determined at $\alpha = 0.05$ corrected for multiple comparisons by the Holm-Bonferonni method.

(high potassium concentrations in the blood). Integrating these results with those reported by others [7,9-12,21], we propose a mechanistic multi-stage disease progression model for WNS that encompasses our current knowledge of disease pathology and physiologic sequelae, including death, that result following infection by *P. destructans* (Figure 2).

As shown in this study, early stages of WNS involving fungal colonization of the wing membrane with progression to erosion and ulceration of the epidermis, are characterized by increased CO_2 levels in blood, resultant acidemia, and hyperkalemia. The accumulation of CO_2 may stem from either increased CO_2 production from an elevated metabolic rate associated with infection, decreased CO_2 expiration, possibly due to inhibition of diffusion across the damaged wing epithelium [7], and/or a compensatory response by the host to attempt to further lower torpor metabolic rates (and conserve fat reserves) by inducing a hypercapnic (high pCO_2) acidosis [15,22-24]. This acidosis may then contribute to the observed hyperkalemia by an acidosis-induced extracellular shift of potassium. Intracellular potassium ions may also leak into the blood through damaged and necrotic cell membranes caused by hyphal invasion of the

Table 2 Body composition measurements

Parameter	Pd infected bats	Control bats
All data	n = 22	n = 10
Initial TBW % BM	53.4 (4.3)	58.8 (2.4)
Final TBW % BM	60.5 (3.9)	61.0 (4.6)
Initial BM (g)	7.64 (0.75)	7.48 (0.58)
Final BM (g)	6.60 (0.68)	6.41 (0.57)
Paired data	n = 14	n = 4
Change in TBW % BM	+ 9.1 (3.5)	+ 4.0 (3.9)
Fat energy use (kJ)	43.9 (13.6)	20.5 (14.7)

Values of body mass (BM) and total body water as percentage of body mass (TBW % BM) were used to estimate net fat energy use over 67 d for individual little brown bats (*Myotis lucifugus*) experimentally infected with *Pseudogymnoascus destructans* and negative control (non-infected) bats. Values in the table are mean (SD) and n = sample size. Initial TBW % BM was significantly different between treatment groups. Over the course of the experiment, infected bats demonstrated a significant increase in TBW % BM and used significantly more fat energy than non-infected bats. Body mass decreased significantly over the experiment in infected and control bats but there was no difference between groups.

Table 3 Doubly labeled water comparisons

Measurement	k	df	Unadjusted p-value α = 0.05	Holm-Bonferroni corrected p-value (α/k)
Fat energy use (I)	8	13	<0.0001*	0.0063
Change in TBW % BM (I)	7	13	<0.0001*	0.0071
Initial TBW % BM (I vs C)	6	25	0.0041*	0.0083
Fat energy use (I vs C)	5	16	0.0088*	0.01
Change in TBW % BM (I vs C)	4	16	0.0243	0.0125
Fat energy use (C)	3	3	0.0687	0.0167
Change in TBW % BM (C)	2	3	0.1353	0.025
Final TBW % BM (I vs C)	1	22	0.7841	0.05

Results of *t*-tests used to compare doubly labeled water measurements for little brown bats (*Myotis lucifugus*) either experimentally infected with *Pseudogymnoascus destructans* (I) or non-infected controls (C). Total body water is represented as percentage of body mass (TBW % BM). Significant differences between treatment groups (*) were determined by p-values < Holm-Bonferroni p-values corrected by the index of comparison (*k*).

epidermis. Overall, these physiologic effects result in a chronic respiratory acidosis, hyperkalemia, and reduction of fat reserves among bats during early stages of WNS.

Consistent with results observed in bats at later and more severe stages of WNS [9,10], we propose that once pCO_2 elevates beyond a tolerance threshold, chemoreceptors stimulate hyperventilation, and resulting increased arousals from torpor serve to remove excess CO_2, returning blood pH to normal [22,25-28]. The high energy demand of these arousals then likely further contributes to accelerated depletion of fat reserves. Additionally, increased ventilatory rates and greater vapor pressure difference with increased body temperatures during arousals would contribute to greater evaporative water loss [29] and dehydration. Together, these outcomes are consistent with data previously published for little brown bats with

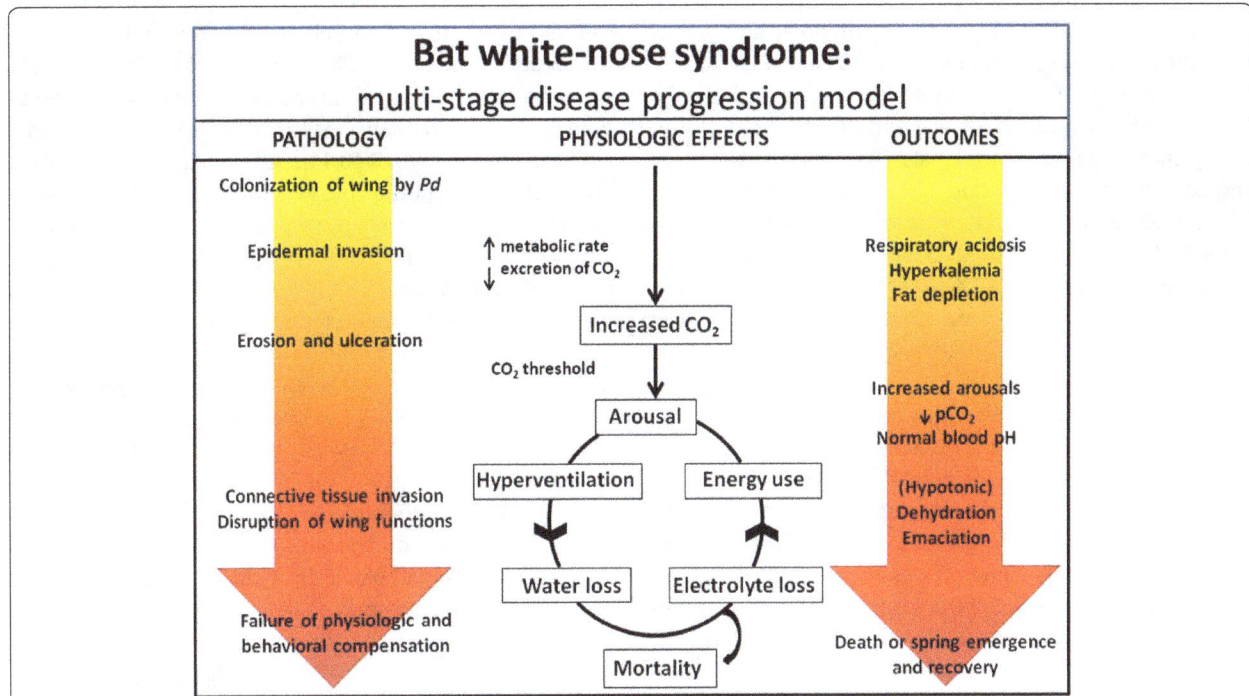

Figure 2 Disease progression model for bat white-nose syndrome (WNS). We propose a mechanistic multi-stage disease model for WNS in a hibernating bat that encompasses current knowledge on the progression of fungal-induced wing pathology and physiologic sequelae leading to mortality from disease. Initial colonization and invasion of the wing epidermis by *Pseudogymnoascus destructans* (*Pd*) results in increased energy expenditure, chronic respiratory acidosis (elevated blood pCO_2 and bicarbonate), and hyperkalemia (elevated blood potassium). Erosion and ulceration of the epidermis stimulate increased frequencies of arousal from torpor, which remove excess CO_2 and normalize blood pH, but contribute to dehydration and depletion of fat reserves. As wing pathology becomes more extensive and severe, these effects are exacerbated by water and electrolyte loss across the epidermis (hypotonic dehydration), which stimulate more frequent arousals and create a positive feedback loop that ultimately leads to mortality when energy reserves and compensatory mechanisms become exhausted.

more severe WNS pathology that exhibited increased frequency of arousal from torpor, decreased pCO_2, normal blood pH, and dehydration [10].

As WNS progresses towards more extensive and severe wing lesions, dehydration may be further exacerbated by water and electrolyte loss across the damaged epidermis of the wing [9,30], further stimulating arousal from hibernation to drink [29,31,32]. Positive feedback loops are then established that link worsening disease-associated wing pathology to further increases in arousal frequency, water loss, and energy use resulting in additional observed acute physiologic changes, including hypocapnia, hypoglycemia, hyponatremia, hypochloremia, and emaciation [9-11]. Once compensatory mechanisms such as cellular buffering, respiratory and metabolic regulation, and/or behavioral adaptations are exhausted, this suite of disturbances ultimately leads to mortality unless the bat has sufficient energy reserves to persist until spring emergence and clear the infection following a return to a metabolically active state [33].

Although normal reference ranges for blood chemistry values in microchiropteran species are generally lacking [34], deviations of measured parameters in infected bats from the negative controls in this study, together with published information for apparently healthy hibernating little brown bats [10,34-39], suggest pathologic and potentially life-threatening physiological disturbances associated with early-stage WNS infections [see Additional file 1]. Bats with WNS in this study had almost 40% higher mean pCO_2 than negative control bats (99.4 and 37.1 mmHg respectively), and pCO_2 values above 90 mmHg are generally considered to be lethal in other non-hibernating animals and humans. Elevated pCO_2 levels and associated acidemia are known to interfere with enzymatic functions, reduce metabolic activity, and cause central depression of respiration; in severe cases, such elevated levels can lead to coma and death.

Direct calculations of energy expenditure could not be determined for most bats in this study because final isotope concentrations were indistinguishable from background levels. However, the increase in TBW as a percent of body mass observed in infected bats indicated that bats with WNS had higher proportions of lean tissue mass to fat tissue mass at the end of the study. This finding implies that bats with WNS used significantly more fat energy reserves compared to negative controls despite hibernating under equivalent conditions. From the estimated changes in fat content over the 67-d measurement period, infected bats utilized 0.65 kJ/d, while control bats utilized 0.31 kJ/d. These results indicate that bats with WNS expended approximately twice as much energy during hibernation as non-infected control bats. Some caution must be taken in interpreting these results due to the small number of control bats for which paired TBW

measurements were available to calculate estimates of fat use. However, the range of expected daily energy use of 0.27 to 0.51 kJ/d predicted for healthy hibernating *M. lucifugus* at the mean temperature of our study [40] is consistent with the daily rates of energy use observed in control bats in this experiment, and lower than rates observed in infected bats. There were no differences in torpor-arousal patterns between treatment groups in this study suggesting that WNS causes an increase in metabolism that is not directly associated with arousal from torpor and occurs at early stages in disease progression. Additionally, there were no differences between infected and control bats in T_{skin} maintained during torpor or arousal bouts. Alternatively, metabolic costs associated with infection and development of wing pathology may be linked to increased costs of thermoregulation caused by inhibition of peripheral vasoconstriction during torpor and arousal [25], catabolism of fat to generate metabolic water in response to increased water loss, or additional energetic costs associated with the host-pathogen interaction.

Rising concentrations of pCO_2 in a mammal would normally stimulate increased respiration to release excess CO_2. However, the unique physiology of mammalian hibernators allows for active suppression of respiration during torpor, and under these conditions, blood pCO_2 increases to levels higher than those observed in metabolically active mammals [22,28,41,42]. This elevation of pCO_2 is thought to be an integral part of hibernation physiology as induction of an acidotic state serves to reduce metabolic rate and thermogenesis [25,43,44]. Additionally, the resultant high pCO_2 gradient improves ventilation efficiency, thereby minimizing energy costs of respiration during torpor [23]. Despite this tolerance for a respiratory acidosis [45], a hibernating mammal must still be able to regulate pCO_2 for proper physiologic function. If CO_2 elimination routes, such as passive diffusion of CO_2 across the wing epithelium [46,47] are compromised by disease, as hypothesized for bats with WNS [7], persistently rising blood pCO_2 levels would cause the severe chronic respiratory acidosis we have observed. Thus, underlying causes for the high pCO_2 levels in bats with WNS are likely a combination of the uniquely adapted physiology of a hibernating mammal compounded by pathologically induced insult(s) to these physiological mechanisms.

Bat WNS presents a new paradigm for the study of infectious disease. Never before has a fungal skin pathogen been known to specifically infect a hibernating mammal, causing severe physiologic disturbances and mortality. Although substantial efforts have been devoted to understanding chytridiomycosis, a lethal fungal skin disease of amphibians, prior to WNS there had been no in-depth study of disease processes in a metabolically repressed animal caused by a psychrophilic and metabolically active pathogen. The poorly characterized capacity of bats to compensate for and respond to infection during hibernation demonstrates the difficulty of understanding how host-pathogen interactions influence disease manifestation and mortality.

Conclusions

This study demonstrated that infection with *P. destructans* and subsequent development of WNS increased energy (fat) use in hibernating bats prior to the onset of altered arousal patterns associated with later stages of WNS. Severe, chronic respiratory acidosis and hyperkalemia were also apparent in bats that developed mild WNS. With these results, we present a multi-stage disease progression model for WNS as a framework for understanding the pathogenesis and underlying causes of mortality due to WNS (Figure 2). This model integrates a range of published work [7,9-12,21] with data from this study into the first attempt to mechanistically define a comprehensive conceptual model of what may occur during development of WNS in a hibernating bat from initial colonization of wing skin by *P. destructans* until the death of the animal. This model identifies key testable hypotheses necessary to develop a comprehensive understanding of the physiologic effects of WNS on hibernating bats. Ultimately, this knowledge will be critical for guiding effective and properly timed management actions to moderate physiologic effects of WNS and minimize morbidity and mortality from this devastating disease.

Methods

Bats

This study was conducted in accordance with experimental protocol #110921 approved by the Institutional Animal Care and Use Committee of the USGS National Wildlife Health Center (NWHC). Sixty (30 male and 30 female) little brown bats (*Myotis lucifugus*) were collected from a hibernaculum in Wisconsin on December 21, 2012 and transported to NWHC. Bats were held individually within tube socks maintained in coolers at approximately 7C during transport. Body mass and right forearm length were recorded for each bat, and both wings of each bat were evaluated for pre-existing injuries. All animals were confirmed negative for *P. destructans* by polymerase chain reaction (PCR) [48] analysis of wing-skin swab samples (PurFlock nylon-flocked swabs, Puritan, Guilford, ME) collected from each bat. An archival temperature logger (iBBat, Alpha Mach) was affixed between the scapulae of each bat using a latex-based adhesive (Ostobond, M.O.C., Vaudreuil, Quebec, Canada) after trimming a 1 cm 1 cm patch of fur to within 1 mm of the skin surface. Loggers were programmed to record skin temperature (T_{skin}) every 15 minutes starting at the time of DLW injection until the end of the experiment. Torpor-arousal patterns were assessed using T_{skin} data downloaded from

iBBat temperature loggers following termination of the experiment. Arousal thresholds were defined as 10% of maximum T_{skin} for each individual [11].

Bats were sorted by sex and randomly assigned to infected (n = 39; 19 males, 20 females) and control (n = 21; 11 males, 10 females) groups. Conidia of *P. destructans* (5 10 ^{5} in 20 µl of PBS with 0.5% Tween-20) were applied to the skin of the dorsal surface of both wings of each bat in the infected group as previously described [49]. PBS Tween-20 lacking conidia was similarly applied to the wings of control (non-infected) bats. Each group was placed into a mesh enclosure (22 H 14 W 14 D; Apogee Reptaria, Reptiledirect.com) within separate environmental incubators (Percival Scientific, Perry, IA) and maintained at 7.5C and 90% RH for 98 days. Bats were monitored every other day for the duration of the experiment and any dead animals removed.

At the end of the experiment, all remaining bats were euthanized. Polymerase chain reaction (PCR) analyses of wing skin were performed as previously described [48] to confirm the presence of *P. destructans*. Additionally, the entire membrane of one wing was examined by histology to identify lesions diagnostic for WNS [21] and to assign severity scores [from 0 (no lesions) to 4 (severe, extensive lesions)] based on extent of fungal infection [11].

Doubly labeled water

The DLW method used a two-sample approach by measuring isotopic concentrations at equilibrium (1 h following DLW injection) and once more at the end of the experiment [17]. The duration of the elimination period was determined from estimates of isotope washout rates modeled using parameters of energy expenditure for hibernating little brown bats [40], assuming torpor bouts of 8 to 16 d interspersed by 0.5 to 1.5 h arousals, as recorded for little brown bats with and without WNS in previous experiments [12]. One additional arousal and a 3-h euthermic period were included in the model to account for initial DLW injection and blood collection at the end of the experiment. Based upon an energy expenditure budget of approximately 60 kJ, isotope washout was predicted to occur 89 to 171 d post-administration of DLW. To increase the likelihood that labeled isotope concentrations would remain measurable over a duration of time sufficient for development of experimentally induced WNS (90 to 120 d; [12,49]), we administered the first dose of DLW 28 d after treatment of bats with fungal conidia.

For administration of DLW, bats were removed from incubators and aroused at room temperature for 20 to 30 min. Once fully aroused, both infected (n = 34) and negative control (n = 16) bats were injected intraperitoneally with approximately 70 µl of a mixture of enriched ^{18}O (approximately 19 atom %) and ^2H (approximately 11 atom %). Dose enrichments were quantified using a standard dilution experiment [50]. Bats were then held at room temperature for approximately 1 h to allow for isotopic equilibration [20]. Following 1 h at euthermic temperatures, 50 to 75 μl of blood was collected from the ventral aspect of the uropatagial vein of each bat [51] into two heparinized 100 μl capillary tubes for determination of initial isotope concentrations and TBW. Ends of the capillary tubes were immediately flame-sealed, dipped in sealing wax, and stored at 4C until analysis. Bats were then returned to incubators and left undisturbed for the duration of the experiment. Additionally, five bats from each treatment group were used to measure background isotope levels [52]; these bats were treated identically as those described above, but they did not receive injections of DLW.

At 95 days post-treatment with conidia (67 d after injection of DLW) bats were removed from hibernation chambers, aroused to euthermic body temperatures, and blood was collected (as above) to determine final isotope concentrations. Blood from bats that did not receive initial DLW injections was also sampled at this time to obtain a concurrent measure of background isotope levels. Since TBW content of each bat was assumed to have changed since sampling at the beginning of the experiment, a dose of the DLW solution used previously was administered to each bat, for which a non-terminal blood sample was collected, to determine TBW at the end of the experiment for infected (n = 22) and control (n = 12) bats. Following the injection with DLW, bats were held at room temp for 1 h for isotopic equilibration, after which time they were anesthetized with 5% isoflurane and decapitated. Whole blood was collected into heparinized capillary tubes, and 50 to 75 μl of blood was immediately sealed in capillary tubes (as described above) for isotope analysis. Rectal temperature was recorded at the time of euthanasia using a miniature probe and digital thermometer (Models RET-4 & BAT7001H, Physitemp Instruments, Inc., Clifton, NJ).

Blood chemistry

Following euthanasia, blood chemistry parameters were analyzed for each bat as previously described [9]. Briefly, 95 μl of whole blood was collected following decapitation and analyzed within one minute using an i-STAT portable clinical analyzer (EC8$^+$ diagnostic cartridge, Abaxis, Union City, California, USA) to assess sodium (Na^+, mmol l^{-1}), potassium (K^+, mmol l^{-1}), chloride (Cl^-, mmol l^{-1}), pH, dissolved carbon dioxide (pCO_2, mmHg), bicarbonate (HCO_3^-, mmol l^{-1}), base excess (BE, mmol l^{-1}), anion gap (AG, mmol l^{-1}), blood urea nitrogen (BUN, mgdL^{-1}), hematocrit (Hct, % PCV), and glucose (mgdL^{-1}). Remaining blood was centrifuged in microtubes (Stat-Spin, Iris Sample Processing, Westwood, MA) for 90 s, and plasma protein (gdL^{-1}) of the serum was measured using a hand-held refractometer (Pulse Instruments, Van Nuys, CA). Temperature-corrected values

for pH and pCO_2 were calculated using rectal temperature of the bat at the time of blood collection, and HCO_3^-, AG, and BE were then calculated using these temperature-corrected values according to the i-STAT manual [53] and specifications of the Clinical Laboratory Standards Institute for Blood Gas and pH Analysis and Related Measurements [54] (see also Additional file 3 for equations).

Isotope analysis

Capillary tubes containing the blood samples were vacuum distilled [55], and water from the resulting distillate was used to produce CO_2 and H_2 (methods in [56] for CO_2 and [57] for H_2). The isotope ratios ^{18}O: ^{16}O and ^2H: ^1H were analyzed using gas source isotope ratio mass spectrometry (Optima, Micromass IRMS and Isochrom μG, Manchester, UK). Samples were run alongside three lab standards for each isotope (calibrated to International standards) to correct delta values to ppm. Isotope enrichments were converted to values of daily energy expenditure using a single pool model as recommended for this size of animal [58].

Dilution spaces for oxygen (N_0) and hydrogen (N_d) were calculated by the plateau method (Speakman and Krol, [59]). CO_2 production was calculated using equation 7.17 of Speakman [50] and used to estimate DEE according to the Weir equation [59] (see Additional file 2 for details).

Statistical analyses

Normality of measured parameters was assessed visually using histograms and Q-Q plots for each parameter. Assumptions of normality and homogeneity of variance were satisfied so no transformations were performed. Mean values of measured parameters for infected bats were compared to control bats using independent two-sample t-tests. Paired data sets from TBW estimates were compared using paired t-tests. All t-tests were two-tailed with $\alpha = 0.05$, and critical values for significance were adjusted to control the family-wise error rate using the Holm-Bonferonni method [60] applied separately to each data set: blood chemistry parameters (12 comparisons), DLW measurements (8 comparisons), and torpor profiles (2 comparisons). All statistical analyses were conducted in R [61]. Data in the text are presented as means (SD).

Competing interests

The authors declare that they have no competing interests.

Authors contributions

MLV, PMC, JML, and DSB conceived and designed the study. MLV coordinated and conducted the experiment, performed molecular analyses, and analyzed the data. JRS formulated the doubly labeled water (DLW), supervised analyses of DLW samples, and provided expert consult on study design and interpretation of results. MLV, PMC, JML, CUM, and DSB participated in data collection. CUM performed the histopathology examinations for disease confirmation. MLV wrote the manuscript, all co-authors provided input, and DSB edited the manuscript. All authors read and approved the manuscript.

Acknowledgments

This project was financially supported by the US Geological Survey through a cooperative agreement with the University of Wisconsin Madison. We are indebted to Dave and Jennifer Redell and Paul White from the Wisconsin Department of Natural Resources for collecting the animals used to complete this study and for assisting with data collection. We thank Melissa Behr for assistance with necropsies and NWHC Animal Care Staff for their help with set-up and maintenance of animals. We thank Lobke Vaanholt and Catherine Hambly (University of Aberdeen, Scotland) for their expertise and coordination in the analyses of the DLW blood samples. Funds were used for direct project costs only. Use of trade, product, or firm names is for descriptive purposes only and does not imply endorsement by the US Government.

Author details

[1]Department of Pathobiological Sciences, School of Veterinary Medicine, University of Wisconsin-Madison, 2015 Linden Dr., Madison, Wisconsin, USA. [2]US Geological Survey National Wildlife Health Center, 6006 Schroeder Rd., Madison, Wisconsin, USA. [3]Institute of Biological and Environmental Sciences, University of Aberdeen, Aberdeen, Scotland, UK. [4]US Geological Survey Fort Collins Science Center, 2150 Centre Ave. Building C, Fort Collins, Colorado, USA. [5]US Geological Survey National Center, Environmental Health, 12201 Sunrise Valley Dr., Reston, Virginia, USA.

References

1. Blehert DS, Hicks AC, Behr MJ, Meteyer CU, Berlowski-Zier BM, Buckles EL, Coleman JTH, Darling SR, Gargas A, Niver R, Okoniewski JC, Rudd RJ, Stone WB: Bat white-nose syndrome: an emerging fungal pathogen? Science 2009, 323:227.
2. Frick WF, Pollock JF, Hicks AC, Langwig K, Reynolds DS, Turner GG, Butchkoski CM, Kunz TH: An emerging disease causes regional population collapse of a common North American bat species. Science 2010, 329:679 682.
3. Turner GG, Reeder DM, Coleman JC: A five-year assessment of mortality and geographic spread of white-nose syndrome in North American bats and a look to the future. Bat Res News 2011, 52:13 27.
4. Gargas A, Trest MT, Christensen M, Volk TJ, Blehert DS: Geomyces destructans sp. nov. asssociated with bat white-nose syndrome. Mycotaxon 2009, 108:147 154.
5. Minnis AM, Lindner DL: Phylogenetic evaluation of Geomyces and allies reveals no close relatives of Pseudogymnoascus destructans, comb. nov., in bat hibernacula of eastern North America. Fungal Biol 2013, 117:638 649.
6. Lorch JM, Muller LK, Russell RE, O Connor M, Lindner DL, Blehert DS: Distribution and environmental persistence of the causative agent of white-nose syndrome, Geomyces destructans, in bat hibernacula of the eastern United States. Appl Environ Microbiol 2012, 79:1293 2839.
7. Cryan PM, Meteyer CU, Boyles JG, Blehert DS: Wing pathology of white-nose syndrome in bats suggests life-threatening disruption of physiology. BMC Biol 2010, 8:135.
8. Willis CKR, Menzies AK, Boyles JG, Wojciechowski MS: Evaporative water loss is a plausible explanation for mortality of bats from white-nose syndrome. Integr Comp Biol 2011, 51:364 373.
9. Cryan PM, Meteyer CU, Blehert DS, Lorch JM, Reeder DM, Turner GG, Webb J, Behr M, Verant ML, Russell RE, Castle KT: Electrolyte depletion in white-nose syndrome bats. J Wildlife Dis 2013, 49:398 402.
10. Warnecke L, Turner JM, Bollinger TK, Misra V, Cryan PM, Blehert DS, Wibbelt G, Willis CKR: Pathophysiology of white-nose syndrome in bats: a mechanistic model linking wing damage to mortality. Biol Lett 2013, 9:20130177.

11. Reeder DM, Frank CL, Turner GG, Meteyer CU, Kurta A, Britzke ER, Vodzak ME, Darling SR, Stihler CW, Hicks AC, Jacob R, Grieneisen LE, Brownlee SA, Muller LK, Blehert DS: Frequent arousal from hibernation linked to severity of infection and mortality in bats with white-nose syndrome. PloS One 2012, 7:e38920.
12. Warnecke L, Turner JM, Bollinger TK, Lorch JM, Misra V, Cryan PM, Wibbelt G, Blehert DS, Willis CKR: Inoculation of bats with European Geomyces destructans supports the novel pathogen hypothesis for the origin of white-nose syndrome. Proc Natl Acad Sci U S A 2012, 109:6999 7003.
13. Kayser C: The Physiology of Natural Hibernation. Oxford: Pergamon Press; 1961.
14. Thomas DW, Dorais M, Bergeron JM: Winter energy budgets and cost of arousals for hibernating little brown bats, Myotis lucifugus. J Mammal 1990, 71:475 479.
15. Geiser F: Metabolic rate and body temperature reduction during hibernation and daily torpor. Annu Rev Physiol 2004, 66:239 274.
16. Butler PJ, Green JA, Boyd IL, Speakman JR: Measuring metabolic rate in the field: the pros and cons of the doubly labelled water and heart rate methods. Funct Ecol 2004, 18:168 183.
17. Lifson N, Gordon GB, McClintock R: Measurement of total carbon dioxide production by means of D_2O^{18}. J Appl Physiol 1955, 7:704 710.
18. Speakman JR, Visser GH, Ward SE, Krl E: The Isotope Dilution Method for the Evaluation of Body Composition. In Body Composition Analysis of Animals. Edited by Speakman JR. Cambridge: Cambridge University Press; 2001:56 98.
19. Kurta A, Bell GP, Nagy KA, Kunz TH: Energetics of pregnancy and lactation in free-ranging little brown bats (Myotis lucifugus). Physiol Zool 1989, 62:804 818.
20. Kurta A, Kunz TH, Nagy KA: Energetics and water flux of free-ranging big brown bats (Eptesicus fuscus) during pregnancy and lactation. J Mammal 1990, 71:59 65.
21. Meteyer CU, Buckles EL, Blehert DS, Hicks AC, Green DE, Shearn-Bochsler V, Thomas NJ, Gargas A, Behr MJ: Histopathologic criteria to confirm white-nose syndrome in bats. J Vet Diagn Invest 2009, 21:411 414.
22. Malan A, Arens H, Waechter A: Pulmonary respiration and acid base state in hibernating marmots and hamsters. Respir Physiol 1973, 17:45 61.
23. Szewczak JM: Matching gas exchange in the bat from flight to torpor. Am Zool 1997, 37:92 100.
24. Malan A, Mioskowski E, Calgari C: Time-course of blood acid base state during arousal from hibernation in the European hamster. J Comp Physiol B 1988, 158:495 500.
25. Snapp BD, Heller HC: Suppression of metabolism during hibernation in ground squirrels (Citellus lateralis). Physiol Zool 1981, 54:297 307.
26. Bickler PE: CO_2 balance of a heterothermic rodent: comparison of sleep, torpor, and awake states. Am J Physiol 1984, 246:49 55.
27. Szewczak JM, Jackson DC: Acid base state and intermittent breathing in the torpid bat, Eptesicus fuscus. Respir Physiol 1992, 88:205 215.
28. Thomas DW, Cloutier D, Gagne D: Arrhythmic breathing, apnea and non-steady state oxygen uptake in hibernating little brown bats (Myotis lucifugus). J Exp Biol 1990, 149:395 406.
29. Thomas DW, Cloutier D: Evaporative water-loss by hibernating little brown bats, Myotis lucifugus. Physiol Zool 1992, 65:443 456.
30. Munoz-Garcia A, Ben-Hamo M, Pinshow B, Williams JB, Korine C: The relationship between cutaneous water loss and thermoregulatory state in Kuhl s pipistrelle Pipistrellus kuhlii, a Vespertillionid bat. Physiol Biochem Zool 2012, 85:516 525.
31. Speakman JR, Racey PA: Hibernal ecology of the Pipistrelle bat - energy-expenditure, water requirements and mass-loss, implications for survival and the function of winter emergence flights. J Anim Ecol 1989, 58:797 813.
32. Ben-Hamo M, Munoz-Garcia A, Williams JB, Korine C, Pinshow B: Waking to drink: rates of evaporative water loss determine arousal frequency in hibernating bats. J Exp Biol 2013, 216:573 577.
33. Meteyer CU, Valent M, Kashmer J, Buckles EL, Lorch JM, Blehert DS, Lollar A, Berndt D, Wheeler E, White CL, Ballmann AE: Recovery of little brown bats (Myotis lucifugus) from natural infection with Geomyces destructans, white-nose syndrome. J Wildlife Dis 2011, 47:618 626.
34. Riedesel ML: Blood Physiology. In Biology of Bats. Volume 3. Edited by Wimsatt W. New York: Academic Press; 1977:651.
35. Cryan PM, Wolf BO: Sex differences in the thermoregulation and evaporative water loss of a heterothermic bat, Lasiurus cinereus, during its spring migration. J Exp Biol 2003, 206:3381 3390.
36. Riedesel ML, Folk GE Jr: Serum electrolyte levels in hibernating mammals. Am Nat 1958, 92:307 312.

37. Riedesel ML: **Serum magnesium levels in mammalian hibernators.** *Trans Kans Acad Sci* 1957, **60**:99 141.

38. Kallen FC: **Plasma and blood volumes in the little brown bat.** *Am J Physiol* 1960, **198**:999 1005.

39. Blood FR, Dodgen CL: **Energy sources in the bat.** *Am J Physiol* 1956, **187**:151 154.

40. Humphries MM, Thomas DW, Speakman JR: **Climate-mediated energetic constraints on the distribution of hibernating mammals.** *Nature* 2002, **418**:313 316.

41. Malan A: **Respiration and Acid Base State in Hibernation.** In *Hibernation and Torpor in Mammals and Birds.* Edited by Lyman CP, Willis JS, Malan A, Wang LCH. New York: Academic Press; 1982:237 282.

42. Hochachka PW, Guppy M: *Metabolic arrest and the control of biological time.* Cambridge, MA: Harvard University Press; 1987.

43. Malan A: **pH and hypometabolism in mammalian hibernation.** *Can J Zool* 1988, **66**:95 98.

44. Schaefer KE, Wunnenberg W: **Threshold temperatures for shivering in acute and chronic hypercapnia.** *J Appl Physiol* 1976, **41**:67 70.

45. Studier EM, Fresquez AA: **Carbon dioxide retention: a mechanism of ammonia tolerance in mammals.** *Ecology* 1969, **50**:492 494.

46. Herreid CF 2nd, Bretz WL, Schmidt-Nielsen K: **Cutaneous gas exchange in bats.** *Am J Physiol* 1968, **215**:506 508.

47. Makanya AN, Mortola JP: **The structural design of the bat wing web and its possible role in gas exchange.** *J Anat* 2007, **211**:687 697.

48. Muller LK, Lorch JM, Lindner DL, O Connor M, Gargas A, Blehert DS: **Bat white-nose syndrome: a real-time TaqMan polymerase chain reaction test targeting the intergenic spacer region of *Geomyces destructans*.** *Mycologia* 2012, **105**:253 259.

49. Lorch JM, Meteyer CU, Behr MJ, Boyles JG, Cryan PM, Hicks AC, Ballmann AE, Coleman JTH, Redell D, Reeder DM, Blehert DS: **Experimental infection of bats with *Geomyces destructans* causes white-nose syndrome.** *Nature* 2011, **480**:376 378.

50. Kunz TH, Nagy KA: **Methods of Energy Budget Analysis.** In *Ecological and Behavior Methods for the Study of Bats.* Edited by Kunz TH. Washington, D.C: Smithsonian Institution Press; 1988:277 302.

51. Speakman JR: *Doubly Labelled Water- Theory and Practice.* London: Chapman and Hall; 1997.

52. Speakman JR, Racey PA: **The equilibrium concentration of O-18 in body-water: implications for the accuracy of the doubly-labeled water technique and a potential new method of measuring RQ in free-living animals.** *J Theor Biol* 1987, **127**:79 95.

53. Abbott Point of Care Inc: *iStat Instruction Manual.* Abbott Park, IL: Abbott Point of Care Inc; 2008.

54. Clinical Laboratory Standards Institute: *Blood gas and pH Analysis and Related Measurements: Approved Guideline - Second Edition.* Wayne, PA: CLSI; 2009.

55. Nagy KA: *The Doubly Labeled Water $^{3}HH^{18}O$ Method: A Guide to its use.* Los Angeles: University of California; 1983.

56. Speakman JR, Nagy KA, Masman D, Mook WG, Poppitt SD, Strathearn GE, Racey PA: **Interlaboratory comparison of different analytical techniques for the determination of oxygen-18 abundance.** *Anal Chem* 1990, **62**:703 708.

57. Speakman JR, Krol E: **Comparison of different approaches for the calculation of energy expenditure using doubly labeled water in a small mammal.** *Physiol Biochem Zool* 2005, **78**:650 667.

58. Speakman JR: **How should we calculate CO_2 production in doubly labelled water studies of animals?** *Funct Ecol* 1993, **7**:746 750.

59. Weir JB: **New methods for calculating metabolic rate with special reference to protein metabolism.** *J Physiol* 1949, **109**:1 9.

60. Holm S: **A simple sequentially rejective multiple test procedure.** *Scand J Stat* 1979, **6**:65 70.

61. R: **A Language and Environment for Statistical Computing.**

13

Importance of uncharged polar residues and proline in the proximal two-thirds (Pro^{107}–Ser^{128}) of the highly conserved region of mouse ileal Na$^+$-dependent bile acid transporter, Slc10a2, in transport activity and cellular expression

Tohru Saeki[1*], Kosuke Sato[1], Shiho Ito[1], Keisuke Ikeda[1] and Ryuhei Kanamoto[1,2]

Abstract

Background: SLC10A2-mediated reabsorption of bile acids at the distal end of the ileum is the first step in enterohepatic circulation. Because bile acids act not only as detergents but also as signaling molecules in lipid metabolism and energy production, SLC10A2 is important as the key transporter for understanding the *in vivo* kinetics of bile acids. SLC10A family members and the homologous genes of various species share a highly conserved region corresponding to Gly^{104}–Pro^{142} of SLC10A2. The functional importance of this region has not been fully elucidated.

Results: To elucidate the functional importance of this region, we previously performed mutational analysis of the uncharged polar residues and proline in the distal one-third (Thr^{130}–Pro^{142}) of the highly conserved region in mouse Slc10a2. In this study, proline and uncharged polar residues in the remaining two-thirds of this region in mouse Slc10a2 were subjected to mutational analysis, and taurocholic acid uptake and cell surface localization were examined. Cell surface localization of Slc10a2 is necessary for bile acid absorption. Mutants in which Asp or Leu were substituted for Pro^{107} (P107N or P107L) were abundantly expressed, but their cell surface localization was impaired. The S126A mutant was completely impaired in cellular expression. The T110A and S128A mutants exhibited remarkably enhanced membrane expression. The S112A mutant was properly expressed at the cell surface but transport activity was completely lost. Replacement of Tyr^{117} with various amino acids resulted in reduced transport activity. The degree of reduction roughly depended on the van der Waals volume of the side chains.

Conclusions: The functional importance of proline and uncharged polar residues in the highly conserved region of mouse Slc10a2 was determined. This information will contribute to the design of bile acid-conjugated prodrugs for efficient drug delivery or SLC10A2 inhibitors for hypercholesterolemia treatment.

Keywords: Bile acid, Enterohepatic circulation, Ileal sodium-dependent bile acid transporter

* Correspondence: tsaeki@kpu.ac.jp
[1]Laboratory of Molecular Nutrition, Kyoto Prefectural University, Nakaragi, Shimogamo, Sakyo-ku, Kyoto 606-8522, Japan
Full list of author information is available at the end of the article

Background

Bile acids are synthesized from cholesterol in the liver and secreted into the small intestine as components of bile for the digestion and absorption of lipids and lipid-soluble vitamins. In addition to the detergent action of bile acids, which aids in the digestion and absorption of lipid and lipid-soluble nutrients by forming micelles with biliary phospholipids and cholesterol, bile acids are now appreciated as signaling molecules that control lipid metabolism and energy production [1-6]. At the distal end of the ileum, 95%–98% of bile acids are effectively reabsorbed by an ileal sodium-dependent bile acid transporter (SLC10A2, also designated ASBT, ISBT, or IBAT) and returned to the liver *via* portal circulation. Among the transporters that are expressed in the liver, intestine, and bile duct and are involved in enterohepatic circulation of bile acids, SLC10A2 is the key transporter for understanding the *in vivo* kinetics of bile acids given that reabsorption of bile acids by SLC10A2 is the first step in enterohepatic circulation. SLC10A2 is the second member of the solute carrier family 10, and consists of 348 amino acids. SLC10A2 is expressed in the ileum, cholangiocytes, and kidney, and contributes to the maintenance of the bile acid pool and cholesterol homeostasis [7-9]. Transport of bile acids by SLC10A2 is facilitated by sodium symport in an electrogenic process with a 2:1 Na^+/bile acid stoichiometry [10]. Given that bile acids are synthesized from cholesterol, inhibition of bile acid reabsorption *via* SLC10A2 inhibition has been used as a cholesterol-lowering therapy. Moreover, due to its high transport capacity in the ileum, SLC10A2 is also an attractive target for the prodrug strategy to enhance drug bioavailability [11,12].

The membrane topology and detailed transport mechanism of SLC10A2 have been studied. Hydropathy analysis and membrane insertion scanning revealed that SLC10A2 has an extracellular N-terminus and a cytoplasmic C-terminus [13,14]. The exact membrane topology remains controversial: *in vitro* translation studies using membrane insertion scanning suggested a 9-transmembrane (TM) topology, whereas N-glycosylation scanning mutagenesis and dual-label epitope insertion scanning mutagenesis support a 7-TM topology [13-19]. The recently published crystal structure of a bacterial homolog of SLC10A2 from *Neisseria meningitidis* (designated $ASBT_{NM}$) supports the 9-TM topology [20].

Protein regions and amino acid residues of SLC10A2 involved in membrane trafficking, substrate recognition, and substrate permeation have been identified. The cytoplasmic tail of rat Slc10a2 acts as a sorting signal for apical trafficking, and Ser^{335} and Thr^{339} phosphorylations are crucial for apical targeting [21]. Computational analysis based on homology-modeling and remote-threading techniques revealed that Asp^{282} and Leu^{283} of human SLC10A2 are involved in hydrogen bond formation with the 12α-hydroxyl group of bile acids [19]. A series of analyses using the substituted-cysteine accessibility method revealed that in the 7-TM model TM7 (Phe^{287}–Tyr^{308}) lines the substrate translocation pathway, TM4 (Ile^{160}–Met^{180}) forms part of the pathway, Asp^{124} interacts with the 7α-hydroxyl group of bile acids, and the extracellular loop (EL) 1 corresponding to Val^{99}–Ser^{126} acts as a Na^+ sensor [22-24]. Glu^{261} in EL3 has also been shown to act as a Na^+ sensor, and EL1 and EL3 have been proposed to act as re-entrant loop segments [25,26]. Despite such extensive studies, the mechanisms underlying the binding and transport of bile acids remain unclear.

Genes homologous to the mammalian SLC10 family are widespread in various species [25,27]. In the alignment of the deduced sequences of these genes, conserved residues are scattered throughout the entire sequences, and some of them are clustered in a region spanning approximately 40 residues corresponding to Gly^{104}–Pro^{142} of SLC10A2 (Figure 1). The high-level conservation indicates that this region may play an important role in substrate interaction, conformational change necessary for function, or interaction with cellular cofactors. As mentioned above, a part of this region corresponding to EL1 has been proposed to function as a dynamic re-entrant loop, but the importance of this region has not yet been fully elucidated. To determine the importance of this region, we previously performed mutational analysis of the uncharged polar residues in the distal one-third (Thr^{130}–Pro^{142}) of the highly conserved region of mouse Slc10a2 (mSlc10a2) and identified residues that may be involved in substrate recognition, transport activity, and cellular localization [28]. In this study, we focused on the uncharged polar residues (Thr^{110}, Ser^{113}, Tyr^{117}, Ser^{126}, and Ser^{128}) and proline (Pro^{107}) in the remaining part of the highly conserved region. The hydroxyl group of the side chains could form hydrogen bonds with the substrate and/or other residues and contribute to the transport process and/or formation of higher-order structures, and proline is expected to contribute to the formation of higher-order structure.

To determine the involvement of these residues in substrate recognition, transport, and intracellular sorting and/or stability of mSlc10a2, taurocholic acid (TCA) transport and cell surface localization were analyzed.

Results

Wild-type mSlc10a2 and Pro^{107} mutants (P107N and P107L) were stably expressed as enhanced green fluorescent protein (EGFP) fusion proteins in LLC-PK_1 cells, and TCA uptake and cellular localization were analyzed. Cells expressing wild-type Slc10a2 exhibited Na^+-dependent uptake of TCA, but this transport activity was completely

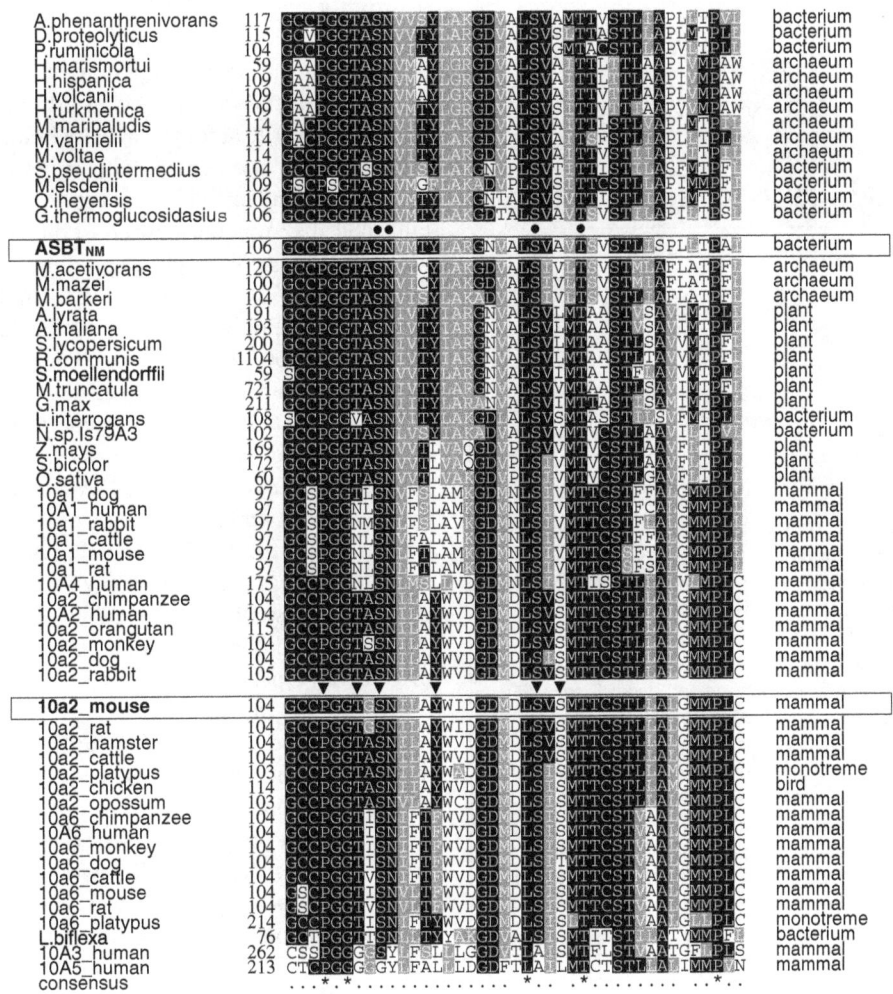

Figure 1 Alignment of amino acid sequences of SLC10A family members and related proteins. The amino acid sequences of 10 of the related genes from bacteria, archaea, and plants that yielded the highest score by a BLAST search using the amino acid sequence corresponding to Gly^{104}–Pro^{142} of mouse Slc10a2 (mSlc10a2) as a query sequence and the amino acid sequence of ASBT$_{NM}$ were compared with the amino acid sequences of SLC10A family members using the ClustalW software, and shading was rendered by the BoxShade program (http://www.ch.embnet.org/software/BOX_form.html). The alignments of the region corresponding to the query sequence are shown. The ASBT$_{NM}$ and mSlc10a2 sequences are boxed and the residues subjected to mutational analysis in this study and residues that have been reported to bind sodium *via* their side chains [20] are indicated by arrowheads and circles, respectively.

abolished in both P107N- and P107L-expressing cells (Figure 2A). Western blot analysis of whole cell lysates revealed that wild-type and mutant mSlc10a2 were abundantly expressed as 55-kDa bands, and an additional band with a lower migration rate at approximately 75 kDa was observed only in the wild type (Figure 2B, left panel). Because the latter band is considered to represent a fully glycosylated protein that is localized to the plasma membrane, we concluded that the mutant Slc10a2 proteins were likely detained in the endoplasmic reticulum (ER) and did not reach the cell surface. This was confirmed by analyzing plasma membrane proteins (Figure 2B, right panel). The glycosylated form was detected only in the wild-type plasma membrane fraction.

Next, we examined the transient expression of wild-type mSlc10a2 and uncharged polar residue mutants (T110A, S112A, Y117F, S126A, and S128A) in COS-7 cells by western blot analysis (Figure 3A). Wild-type mSlc10a2 and all the mutants except S126A were expressed as 55-kDa proteins. A broad band ranging from 60–80 kDa, the fully glycosylated form, was also detected in each lane.

To evaluate the ability of the mutants to transport bile acids, TCA uptake by the wild-type and mutant mSlc10a2 was compared (Figure 3B). Because cellular expression of S126A was not detected, this mutant was omitted from further analysis. The S128A mutant exhibited uptake levels comparable to that of wild type, and

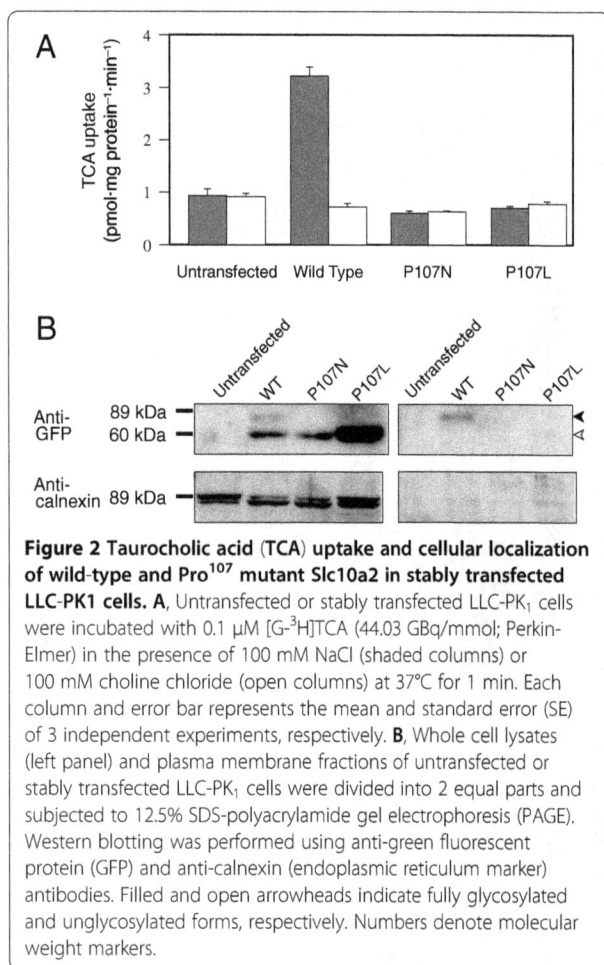

Figure 2 Taurocholic acid (TCA) uptake and cellular localization of wild-type and Pro[107] mutant Slc10a2 in stably transfected LLC-PK1 cells. A, Untransfected or stably transfected LLC-PK$_1$ cells were incubated with 0.1 μM [G-^{3}H]TCA (44.03 GBq/mmol; Perkin-Elmer) in the presence of 100 mM NaCl (shaded columns) or 100 mM choline chloride (open columns) at 37°C for 1 min. Each column and error bar represents the mean and standard error (SE) of 3 independent experiments, respectively. **B**, Whole cell lysates (left panel) and plasma membrane fractions of untransfected or stably transfected LLC-PK$_1$ cells were divided into 2 equal parts and subjected to 12.5% SDS-polyacrylamide gel electrophoresis (PAGE). Western blotting was performed using anti-green fluorescent protein (GFP) and anti-calnexin (endoplasmic reticulum marker) antibodies. Filled and open arrowheads indicate fully glycosylated and unglycosylated forms, respectively. Numbers denote molecular weight markers.

TCA uptake by the T110A mutant was significantly higher than that of wild type. TCA uptake by the Y117F mutant was approximately half that by the wild type, but the difference was not statistically significant. S112A did not exhibit Na$^+$-dependent TCA uptake.

The kinetics of TCA transport by the wild type and the 3 functional mutants were examined (Figure 3C and Table 1). The V_{max} of Y117F was approximately half that of the wild type, and those of T110A and S128A were 2.5- and 5-fold higher than that of the wild type, respectively; interestingly, the K_m values of the 3 mutants were comparable to that of the wild type, suggesting that the differences in the apparent TCA transport activities of the polar residue mutants were not due to altered affinity for TCA.

The cellular localization of the expressed transporters was investigated by cell surface biotinylation (Figure 3D). The fully glycosylated form was predominantly detected in the biotinylated fraction. Membrane expression of Y117F was similar to that of wild type, and the membrane expression of T110A and S128A was significantly higher than that of wild type, suggesting that removal of the polar

hydroxyl group from Thr^{110} and Ser^{128} improved membrane sorting and/or stability of mSlc10a2. Although S112A was a loss-of-function mutation, membrane expression of the mutant was clearly detected, indicating that Ser^{112} is critical for the activity of mSlc10a2.

To compare the activities of the mutant transporters, the Na$^+$-dependent TCA uptake by wild-type and mutant mSlc10a2 was normalized to the cell surface expression of the corresponding proteins (Figure 3E). The normalized V_{max} of the T110A mutant (1600 [70] pmol·mg protein^{-1}·min^{-1}) was similar to that of the wild type (1620 [50] pmol·mg protein^{-1}·min^{-1}), indicating that the difference in the apparent TCA transport activity of this mutant was mainly due to the different level of its expression at the cell surface. By contrast, the apparently higher activity of S128A could not be explained by abundant membrane expression because the normalized V_{max} of the S128A mutant (2410 [100] pmol·mg protein^{-1}·min^{-1}) was remarkably higher than that of wild type. The normalized V_{max} value of the Y117F mutant (1170 [90] pmol·mg protein^{-1}·min^{-1}) was lower than that of wild type.

The Y117C mutation in human SLC10A2 has been reported to be a loss-of-function mutation due to its impaired membrane expression [23]. This is in striking contrast to our finding that the Y117F mutant of mSlc10a2 was properly expressed on the plasma membrane and that transport activity was preserved even though its apparent activity was lower. Because the Tyr to Phe mutation used in the present study removed only the polar hydroxyl group from the benzene ring of the side chain, we infer that what is important at this position is not polarity but the bulkiness required for higher-order structure or stability of SLC10A2/Slc10a2. The complete conservation of bulky residues, i.e., Tyr, Phe, or Leu, at this position in the related genes (Figure 1) supports this view. Therefore, we next examined the cell surface expression and transport activities of mSlc10a2 mutants in which various residues were substituted for Tyr^{117}. For this purpose, a T7 tag was attached at the N-terminus of mSlc10a2, which is exposed on the cell surface. Western blot analysis revealed that the wild-type and Tyr^{117} mutants were expressed as 40-kDa bands; additional bands with lower migration rates, ranging from 50–60 kDa, were also detected in each lane, indicating that all the Tyr^{117} mutants as well as the wild type were properly expressed on the plasma membrane (Figure 4A). Cell surface expression was confirmed with immunofluorescence. Under nonpermeabilized conditions, the plasma membrane was predominantly stained, whereas additional intracellular compartments were also stained under permeabilized conditions (Figure 5). Cell surface expression levels were examined by surface enzyme-linked immunosorbent assay. The cell-surface expression of the

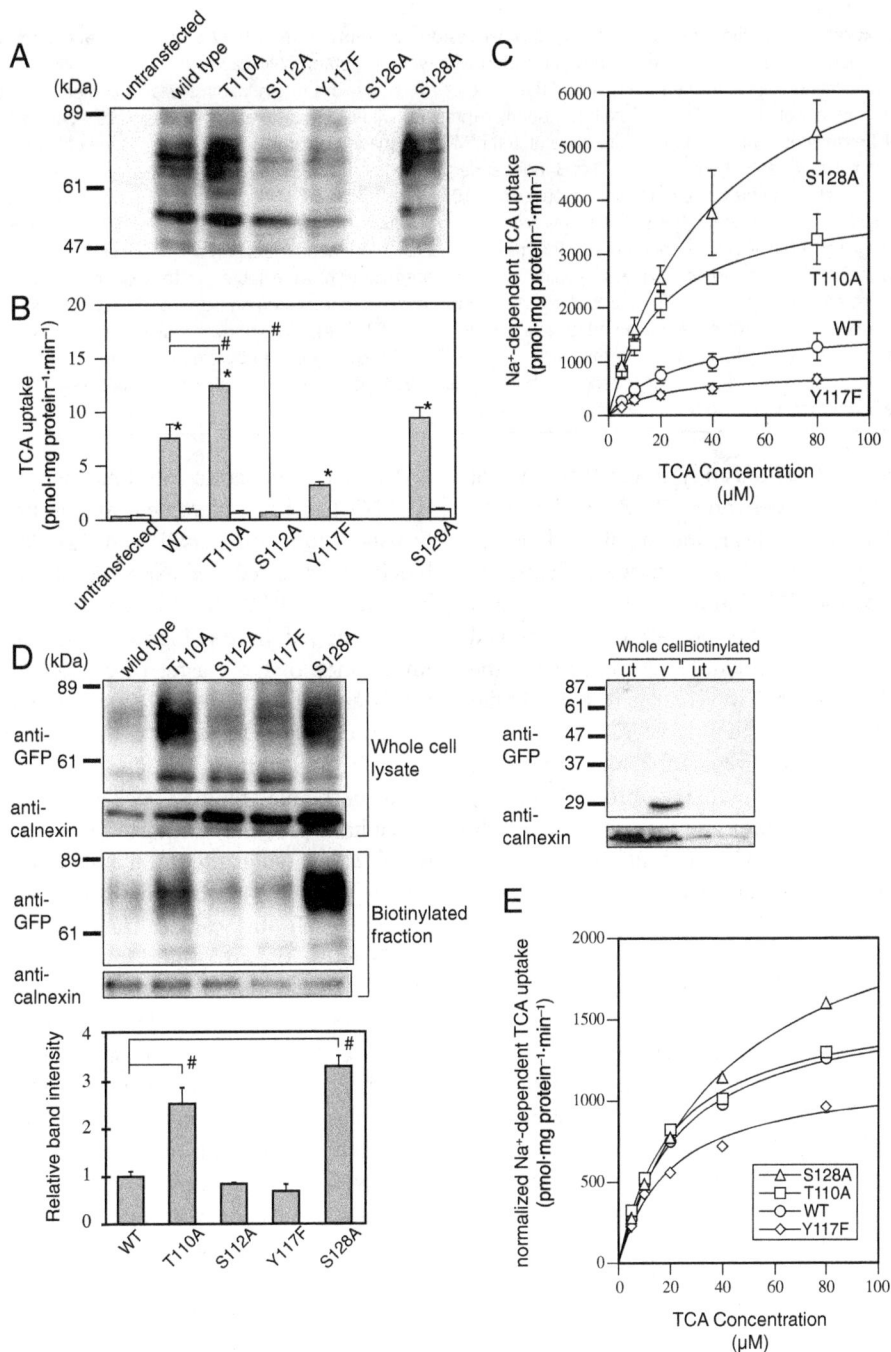

Figure 3 (See legend on next page.)

(See figure on previous page.)

Figure 3 Transient expression of wild-type and uncharged polar residue mutants of mSlc10a2 and cell surface biotinylation. A, Twenty micrograms of whole cell lysates of COS-7 cells transiently expressing wild-type or mutant mSlc10a2 fused with EGFP were subjected to 7.5% SDS-PAGE and western blotting was performed using anti-GFP antibody. Consistency of protein loading was confirmed by Ponceau S staining of the blotted PVDF membrane (not shown). **B**, COS-7 cells transiently expressing wild-type or mutant mSlc10a2 were incubated with 0.1 μM ^{3}H-TCA (185 GBq/mmol; Perkin-Elmer) for 5 min in the presence of 100 mM NaCl (shaded columns) or 100 mM choline chloride (open columns). Each column and error bar represents the mean and SE of 3 independent experiments, respectively. *, Uptake in the presence of NaCl is significantly higher than that in the presence of choline chloride ($p < 0.05$); #, Na$^+$-dependent uptake is significantly different from that of wild-type Slc10a2 ($p < 0.05$). **C**, Na$^+$-dependent uptake of TCA was calculated by subtracting the uptake in the presence of 100 mM choline chloride from that in the presence of 100 mM NaCl. Data represent the mean and SE of 3 independent experiments. **D**, Left panel, Whole cell lysates and biotinylated fractions of COS-7 cells transiently expressing wild-type or mutant mSlc10a2 were subjected to western blot analysis. The image is representative of 3 independent experiments. The graph shows the densitometry of bands ranging from 65–90 kDa expressed as the mean and SE of 3 independent experiments. Right panel, Western blot analysis of whole cell lysates and biotinylated fractions of untransfected (ut) and empty vector-transfected (v) COS-7 cells. Because the migration rate of EGFP (26.9 kDa) encoded by empty vector is smaller than that of EGFP-fused mSlc10a2, proteins were resolved on a higher concentration (12.5%) of SDS-polyacrylamide gel. **E**, Na$^+$-dependent TCA uptake by wild-type and mutant mSlc10a2 were normalized to their cell surface expression.

Tyr^{117} mutants was not significantly lower than that of wild type (Figure 4B). Na$^+$-dependent TCA uptake by all the Tyr^{117} mutants, except Y117F, was significantly lower than that of wild type (Figure 4C). Next, we analyzed the kinetic properties of the Y117S mutant, which exhibited remarkably reduced TCA uptake compared to that of wild type. The K_m for Na$^+$-dependent TCA uptake by the Y117S mutant (19.1 [2.4] μM) was similar to that of wild type (19.8 [4.7] μM), whereas the V_{max} of Y117S (216 [10] pmol·mg protein^{-1}·min^{-1}) was remarkably lower than that of wild type (2965 [263] pmol·mg protein^{-1}·min^{-1}) (Figure 4D). These results indicate that the apparently decreased activities of the Tyr^{117} mutants are probably due to their decreased molecular activities.

Discussion

Optimal function of SLC10A2 is required for bile acid reabsorption in the ileum. Impairment of this function not only affects cholesterol homeostasis but may also increase the possibility of colorectal tumorigenesis due to increased flow of bile acids into the large intestine. Indeed, prevention of bile acid reabsorption by surgical removal of the ileum increased colonic tumorigenesis in rats fed deoxycholic acid [29]. The C to T polymorphism at codon 169 of the human *SLC10A2* gene is associated with colorectal adenomas, indicating the role of bile acids in the etiology of this disease [30]. A genetic polymorphism associated with primary bile acid malabsorption

(PBAM) or idiopathic intestinal bile acid malabsorption (IBAM) has been identified, and mutations that abolish transport function (L243P and T262M) and a haplotype block linked to reduced expression have been reported for human SLC10A2 [31,32]. This polymorphism has not been mapped in the highly conserved region, and the importance of the cluster of conserved residues has not yet been fully clarified. Toward the end of the study presented here, the crystal structure of ASBT$_{NM}$ was reported, and some of the residues were indicated to form a part of the Na$^+$-binding pocket [20].

We have previously reported the importance of Pro^{142}, which is located at the distal end of the highly conserved region [28]. Substitution of Pro^{142} with Val completely impaired cell surface localization of mSlc10a2. This is consistent with our results from the mutational analysis of Pro^{107} showing that Asn or Leu substitution for Pro^{107} impaired cell surface expression of mSlc10a2, resulting in the loss of transport activity. In the 9-TM model, Pro^{107} is located in the middle of TM3. Proline acts as a "helix breaker" due to its inability to form hydrogen bonds with neighboring residues; therefore, TM3 would be bent at Pro^{107}, forming hydrophobic and amphipathic half helices. Indeed, the crystal structure of ASBT$_{NM}$ suggests that the helix that contains Pro^{107} is broken precisely at this residue [20]. In the 7-TM model, Pro^{107} is located in the EL between TM2 and TM3. In the ER, immediately after the synthesis of the nascent protein, this loop faces the lumen. Substitution of Pro^{107} with Asn or Leu may have introduced an interaction of this loop with other ELs or ER factors, resulting in detention of the mutant Slc10a2. In either case, failure of the Pro^{107} mutants to localize to the cell surface suggests that the peculiar nature of proline, an imino acid, and not the hydrophobicity or bulkiness of the side chain is important for intracellular sorting. Given that proline at this position is highly conserved in the related proteins, it is expected to be crucial for function through correct secondary structure formation and cellular localization.

Table 1 Kinetic values for taurocholic acid transport by wild-type and polar-residue mutant mouse Slc10a2 proteins

	K_m (μM)	V_{max} (pmol·mg protein^{-1}·min^{-1})
Wild type	24.0 (2.0)	1620 (50)
T110A	20.2 (2.3)	4010 (170)
Y117F	20.7 (4.1)	806 (61)
S128A	42.0 (3.7)	7930 (340)

Data are expressed as mean (standard error).

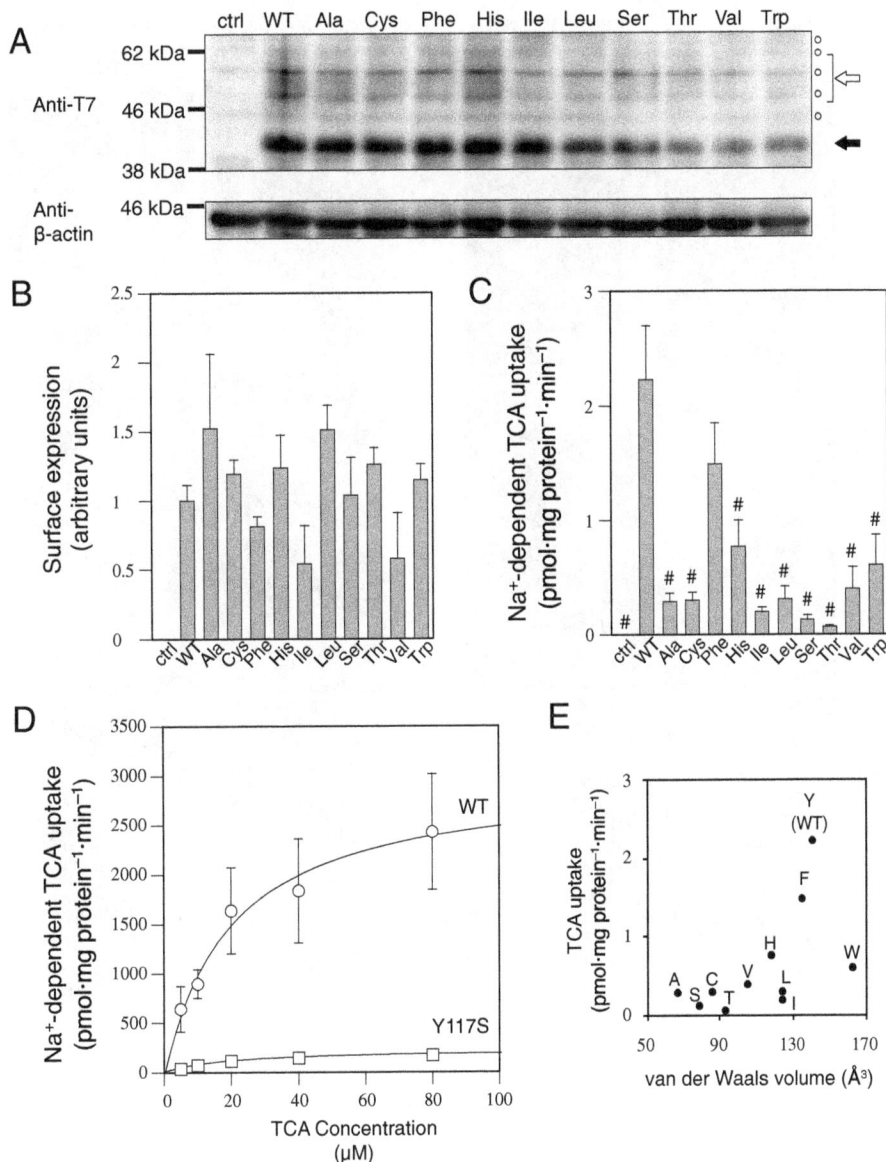

Figure 4 Expression and transport activities of Tyr[117] mutants. A, COS-7 cells were transiently transfected with expression vectors for T7-tagged wild-type or mutant mSlc10a2. Whole cell lysates were examined by western blotting using anti-T7 antibody (upper). Whole cell lysate of untransfected cells was loaded as a control (ctrl). Filled and open arrows indicate core-glycosylated and fully glycosylated forms of T7-mSlc10a2, respectively. T7-tag constructs yield lower levels of the fully glycosylated form compared to EGFP-fusion constructs. Circles indicate apparently nonspecific bands. The membrane was stripped and reprobed with anti-β-actin antibody (lower). **B**, Cell surface expression was measured by surface enzyme-linked immunosorbent assay. Data are expressed as mean and SE of a sextuplicate experiment. **C**, COS-7 cells transiently expressing wild-type or mutant mSlc10a2 were incubated with 0.02 μM ^{3}H-TCA (370 GBq/mmol; American Radiolabeled Chemicals) for 5 min in the presence of 100 mM NaCl or 100 mM choline chloride, and Na$^+$-dependent uptake was calculated by subtracting the uptake in the presence of 100 mM choline chloride from that in the presence of 100 mM NaCl. Na$^+$-dependent uptake data are expressed as mean and SE of 3 independent experiments. #, Na$^+$-dependent uptake is significantly different from that of wild-type Slc10a2 ($p < 0.05$). **D**, Kinetic analysis of Na$^+$-dependent TCA transport by wild-type and Y117S. Data are expressed as the mean and SE of 3 independent experiments. Circles, wild type; squares, Y117S. **E**, Na$^+$-dependent TCA uptake by the wild-type mSlc10a2 and Tyr[117] mutants are plotted against the van der Waals volume of the residue at position 117.

Ser[112] was considered indispensable for the synthesis or stability of human SLC10A2 because replacement of Ser[112] with Cys completely abolished expression [23]. In this study, however, Ala substitution of Ser[112] did not impair membrane expression of mSlc10a2, whereas TCA transport activity was completely lost. This suggests that Ser[112] is not critical for mSlc10a2 expression but is essential for TCA transport activity. Based on the crystal structure of ASBT$_{NM}$, Ser[112] of mSlc10a2 is thought to bind Na$^+$ with its side chain [20]. Ser is conserved at this

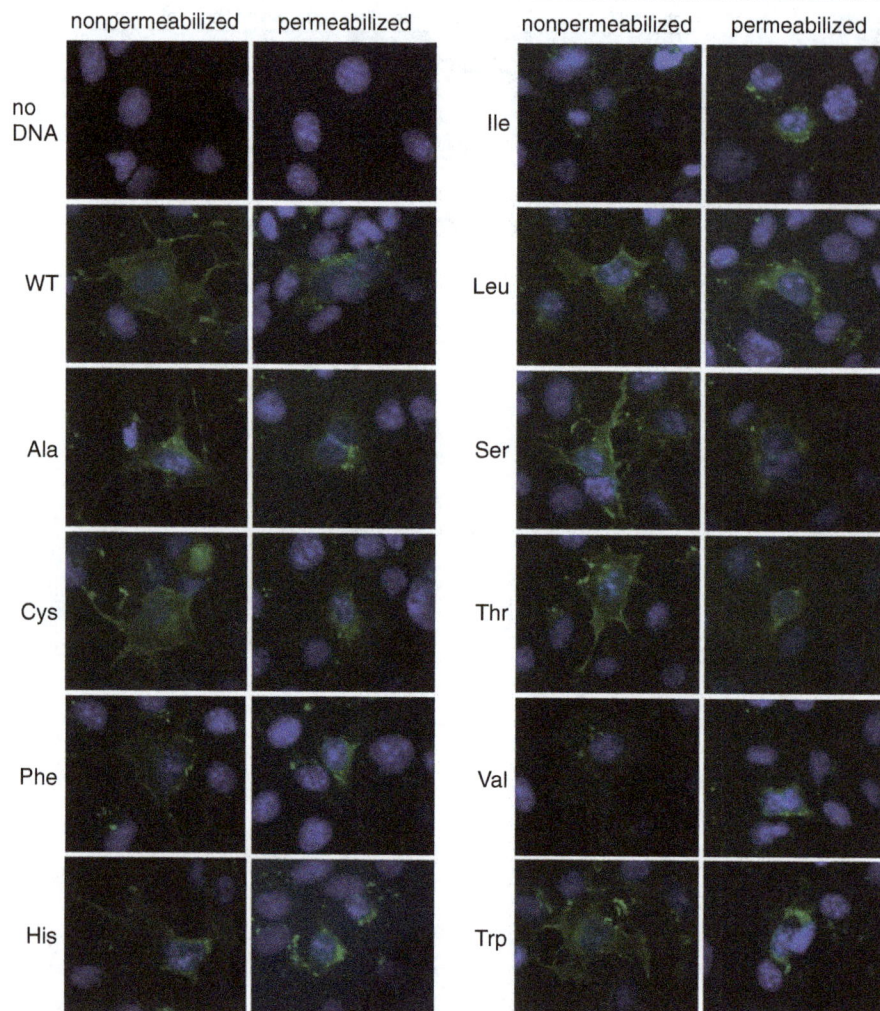

Figure 5 Immunofluorescence microscopy of wild-type and Tyr117 mutant mSlc10a2. COS-7 cells transiently expressing T7-tagged mSlc10a2 proteins were incubated with anti-T7 antibody under nonpermeabilized (left panel) or permeabilized (right panel) conditions, followed by fluorescein-conjugated secondary antibody. The merged image of mSlc10a2 immunofluorescence (green) and nuclear staining (blue) is shown.

position in all the related proteins except SLC10A5 (Figure 1), suggesting that this residue is also critical in all the other members.

Expression of the S126A mutant was undetectable even in whole cell lysates. This is consistent with a previous report showing the failure of expression of the human SLC10A2 S126C mutant [23]. This residue has been suggested to bind Na^+ [20], and it is likely that Ser^{126} plays an important role in the other members as well, given that this residue is conserved in all the genes except those encoding SLC10A3 and SLC10A5.

Because Thr^{110} and Ser^{128} are not conserved in the related proteins, particularly in the Na^+-dependent bile acid transporter SLC10A1 (also designated NTCP or BSBT), which is expressed on the sinusoidal membrane of hepatocytes, it is unlikely that these residues are involved

in the interaction with bile acids. The apparently higher membrane expression of the T110A and S128A mutants suggests that these residues may be involved in the negative regulation of stability or intracellular sorting *via* formation of higher-order structures or interaction with cellular cofactors.

The Phe substitution for Tyr^{117}, which removes a polar hydroxyl group, reduced the transport activity of mSlc10a2; however, substrate affinity was not affected. This result was inconsistent with the previous finding that the Y117C mutation completely impaired membrane expression of human SLC10A2. To resolve this discrepancy, we replaced Tyr^{117} of mSlc10a2 with various amino acids and examined cellular localization and transport activities. None of the residues substituted for Tyr^{117} affected cell surface expression of mSlc10a2;

however, the apparent transport activities were reduced. The reason for the contradiction between our results and the results of the Y117C mutation in human SLC10A2 is not clear, but a difference in the amino acid sequence context between mSlc10a2 and the human counterpart or undefined differences in experimental conditions may have affected the results. The relationship between the apparent activities and physicochemical properties of the residues were analyzed. Hydrophobicity and polarity did not correlate with activity (data not shown), but a weak correlation was observed between the van der Waals volumes of the residues and the activities of the mutants (Figure 4E). However, the correlation was not statistically significant (p = 0.0705), because the Y117W mutant with the bulkiest side chain exhibited moderate activity, and substitution with Ile and Leu, which have relatively bulky side chains, elicited low transport activities, suggesting that the volume of the side chain as well as its shape are important at this position. Although the crystal structure of ASBT$_{NM}$ indicated that Tyr^{117} does not directly interact with Na$^+$ or taurocholate, it is obvious that this residue is important for the molecular activity of the transporter. Tyr^{117} may be involved in conformational changes during TCA transport.

Conclusions

In this study, residues critical for transport activity, expression, and stability and/or intracellular trafficking, but not substrate recognition, were identified within the proximal two-thirds of the highly conserved region. Functionally important residues are clustered in the highly conserved region. Due to the specific and high transport capacity of SLC10A2 in the ileum, bioavailability of drugs may be enhanced by designing them as bile acid-conjugated prodrugs. The information on functionally critical residues will contribute to the design of prodrugs for efficient drug delivery and SLC10A2 inhibitors for treatment of hypercholesterolemia.

Methods
Materials
[G-^{3}H]TCA was purchased from Perkin-Elmer (Waltham, MA) and American Radiolabeled Chemicals (St. Louis, MO). Unlabeled sodium taurocholate was purchased from Nacalai Tesque (Kyoto, Japan). The Cell Surface Protein Isolation Kit, which included sulfosuccinimidyl 2-(biotinamido)ethyl-1,3-dithiopropionate (sulfo-NHS-SS-biotin), was purchased from Pierce (Rockford, IL). Streptavidin agarose was purchased from Merck (Darmstadt, Germany). The anti-green fluorescent protein (GFP) monoclonal antibody was purchased from Nacalai Tesque. The anti-T7 tag monoclonal antibody was purchased from Merck. The anti-calnexin rabbit polyclonal antibody was from Novus Biologicals (Littleton, CO). Secondary antibodies

(horseradish peroxidase (HRP)-conjugated anti-mouse, anti-rat, and anti-rabbit IgG) were purchased from Nacalai Tesque. Fluorescein-labeled anti-mouse secondary antibody was purchased from Kirkegaard & Perry Laboratories (Gaithersburg, MD). The cloning vector pUC119 was purchased from Takara Bio (Shiga, Japan). The mammalian expression vectors pEGFP-N1 and pZeoSV2(+) were purchased from Clontech (Shiga, Japan) and Invitrogen (Tokyo, Japan), respectively. Mutagenic oligonucleotide primers for site-directed mutagenesis were custom synthesized and purchased from Invitrogen. Site-directed mutagenesis of Pro^{107} and uncharged polar residues was performed using the Quickchange II Site-Directed Mutagenesis Kit purchased from Stratagene (La Jolla, CA). Site-directed mutagenesis of Tyr^{117} was performed using the PrimeSTAR Mutagenesis Basal Kit purchased from Takara Bio.

Cell culture
The simian kidney fibroblast cell line COS-7 was grown in Dulbecco's modified Eagle's medium supplemented with 10% fetal bovine serum (FBS), 4 mM L-Gln, and 0.1 mg/mL kanamycin sulfate. The porcine kidney cell line LLC-PK$_1$ was grown in M199 medium supplemented with 10% FBS and 0.1 mg/mL kanamycin. Cells were cultured at 37°C in a humidified atmosphere of 5% CO$_2$.

Construction of expression vectors
The mSlc10a2 cDNA encoding the full-length transporter (molecular weight, 38 kDa) was cloned in our laboratory [33]. Wild-type or mutant mSlc10a2 was expressed as a fusion protein with enhanced green fluorescent protein (EGFP) or a T7 tag. The expression vectors for EGFP-fused mSlc10a2 were constructed as previously reported [28]. To construct the expression vector for T7-tagged mSlc10a2, an EcoRI recognition site was introduced at the start codon by polymerase chain reaction (PCR) using the 5′ primer 5′-CGAATTCAG<u>ATG</u>GATAACTCCTCTGTC TG-3′, in which the underlined portion represents the start codon, and the 3′ primer 5′-GAAGGATCCCCATGG TCTCTTTATATGTCC-3′ corresponding to nucleotides 178–207 of the coding region in which a BamHI site was introduced without affecting the amino acid sequence. The amplified fragment was cloned into pUC119 and sequenced to confirm the absence of PCR-derived mutations. The EcoRI-BamHI fragment obtained from the amplified clone and the remaining part of the coding region were cloned into pZeoSV2(+), and a double-stranded synthetic oligonucleotide encoding the T7 tag next to the start codon (top strand, 5′-CTAGCATGGGGATG<u>GCT AGCATGACTGGTGGACAACAGATGGGT</u>GG-3′; bottom strand, 5′-AATTCC<u>ACCCATCTGTTGTCCACCA GTCATGCTAGCCATCCCCATG</u>-3′, where the underlined portions represent the T7 tag) was inserted at the

*Nhe*I and *Eco*RI sites to construct an expression vector designated pSV40-T7-mSLC10A2.

Site-directed mutagenesis

An *Eco*RI-*Bam*HI restriction fragment corresponding to nucleotides 1–589 of the coding region of mSlc10a2 cDNA was cloned into pUC119, and site-directed mutagenesis was performed according to the manufacturer's instructions. Mutagenesis of Pro[107] was performed using synthetic double-stranded primers (sense primer, 5'-G CTAATTATGGGTTGCTGCNNNGGAGGAACTGGC TCC-3'; and antisense primer, 5'-GGAGCCAGTTCC TCCNNNGCAGCAACCCATAATTAGC-3'; where the underlined portions represent the Pro[107] codon, and N indicates a randomized nucleotide). Following nucleotide sequence analysis, 2 clones with Asn and Leu substitutions for Pro[107] were obtained. Mutagenesis of uncharged polar residues was performed using synthetic double-stranded primers (T110A sense primer, 5'-GCTGCCCTG GAGGAGCTGGCTCCAATATCC-3', and antisense primer, 5'-GGATATTGGAGCCAGCTCCTCCAGGGCAG C-3'; S112A sense primer, 5'-CTGGAGGAACTGGCGCC AATATCCTGGCC-3', and antisense primer, 5'-GGCCA GGATATTGGCGCCAGTTCCTCCAG-3'; Y117F sense primer, 5'-GCTCCAATATCCTGGCCTTTTGGATAGA TGGCG-3', and antisense primer, 5'-CGCCATCTATCCA AAAGGCCAGGATATTGGAGC-3'; S126A sense primer, 5'-GGCGACATGGACCTCGCTGTTAGCATGACCACT TGC-3', and antisense primer, 5'-GCAAGTGGTCATG CTAACAGCGAGGTCCATGTCGCC-3'; S128A sense primer, 5'-CATGGACCTCAGTGTTGCCATGACCACT TGCTCCAC-3', and antisense primer, 5'-GTGGAGCA AGTGGTCATGGCAACACTGAGGTCCATG-3'; where the underlined portions represent the target codons). Mutagenesis of Tyr[117] was performed using synthetic double-stranded primers (sense primer, 5'-CTGGCCTATTGGAT AGATGGCGACAT-3'; and antisense primer, 5'-TATCCA ATAGGCCAGGATATTGGAGCC-3'; the underlined portions represent the Tyr[117] codon of wild-type mSlc10-a2, and this codon was replaced with the following sequences: Y117A, GCT; Y117C, TGT; Y117H, CAT; Y117I, ATT; Y117L, CTT; Y117S, TCT; Y117T, ACT; Y117V, GTT; Y117W, TGG). All the mutations were verified by DNA sequencing. The corresponding segment of the expression vector was replaced with the restriction fragment containing the expected mutation.

Transient expression and TCA uptake

On the day before transfection, 2.4×10^5 COS-7 cells were seeded in a 3.5-cm dish. The cells were transfected with appropriate expression vectors using Lipofectamine and Plus reagent (both purchased from Invitrogen), according to the manufacturer's instructions. Two days after transfection, uptake of ^{3}H-TCA was measured as previously described with slight modifications [34]. The cells were washed twice with a wash buffer (10 mM Tris-HCl, pH 7.4, 200 mM mannitol), and were then covered with 1 mL of uptake buffer (10 mM Tris-HCl, pH 7.4, 100 mM NaCl or choline chloride, 3 mM K_2HPO_4) containing the indicated concentration of ^{3}H-TCA and incubated at 37°C. The reaction was stopped by washing cells twice with 1 mL of ice-cold wash buffer, and cells were lysed in 1 mL of 0.2 M NaOH. Cell-associated radioactivity was measured using a liquid scintillation counter (Perkin-Elmer) and normalized to the total protein content determined using the Bradford method with bovine serum albumin as a concentration standard. For quantitative transport analysis, TCA was used at a concentration range much lower than the critical micellar concentration.

Apparent K_m and V_{max} values for TCA uptake were determined by measuring the initial rates of uptake at various concentrations of taurocholate. The TCA concentration was adjusted by adding unlabeled TCA. The data were fitted to the Michaelis-Menten equation by nonlinear regression using the KaleidaGraph 4.0 software (Synergy Software, Reading, PA).

Cell surface biotinylation

Biotinylation of cell surface proteins was performed using the Cell Surface Protein Isolation Kit according to the manufacturer's instructions with modifications. COS-7 cells were transfected with pZmISBT-EGFP2, as described above, and incubated for 2 days. The cells were washed twice with ice-cold phosphate-buffered saline (PBS; 0.1 M sodium phosphate, 0.15 M NaCl, pH 7.2) and then covered with a membrane-impermeable biotinylating reagent (2.0 mL of 1.5 mg/mL sulfo-NHS-SS-biotin dissolved in ice-cold PBS) at 4°C for 30 min with constant agitation. The reaction was stopped by adding 100 µL of quenching solution (provided as a component of the kit) and washed with Tris-buffered saline (0.025 M Tris-HCl, 0.15 M NaCl, pH 7.2). The cells were then covered with 700 µL of lysis buffer (150 mM NaCl, 1 mM EDTA, 0.1% SDS, 1% Triton X-100, 10 mM Tris-HCl, pH 7.4) supplemented with protease inhibitors (2 mM phenylmethylsufonyl fluoride, 0.022 trypsin inhibitor units/mL aprotinin, 5 µg/mL leupeptin, 0.1 µg/mL pepstatin) at 4°C for 1 h with constant agitation. The lysate was centrifuged at 13,000 rpm at 4°C for 10 min, and 600 µL of the supernatant was collected. The supernatant was incubated with 40 µL of 50% (vol/vol) streptavidin-agarose beads for 1 h with constant agitation. The mixture was centrifuged at 13,000 rpm for 2 min, and the supernatant was discarded. The beads were washed 4 times with ice-cold lysis buffer and suspended in 20 µL of 2 × SDS sample buffer (30% glycerol, 1% SDS, 0.093 g/mL DTT, 0.12 mg/mL bromophenol blue, 0.35 M Tris-HCl, pH 6.8). Ten microliters of the samples was subjected to 7.5% SDS-polyacrylamide gel electrophoresis, and western blotting was performed using anti-GFP antibody. The blots were then immersed in 0.2 M NaOH for 5 min to remove antibodies, and washed with distilled water for 5 min. The blots were reprobed with anti-calnexin antibody. The relative intensities of the protein bands were analyzed using Image J software (http://rsb.info.nih.gov/ij/).

Plasma membrane fractionation

The plasma membrane fraction was extracted from cells cultured in a 10-cm dish using the Plasma Membrane Protein Extraction Kit (Biovision, Milpitas, CA), according to the manufacturer's instructions.

Immunofluorescence microscopy and surface ELISA

COS-7 cells were transfected with pSV40-T7-mSLC10A2. Two days after transfection, the cells were washed 3 times with PBS and incubated with 4% paraformaldehyde dissolved in PBS for 20 min at room temperature. The cells were then washed 3 times with PBS. For immunofluorescence under permeabilized conditions, the cells were incubated with 0.2% Triton X-100 for 20 min and blocked with 1% BSA in PBS for 30 min at room temperature. For nonpermeabilized conditions, incubation with Triton X-100 was omitted. The cells were incubated with anti-T7 tag monoclonal antibody at 1/2000 dilution for 30 min at room temperature. The cells were washed 3 times with PBS and incubated with fluorescein-conjugated anti-mouse antibody at 1/500 dilution for 1 h in the dark. The cells were stained with 10 μg/mL Hoechst 33342 for 5 min and washed 3 times with PBS in the dark. The cells were examined under a microscope (Axio Imager M1; Carl Zeiss, Tokyo, Japan), and images were captured using a digital camera (AxioCam MRm; Carl Zeiss). For surface ELISA, the cells were incubated with HRP-conjugated anti-T7 tag monoclonal antibody at 1/2000 dilution for 1 h at room temperature. The cells were washed 3 times with PBS, and incubated with SuperSignal ELISA Femto Maximum Sensitivity Substrate (Pierce) for 1 min at room temperature. Luminescence was measured using a plate reader (2030 ARVO X3; PerkinElmer).

Alignment of amino acid sequences

The nucleotide sequences of the related genes were retrieved by a BLAST search (tblastn program provided at http://blast.ncbi.nlm.nih.gov/) using the amino acid sequence "GCCPGGTGSNILAYWIDGDMDLSVSMTT CSTLLALGMMP" corresponding to Gly^{104}–Pro^{142} of mouse Slc10a2 (mSlc10a2) as a query sequence. The deduced amino acid sequences of 10 of the identified genes from bacteria, archaea, and plants that yielded the highest score and the amino acid sequence of $ASBT_{NM}$ were compared with the amino acid sequences of SLC10A family members using the ClustalW software. The amino acid sequences were deduced from GenBank nucleotide sequences with the following accession numbers: *Arthrobacter phenanthrenivorans*, [CP002379]; *Deinococcus proteolyticus*, [CP002537]; *Prevotella ruminicola*, [CP002006]; *Haloarcula marismortui*, [AY596296]; *Haloarcula hispanica*, [CP002923]; *Haloferax volcanii*, [CP001956]; *Haloterrigena turkmenica*, [CP001860]; *Methanococcus maripaludis*, [CP000609]; *Methanococcus vannielii*, [CP000742]; *Methanococcus voltae*, [CP002057]; *Staphylococcus pseudintermedius*, [CP002439]; *Megasphaera elsdenii*, [HE576794]; *Oceanobacillus iheyensis*, [BA000028]; *Geobacillus thermoglucosidasius*, [CP002835]; *Methanosarcina acetivorans*, [AE010299]; *Methanosarcina mazei*, [AE008384]; *Methanosarcina barkeri*, [CP000099]; *Arabidopsis lyrata*, [XM_002889153]; *Arabidopsis thaliana*, [BX816582]; *Solanum lycopersicum*, [AK320352]; *Ricinus communis*, [XM_002531199]; *Selaginella moellendorffii*, [FJ51633]; *Medicago truncatula*, [XM_003638354]; *Glycine max*, [XM_003543135]; *Leptospira interrogans*, [AE010301]; *Nitrosomonas* sp. Is79A3, [CP002876]; *Zea mays*, [NM_001158879]; *Sorghum bicolor*, [XM_002442850]; *Oryza sativa*, [NM_001189880]; *Leptospira biflexa*, [CP000786]; SLC10A1/Slc10a1, dog, [XM_537494]; human, [NM_003049]; rabbit, [NM_001082768]; cattle, [BC105471]; mouse, [NM_011387]; rat, [NM_017047]; SLC10A2/Slc10a2, chimpanzee, [XM_522716]; human, [NM_000452]; orangutan, [NM_001131608]; *Macaca mulatta* (rhesus monkey), [XM_001095212]; dog, [NM_001002968]; rabbit, [NM_001082764]; mouse, [NM_011388]; rat, [NM_017222]; hamster, [NM_001246820]; cattle, [XM_604179]; platypus, [XM_001513315], chicken, [XM_425589]; opossum, [XM_001376304]; human SLC10A3, [NM_019848]; SLC10A4, [NM_152679]; SLC10A5, [NM_001010893]; SLC10A6/Slc10a6, chimpanzee, [XM_526626]; human, [NM_197965]; monkey, [XM_001092284]; dog, [XM_846210]; cattle, [NM_001081738]; mouse, [NM_029415]; rat, [NM_198049]; platypus, [XM_001515822]. The amino acid sequence of $ASBT_{NM}$ was obtained from UniProt [Q9K0A9].

Statistical analysis

TCA uptake and biotinylation results were analyzed by Dunnett's test and Student's t-test using the JMP software (SAS Institute, Tokyo, Japan).

Abbreviations

EGFP: Enhanced green fluorescent protein; EL: Extracellular loop; mSlc10a2: Mouse solute carrier family 10 member 2; Sulfo-NHS-SS-biotin: Sulfosuccinimidyl 2-(biotinamido)ethyl-1,3-dithiopropionate; TCA: Taurocholic acid; TM: Transmembrane.

Competing interests

The authors declare that they have no competing interests.

Authors' contributions

TS designed and supervised the study, performed all the experiments except those mentioned below, and drafted the manuscript. KS constructed the expression vectors for T7-tagged Tyr[117] mutants and performed surface ELISA (Figure 4B) and fluorescence microscopy (Figure 5). SI performed kinetic analysis of TCA uptake by the Y117S mutant (Figure 4D). KI constructed the expression vectors for EGFP-fused uncharged polar residue mutants, measured TCA uptake by these mutants, and performed western blot analyses (Figure 3). RK was the principal supervisor. All authors approved the final manuscript.

Author details

[1]Laboratory of Molecular Nutrition, Kyoto Prefectural University, Nakaragi, Shimogamo, Sakyo-ku, Kyoto 606-8522, Japan. [2]Current affiliation: Laboratory of Physiological Function of Food, Division of Food Science and Biotechnology, Graduate School of Agriculture, Kyoto University, Gokasho, Uji city, Kyoto Prefecture 611-0011, Japan.

References

1. Houten SM, Watanabe M, Auwerx J: **Endocrine functions of bile acids.** *EMBO J* 2006, **25**:1419–1425.
2. Jung D, Inagaki T, Gerard RD, Dawson PA, Kliewer SA, Mangelsdorf DJ, Moschetta A: **FXR agonists and FGF15 reduce fecal bile acid excretion in a mouse model of bile acid malabsorption.** *J Lipid Res* 2007, **48**:2693–2700.
3. Kim I, Ahn SH, Inagaki T, Choi M, Ito S, Guo GL, Kliewer SA, Gonzalez FJ: **Differential regulation of bile acid homeostasis by the farnesoid X receptor in liver and intestine.** *J Lipid Res* 2007, **48**:2664–2672.
4. Makishima M, Okamoto AY, Repa JJ, Tu H, Learned RM, Luk A, Hull MV, Lustig KD, Mangelsdorf DJ, Shan B: **Identification of a nuclear receptor for bile acids.** *Science* 1999, **284**:1362–1365.
5. Parks DJ, Blanchard SG, Bledsoe RK, Chandra G, Consler TG, Kliewer SA, Stimmel JB, Willson TM, Zavacki AM, Moore DD, Lehmann JM: **Bile acids: natural ligands for an orphan nuclear receptor.** *Science* 1999, **284**:1365–1368.
6. Watanabe M, Houten SM, Mataki C, Christoffolete MA, Kim BW, Sato H, Messaddeq N, Harney JW, Ezaki O, Kodama T, Schoonjans K, Bianco AC, Auwerx J: **Bile acids induce energy expenditure by promoting intracellular thyroid hormone activation.** *Nature* 2006, **439**:484–489.
7. Craddock AL, Love MW, Daniel RW, Kirby LC, Walters HC, Wong MH, Dawson PA: **Expression and transport properties of the human ileal and renal sodium-dependent bile acid transporter.** *Am J Physiol* 1998, **274**:G157–G169.
8. Shneider BL: **[Intestinal bile acid transport: biology, physiology, and pathophysiology.** *J Pediatr Gastroenterol Nutr* 2001, **32**:407–417.
9. Wong MH, Oelkers P, Craddock AL, Dawson PA: **Expression cloning and characterization of the hamster ileal sodium-dependent bile acid transporter.** *J Biol Chem* 1994, **269**:1340–1347.
10. Weinman SA, Carruth MW, Dawson PA: **Bile acid uptake via the human apical sodium-bile acid cotransporter is electrogenic.** *J Biol Chem* 1998, **273**:34691–34695.
11. Balakrishnan A, Wring SA, Polli JE: **Interaction of native bile acids with human apical sodium-dependent bile acid transporter (hASBT): influence of steroidal hydroxylation pattern and C-24 conjugation.** *Pharm Res* 2006, **23**:1451–1459.
12. Tolle-Sander S, Lentz KA, Maeda DY, Coop A, Polli JE: **Increased acyclovir oral bioavailability via a bile acid conjugate.** *Mol Pharm* 2004, **1**:40–48.
13. Hagenbuch B, Meier PJ: **Molecular cloning, chromosomal localization, and functional characterization of a human liver Na+/bile acid cotransporter.** *J Clin Invest* 1994, **93**:1326–1331.
14. Hallén S, Branden M, Dawson PA, Sachs G: **Membrane insertion scanning of the human ileal sodium/bile acid co-transporter.** *Biochemistry* 1999, **38**:11379–11388.
15. Banerjee A, Ray A, Chang C, Swaan PW: **Site-directed mutagenesis and use of bile acid-MTS conjugates to probe the role of cysteines in the human apical sodium-dependent bile acid transporter (SLC10A2).** *Biochemistry* 2005, **44**:8908–8917.
16. Banerjee A, Swaan PW: **Membrane topology of human ASBT (SLC10A2) determined by dual label epitope insertion scanning mutagenesis. New evidence for seven transmembrane domains.** *Biochemistry* 2006, **45**:943–953.

17. Hallén S, Mareninova O, Branden M, Sachs G: **Organization of the membrane domain of the human liver sodium/bile acid cotransporter.** *Biochemistry* 2002, **41**:7253–7266.
18. Mareninova O, Shin JM, Vagin O, Turdikulova S, Hallen S, Sachs G: **Topography of the membrane domain of the liver Na+-dependent bile acid transporter.** *Biochemistry* 2005, **44**:13702–13712.
19. Zhang EY, Phelps MA, Banerjee A, Khantwal CM, Chang C, Helsper F, Swaan PW: **Topology scanning and putative three-dimensional structure of the extracellular binding domains of the apical sodium-dependent bile acid transporter (SLC10A2).** *Biochemistry* 2004, **43**:11380–11392.
20. Hu NJ, Iwata S, Cameron AD, Drew D: **Crystal structure of a bacterial homologue of the bile acid sodium symporter ASBT.** *Nature* 2011, **478**:408–411.
21. Sun AQ, Salkar R, Sachchidanand, Xu S, Zeng L, Zhou MM, Suchy FJ: **A 14-amino acid sequence with a beta-turn structure is required for apical membrane sorting of the rat ileal bile acid transporter.** *J Biol Chem* 2003, **278**:4000–4009.
22. Hussainzada N, Banerjee A, Swaan PW: **Transmembrane domain VII of the human apical sodium-dependent bile acid transporter ASBT (SLC10A2) lines the substrate translocation pathway.** *Mol Pharmacol* 2006, **70**:1565–1574.
23. Hussainzada N, Da Silva TC, Zhang EY, Swaan PW: **Conserved Aspartic Acid Residues Lining the Extracellular Loop I of Sodium-coupled Bile Acid Transporter ASBT Interact with Na+ and 7α-OH Moieties on the Ligand Cholestane Skeleton.** *J Biol Chem* 2008, **283**:20653–20663.
24. Khantwal CM, Swaan PW: **Cytosolic half of transmembrane domain IV of the human bile acid transporter hASBT (SLC10A2) forms part of the substrate translocation pathway.** *Biochemistry* 2008, **47**:3606–3614.
25. Geyer J, Wilke T, Petzinger E: **The solute carrier family SLC10: more than a family of bile acid transporters regarding function and phylogenetic relationships.** *Naunyn Schmiedebergs Arch Pharmacol* 2006, **372**:413–431.
26. Zahner D, Eckhardt U, Petzinger E: **Transport of taurocholate by mutants of negatively charged amino acids, cysteines, and threonines of the rat liver sodium-dependent taurocholate cotransporting polypeptide Ntcp.** *Eur J Biochem* 2003, **270**:1117–1127.
27. Rzewuski G, Sauter M: **The novel rice (Oryza sativa L.) gene OsSbf1 encodes a putative member of the Na+/bile acid symporter family.** *J Exp Bot* 2002, **53**:1991–1993.
28. Saeki T, Mizushima S, Ueda K, Iwami K, Kanamoto R: **Mutational analysis of uncharged polar residues and proline in the distal one-third (Thr[130]–Pro[142]) of the highly conserved region of mouse Slc10a2.** *Biosci Biotechnol Biochem* 2009, **73**:1535–1540.
29. Kanamoto R, Azuma N, Suda H, Saeki T, Tsuchihashi Y, Iwami K: **Elimination of Na+-dependent bile acid transporter from small intestine by ileum resection increases [correction of increase] colonic tumorigenesis in the rat fed deoxycholic acid.** *Cancer Lett* 1999, **145**:115–120.
30. Wang W, Xue S, Ingles SA, Chen Q, Diep AT, Frankl HD, Stolz A, Haile RW: **An association between genetic polymorphisms in the ileal sodium-dependent bile acid transporter gene and the risk of colorectal adenomas.** *Cancer Epidemiol Biomarkers Prev* 2001, **10**:931–936.
31. Oelkers P, Kirby LC, Heubi JE, Dawson PA: **Primary bile acid malabsorption caused by mutations in the ileal sodium-dependent bile acid transporter gene (SLC10A2).** *J Clin Invest* 1997, **99**:1880–1887.
32. Renner O, Harsch S, Schaeffeler E, Schwab M, Klass DM, Kratzer W, Stange EF: **Mutation screening of apical sodium-dependent bile acid transporter (SLC10A2): novel haplotype block including six newly identified variants linked to reduced expression.** *Hum Genet* 2009, **125**:381–391.
33. Saeki T, Matoba K, Furukawa H, Kirifuji K, Kanamoto R, Iwami K: **Characterization, cDNA cloning, and functional expression of mouse ileal sodium-dependent bile acid transporter.** *J Biochem (Tokyo)* 1999, **125**:846–851.
34. Saeki T, Munetaka Y, Ueda K, Iwami K, Kanamoto R: **Effects of Ala substitution for conserved Cys residues in mouse ileal and hepatic Na+-dependent bile acid transporters.** *Biosci Biotechnol Biochem* 2007, **71**:1865–1872.

14

Contribution of transient and sustained calcium influx, and sensitization to depolarization-induced contractions of the intact mouse aorta

Paul Fransen[1*], Cor E Van Hove[2], Johanna van Langen[2], Dorien M Schrijvers[1], Wim Martinet[1], Guido R Y De Meyer[1] and Hidde Bult[2]

Abstract

Background: Electrophysiological studies of L-type Ca^{2+} channels in isolated vascular smooth muscle cells revealed that depolarization of these cells evoked a transient and a time-independent Ca^{2+} current. The sustained, non-inactivating current occurred at voltages where voltage-dependent activation and inactivation overlapped (voltage window) and its contribution to basal tone or active tension in larger multicellular blood vessel preparations is unknown at present. This study investigated whether window Ca^{2+} influx affects isometric contraction of multicellular C57Bl6 mouse aortic segments.

Results: Intracellular Ca^{2+} (Ca_i^{2+}, Fura-2), membrane potential and isometric force were measured in aortic segments, which were clamped at fixed membrane potentials by increasing extracellular K^+ concentrations. K^+ above 20 mM evoked biphasic contractions, which were not affected by inhibition of IP_3- or Ca^{2+} induced Ca^{2+} release with 2-aminoethoxydiphenyl borate or ryanodine, respectively, ruling out the contribution of intracellular Ca^{2+} release. The fast force component paralleled Ca_i^{2+} increase, but the slow contraction coincided with Ca_i^{2+} decrease. In the absence of extracellular Ca^{2+}, basal tension and Ca_i^{2+} declined, and depolarization failed to evoke Ca_i^{2+} signals or contraction. Subsequent re-introduction of external Ca^{2+} elicited only slow contractions, which were now matched by Ca_i^{2+} increase. After Ca_i^{2+} attained steady-state, isometric force kept increasing due to Ca^{2+}- sensitization of the contractile elements. The slow force responses displayed a bell-shaped voltage-dependence, were suppressed by hyperpolarization with levcromakalim, and enhanced by an agonist of L-type Ca^{2+} channels (BAY K8644).

Conclusion: The isometric response of mouse aortic segments to depolarization consists of a fast, transient contraction paralleled by a transient Ca^{2+} influx via Ca^{2+} channels which completely inactivate. Ca^{2+} channels, which did not completely inactivate during the depolarization, initiated a second, sustained phase of contraction, which was matched by a sustained non-inactivating window Ca^{2+} influx. Together with sensitization, this window L-type Ca^{2+} influx is a major determinant of basal and active tension of mouse aortic smooth muscle.

Keywords: Vascular smooth muscle, L-type Ca^{2+} channel, Vasoconstriction, Intracellular Ca^{2+}, Depolarization, Window Ca^{2+} influx

* Correspondence: paul.fransen@ua.ac.ac
[1]Laboratory of Physiopharmacology, University of Antwerp, Universiteitsplein 1 Building T, 2.18, Wilrijk B-2610, Belgium
Full list of author information is available at the end of the article

Background

Transcripts and protein expression of the Ca^{2+} channel gene are found widely in the cardiovascular system, where the channels play a dominant role in blood pressure regulation [1-5]. This regulation not only occurs via modulation of peripheral resistance, but also via determination of the arterial compliance, especially in old age (systolic) hypertension [6-8]. It has been shown that L-type Ca^{2+} channel blockers increase vascular compliance of large elastic vessels. As such, they may also be of importance for the pathogenesis and prognosis of cardiovascular complications such as atherosclerosis, left ventricular hypertrophy and heart failure [8-14]. Vascular reactivity via L-type Ca^{2+} influx is often studied by increasing the extracellular K^+ and depolarizing the cell's membrane potential (V_m). High K^+ induces biphasic contractions in rabbit arteries [15], rat basilar arterial rings [16] and mouse aorta [17], whereby the tonic rise in force is actually accompanied by a decline of intracellular Ca^{2+}. This is often attributed to Ca^{2+}-sensitization, whereby suppression of myosin light chain phosphatase activity raises contractile force independently of further increases or even decrease in intracellular Ca^{2+} [15,18-21]. In those studies, however, relationships between force and continuous background Ca^2 influx via non-inactivating L-type Ca^{2+} channels were not explored.

Indeed, (electro)physiological characteristics of L-type Ca^{2+} channels, which have been studied extensively in isolated cardiomyocytes and vascular smooth muscle cells (VSMCs), are such that voltage-dependent activation and inactivation curves show substantial overlap between –40 and –15 mV revealing a time-independent, but voltage-dependent Ca^{2+} influx (window current) in isolated cells [22-26]. Although pharmacological evidence suggested that this window may at least serve as a background Ca^{2+} influx pathway responsible for myogenic tone of small arteries, coronary arteries and microvascular resistance vessels [27-29], window Ca^{2+} currents and related window intracellular Ca^{2+} signals have only been determined in voltage-clamped isolated SMCs and not in multicellular vascular tissue [24]. The present study used aortic segments of C57Bl6 mice to investigate relationships between VSMC Ca^{2+} mobilization and isometric contraction with focus on the L-type Ca^{2+} channel window. Since electrophysiological voltage-clamp of intact aorta segments was impossible, we decided to clamp the membrane potential at fixed potentials by increasing external K^+ concentration. By modulating influx of Ca^{2+} before and during depolarization, we show that not only basal tension, but also the tonic contractile component of C57Bl6 mouse aortic VSMCs depends on the window L-type Ca^{2+} influx and subsequent Ca^{2+} sensitization mechanisms. These observations may have important consequences

for the effects of nitric oxide (NO) on L-type Ca^{2+} influx. Recently, we showed that the relaxing efficacy of NO in mouse aorta was dependent on the contractile agonist, and more specifically, decreased when the contraction was mainly elicited via L-type Ca^{2+} influx as with elevated extracellular K^+, but increased when Ca^{2+} influx was partially inhibited with L-type Ca^{2+} channel blockers [30].

Results

Contraction at depolarized potentials

Membrane potentials (V_m) in intact mouse aortic VSMCs were K^+-dependent and depolarised from –60 mV at 5.9 mM K^+ to –30 mV at 50 mM K^+ (see Additional file 1). Hence, elevation of extracellular K^+ is a good method to clamp multicellular aortic segments from resting potentials at 5.9 mM K^+ to depolarized potentials. Two K^+ clamp protocols, as shown in Figure 1, were used; they differed in the relative number of L-type Ca^{2+} channels that can be activated with the subsequent depolarization. In the repetitive protocol (Figure 1 A-C), which mimics the depolarizing voltage steps in voltage-clamp experiments of single VSMCs, segments at 5.9 mM K^+ were repetitively exposed to elevated K^+ followed by return to 5.9 mM K^+. In this protocol, the number of channels that can be activated by the depolarization step is always the same at the start of the depolarization. In the cumulative protocol (Figure 1 D-F), which mimics the variable holding potentials in voltage-clamp experiments in single VSMCs, the segments were depolarized to the subsequent higher K^+ concentration without return to 5.9 mM K^+. Therefore, with this protocol the relative number of Ca^{2+} channels that can be activated with the subsequent depolarization decreases with higher K^+.

Isometric force by the repetitive protocol followed a bi-exponential time course, except at 10 mM K^+ (Figure 1A). Amplitude (Figure 1B) and velocity of the fast component increased with the K^+ concentration (time constant 27.1 ± 6.0 s at 20 mM K^+, 3.8 ± 0.7 s at 124 mM K^+, P<0.001). The amplitude of the slow component showed a maximum around 50 mM K^+, but then significantly decreased at 90 and 124 mM K^+ (Figure 1C). Remarkably, its time constant was independent of external K^+ (258 ± 34 s at 20 mM K^+ and 253 ± 27 s at 124 mM K^+). [K^+]-force relationships (Figure 1C) revealed E_{max}-values of 6.1 ± 0.5, 9.4 ± 1.3 and 14.4 ± 1.6 mN for fast, slow and steady-state force. EC_{50} values were respectively 23.5 ± 1.2, 22.2 ± 0.3 and 22.0 ± 0.3 mM K^+ and were not significantly different.

In the cumulative protocol, two force signals were seen at 15 and 20 mM K^+: on top of a tonic rise upon depolarization, transient force spikes were observed (Figure 1D and E). These spikes faded away as time

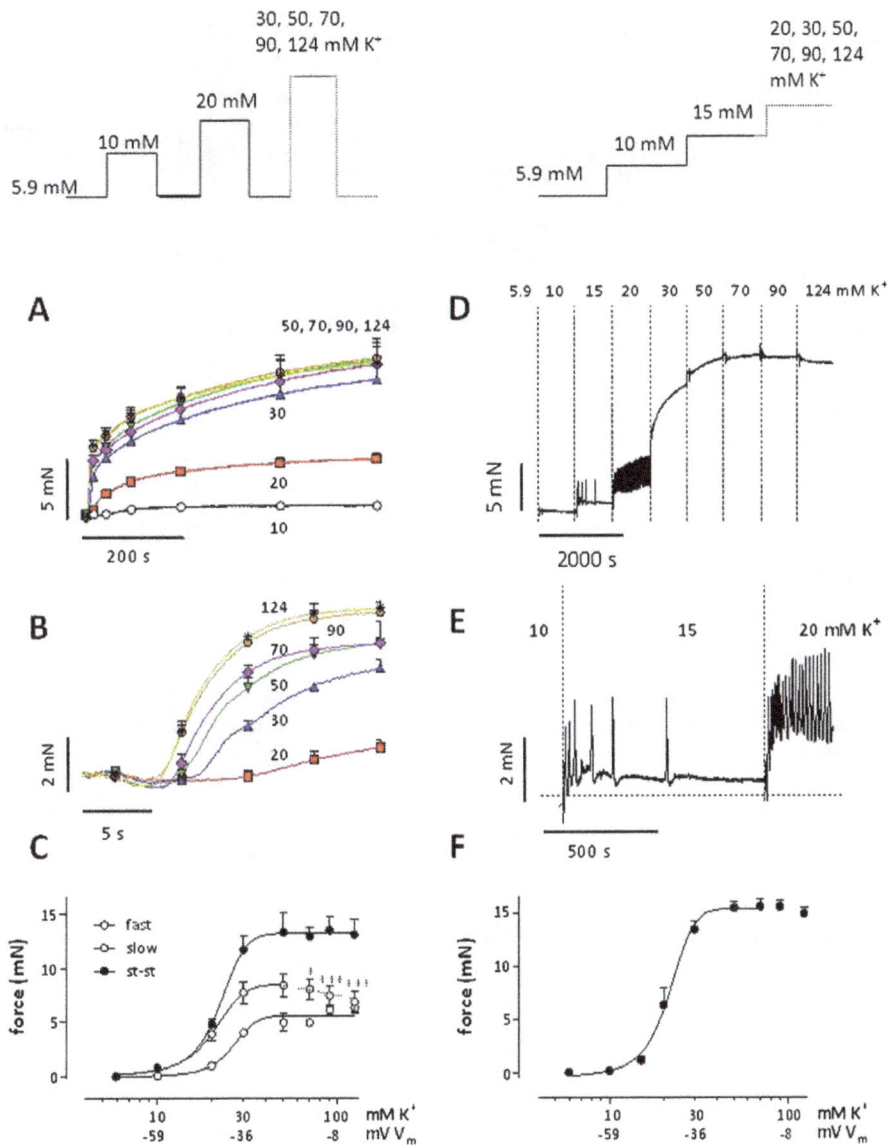

Figure 1 Isometric contractions by elevation of external K⁺ in mouse aorta. K⁺ was elevated from 5.9 mM to 10, 20, 30, 50, 70, 90 or 124 mM K⁺ according to the protocols shown in the top panels. For the repetitive protocol (**A-C**), traces, shown on condensed (**A**) and expanded (**B**) time scales, were analyzed with a bi-exponential function revealing [K⁺]-force curves for the fast, slow and steady-state (st-st) force components (**C**). For the cumulative protocol (**D-F**), **D** shows a representative example of isometric force elicited by gradual elevations of extracellular K⁺. **E** displays the 5.9 to 10, 10 to 15 and 15 to 20 mM K⁺ depolarizations on an expanded time scale. In **F** "steady-state" force at each step was plotted in function of [K⁺]. Results show mean ± s.e.m, n = 4 (**A-C**) or n = 5 (**F**). *, ***: P<0.05, 0.001 decrease of slow component amplitude versus maximum at 50 mM K⁺. The estimated values of V_m at 10, 30 and 100 mM [K⁺] are indicated. These values are respectively −59, -36 and −8 mV (see Additional file 1).

progressed (15 mM K⁺), and showed increased frequency, but similar amplitudes at 20 mM K⁺. At 30 and 50 mM K⁺ these spikes disappeared, but force developed with a fast and slow component. Above 50 mM K⁺ only a small increase (50–70 mM K⁺) or even a decrease (90–124 mM K⁺) of force was observed (Figure 1D). E_{max} (15.5 ± 0.6 mN, Figure 1F) and EC_{50} (21.8 ± 1.2 mM K⁺) were not significantly different from the steady state values measured with repetitive depolarization (*vide supra*).

Neurotransmitter release from perivascular nerves did not contribute to the biexponential nature of high K⁺ contractions or to the K⁺-dose–response relationships in aortic segments (see Additional file 1). There was also no evidence of involvement of sarcoplasmic reticulum (SR) Ca^{2+} store Ca^{2+} release. Although inhibition of Ca^{2+}-induced Ca^{2+} release with 15 μM ryanodine raised basal tension (Figure 2A), and inhibited the transient caffeine-induced contraction by more than 50%

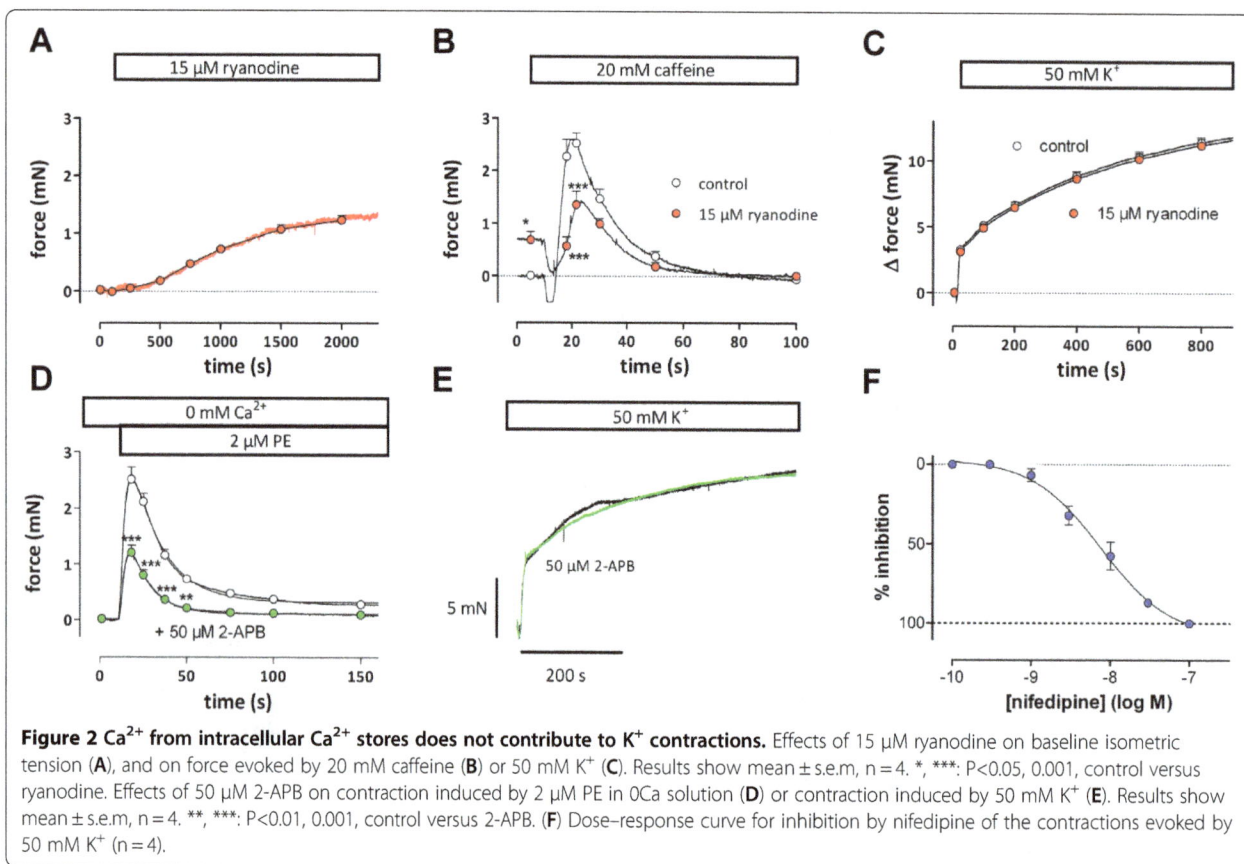

Figure 2 Ca^{2+} from intracellular Ca^{2+} stores does not contribute to K$^+$ contractions. Effects of 15 μM ryanodine on baseline isometric tension (**A**), and on force evoked by 20 mM caffeine (**B**) or 50 mM K$^+$ (**C**). Results show mean ± s.e.m, n = 4. *, ***: P<0.05, 0.001, control versus ryanodine. Effects of 50 μM 2-APB on contraction induced by 2 μM PE in 0Ca solution (**D**) or contraction induced by 50 mM K$^+$ (**E**). Results show mean ± s.e.m, n = 4. **, ***: P<0.01, 0.001, control versus 2-APB. (**F**) Dose–response curve for inhibition by nifedipine of the contractions evoked by 50 mM K$^+$ (n = 4).

(Figure 2B), 50 mM K$^+$-induced contractions were not affected (Figure 2C). Similar observations were made for inositoltriphosphate (IP$_3$)-mediated Ca^{2+} release. Contractions by 2 μM phenylephrine (PE) in the absence of extracellular Ca^{2+} were significantly reduced by 50 μM 2-aminoethoxydiphenyl borate (2-APB), a blocker of IP$_3$-induced Ca^{2+} release [31] (Figure 2D), whereas contractions by 50 mM K$^+$ were not affected (Figure 2E).

Moreover, K$^+$ in Ca^{2+}-free KR (0Ca) or in the presence of 3 μM nifedipine, an inhibitor of L-type Ca^{2+} channels, failed to elicit tension, and addition of nifedipine (3 to 300 nM) to segments constricted with 50 mM K$^+$ caused complete relaxation (E$_{max}$ 107 ± 3%, logEC$_{50}$ -8.12 ± 0.12, n = 4, Figure 2F). Finally, inhibition of SERCA and emptying the intracellular Ca^{2+} stores with 1 μM cyclopiazonic acid (CPA) did not affect the contraction by 50 mM K$^+$.

These results indicated that SR Ca^{2+} is not involved in K$^+$-evoked contractions and that fast and slow force components evoked by high K$^+$ were both initiated and sustained by Ca^{2+} influx via VSMC L-type Ca^{2+} channels only.

Relationship between force and Ca^{2+} influx

Temporal relationships between intracellular Ca^{2+} and isometric force were explored using the cumulative protocol. For K$^+$ elevations from 15 to 20, from 20 to 25 and from 25 to 30 mM K$^+$, there was a strict temporal relationship between Ca^{2+} and force (Figure 3). Again, there were tonic and phasic contractions (cf Figure 1D and E), though at slightly higher K$^+$ concentrations (20–30 mM K$^+$). They coincided with phasic Ca^{2+} spikes on top of a tonic rise of Ca^{2+} (Figure 3). Both Ca^{2+} and force spikes faded away as time progressed (15 to 20 mM K$^+$), displayed higher frequency at the subsequent step (25 mM K$^+$) and disappeared at holding potentials above 30 mM K$^+$. From 35 up to 124 mM K$^+$ the temporal relationships between Ca^{2+} (transient peak tapering off to lower plateau) and force (biphasic increase) were not clear and during these depolarizations Ca^{2+} decreased whereas force increased (arrows in Figure 3).

The deviations between Ca^{2+} and force above 30 mM K$^+$ were studied in greater detail by depolarizing the segments from 5.9 mM K$^+$ to 50 or 124 mM K$^+$. The initial, fast contraction was accompanied by a fast rise in Ca^{2+} (Figure 4). Amplitude and velocity of the fast Ca^{2+} (7.2 ± 1.5 s) and force (7.7 ±1.2 s) components were greater at 124 mM K$^+$ as compared with 50 mM K$^+$ (16.8 ± 3.7 s and 14 ± 3 s respectively). After reaching a maximum, Ca^{2+} declined faster (50 ± 6 s versus 137 ± 24 s, P<0.01) and to a lower level at 124 mM K$^+$

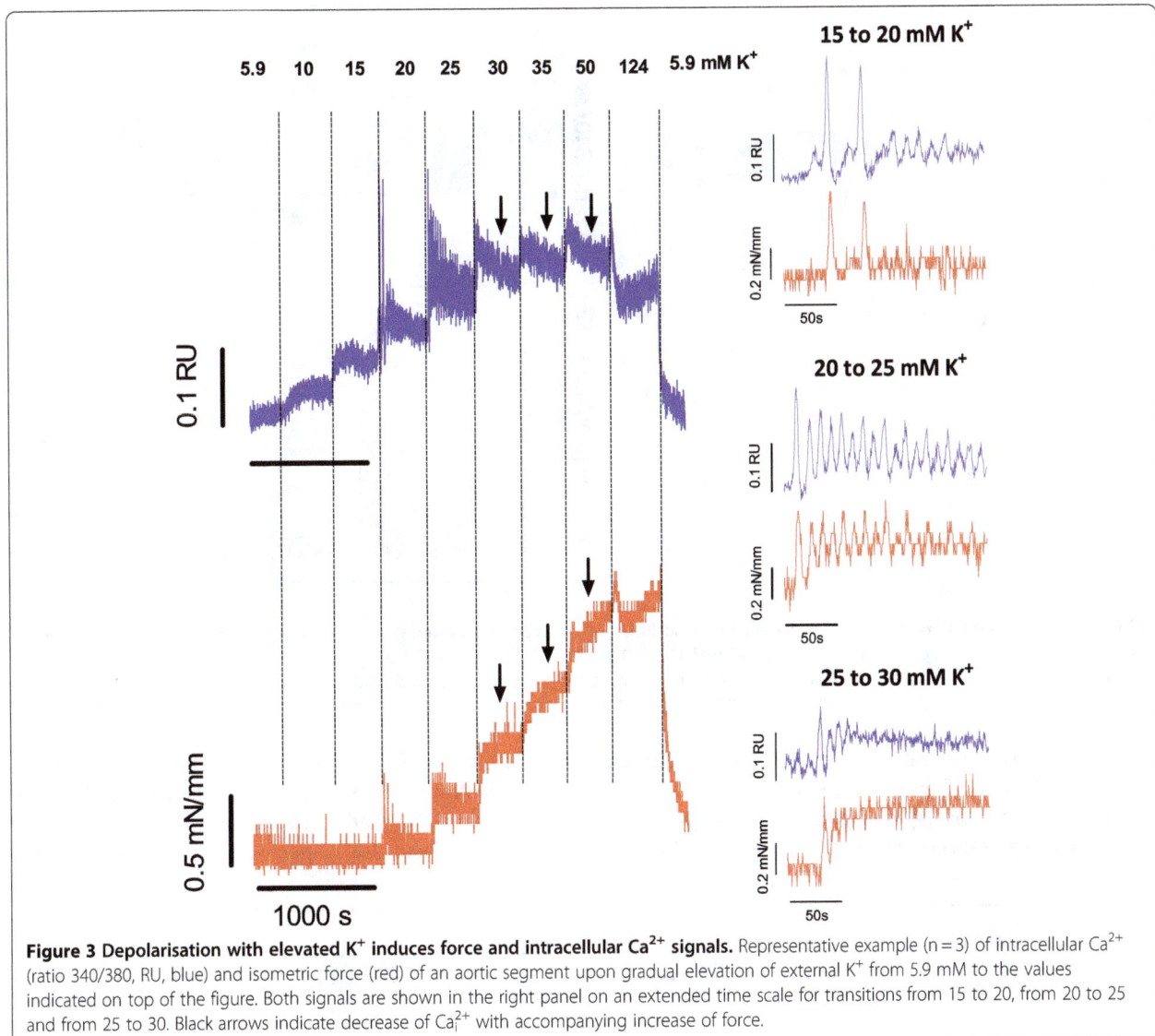

Figure 3 Depolarisation with elevated K⁺ induces force and intracellular Ca²⁺ signals. Representative example (n = 3) of intracellular Ca²⁺ (ratio 340/380, RU, blue) and isometric force (red) of an aortic segment upon gradual elevation of external K⁺ from 5.9 mM to the values indicated on top of the figure. Both signals are shown in the right panel on an extended time scale for transitions from 15 to 20, from 20 to 25 and from 25 to 30. Black arrows indicate decrease of Ca$_i^{2+}$ with accompanying increase of force.

than at 50 mM K⁺, and the slow force increase during the plateau phase was slightly smaller at 124 mM K⁺.

These results indicate that at 50 or 124 mM K⁺ the slow contraction was actually accompanied by a decline of Ca²⁺, but that there was a good temporal relationship between intracellular Ca²⁺ and force development immediately after the depolarization.

Experimental dissection of the Ca²⁺ and force components

At 5.9 mM K⁺, removal of extracellular Ca²⁺ (0Ca) decreased basal intracellular Ca²⁺ and force from 0.91 ± 0.03 to 0.81 ± 0.02 RU ($p < 0.005$, n = 6) and from 0.52 ± 0.02 to 0.40 ± 0.05 mN/mm ($p < 0.05$, n = 6), indicating baseline Ca²⁺ influx via Ca²⁺ channels in normal conditions. Depolarizing the segments with 124 mM K⁺ in 0Ca abrogated Ca²⁺ influx via L-type Ca²⁺ channels and

neither contraction nor Ca²⁺ influx was observed. Because in the absence of extracellular Ca²⁺ L-type Ca²⁺ channels display normal gating currents [32], subsequent addition of external Ca²⁺ can evoke Ca²⁺ influx and contraction only if a subpopulation of L-type Ca²⁺ channels is not completely inactivated during the preceding depolarization in 0Ca. Indeed, re-addition of Ca²⁺ to 0Ca caused intracellular Ca²⁺ and force to increase (Figure 5B). Contrary to the control situation (Figure 5A), intracellular Ca²⁺ did not decline during the contraction plateau in the Ca²⁺ re-addition experiments. As a consequence, a clear temporal relationship between the slow Ca²⁺ and force signals was observed (Figure 5B) and the force and Ca²⁺ signals could now be dissected in parallel fast and slow components.

The fast Ca²⁺ and force components that were eliminated in the Ca²⁺ re-addition experiments, could be

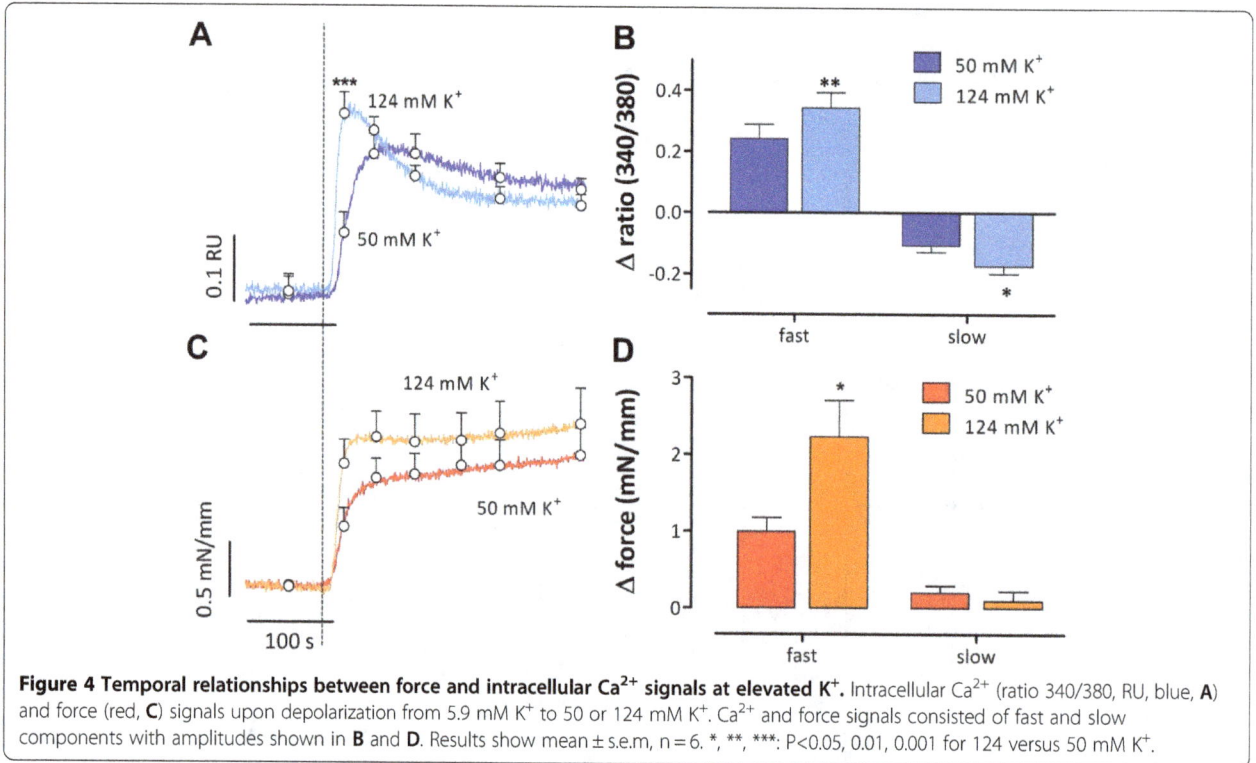

Figure 4 Temporal relationships between force and intracellular Ca²⁺ signals at elevated K⁺. Intracellular Ca²⁺ (ratio 340/380, RU, blue, **A**) and force (red, **C**) signals upon depolarization from 5.9 mM K⁺ to 50 or 124 mM K⁺. Ca²⁺ and force signals consisted of fast and slow components with amplitudes shown in **B** and **D**. Results show mean ± s.e.m, n = 6. *, **, ***: P<0.05, 0.01, 0.001 for 124 versus 50 mM K⁺.

visualized by pair-wise subtracting Ca²⁺ and force traces from control traces (Figure 5C, D). The differential Ca²⁺ and force signals displayed a similar time-dependency (time constants respectively 15 ± 2 s and 9 ± 2 s for rise,

and 57 ± 4 s and 54 ± 4 s for fall). Therefore, Figures 4 and 5 illustrate the strict temporal relationships between fast and slow Ca²⁺ and force signals upon depolarization: the fast transient Ca²⁺ increase during depolarization

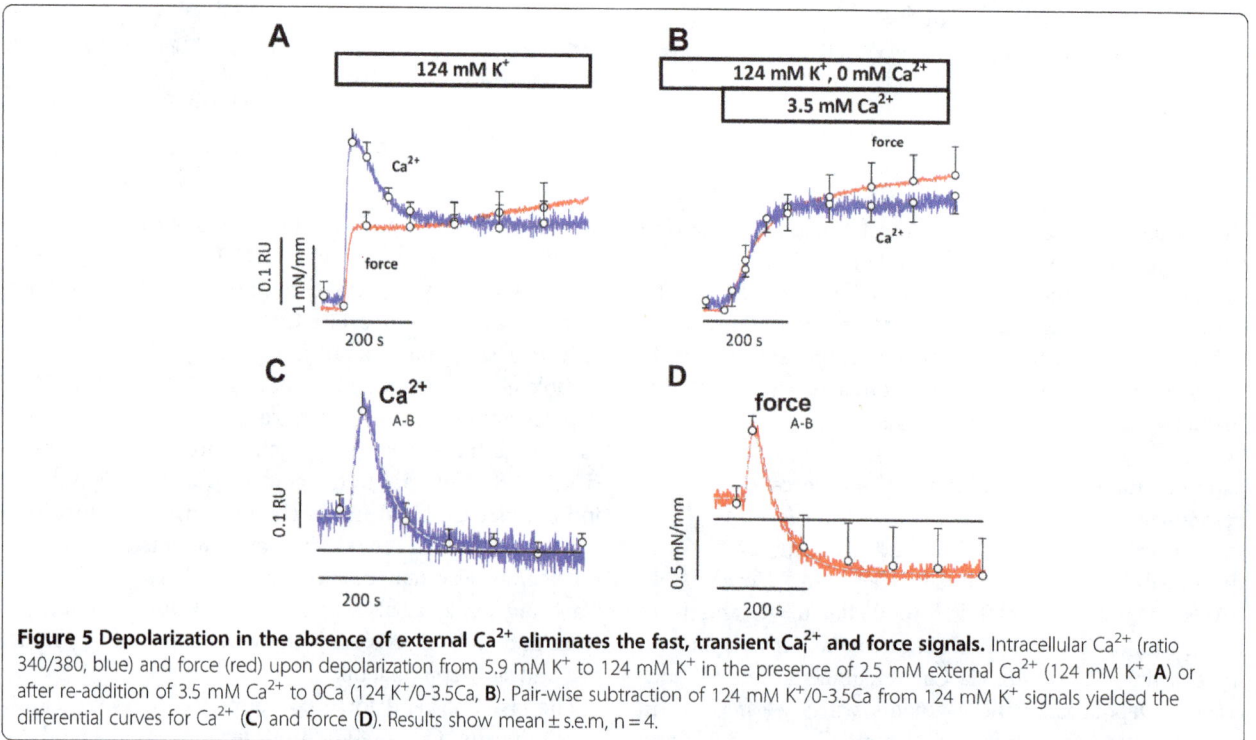

Figure 5 Depolarization in the absence of external Ca²⁺ eliminates the fast, transient Ca$_i$²⁺ and force signals. Intracellular Ca²⁺ (ratio 340/380, blue) and force (red) upon depolarization from 5.9 mM K⁺ to 124 mM K⁺ in the presence of 2.5 mM external Ca²⁺ (124 mM K⁺, **A**) or after re-addition of 3.5 mM Ca²⁺ to 0Ca (124 K⁺/0-3.5Ca, **B**). Pair-wise subtraction of 124 mM K⁺/0-3.5Ca from 124 mM K⁺ signals yielded the differential curves for Ca²⁺ (**C**) and force (**D**). Results show mean ± s.e.m, n = 4.

initiates fast force development, whereas a simultaneously activated slower influx of Ca^{2+} is responsible for sustained force development during the plateau phase.

Is L-;type Ca^{2+} window current responsible for the slow contraction phase?

An important electrophysiological property of L-type Ca^{2+} channels is that in the voltage range where activation and inactivation curves overlap, they allow a continuous, time-independent Ca^{2+} influx, the so-called window L-type Ca^{2+} channel current [24,26]. If this current is responsible for the slow contraction phase following addition of external Ca^{2+} to segments depolarized in 0Ca, then force should display a bell-shaped concentration-response relationship. Figure 6 shows the contractions evoked by re-introduction of Ca^{2+} to 0Ca at different K^+ concentrations. After 200 s the slow component showed a linear rather than exponential increase with time. Force measured at 600 s was maximal at 50 mM K^+ and declined at higher K^+ concentrations (Figure 6A).

[K^+]-contraction curves were determined after 200, 400 and 600 s (Figure 6B and C). At these time intervals, the [K^+]-contraction curve indeed became bell-shaped. The bell-shape and the complete inhibition with the L-type Ca^{2+} channel blocker, nifedipine (data not shown) are typical characteristics of the window L-type Ca^{2+}

current. The EC_{50} for K^+ was time-independent and was respectively 20.9 ± 0.4 mM, 20.4 ± 0.2 mM and 20.5 ± 0.2 mM (n = 6). The continuous increase of force with time is presumably due to Ca^{2+} sensitization as intracellular Ca^{2+} reached steady-state after 200 s (Figure 5). Further evidence for Ca^{2+} sensitization was provided by Rho kinase inhibition with Y-27632 (1 and 3 µM). Y-27632 attenuated depolarization-induced contractions, but inhibition of Ca^{2+} sensitization emphasized the bell shape of the [K^+]-contraction curve even more. This suggests that the decrease of force at 90 and 124 mM K^+ was not due to a reduction in sensitivity to Ca^{2+}, but was proportional to the window influx of Ca^{2+} via L-type Ca^{2+} channels (Figure 7). Similar results were obtained with HA 1077 (5 µM, not shown).

Modulation of L-type window Ca^{2+} influx

Changes of V_m of the VSMCs or changes of the voltage-dependent parameters of L-type Ca^{2+} channel gating (activation or inactivation) are expected to affect Ca^{2+} influx and contraction of the segments. Segments could be hyperpolarized from –60 mV to the K^+ equilibrium potential (V_K) of –86 mV at 5.9 mM K^+ with levcromakalim (200 nM), an opener of ATP-dependent K^+ channels (see Additional file 1, Figure 1). The L-type Ca^{2+} channel activation curve can be shifted to hyperpolarized potentials with BAY K8644 (30 nM), an activator of L-type

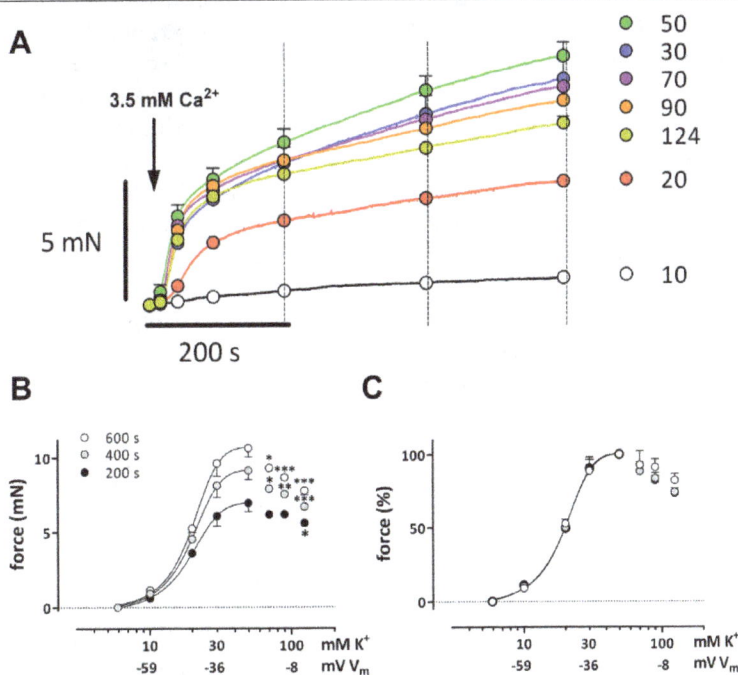

Figure 6 K^+-dependent development of window contraction. Isometric contractions induced by addition of 3.5 mM Ca^{2+} to 0Ca containing 10 up to 124 mM K^+ (**A**). Absolute (**B**) and relative (50 mM K^+ set to 100%, **C**) [K^+]-force curves were determined at 200, 400 and 600 s (see dotted lines in **A**), were bell-shaped and could only be fitted up to 50 mM K^+ (**B, C**). Results show mean ± s.e.m, n = 6. *, **, ***: P<0.05, 0.01, 0.001 versus 50 mM K^+.

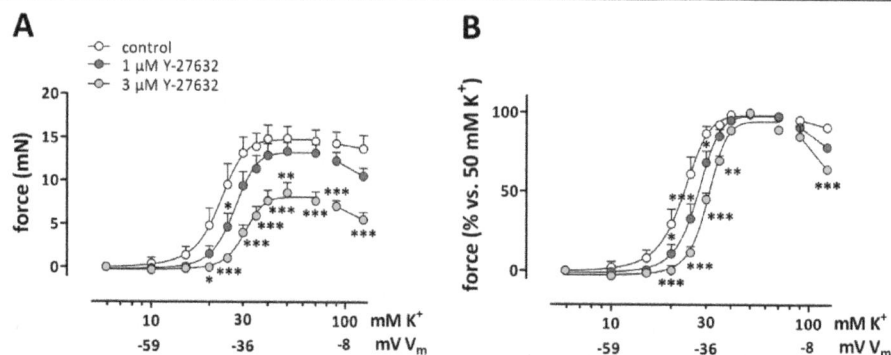

Figure 7 Effects of Rho kinase inhibition with Y-27632 on window contractions. A: "Steady-state" isometric contractions induced by depolarizations with cumulative K$^+$ concentrations in the absence (control) and in the presence of 1 and 3 µM Y-27632. In **B**, force was normalized with values at 50 mM K$^+$ as 100%. Results show mean ± s.e.m, n = 4. *, **, ***: P<0.05, 0.01, 0.001 versus control.

Ca^{2+} channels [30,33,34]. When segments were subjected to increasing K$^+$ concentrations in the presence of levcromakalim, BAY K8644, or their combination (Figure 8A and B), levcromakalim shifted the curve to higher K$^+$ concentrations (+5.93 ± 0.87 mM), whereas BAY K8644 caused a shift to lower K$^+$ concentrations (-7.98 ± 1.09 mM). Both effects were fully additive, indicating independent effects of V$_m$ (levcromakalim) and L-type Ca^{2+} channel gating (BAY K8644) on window contractions.

At normal extracellular K$^+$, levcromakalim caused a glibenclamide (inhibitor of ATP-sensitive K$^+$ channels)-sensitive decline of intracellular Ca^{2+} (-0.042 ± 0.012 RU, n = 3) and baseline tension (-0.56 ± 0.28 mN, n = 4), whereas BAY K8644 raised resting intracellular Ca^{2+} (+0.016 ± 0.008 RU) and force (+1.77 ± 0.51 mN, n = 4). The BAY effect could be reversed by addition of levcromakalim or nifedipine (data not shown). To illustrate the physiological importance of the window Ca^{2+} influx for basal contraction of mouse aortic segments, the external K$^+$ concentration was changed to obtain depolarizations or repolarizations within the physiological range of V$_m$ for VSMCs (Figure 8C). Changes of the extracellular K$^+$ between 2 and 15 mM and V$_m$ between -77 and -51 mV caused significant alterations of basal force in control, which could be amplified by adding 30 nM BAY K8644 or removed by adding 200 nM levcromakalim (data not shown). These data provide further evidence for the importance of window Ca^{2+} influx within the physiological range of V$_m$ or K$^+$ concentrations [35,36].

Discussion and conclusions

The present study showed that the main determinant of depolarization-induced contractions of the mouse aorta was the influx of extracellular Ca^{2+} via L-type Ca^{2+} channels. Thereby, both Ca^{2+} influx and contraction depended on the amplitude of depolarization (reflected by the increase of external K$^+$) and on the resting potential of the VSMC (concentration of external K$^+$ at the start of depolarization). At resting membrane potentials, elevation of extracellular K$^+$ above 10–20 mM caused biphasic contractions and Ca^{2+} signals. Although the relationships between intracellular Ca^{2+} and force appeared to be complex and sometimes non-linear (slow component), we demonstrated that the fast, phasic force component was related to a transient Ca^{2+} influx, presumably via a population of L-type Ca^{2+} channels which activated and completely inactivated during the depolarization. On the other hand, the slow, tonic force component displayed a bell-shaped voltage (K$^+$)-dependence and could be attributed to voltage-dependent, "steady state" Ca^{2+} influx via a population of L-type Ca^{2+} channels. These channels did not completely inactivate during sustained depolarization and gave rise to a window contraction. In addition to the Ca^{2+} influx via both populations of L-type Ca^{2+} channels, a time-dependent Ca^{2+} sensitization contributed to the depolarization-induced contractions of the mouse aorta.

Depolarization-induced contraction is due to activation of L-type Ca^{2+} channels and not to Ca^{2+} release from the SR

As expected [37], contractions induced by high K$^+$ were mainly due to influx of extracellular Ca^{2+} via L-type Ca^{2+} channels in the mouse aorta. Firstly, depolarization in the absence of external Ca^{2+} did not elicit intracellular Ca^{2+} signals or contractions. Secondly, selective L-type Ca^{2+} channel blockade (3 µM nifedipine) completely inhibited K$^+$-induced contractions. Thirdly, BAY K8644, an agonist of L-type Ca^{2+} channels, increased the K$^+$-sensitivity of the contractions. Finally, although intracellular Ca^{2+} release or Ca^{2+}-induced Ca^{2+} release through activation of IP$_3$ or ryanodine receptors or Ca^{2+} re-uptake to the SR have been shown to contribute to K$^+$-induced contractions [16,37,38], this was not observed in mouse aorta segments (see also [24]). Hence, intracellular Ca^{2+} release

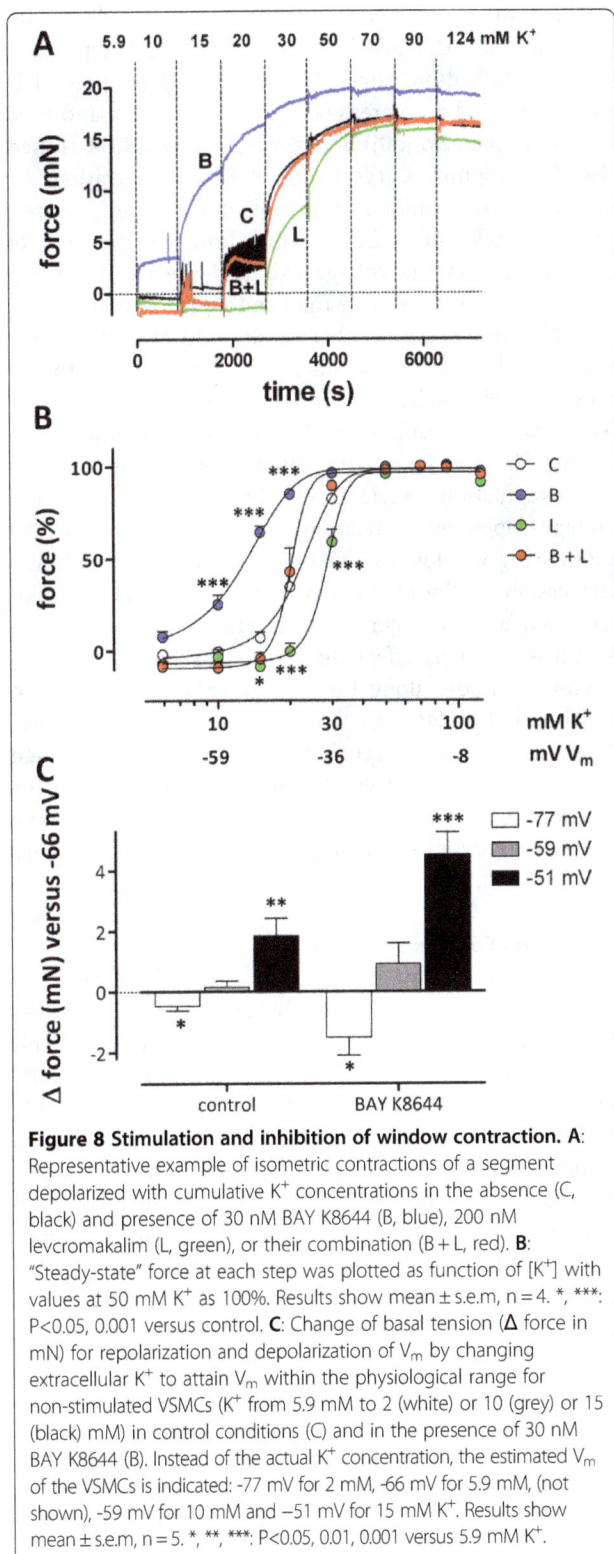

Figure 8 Stimulation and inhibition of window contraction. A: Representative example of isometric contractions of a segment depolarized with cumulative K$^+$ concentrations in the absence (C, black) and presence of 30 nM BAY K8644 (B, blue), 200 nM levcromakalim (L, green), or their combination (B + L, red). **B**: "Steady-state" force at each step was plotted as function of [K$^+$] with values at 50 mM K$^+$ as 100%. Results show mean ± s.e.m, n = 4. *, ***: P<0.05, 0.001 versus control. **C**: Change of basal tension (Δ force in mN) for repolarization and depolarization of V$_m$ by changing extracellular K$^+$ to attain V$_m$ within the physiological range for non-stimulated VSMCs (K$^+$ from 5.9 mM to 2 (white) or 10 (grey) or 15 (black) mM) in control conditions (C) and in the presence of 30 nM BAY K8644 (B). Instead of the actual K$^+$ concentration, the estimated V$_m$ of the VSMCs is indicated: -77 mV for 2 mM, -66 mV for 5.9 mM, (not shown), -59 mV for 10 mM and −51 mV for 15 mM K$^+$. Results show mean ± s.e.m, n = 5. *, **, ***: P<0.05, 0.01, 0.001 versus 5.9 mM K$^+$.

Relationships between fast and slow contraction phases and Ca^{2+} influx

The contraction elicited by depolarization of VSMCs has been studied extensively [39], but has never been directly correlated with the known electrophysiological properties of L-type Ca^{2+} channels. L-type Ca^{2+} currents in isolated SMCs of various tissues and species display a bell-shaped voltage-dependence with maximal currents at 0 to +20 mV [1,2,14,22,23,25,40]. Activation (opening) of L-type Ca^{2+} channels starts at −50 to −40 mV with half-maximal activation at −30 mV [25,41], whereas inactivation starts at −60 mV, is half maximal at about −30 mV and complete at 0 mV [23,25,41,42]. As a consequence, at voltages between current activation (around −45 mV, 20 to 25 mM K$^+$) and complete current inactivation (around 0 mV, 124 mM K$^+$), two populations of L-type Ca^{2+} channels are expected to contribute to Ca^{2+} influx and contraction. One population of channels will activate and completely inactivate during the depolarization leading to a transient Ca^{2+} influx and concomitant contraction (see Figure 5C and D). This contraction corresponds with the fast phase of contraction as described in Figure 1C, where it was elicited by step depolarizations of V$_m$ by sudden increase of K$^+$ from 5.9 mM to values above 20 mM. The physiological importance of these events in VSMCs can be questioned. However, in some experiments (Figure 3), fast time- and voltage-dependent intracellular Ca^{2+} and force spikes appeared on top of a slow rise in tone or Ca^{2+} at 15 to 20 mM K$^+$ (−50 to −44 mV), which is near the activation voltage of L-type Ca^{2+} channels and within the physiological range of VSMCs V$_m$. As their spiking frequency increased with the amplitude of the depolarization step, fusing to a single fast component at 30 and 50 mM K$^+$ (−36 and −24 mV) similar to the fast component in the step protocol, these events might be related with activation and complete inactivation of L-type Ca^{2+} channels. Because they occur at physiological V$_m$ of VSMCs, they may have physiological importance. They may be related with the persistent calcium sparklets that are increased in hypertension [43], with artery vasospasm [44] or other pathophysiological processes.

However, at all K$^+$ concentrations studied, a variable population of channels will not completely inactivate and will permit "time-independent" Ca^{2+} influx via the so-called voltage window [24]. Hence, every depolarization positive to −45 mV (± 20 mM K$^+$) should activate a time-independent, non-inactivating Ca^{2+} influx. Following removal of the fast force component by depolarization in the absence of external Ca^{2+} and, then, re-adding Ca^{2+} (Figures 5 and 6) we demonstrated that this "window" contraction showed a close temporal relationship with the increase of intracellular Ca^{2+} via window L-type Ca^{2+} influx. The electrophysiological

did not account for the biphasic pattern of high K$^+$-induced force and Ca$_i^{2+}$ and either phase was solely initiated by L-type Ca^{2+} influx.

characteristics of the L-type Ca^{2+} channel window, i.e. maximal Ca^{2+} influx at -30 mV (40 to 50 mM K^+) and a bell-shaped voltage-dependence are paralleled by a tonic force component which increased with $[K^+]$ up to 50 or 70 mM ($V_m = -20$ to -30 mV), but decreased again above 70 mM K^+, leading to a bell-shaped $[K^+]$-contraction curve. Its voltage range is bounded at negative potentials by channel activation and at more positive potentials by channel inactivation. This agrees with the K^+-dependence of the slow force component described in Figure 1C and Figure 6.

Manipulation of the window Ca^{2+} influx and contraction

Our experiments predict that basal force by aortic segments will depend on V_m and that changes of V_m within the voltage range of the L-type Ca^{2+} channel window will stimulate or inhibit Ca^{2+} influx via L-type Ca^{2+} channels and the concomitant contraction. Since removal of extracellular Ca^{2+} led to a decline of intracellular Ca^{2+} and basal tension in the VSMC of the mouse aorta, a "window" Ca^{2+} influx appeared to be operative and functional at resting potentials, which are between -40 to -60 mV [45,46]. As a consequence, a small decrease (2 mM K^+, repolarization) or increase (10 mM K^+, depolarization) of external K^+ modulates basal tension of the mouse aortic segments, probably via closing and opening of L-type Ca^{2+} channels because the effects of K^+ changes are emphasized by applying BAY K8644 (Figure 8C).

Hyperpolarization of V_m, as with EDHF [35,36,47-49] or with K_{ATP} channel openers such as levcromakalim (present study) or cromakalim [45], or with reduction of extracellular K^+ might pull V_m out of the window, thereby decreasing L-type Ca^{2+} influx, inducing vasodilatation, elevated arterial compliance [50], and hypotension. For example, in the present study, levcromakalim, which causes hyperpolarization to V_K of -85 mV at 5.9 mM K^+ [47], caused a decline of resting intracellular Ca^{2+} and baseline tension, and shifted the $[K^+]$-contraction curve to higher K^+ concentrations by $+6$ mM K^+ at midpoint.

On the other hand, it is expected that factors causing depolarization of the membrane potential such as intravascular pressure [51], hypertension [2,52], a deficient NO release as in $eNOS^{-/-}$ mice [45], the absence of TRPC6 channels [46] might force the VSMC V_m in the L-type Ca^{2+} channel window leading to increased window L-type Ca^{2+} influx, basal constriction, decreased arterial compliance, increased myogenic responses and hypertension.

Therefore, results of the present study indicate that the position of the L-type Ca^{2+} channel window along the voltage axis may have profound effects on basal and stimulated Ca^{2+} influx in VSMC, but also predict that shifts of the activation or inactivation curves of L-type Ca^{2+} channels affect vasoconstriction and/or dilatation. For example, BAY K8644, which shifts the L-type Ca^{2+} channel activation curve to hyperpolarized potentials [33,34], caused an increase of basal Ca^{2+} influx and tone (Figure 8, see also [30]). Furthermore, Bay K8644 shifted the $[K^+]$-response curve to lower K^+ concentrations by about 8 mM at midpoint, independent of the presence of levcromakalim, indicating that both the position of the window on the voltage axis and the resting membrane potential determine the window contraction.

Finally, because a number of alternatively spliced isoforms of the calcium channel gene protein exist, the L-type Ca^{2+} channel population is not homogeneous. The isoforms display differences in tissue distribution, physiology, pharmacology and disease-related up- and/or down-regulation [14,41,42,53], but also show altered voltage-dependent activation and inactivation, thereby influencing window currents [54]. Hence, changes in the expression of the channel isoforms within the vascular tree [55] as can occur in hypertension [53] or atherosclerosis [14] may affect the position of the L-type Ca^{2+} channel window along the voltage axis with effects on basal and stimulated Ca^{2+} influx and blood vessel tone. Moreover, different splice variants can be expressed within a single blood vessel type and depending on the dominance of one or more isoforms, this may determine the electrophysiological properties of the Ca^{2+} channels [42,53,55,56].

K^+-induced Ca^{2+} sensitization

The "window" intracellular Ca^{2+} signal elicited by depolarization reached a steady-state at 200 s, whereas tension increased further at later time intervals. This pointed to a time-dependent and Ca^{2+}-dependent Ca^{2+} sensitization, but after normalization of the contractile responses, there was no shift of the curves with time. Hence, the time-dependent Ca^{2+} sensitization was proportional to intracellular Ca^{2+}, which is mainly determined by the extent of "steady-state" Ca^{2+} influx at each $[K^+]$. This is in line with recent data indicating that the depolarization-induced Ca^{2+} sensitization depends on Ca^{2+} entry [15,18-21] and with the results obtained with the Rho kinase inhibitors Y-27632 and HA 1077. Rho-kinase inhibition did not eliminate the bell-shape of the $[K^+]$-force curves, but emphasized its voltage-dependence. Therefore, both continuous Ca^{2+} influx and Ca^{2+}-dependent Ca^{2+} sensitization are necessary to maintain contraction, whereby Ca^{2+} influx occurs independently from Ca^{2+} sensitization, but not vice versa.

Limitations of the study

Voltage-clamp of multicellular aortic segments with electrophysiological techniques is impossible with current methods because of temporal and spatial voltage heterogeneity. Therefore, we clamped the aortic rings with extracellular K^+ although the resting V_m is not solely determined by the K^+ equilibrium potential (V_K), especially at low K^+ [51] (see Additional file 1). Taking into account that levcromakalim hyperpolarized V_m of rat mesenteric arteries from −58 to −82 mV (hyperpolarization to V_K) [47] and that in the present study levcromakalim shifted the [K^+]-force curve by +5.9 mM K^+ at midpoint, V_m at normal K^+ of 5.9 mM was calculated to be 19 mV less polarized than V_K (−66 mV instead of the Nernstian −85 mV); this is in good agreement with resting V_m of arterial SMCs mentioned in the literature [28,47] (see Additional file 1). At 20 and 50 mM K^+, the difference between V_m and V_K further diminished from 19 to 7 and 3 mV. Therefore, clamping the segments with K^+ was, in our hands, a good technique to restrain the resting V_m of the SMCs.

Conclusions

Besides a phasic, fast transient Ca^{2+} and force component, depolarization of aortic segments of C57Bl6 mice with elevated extracellular K^+ causes a tonic, slow Ca^{2+} and force component. Both components reflect the electrophysiological properties of L-type Ca^{2+} channels. The tonic force component could be attributed to window L-type Ca^{2+} influx, plays a prominent role in maintaining basal and stimulated intracellular Ca^{2+} and tension in mouse aorta, and together with Rho-kinase-mediated Ca^{2+} sensitizing may be of great importance for the (patho)physiology of conduit blood vessels. Hence, any modulation of L-type Ca^{2+} influx in VSMC is expected to affect endothelium-dependent and -independent Ca^{2+} mobilization and related vasomotor responses of blood vessels or arterial compliance. Window L-type Ca^{2+} influx may underlie the reduced relaxing efficacy of NO in mouse aorta when the contraction is elicited mainly via L-type Ca^{2+} influx [30]. Therefore, we conclude that every intervention (short or long term) that changes the resting V_m of the VSMC or the expression/properties of the population of L-type Ca^{2+} channels, favoring one or another isoform, might have implications for the window Ca^{2+} current, influx and contraction, for the sensitivity to L-type Ca^{2+} channel blockers and NO, for the arterial compliance and for the effects of hypertension on the cardiovascular system.

Methods

Aortic segments

The studies were approved by the Ethical Committee of the University of Antwerp, and the investigations conform to the Guide for the Care and Use of Laboratory Animals published by the US National Institutes of Health (NIH Publication No. 85–23, revised 1996). C57Bl6 mice (n = 72, food and water ad libitum, 12/12

light–dark cycle) were used at the age of 4 to 7 months. Animals were euthanized under pentobarbital anesthesia (sodium pentobarbital, 75 mg kg^{-1}, i.p.). The thoracic aorta was carefully removed, stripped of adherent tissue and dissected systematically. Starting at the diaphragm, the ascending thoracic aorta was cut in segments of 2 mm width (5 to 6 segments). Vessels were immersed in Krebs Ringer solution (KR 37°C, 95% O_2/5% CO_2, pH 7.4) with (in mM): NaCl 118, KCl 4.7, $CaCl_2$ 2.5, KH_2PO_4 1.2, $MgSO_4$ 1.2, $NaHCO_3$ 25, CaEDTA 0.025, and glucose 11.1. When Ca^{2+} was omitted from the KR, 1 mM EGTA was added (further named 0Ca) and, hence, to restore 2.5 mM free Ca^{2+}, 3.5 mM Ca^{2+} was added to 0Ca (further named 0–3.5Ca) from a 1.75 M $CaCl_2$ stock. High K^+- solutions were prepared by replacing NaCl with equimolar KCl.

To measure resting membrane potentials (V_m) inverted (inside out) endothelium-denuded segments were mounted in the wire myograph, incubated with HEPES-buffered bathing solution (5.4 mM KCl, 141 mM NaCl, 10 mM HEPES, 0.8 mM $MgCl_2$, 10 mM glucose, 1.8 mM $CaCl_2$, 1 μM amlodipine, pH = 7.4 at 37°C with 1 M NaOH) and impaled with glass intracellular microelectrodes (filled with 2 mM KCl and tip resistances between 65 and 90 MΩ). V_m was measured with a HEKA EPC9 amplifier (HEKA Electroniks, Germany) in the zero current clamp mode and recorded on paper (Gould pen writer). Only measurements of V_m starting with a sharp decrease of V_m upon impalement and a sharp return to approximately 0 mV upon withdrawal of the electrode were considered.

To simulate voltage clamp protocols used in electrophysiological studies, extracellular K^+ was used to clamp the aortic segments at certain estimated potentials. Depolarizing voltage steps were mimicked by graded elevation of extracellular K^+ starting from and returning to a normal resting potential at 5.9 mM K^+ (repetitive depolarization protocol). The holding potential from which voltage steps would be applied was mimicked by holding the segments at each K^+ concentration before a subsequent challenge with higher K^+ (cumulative depolarization protocol).

Isometric tension measurements

Aortic segments were mounted in 10 ml organ baths, tension (mN) was measured isometrically with a Statham UC2 force transducer (Gould) connected to a data acquisition system (Powerlab 8/30, ADInstruments, Spechbach, Germany) as described [30]. Segments were gradually stretched until a stable loading tension of 16 mN, the optimal preload to attain maximal force development by 50 or 124 mM K^+. Isometric force was reported in mN. Nitric oxide (NO) formation was inhibited with a combination of 300 μM N^Ω-nitro-L-arginine methyl ester (L-NAME) and 300 μM N^{Ω}-nitro-L-argin-ine (L-NNA) and to avoid any vasomotor interference due to prostanoids, 10 μM indomethacin was present.

Combined assay of isometric tension and VSMC Ca$_i^{2+}$

Segments were mounted in a wire (40 μm) myograph above an inverted microscope (Axiovert 200, Carl Zeiss, Zaventem, Belgium) after removal of the endothelium by rubbing their interior with a braided silk wax to avoid interference by endothelial Ca^{2+} signals. Segments were loaded for 120 minutes with aerated (95% O_2/5% CO_2, pH 7.4) KR containing 10 μM Fura-2 AM, 1 mg/ml bovine serum albumin and 0.02% Pluronic at room temperature. Then, temperature was raised to 37°C and the segment was set to its normalized diameter [30]. The single emission (510 nm) ratio at dual excitation (340 and 380 nm) was used as a relative measure of free Ca$_i^{2+}$ (relative units, RU) after subtraction of background emission values, which were determined by adding 2 mM $MnCl_2$ at the end of each experiment. Contractile force was measured simultaneously and reported in mN mm^{-1} [30].

Data analysis

All results are expressed as mean ± sem; n represents the number of mice. Time-force curves were fitted with a bi-exponential function revealing amplitudes and time constants of first (fast) and second (slow) components. Concentration-response curves were fitted with sigmoidal concentration-response equations with variable slope, which revealed maximal responses (E$_{max}$) and the negative logarithm of the concentration resulting in 50% of the maximal effect (pEC$_{50}$) for each vessel segment. Two-way ANOVA with Bonferroni post-test (concentration-response curves) and paired or unpaired t-test (GraphPad Prism, version 5, GraphPad Software, San Diego California USA) were used to compare means of the different experimental groups. A 5% level of significance was selected.

Materials

Sodium pentobarbital (Nembutal®) was obtained from Sanofi (Brussels, Belgium), indomethacin from CERTA (Belgium), L-NNA, L-NAME, nifedipine, ryanodine, 2-APB, HA-1077 dihydrochloride from Sigma (Bornem, Belgium), Fura 2-AM from Molecular Probes (Invitrogen, Merelbeke, Belgium), (±) BAY K8644, levcromakalim, glibenclamide from TOCRIS (Bristol, United Kingdom), Y-27632 dihydrochloride from Abcam Biochemicals (Cambridge, UK).

Abbreviations

Ca^{2+}: Calcium; VSMC: Vascular smooth muscle cell; K$^+$: Potassium; 2-APB: 2-aminoethoxydiphenyl borate; L-NAME: N^{Ω}-nitro-L-arginine methyl ester; L-NNA: N^{Ω}-nitro-L-arginine; NO: Nitric oxide; SERCA: Sarco-endoplasmic reticulum calcium ATPase; SR: Sarcoplasmic reticulum; eNOS: Endothelial nitric oxide synthase; V$_K$: Equilibrium potential for K$^+$ ions; V$_m$: Membrane potential.

Competing interests

The authors declare that they have no competing interests.

Authors' contributions

All authors read and approved the final manuscript. PF and CVH conceived of the study, designed the experiments, collected and analyzed the data; PF and HB drafted the manuscript, PF, CVH, JVL, DS, WM, GDM and HB participated in interpretation of the results and final draft of the manuscript.

Acknowledgements

This work was supported by grants from the Research Foundation - Flanders (Fonds voor Wetenschappelijk Onderzoek, FWO, Vlaamse Gemeenschap, project G.0174.06 and G.0293.10 N). Johanna Van Langen is supported by a Ph. D. fellowship (Aspirant) of the FWO-Flanders. With special thanks to Francois Pittoors and Pierre-Paul Van Bogaert (Faculty of Medicine, Department Physiology, University of Antwerp) for help with electrophysiological measurements.

Author details

[1]Laboratory of Physiopharmacology, University of Antwerp, Universiteitsplein 1 Building T, 2.18, Wilrijk B-2610, Belgium. [2]Laboratories of Pharmacology, University of Antwerp, Antwerp, Belgium.

References

1. Moosmang S, Schulla V, Welling A, Feil R, Feil S, Wegener JW, Hofmann F, Klugbauer N: Dominant role of smooth muscle L-type calcium channel Ca$_v$1.2 for blood pressure regulation. *EMBO J* 2003, **22**:6027–6034.
2. Pesic A, Madden JA, Pesic M, Rusch NJ: High blood pressure upregulates arterial L-type Ca^{2+} channels: is membrane depolarization the signal? *Circ Res* 2004, **94**:e97–e104.
3. Rhee SW, Stimers JR, Wang W, Pang L: Vascular smooth muscle-specific knockdown of the noncardiac form of the L-type calcium channel by microRNA-based short hairpin RNA as a potential antihypertensive therapy. *J Pharmacol Exp Ther* 2009, **329**:775–782.
4. Zhou ZH, Wang J, Xiao H, Chen ZJ, Wang M, Cheng X, Liao YH: A novel autoantibody in patients with primary hypertension: antibody against L-type Ca^{2+} channel. *Chin Med J (Engl)* 2008, **121**:1513–1517.
5. Mancia G, De BG, Dominiczak A, Cifkova R, Fagard R, Germano G, Grassi G, Heagerty AM, Kjeldsen SE, Laurent S, et al: 2007 Guidelines for the Management of Arterial Hypertension: The Task Force for the Management of Arterial Hypertension of the European Society of Hypertension (ESH) and of the European Society of Cardiology (ESC). *J Hypertens* 2007, **25**:1105–1187.
6. Westerhof N, Lankhaar JW, Westerhof BE: The arterial Windkessel. *Med Biol Eng Comput* 2009, **47**:131–141.
7. Mitchell GF: Pulse pressure, arterial compliance and cardiovascular morbidity and mortality. *Curr Opin Nephrol Hypertens* 1999, **8**:335–342.
8. Belz GG: Elastic properties and Windkessel function of the human aorta. *Cardiovasc Drugs Ther* 1995, **9**:73–83.
9. Bellien J, Favre J, Iacob M, Gao J, Thuillez C, Richard V, Joannides R: Arterial stiffness is regulated by nitric oxide and endothelium-derived hyperpolarizing factor during changes in blood flow in humans. *Hypertension* 2010, **55**:674–680.
10. Safar ME, Pannier B, Laurent S, London GM: Calcium-entry blockers and arterial compliance in hypertension. *J Cardiovasc Pharmacol* 1989, **14**(Suppl 10):S1–S6.
11. Slama M, Safavian A, Tual JL, Laurent S, Safar ME: Effects of antihypertensive drugs on large artery compliance. *Neth J Med* 1995, **47**:162–168.

12. Essalihi R, Zandvliet ML, Moreau S, Gilbert LA, Bouvet C, Lenoel C, Nekka F, McKee MD, Moreau P: Distinct effects of amlodipine treatment on vascular elastocalcinosis and stiffness in a rat model of isolated systolic hypertension. *J Hypertens* 2007, 25:1879–1886.

13. Vayssettes-Courchay C, Ragonnet C, Isabelle M, Verbeuren TJ: Aortic stiffness in vivo in hypertensive rat via echo-tracking: analysis of the pulsatile distension waveform. *Am J Physiol Heart Circ Physiol* 2011, 301:H382–H390.

14. Tiwari S, Zhang Y, Heller J, Abernethy DR, Soldatov NM: Atherosclerosis-related molecular alteration of the human Cav1.2 calcium channel alpha1C subunit. *Proc Natl Acad Sci USA* 2006, 103:17024–17029.

15. Ratz PH, Miner AS: Role of protein kinase Czeta and calcium entry in KCl-induced vascular smooth muscle calcium sensitization and feedback control of cellular calcium levels. *J Pharmacol Exp Ther* 2009, 328:399–408.

16. Fernandez-Tenorio M, Porras-Gonzalez C, Castellano A, del Valle-Rodriguez A, Lopez-Barneo J, Urena J: Metabotropic regulation of RhoA/Rho-associated kinase by L-type Ca2+ channels: new mechanism for depolarization-evoked mammalian arterial contraction. *Circ Res* 2011, 108:1348–1357.

17. Van Assche T, Fransen P, Guns PJ, Herman AG, Bult H: Altered Ca^{2+} handling of smooth muscle cells in aorta of apolipoprotein E-deficient mice before development of atherosclerotic lesions. *Cell Calcium* 2007, 41:295–302.

18. Villalba N, Stankevicius E, Simonsen U, Prieto D: Rho kinase is involved in Ca^{2+} entry of rat penile small arteries. *Am J Physiol Heart Circ Physiol* 2008, 294:H1923–H1932.

19. Sakurada S, Takuwa N, Sugimoto N, Wang Y, Seto M, Sasaki Y, Takuwa Y: Ca^{2+}-dependent activation of Rho and Rho kinase in membrane depolarization-induced and receptor stimulation-induced vascular smooth muscle contraction. *Circ Res* 2003, 93:548–556.

20. Hirano K: Current topics in the regulatory mechanism underlying the Ca^{2+} sensitization of the contractile apparatus in vascular smooth muscle. *J Pharmacol Sci* 2007, 104:109–115.

21. Mita M, Yanagihara H, Hishinuma S, Saito M, Walsh MP: Membrane depolarization-induced contraction of rat caudal arterial smooth muscle involves Rho-associated kinase. *Biochem J* 2002, 364:431–440.

22. Ganitkevich VY, Isenberg G: Contribution of two types of calcium channels to membrane conductance of single myocytes from guinea-pig coronary artery. *J Physiol* 1990, 426:19–42.

23. Matsuda JJ, Volk KA, Shibata EF: Calcium currents in isolated rabbit coronary arterial smooth muscle myocytes. *J Physiol* 1990, 427:657–680.

24. Fleischmann BK, Murray RK, Kotlikoff MI: Voltage window for sustained elevation of cytosolic calcium in smooth muscle cells. *Proc Natl Acad Sci U S A* 1994, 91:11914–11918.

25. Curtis TM, Scholfield CN: Nifedipine blocks Ca^{2+} store refilling through a pathway not involving L-type Ca^{2+} channels in rabbit arteriolar smooth muscle. *J Physiol* 2001, 532:609–623.

26. Smirnov SV, Aaronson PI: Ca^{2+} currents in single myocytes from human mesenteric arteries: evidence for a physiological role of L-type channels. *J Physiol* 1992, 457:455–475.

27. Zhang J, Berra-Romani R, Sinnegger-Brauns MJ, Striessnig J, Blaustein MP, Matteson DR: Role of $Ca_v1.2$ L-type Ca^{2+} channels in vascular tone: effects of nifedipine and Mg^{2+}. *Am J Physiol Heart Circ Physiol* 2007, 292:H415–H425.

28. Cobine CA, Callaghan BP, Keef KD: Role of L-type calcium channels and PKC in active tone development in rabbit coronary artery. *Am J Physiol Heart Circ Physiol* 2007, 292:H3079–H3088.

29. Sonkusare S, Palade PT, Marsh JD, Telemaque S, Pesic A, Rusch NJ: Vascular calcium channels and high blood pressure: pathophysiology and therapeutic implications. *Vascul Pharmacol* 2006, 44:131–142.

30. Van Hove CE, Van der Donckt C, Herman AG, Bult H, Fransen P: Vasodilator efficacy of nitric oxide depends on mechanisms of intracellular calcium mobilization in mouse aortic smooth muscle cells. *Br J Pharmacol* 2009, 158:920–930.

31. Bootman MD, Collins TJ, Mackenzie L, Roderick HL, Berridge MJ, Peppiatt CM: 2-aminoethoxydiphenyl borate (2-APB) is a reliable blocker of store-operated Ca^{2+} entry but an inconsistent inhibitor of InsP3-induced Ca^{2+} release. *FASEB J* 2002, 16:1145–1150.

32. Barrett CF, Cao YQ, Tsien RW: Gating deficiency in a familial hemiplegic migraine type 1 mutant P/Q-type calcium channel. *J Biol Chem* 2005, 280:24064–24071.

33. Saponara S, Sgaragli G, Fusi F: Quercetin antagonism of Bay K 8644 effects on rat tail artery L-type Ca(2+) channels. *Eur J Pharmacol* 2008, 598:75–80.

34. Teramoto N, Tomoda T, Ito Y: Mefenamic acid as a novel activator of L-type voltage-dependent Ca^{2+} channels in smooth muscle cells from pig proximal urethra. *Br J Pharmacol* 2005, 144:919–925.

35. Edwards G, Dora KA, Gardener MJ, Garland CJ, Weston AH: K^+ is an endothelium-derived hyperpolarizing factor in rat arteries. *Nature* 1998, 396:269–272.

36. Edwards G, Weston AH: Potassium and potassium clouds in endothelium-dependent hyperpolarizations. *Pharmacol Res* 2004, 49:535–541.

37. Karaki H, Ozaki H, Hori M, Mitsui-Saito M, Amano K, Harada K, Miyamoto S, Nakazawa H, Won KJ, Sato K: Calcium movements, distribution, and functions in smooth muscle. *Pharmacol Rev* 1997, 49:157–230.

38. Urena J, del Valle-Rodriguez A, Lopez-Barneo J: Metabotropic Ca^{2+} channel-induced calcium release in vascular smooth muscle. *Cell Calcium* 2007, 42:513–520.

39. Akata T: Cellular and molecular mechanisms regulating vascular tone. Part 1: basic mechanisms controlling cytosolic Ca^{2+} concentration and the Ca^{2+}-dependent regulation of vascular tone. *J Anesth* 2007, 21:220–231.

40. Navedo MF, Amberg GC, Westenbroek RE, Sinnegger-Brauns MJ, Catterall WA, Striessnig J, Santana LF: Ca(v)1.3 channels produce persistent calcium sparklets, but Ca(v)1.2 channels are responsible for sparklets in mouse arterial smooth muscle. *Am J Physiol Heart Circ Physiol* 2007, 293:H1359–H1370.

41. Liao P, Yong TF, Liang MC, Yue DT, Soong TW: Splicing for alternative structures of $Ca_v1.2$ Ca^{2+} channels in cardiac and smooth muscles. *Cardiovasc Res* 2005, 68:197–203.

42. Liao P, Yu D, Li G, Yong TF, Soon JL, Chua YL, Soong TW: A smooth muscle $Ca_v1.2$ calcium channel splice variant underlies hyperpolarized window current and enhanced state-dependent inhibition by nifedipine. *J Biol Chem* 2007, 282:35133–35142.

43. Nieves-Cintron M, Amberg GC, Navedo MF, Molkentin JD, Santana LF: The control of Ca^{2+} influx and NFATc3 signaling in arterial smooth muscle during hypertension. *Proc Natl Acad Sci U S A* 2008, 105:15623–15628.

44. McNeish AJ, Altayo FJ, Garland CJ: Evidence both L-type and non-L-type voltage-dependent calcium channels contribute to cerebral artery vasospasm following loss of NO in the rat. *Vascul Pharmacol* 2010, 53:151–159.

45. Chataigneau T, Feletou M, Huang PL, Fishman MC, Duhault J, Vanhoutte PM: Acetylcholine-induced relaxation in blood vessels from endothelial nitric oxide synthase knockout mice. *Br J Pharmacol* 1999, 126:219–226.

46. Dietrich A, Mederos YS, Gollasch M, Gross V, Storch U, Dubrovska G, Obst M, Yildirim E, Salanova B, Kalwa H, et al: Increased vascular smooth muscle contractility in TRPC6$^{-/-}$ mice. *Mol Cell Biol* 2005, 25:6980–6989.

47. Weston AH, Richards GR, Burnham MP, Feletou M, Vanhoutte PM, Edwards G: K^+-induced hyperpolarization in rat mesenteric artery: identification, localization and role of Na^+/K^+-ATPases. *Br J Pharmacol* 2002, 136:918–926.

48. Feletou M, Vanhoutte PM: EDHF: an update. *Clin Sci (Lond)* 2009, 117:139–155.

49. Scotland RS, Madhani M, Chauhan S, Moncada S, Andresen J, Nilsson H, Hobbs AJ, Ahluwalia A: Investigation of vascular responses in endothelial nitric oxide synthase/cyclooxygenase-1 double-knockout mice: key role for endothelium-derived hyperpolarizing factor in the regulation of blood pressure in vivo. *Circulation* 2005, 111:796–803.

50. Safar ME, Blacher J, Jankowski P: Arterial stiffness, pulse pressure, and cardiovascular disease-is it possible to break the vicious circle? *Atherosclerosis* 2011, 218:263–271.

51. Knot HJ, Nelson MT: Regulation of arterial diameter and wall [Ca^{2+}] in cerebral arteries of rat by membrane potential and intravascular pressure. *J Physiol* 1998, 508(Pt 1):199–209.

52. Morel N, Godfraind T: Selective interaction of the calcium antagonist amlodipine with calcium channels in arteries of spontaneously hypertensive rats. *J Cardiovasc Pharmacol* 1994, 24:524–533.

53. Tang ZZ, Liao P, Li G, Jiang FL, Yu D, Hong X, Yong TF, Tan G, Lu S, Wang J, et al: Differential splicing patterns of L-type calcium channel $Ca_v1.2$

subunit in hearts of Spontaneously Hypertensive Rats and Wistar Kyoto Rats. *Biochim Biophys Acta* 2008, **1783:**118–130.

54. Liao P, Yu D, Lu S, Tang Z, Liang MC, Zeng S, Lin W, Soong TW: **Smooth muscle-selective alternatively spliced exon generates functional variation in Ca_v1.2 calcium channels.** *J Biol Chem* 2004, **279:**50329–50335.

55. Nystoriak MA, Murakami K, Penar PL, Wellman GC: **Ca(v)1.2 splice variant with exon 9* is critical for regulation of cerebral artery diameter.** *Am J Physiol Heart Circ Physiol* 2009, **297:**H1820–H1828.

56. Cheng X, Pachuau J, Blaskova E, suncion-Chin M, Liu J, Dopico AM, Jaggar JH: **Alternative splicing of Ca_v1.2 channel exons in smooth muscle cells of resistance-size arteries generates currents with unique electrophysiological properties.** *Am J Physiol Heart Circ Physiol* 2009, **297:**H680–H688.

15

Significance of K_{ATP} channels, L-type Ca^{2+} channels and CYP450-4A enzymes in oxygen sensing in mouse cremaster muscle arterioles *In vivo*

Anh Thuc Ngo[1*], Mads Riemann[1], Niels-Henrik Holstein-Rathlou[1], Christian Torp-Pedersen[2] and Lars Jørn Jensen[3]

Abstract

Background: ATP-sensitive K^+ channels (K_{ATP} channels), NO, prostaglandins, 20-HETE and L-type Ca^{2+} channels have all been suggested to be involved in oxygen sensing in skeletal muscle arterioles, but the role of the individual mechanisms remain controversial. We aimed to establish the importance of these mechanisms for oxygen sensing in arterioles in an *in vivo* model of metabolically active skeletal muscle. For this purpose we utilized the exteriorized cremaster muscle of anesthetized mice, in which the cremaster muscle was exposed to controlled perturbation of tissue PO_2.

Results: Change from "high" oxygen tension ($PO_2 = 153.4 \pm 3.4$ mmHg) to "low" oxygen tension ($PO_2 = 13.8 \pm 1.3$ mmHg) dilated cremaster muscle arterioles from 11.0 ± 0.4 μm to 32.9 ± 0.9 μm (n = 28, P < 0.05). Glibenclamide (K_{ATP} channel blocker) caused maximal vasoconstriction, and abolished the dilation to low oxygen, whereas the K_{ATP} channel opener cromakalim caused maximal dilation and prevented the constriction to high oxygen. When adding cromakalim on top of glibenclamide or vice versa, the reactivity to oxygen was gradually restored. Inhibition of L-type Ca^{2+} channels using 3 μM nifedipine did not fully block basal tone in the arterioles, but rendered them unresponsive to changes in PO_2. Inhibition of the CYP450-4A enzyme using DDMS blocked vasoconstriction to an increase in PO_2, but had no effect on dilation to low PO_2.

Conclusions: We conclude that: 1) L-type Ca^{2+} channels are central to oxygen sensing, 2) K_{ATP} channels are permissive for the arteriolar response to oxygen, but are not directly involved in the oxygen sensing mechanism and 3) CYP450-4A mediated 20-HETE production is involved in vasoconstriction to high PO_2.

Keywords: Hypoxic vasodilation, Hyperoxic vasoconstriction, Oxygen sensing, ATP-sensitive K^+ channels, 20-HETE, L-type Ca^{2+} channels, Prostaglandin, NO-synthase, Skeletal muscle, Arterioles

Background

In the microcirculation, the arterioles regulate tissue blood flow to maintain a close relationship between oxygen supply and demand [1]. Changes in oxygen tension due to changes in the metabolic activity of tissues, particularly in skeletal muscle undergoing vast changes in performance, are believed to be crucial in the regulation of local blood flow. For example, skeletal muscle arterioles dilate/constrict when exposed to a decrease/increase in oxygen tension, thereby controlling the local blood flow to the tissue [1,2].

The mechanisms by which changes in oxygen tension are sensed and converted into downstream signals that lead to vasomotor responses is known as *oxygen sensing*. Because of the importance of oxygen sensing for adjusting skeletal muscle blood flow, several studies have sought to determine its underlying molecular mechanisms. A number of studies have provided evidence which suggests the involvement of ATP-sensitive K^+ channels (K_{ATP} channels) in the process [3-6], but a similar number of studies from

* Correspondence: anhngo@sund.ku.dk
[1]Department of Biomedical Sciences, Faculty of Health and Medical Sciences, The Panum institute, University of Copenhagen, Blegdamsvej 3, DK-2200 Copenhagen N, Denmark
Full list of author information is available at the end of the article

other groups have failed to find evidence to support this notion [7-9]. As an alternative it has been suggested that hypoxia may act on the voltage-dependent L-type Ca^{2+} channels reducing the Ca^{2+} influx into the vascular smooth muscle cells (VSMCs) causing hypoxic vasodilation [9,10]. Nitric oxide (NO) and certain prostaglandins are known to be important endothelium-derived vasodilators and may therefore also play a role in hypoxic vasodilation.

Hypoxic vasodilation may be viewed as a single O_2-sensitive effector mechanism operating to continuously modify the basal tone of the vessel. However, the operation of dual control mechanisms, i.e. both hypoxic vasodilation and a separate mechanism primarily activated during high oxygen tension to cause vasoconstriction may contribute to an even more elaborate and efficient regulation of local blood flow. The vasoconstrictor 20-hydroxy-eicosatetraenoic acid (20-HETE), which is a ω-hydroxylation product of arachidonic acid produced by the CYP450-4A enzyme system in the presence of molecular oxygen, may be such a mechanism involved in hyperoxic vasoconstriction [11-14].

Many studies have been performed *in vitro*, and have focused on determining the role of a single mechanism for oxygen sensing. However, by examining several proposed mechanisms in an *in vivo* animal model during controlled physiological conditions we are able to study the integrated roles of the different mechanisms for oxygen sensing.

In the present study, we used the exteriorized cremaster muscle in anesthetized male mice. The influence of experimental procedures was minimized by doing only mild surgery under the influence of neurolept anesthesia, which is not known to have any major effects on cardiovascular function [15], and the diameter responses to local tissue oxygen perturbations were observed by intravital microscopy.

Since considerable controversy remains regarding the specific mechanisms responsible for oxygen sensing in skeletal muscle, the main purpose of this study was to address the specific roles of K_{ATP} channels, NO, prostaglandins, 20-HETE and L-type Ca^{2+} channels in this process.

Methods

Cremaster muscle preparation

All procedures and protocols were approved by the Danish Animal Care and Use Committee. Male C57BL/6J mice (body weight = 27.6 ± 0.7 g, n = 28; Taconic, DK-8680 Ry, Denmark) were anesthetized by *i.p.* injection with a mixture of droperidol (30.8 mg/kg), midazolam (4.0 mg/kg) and fentanyl (0.2 mg/kg) dissolved in saline (total volume given was 20 ml/kg). This same anesthetic mixture was used to maintain anesthesia, by continuous *i.v.* infusion with the rate of 20 ml/kg/h (syringe pump model 100,

serial no. 671, KD Scientific, U.S.A). The mice were tracheotomized to maintain airway patency and the jugular vein was cannulated to allow for infusion of anesthesia and saline, while resting on top of the heated microscope stage. Using gentle dissection, the cremaster muscle with its blood perfusion intact was placed flat on top of a coverslip and fixed by sutures (Prolene 6-0, Ethicon Inc., Somerville, New Jersey, U.S.A.) attached to a silicone bank.

Superfusion of the cremaster muscle

The Krebs' solutions (118.4 mM NaCl, 4.8 mM KCl, 2.5 mM $CaCl_2$, 1.2 mM $MgSO_4$, 25.0 mM $NaHCO_3$ and 1.2 mM KH_2PO_4, pH range 7.35-7.45) were vigorously bubbled with 95% N_2/5% CO_2 or 21% O_2/74% N_2/5% CO_2 gas mixtures to yield low or high oxygen tension Krebs' solutions respectively. To minimize gas exchange between the superfusate in the supply tubing and the atmospheric air, the length of the tubing was kept at a minimum and thick-walled polyurethane tubing was used (Flexible Tubing 85 Durometer Polyurethane AP01T122PENA, Ark-Plas Products, Inc. Flippin, Arkansas). The superfusate was heated through an inline heater system (Inline heater Model SH-27B, automatic temperature controller TC-324B, Warner Instrument Corporation, Hamden, Connecticut) to a temperature of 34-36°C.

Vessel diameter measurement

The microcirculation of the cremaster muscle was visualized using a motorized Olympus BX50WI microscope with a fixed stage enabling free positioning of the 4× air- or 20× water-immersion objectives on top of the exteriorized cremaster muscle. The field was viewed on a monitor (Triniton, PWM 1442 QM, Sony, Tokyo, Japan) using a monochrome CCD camera (CCD72S, Dage-MTI Michigan City, IN), and images were recorded on a HDD-recorder (Pioneer DVD recorder DVR-530H) for later off-line analysis. The final magnification (20× objective) of the image was ~700× and the final pixel size was ~0.6 μm. The vessel diameter of the arteriole was measured offline as the external diameter in micrometers (μm).

Oxygen tension measurement

A fiber-optic oxygen microsensor system (Tapered tip sensor, tip diameter < 50 μm, Microx TX3 Oxygen Meter, PreSens, Regensburg, Germany) was used to measure oxygen tensions in the cremaster muscle microcirculation. The oxygen microsensor consists of a fiber-optic cable with a luminophore at the tip. The luminophore is excited by photons from the oxygen meter. Depending on the presence of molecular oxygen, either photons are reemitted from the luminophore and these are subsequently registered by the oxygen meter, or the energy from the activated luminophore is transferred to the oxygen molecules in the surrounding solution. Thus, the probe does not consume oxygen during the measurements, and consequently, does not by itself affect the oxygen levels within the cremaster muscle tissue. Calibration of the microsensor was performed with a two-point calibration in *oxygen-free water* prepared by diluting 4 g sodium dithionite ($Na_2S_2O_4$) in 60 ml water in a beaker, and *water vapor-saturated air* prepared by placing wet cotton wool in another beaker. The output of the oxygen sensor is given as the partial oxygen tension in mmHg. All oxygen tension measurements were done with the tip of the oxygen microsensor placed on top of the cremaster muscle in the intersection between the cremaster muscle and the superfusate in close proximity (< 100 µm) to the arterioles under study. The tip, which is the active part of the oxygen microsensor, was always covered by Krebs' solution and continuous measurements were done throughout the whole experiment with a 1 Hz sampling rate.

Drugs

To study the mechanisms of oxygen sensing, different drugs were used. Cromakalim (1 and 5 µM), an activator of K_{ATP} channels, glibenclamide (10 and 100 µM), an inhibitor of K_{ATP} channels and nifedipine (3 and 30 µM), a Ca^{2+} antagonist, which inhibits voltage-dependent L-type Ca^{2+} channels, were used to study the role of K_{ATP} channels and L-type Ca^{2+} channels. Dibromo-dodecenyl-methylsulfimide (DDMS, 10 µM), an inhibitor of the cytochrome P450-4A enzyme system (CYP450-4A), was used to study the role of 20-HETE. The role of prostaglandins was studied by using indomethacin (28 µM), an inhibitor of cyclooxygenase. L-NAME (100 µM), an inhibitor of NO-synthases, was used to study the role of NO. Papaverine (100 µM), a smooth muscle cell relaxant, was used to maximally dilate the arterioles to obtain the passive diameter of the arterioles. Cromakalim, glibenclamide and indomethacin were dissolved in dimethyl sulfoxide (DMSO, 0.3%) prior to adding to the Krebs' solution. The other drugs were dissolved directly in Krebs' solution. Cromakalim, glibenclamide, indomethacin, L-NAME, nifedipine and papaverine were bought from Sigma-Aldrich, Copenhagen, Denmark, whereas DDMS was bought from Cayman chemical, Michigan, USA.

Experimental procedures

After preparation of the exteriorized cremaster muscle, the tissue was superfused with low oxygen Krebs' solution and the preparation was allowed to rest for the next 15-20 minutes to obtain steady state. Subsequently, hyperoxic vasoconstriction and hypoxic vasodilation was induced by superfusing the cremaster muscle with Krebs' solution containing high or low oxygen tension, respectively. Among several cremaster muscle arterioles

(diameter < 40 µm) showing both hyperoxic vasoconstriction and hypoxic vasodilation, one or two arterioles were randomly picked for further study.

The experimental protocol was as follows. During the control period the cremaster muscle was exposed to low oxygen tension followed by high oxygen tension two or three times. Then the cremaster muscle was exposed to low oxygen tension and high oxygen tension in the presence of drugs, and this was repeated at least once. In some experiments two different drugs were added, in other experiments cumulative concentrations of the same drug were added. Afterwards the cremaster muscle was exposed to low oxygen and high oxygen tensions without drugs (wash-out period). At the end of the experiments papaverine was superfused to yield the maximal vessel diameter.

Data analysis

One or two arterioles were studied per mouse and the outer vessel diameters (D) were measured. $\Delta D = D_{low\ oxygen} - D_{high\ oxygen}$, where $D_{low\ oxygen}$ is vessel diameter during low oxygen tension and $D_{high\ oxygen}$ is vessel diameter during high oxygen tension. All results are presented as mean ± SEM. Statistical comparisons were performed by paired two-tailed Student's t-test or one-way ANOVA repeated measures with Holm-Sidak method as post-hoc analysis. P-values < 0.05 were considered as statistically significant.

Results

Superfusion with either low or high oxygen Krebs' solutions had a pronounced effect on the arteriolar diameter and hence on local blood flow to the mouse cremaster muscle. The preparations were stable for 2-3 hours, enough time to study vasomotor responses under different experimental conditions. Images in Figure 1A-C show a representative mouse cremaster muscle arteriole during exposure to low (A), high oxygen tensions (B) and during exposure to a 100 µM papaverine (C). During low oxygen tension (PO_2 = 4.6 mmHg) the external diameter of the arteriole was 32.0 µm. During high oxygen tension (PO_2 = 163.4 mmHg) the arteriole was constricted with external diameter of 9.8 µm. Exposure to 100 µM papaverine (PO_2 = 42.6 mmHg) yielded a maximal external diameter of 35.1 µm. Table 1 summarizes the effects on the vasomotor responses during superfusion with low (PO_2 = 13.8 ± 1.3 mmHg) and high oxygen tensions (PO_2 = 153.4 ± 3.4 mmHg) and 100 µM papaverine (PO_2 = 21.5 ± 1.9 mmHg) from all experiments conducted in this study (n = 28).

Vehicle control

DMSO was used to dissolve cromakalim, glibenclamide and indomethacin. DMSO at concentrations up to 0.3%

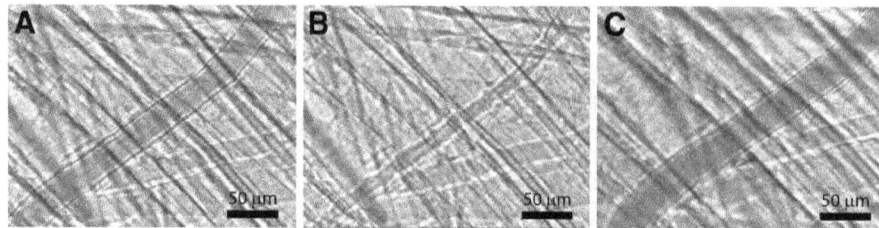

Figure 1 Representative images of a mouse cremaster arteriole during exposure to A) a low oxygen tension, B) a high oxygen tension and C) during application of 100 µM papaverine.

was used in the final Krebs' solution. To ensure that DMSO did not affect the vascular responses, we tested if there was any difference between the control without DMSO vs. superfusion with Krebs' solution containing 0.3% DMSO (See Figure 2) (n = 3). During the control, change from high oxygen ($PO_2 = 147.6 \pm 6.0$ mmHg) to low oxygen tension ($PO_2 = 16.5 \pm 1.7$ mmHg) caused a vasodilation ($\Delta D = 19.9 \pm 0.9$ µm). In the presence of 0.3% DMSO, change from high oxygen ($PO_2 = 145.3 \pm 6.5$ mmHg) to low oxygen tension ($PO_2 = 20.2 \pm 2.2$ mmHg) caused a similar vasodilation ($\Delta D = 19.3 \pm 1.5$ µm) as during the control (p = 0.48, n = 3). Application of 100 µM papaverine yielded the maximal vessel diameter 32.0 ± 1.4 µm.

Role of K$_{ATP}$ channels

Figure 3 shows the effects of pharmacological modification of K$_{ATP}$ channel activity using glibenclamide and cromakalim. During the control period, change from high oxygen ($PO_2 = 148.4 \pm 10.2$ mmHg) to low oxygen tension ($PO_2 = 12.7 \pm 2.6$ mmHg) caused vasodilation ($\Delta D = 21.2 \pm 1.9$ µm). Subsequent application of 5 µM glibenclamide inhibited vasodilation during low oxygen tension ($PO_2 = 9.6 \pm 4.6$ mmHg). This inhibition could be reversed stepwise by additional application of 1 and 5 µM cromakalim. After a wash-out period lasting ~10 minutes, the vessels regained the same degree of responsiveness to low and high oxygen tensions as during the control period. Application of 100 µM papaverine yielded the maximal vessel diameter 36.8 ± 1.7 µm (n = 5).

To examine a potential effect of order of application, cromakalim was now applied prior to glibenclamide. In

Table 1 The summarized effects of exposure to low, high oxygen tension and during application of 100 µM papaverine on arteriolar diameter (Mean ± SEM, *p < 0.05 vs. high oxygen and papaverine, †p < 0.05 vs. low oxygen and papaverine, ‡p < 0.05 vs. low oxygen and high oxygen, n = 28)

n = 28	Low oxygen	High oxygen	100 µM papaverine
Arteriolar diameter	32.9 ± 0.9 µm *	11.0 ± 0.4 µm †	37.5 ± 1.3 µm ‡
Oxygen tension	13.8 ± 1.3 mmHg	153.4 ± 3.4 mmHg	21.5 ± 1.9 mmHg

Figure 4A, during the control period a change from high oxygen ($PO_2 = 143.5 \pm 5.5$ mmHg) to low oxygen tension ($PO_2 = 10.8 \pm 3.1$ mmHg) caused vasodilation ($\Delta D = 24.9 \pm 1.2$ µm). Subsequent application of 1 µM cromakalim inhibited the vasoconstriction during high oxygen tension. The additional application of 10 µM glibenclamide caused reappearance of the vasoconstriction during high oxygen tension ($PO_2 = 153.0 \pm 7.1$ mmHg), whereas the dilation during low oxygen tension ($PO_2 = 7.7 \pm 2.2$ mmHg) was blunted. In a separate series of experiments (See Figure 4B), 100 µM glibenclamide completely reversed the cromakalim-induced vasodilation. In both series of experiments the vessels regained full responsiveness to changes in oxygen tension following wash-out of the drugs.

Role of 20-HETE

Figure 5 shows the effect of application of DDMS, an inhibitor of 20-HETE production, on vasomotor responses during low and high oxygen tensions (n = 5). During the control period, change from high oxygen ($PO_2 = 179.5 \pm 6.5$ mmHg) to low oxygen tension ($PO_2 = 10.3 \pm 3.1$ mmHg) dilated the arterioles ($\Delta D = 19.8 \pm 1.5$ µm). Application of

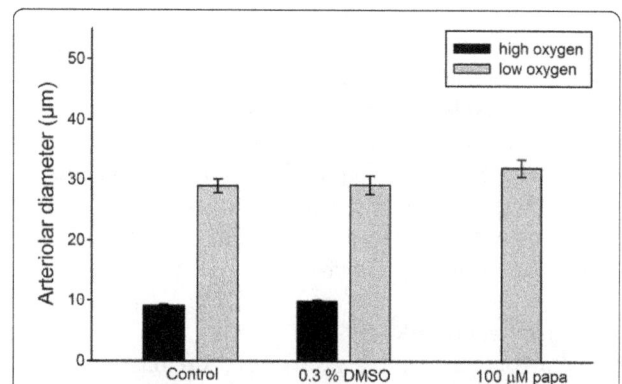

Figure 2 Effects of DMSO were evaluated. During the control, high oxygen tension constricted the arterioles, whereas low oxygen tension dilated them. Vessels responded equally in the presence or absence of 0.3% DMSO. There were no statistically significant difference in arteriolar diameter between the control and 0.3% DMSO during low oxygen tension (p = 0.709) and during high oxygen tension (p = 0.188).

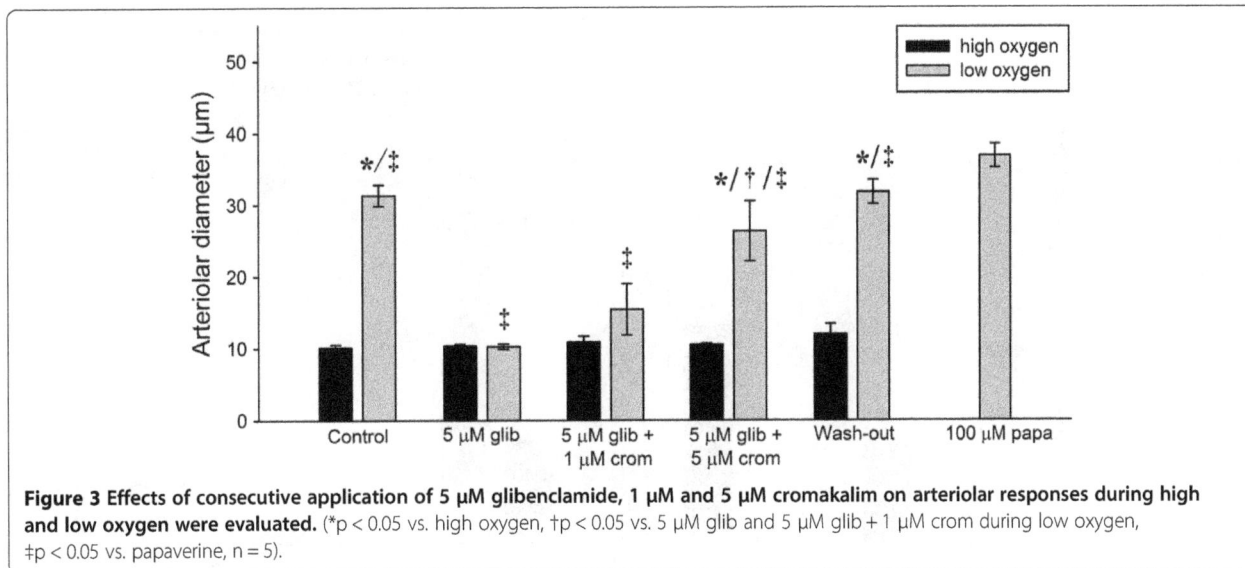

Figure 3 Effects of consecutive application of 5 µM glibenclamide, 1 µM and 5 µM cromakalim on arteriolar responses during high and low oxygen were evaluated. (*p < 0.05 vs. high oxygen, †p < 0.05 vs. 5 µM glib and 5 µM glib + 1 µM crom during low oxygen, ‡p < 0.05 vs. papaverine, n = 5).

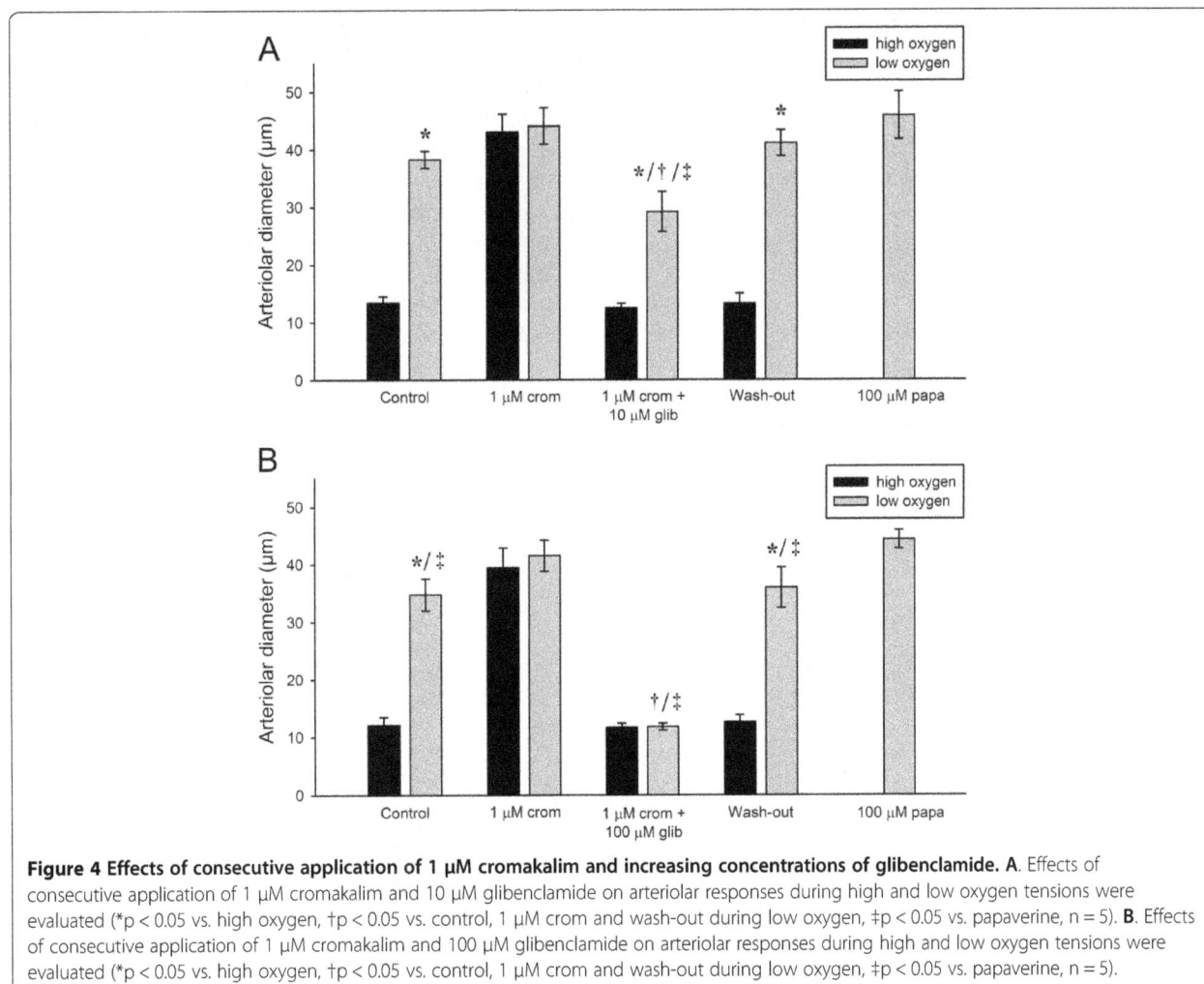

Figure 4 Effects of consecutive application of 1 µM cromakalim and increasing concentrations of glibenclamide. A. Effects of consecutive application of 1 µM cromakalim and 10 µM glibenclamide on arteriolar responses during high and low oxygen tensions were evaluated (*p < 0.05 vs. high oxygen, †p < 0.05 vs. control, 1 µM crom and wash-out during low oxygen, ‡p < 0.05 vs. papaverine, n = 5). **B**. Effects of consecutive application of 1 µM cromakalim and 100 µM glibenclamide on arteriolar responses during high and low oxygen tensions were evaluated (*p < 0.05 vs. high oxygen, †p < 0.05 vs. control, 1 µM crom and wash-out during low oxygen, ‡p < 0.05 vs. papaverine, n = 5).

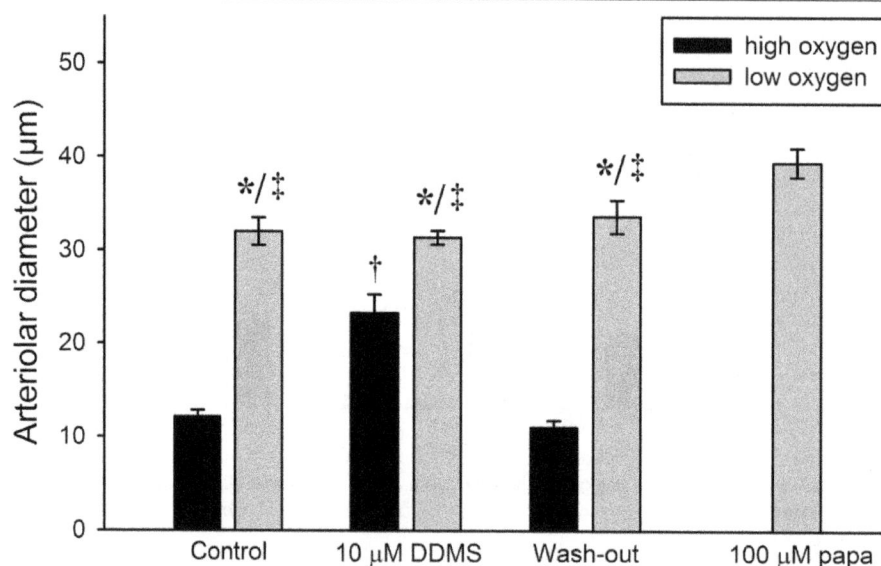

Figure 5 Effects of 10 µM DDMS on the arteriolar responses during high and low oxygen tensions were evaluated (*p < 0.05 vs. high oxygen, †p < 0.05 vs. control high oxygen and wash-out high oxygen, ‡p < 0.05 vs. papaverine, n = 5).

10 µM DDMS significantly inhibited vasoconstriction during high oxygen (PO_2 = 174.2 ± 3.3 mmHg) (p < 0.05, n = 5), but did not have any effect on arteriolar diameter during low oxygen tension (PO_2 = 8.1 ± 2.8 mmHg). After wash-out, vasomotor responses to changes in oxygen tension were similar to control. Application of 100 µM papaverine yielded the maximal vessel diameter 39.4 ± 1.6 µm.

Role of L-type Ca²⁺ channels

Both K_{ATP} channels and 20-HETE [4,11] cause vasomotor responses through changes in VSMC membrane potential and voltage-dependent L-type Ca^{2+} channels are therefore a central part of their signaling pathways.

Moreover, L-type Ca^{2+} channels have been proposed to be sensitive to changes in the oxygen tension [9,10].

Figure 6 shows the effects of blockade of the L-type Ca^{2+} channels by increasing concentrations of nifedipine (3 and 30 µM) on vasomotor responses of the arterioles during both low and high oxygen tensions (n = 5). During the control period, change from high (PO_2 = 167.1 ± 4.3 mmHg) to low oxygen tension (PO_2 = 14.2 ± 3.3 mmHg) caused vasodilation (ΔD = 19.4 ± 1.0 µm). Application of 3 µM nifedipine completely abolished the vasomotor response following the change from high (PO_2 = 159.7 ± 4.6 mmHg) to low oxygen tension (PO_2 = 14.8 ± 1.9 mmHg) in the superfusate. However, the vessels retained a statistically significant basal tone at both

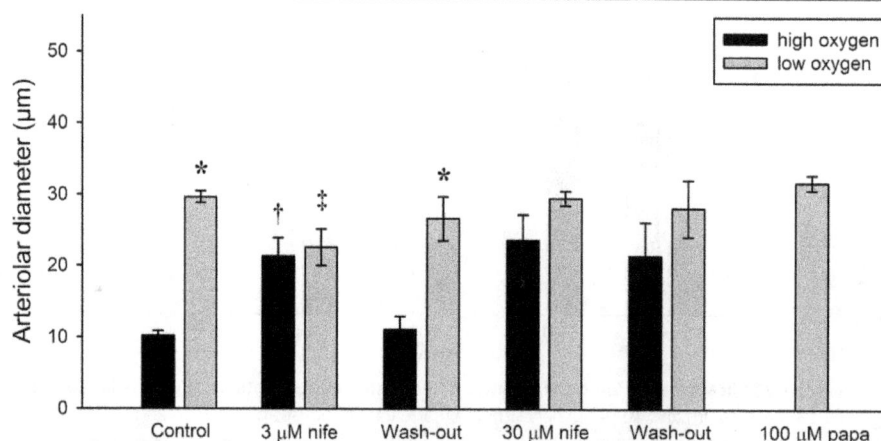

Figure 6 Effects of cumulative stepwise application of 3 µM and 30 µM nifedipine on arteriolar responses were evaluated (*p < 0.05 vs. high oxygen, †p < 0.05 vs. control and washout during high oxygen, ‡p < 0.05 vs. papaverine, n = 5).

low and high oxygen tension. Increasing the concentration of nifedipine to 30 μM abolished basal tone, and a change from high oxygen ($PO_2 = 148.9 \pm 3.4$ mmHg) to low oxygen tension ($PO_2 = 9.3 \pm 2.4$ mmHg) did not cause any significant vasodilation (p = 0.11, n = 5). There were no statistically significant differences between the vessel diameters at high or low oxygen tension at 3 vs. 30 μM nifedipine. Finally, application of 100 μM papaverine yielded a maximal vessel diameter of 31.7 ± 1.0 μm.

Role of prostaglandins and NO-synthase

Prostaglandins and NO are the two major endothelium-derived vasodilators. Figure 7 shows the effects on vasomotor responses of inhibition of both prostaglandin and NO synthesis, by applying indomethacin followed by L-NAME during both low and high oxygen tensions (n = 5). During the control period, change from high ($PO_2 = 148.4 \pm 9.9$ mmHg) to low oxygen tension ($PO_2 = 11.8 \pm 5.0$ mmHg) caused vasodilation ($\Delta D = 23.0 \pm 1.3$ μm). Application of 28 μM indomethacin, a concentration previously shown to effectively block prostaglandin synthesis in hamster cremaster muscle arterioles *in vivo* [16,17], acutely (< 30 sec) inhibited vasodilation during low oxygen tension ($PO_2 = 5.9 \pm 4.1$ mmHg). However, after a period of ~2-3 minutes (steady state) with presence of indomethacin, the vessel regained its responsiveness to low oxygen by dilating again. Additional application of 100 μM L-NAME did not affect vasomotor responses to changes in oxygen tensions.

Discussion

According to a prominent hypothesis for the mechanism of oxygen sensing in the microcirculation, low oxygen tension opens K_{ATP} channels in VSMCs due, at least in part, to an increase in the ADP/ATP concentration ratio.

This leads to efflux of K^+ and hyperpolarization of the cell, which in turn inhibits the influx of Ca^{2+} through the voltage-gated L-type Ca^{2+} channels leading to smooth muscle relaxation and eventually vasodilation [3,18,19]. In apparent agreement with this notion the present study shows that hypoxic vasodilation was completely inhibited by glibenclamide, and the reactivity could be restored gradually by increasing concentrations of the K_{ATP} channel activator cromakalim (1 μM and 5 μM cromakalim). Likewise cromakalim alone caused maximal vasodilation and a complete loss of hyperoxic vasoconstriction, which was gradually restored by application of 10 μM and 100 μM glibenclamide.

Importantly, however, studies by Jackson have provided evidence against the direct involvement of K_{ATP} channels in hypoxic vasodilation [9]. Jackson showed that low oxygen tension, in a glibenclamide sensitive manner, inhibited norepinephrine-induced contraction in VSMCs from hamster cremaster muscle arterioles. However, the effect of low oxygen tension was neither associated with a change of the whole-cell conductance nor of the membrane potential of the VSMCs [9], which clearly argues against the opening of K^+ channels. Instead it was suggested that the reported effect of glibenclamide was unspecific, possibly related to a drug-induced membrane depolarization [9].

The results of the present study are therefore difficult to reconcile with a direct role for K_{ATP} channels in oxygen sensing in cremaster muscle arterioles. The most likely explanation of the present results appears to be that the effects of glibenclamide and cromakalim, both when applied alone and in combination, are mediated indirectly through changes in the membrane potential. In cremaster muscle VSMCs glibenclamide applied alone closes K_{ATP} channels, and depolarizes the cell membrane [9]. This will activate the L-type Ca^{2+} channels, and

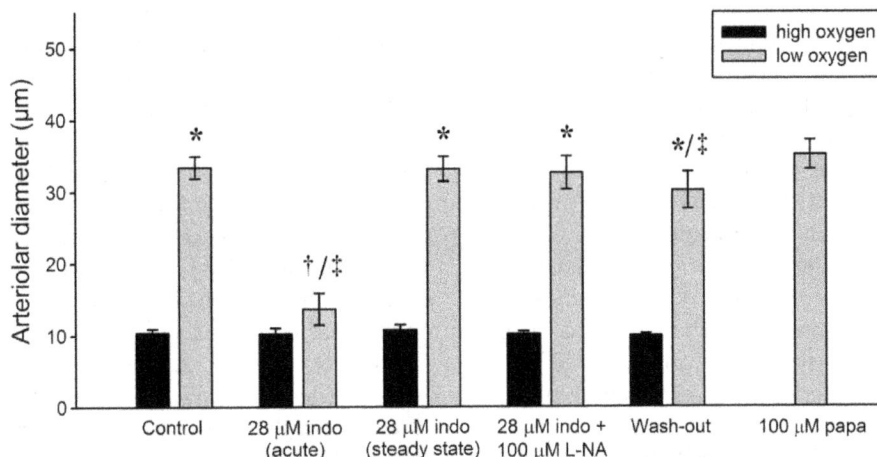

Figure 7 Effects of consecutive application of 28 μM indomethacin and 100 μM L-NAME on arteriolar response during high and low oxygen were evaluated (*p < 0.05 vs. high oxygen, †p < 0.05 vs. control and 28 μm indo (steady state) during low oxygen, ‡p < 0.05 vs. papaverine, n = 5).

constrict the vessels. We hypothesize that if the membrane depolarization is pronounced, the activation of the L-type channels will be sufficient, even in the presence of hypoxia, to elicit maximal vasoconstriction. The addition of cromakalim antagonizes the effect of glibenclamide and the membrane potential will gradually become more negative as the K_{ATP} channels are reactivated [9]. This will partially deactivate the L-type Ca^{2+} channels due to the steep voltage-dependence of their gating behavior in the physiological range of membrane potentials (−60 to −30 mV), and eventually render them responsive towards the effects of hypoxia. When cromakalim is added alone to maximally activate the K_{ATP} channels, the membrane will be hyperpolarized and the L-type Ca^{2+} channels closed. The vessel will therefore be close to maximally dilated, and once more irresponsive to changes in oxygen levels.

These apparently competitive actions of glibenclamide and cromakalim on the K_{ATP} channels are in line with previous *ex vivo* as well as *in vivo* observations. In isolated porcine coronary artery, the concentration-response curve of glibenclamide was right-shifted in the presence of cromakalim demonstrating a competitive action of these drugs on K_{ATP} channels [20]. In an elaborate *in vivo* study in rats, Gardiner et al showed that the hindquarter skeletal muscle blood flow was increased significantly by levcromakalim, and that this was reversibly antagonized by glibenclamide, demonstrating that glibenclamide and a cromakalim analogue have reversible and competitive actions on local blood flow in rat skeletal muscle *in vivo*. Similar effects were obtained in the mesenteric and renal circulations [21]. However, in an early pharmacological study glibenclamide (IC_{50} 148 nM) was able to block cromakalim (0.5 µM) induced relaxation of isolated rabbit superior mesenteric artery [22]. As we have used much higher concentrations of these drugs due to the fact that it was an *in vivo* study, we speculate that only at sufficiently high concentrations are cromakalim able to compete with the actions of glibenclamide on K_{ATP} channels. We find it unlikely that the observed effects represent unspecific effects due to the high concentrations of the respective drugs. However, we cannot rule out this possibility, and it is clearly a limitation of the present *in vivo* study.

The results of the glibenclamide/cromakalim experiments show that oxygen sensing depends critically on the level of the membrane potential, and this suggest that voltage gated L-type Ca^{2+} channels could play a central role in the mechanism. As is apparent from Figure 6, this was indeed the case. In the presence of medium (3 µM) to high (30 µM) concentrations of nifedipine, there was no significant difference in vessel diameter between high and low oxygen tension. The failure to dilate in response to hypoxia was not due to a

complete loss of vessel tone as indicated by the fact that even in the presence of 3 µM nifedipine, the vessels were still able to dilate further when papaverine was added to the superfusate. L-type Ca^{2+} channels are only one of several Ca^{2+} entry mechanisms in VSMCs, and it is therefore not surprising that the vessels are able to retain tone despite the presence of nifedipine. This suggests that the failure to dilate in response to hypoxia was not due to a complete loss of vessel tone, but rather due to the inhibition of the L-type Ca^{2+} channels. When given at a high concentration (30 µM) nifedipine had a more pronounced effect on vascular tone, and this effect was irreversible within the time limit of the washout period. The fact that changes in Ca^{2+} influx through the L-type channels appears to be involved in oxygen sensing does not indicate that the change in influx is mediated by changes in the membrane potential. Previous studies have suggested that hypoxia could induce vasodilation by acting directly on the voltage operated L-type Ca^{2+} channels, reducing Ca^{2+} influx [9,10]. Our findings therefore show that L-type Ca^{2+} channels are central for the oxygen sensing mechanism, but they do not allow us to discriminate between a direct action of oxygen on the channels, and an indirect effect mediated through changes in membrane potential.

20-HETE has been proposed to be involved in oxygen sensing by acting as a vasoconstrictor. It is produced in the VSMCs by the CYP450-4A enzyme system with arachidonic acid as a substrate. In the presence of oxygen, CYP450-4A oxidizes arachidonic acid to 20-HETE. The K_m for oxygen is approximately 55 µM at 37°C [12]. This value corresponds to an oxygen tension of around 40 mmHg, which is above the normal values in skeletal muscle [2,23-25]. The synthesis of 20-HETE is therefore partially limited by the availability of oxygen, and an increased oxygen tension will lead to an increased production rate for 20-HETE. 20-HETE inhibits large-conductance Ca^{2+}-activated K^+ channels (BK_{Ca} channels) located in the plasma membrane of VSMCs, which leads to depolarization of the cell. This in turn activates voltage-dependent L-type Ca^{2+} channels, increasing influx of Ca^{2+} and causing contraction of the VSMCs and eventually vasoconstriction [11,12,14]. Evidence supporting this includes a patch clamp study on cat cerebral microvessel VSMCs [11] and an intravital microscopy study of rat cremaster muscle arterioles, showing inhibition of hyperoxic vasoconstriction by 17-octadecynoic acid (17-ODYA), an inhibitor of CYP450-4A [12]. In our preparation, inhibition of 20-HETE production using 10 µM DDMS inhibited vasoconstriction to high oxygen tension in a reversible manner, but did not affect vasodilation to low oxygen tension (Figure 5). Previous studies have shown that vessels maintain their reactivity to vasoconstrictors (norepinephrine) following addition of DDMS [26], and in the present study the vessels maintained some tone after addition of DDMS. It is therefore unlikely that the lack of response to high oxygen reflects a general failure of the VSMC to contract. The results show that 20-HETE plays a role in vasoconstriction to high oxygen tension in mouse cremaster muscle arterioles, but has no role in hypoxic vasodilation. Since 20-HETE acts as a vasoconstrictor through inhibition of BK_{Ca} channels and/or stimulation of TRPC6 channels [27,28], it is interesting that specific activation of the K_{ATP} channels using cromakalim was able to abolish hyperoxic vasoconstriction (Figure 4A & B). This further strengthens the notion that the effect on oxygen sensing of blocking the K_{ATP} channels is indirect. When the K_{ATP} channels are activated by addition of cromakalim the membrane hyperpolarizes, and we expect that inhibition of the BK_{Ca} channels by 20-HETE will not be able to depolarize the membrane sufficiently to elicit vasoconstriction.

Vasodilator prostaglandins PGE_2 and PGI_2 (prostacyclin) and NO released from the vascular endothelium play important roles in regulating vascular tone in the microcirculation [29-33]. Release of prostaglandins and NO has been proposed to occur during low oxygen tension, and these substances could contribute to oxygen sensing [34-38]. Evidence of prostaglandins as effectors of hypoxic vasodilation comes from *in vitro* studies on isolated arterioles, where inhibition of cyclooxygenase using indomethacin inhibited hypoxic vasodilation [37,38]. Moreover, skeletal muscle contraction-induced vasodilation in hamster cremaster muscle arterioles paired with venules was blocked by indomethacin *in vivo* [16].

In our study, inhibition of prostaglandin synthesis by application of 28 μM indomethacin (Figure 7), acutely inhibited vasodilation during low oxygen, but after ~2-3 minutes (steady state) the arterioles had regained their responsiveness, and dilated to low oxygen with a response comparable to the control. The transient reduction in the vessel diameter was probably due to a sudden disruption of a constitutive release of vasodilator prostaglandins causing a transient vasoconstriction. Alternatively, the rate of vasodilation to hypoxia could be severely slowed by the acute lack of prostaglandins. However the vessels quickly regained their responsiveness to low oxygen tension, indicating that prostaglandins are not involved in the steady state mechanism of hypoxic vasodilation. In a previous *in vivo* study, indomethacin inhibited contraction-induced dilation of 3rd order arterioles paired to venules in the hamster cremaster muscle, but had no effect on unpaired 3rd order arterioles. It was therefore suggested that prostaglandins, released from the venules and diffusing to the arterioles, participate in the vasodilator response during muscular contraction [16]. In our study, only unpaired 3rd order arterioles were examined, and in good agreement with

the findings of Hammer et al., we did not find evidence for the involvement of prostaglandins in unpaired arterioles in hypoxic vasodilation.

In the present study we tested whether NO was released during low oxygen tension by additional application of 100 μM L-NAME, a concentration which we formerly have shown to effectively abolish bradykinin-induced vasodilation in the mouse cremaster muscle microcirculation *in situ* [6]. In the presence of indomethacin and L-NAME the vessels responded with vasodilation and constriction to low and high oxygen tension as during the control, indicating that NO is not involved in hypoxic vasodilation in mouse cremaster muscle arterioles. This is in good agreement with recent studies from our laboratory, where application of L-NAME did not affect vasomotor responses to low or high oxygen tension [6,39].

The exteriorized cremaster muscle preparation is a well-established *in vivo* model for studying the microcirculation of skeletal muscles. Several studies have investigated the effect of tissue oxygen tension perturbations on vascular responses caused by superfusion of the cremaster muscle with physiological salt solutions equilibrated with gas mixtures with different % O_2, balanced with N_2 and 5% CO_2 [40-42]. When the oxygen levels are low the superfusate acts as an "oxygen-sink", and the tissue oxygen tension is reduced. Conversely, the tissue oxygen tension is increased by elevating the PO_2 of the superfusate, which now behaves as an "oxygen-source" [43,44]. We recently showed that, when the oxygen microsensor tip was placed below the cremaster muscle, a decrease or increase in oxygen tension could be measured that mirrored changes in the superfusate oxygen tension above the tissue [39]. This provides an efficient method for studying the influence of tissue oxygen tensions in the microcirculation of a living animal, and allows changing the oxygen tension locally in the cremaster muscle independently of the oxygen supplied by the vessels. The preparation, on the other hand, does not allow us to determine whether the responses are mediated by oxygen acting directly on the proteins in question, or whether the changes in oxygen levels exert their effect through changes in the production of various metabolites. Nor is it possible to determine the specific cellular location of the signaling pathways, i.e. if they are strictly intravascular or whether they involve the parenchymal cells as well.

Conclusions

In conclusion, this *in vivo* study supports the notion that K_{ATP} channels are permissive for the response to oxygen by controlling the membrane potential in cremaster muscle VSMCs, whereas the activity of L-type Ca^{2+} channels are central to the oxygen sensing mechanism. As an additional mechanism, 20-HETE mediates hyperoxic vasoconstriction. Our conclusions are highlighted by the fact that blockade of L-type Ca^{2+} channels, which constitute a common pathway for the two mechanisms, inhibited both vasodilation and constriction to low and high oxygen tensions, respectively. In contrast, the lack of effects of inhibiting two major endothelial-derived vasodilator metabolites, prostaglandins and NO, suggests that these pathways are not involved in hypoxic vasodilation in mouse cremaster muscle arterioles *in vivo*.

Competing interests
The authors declare that they have no competing interests.

Authors' contributions
AN conceived and designed the study, carried out all the *in vivo* experiments, analyzed and interpreted the data and drafted and revised the manuscript. MR contributed to the design of the study and helped revising the manuscript. NH contributed to the design of the study, analyzed and interpreted the data as well as helping to draft and revise the manuscript. CT contributed in the design of the study and contributed to drafting and revising of the manuscript. LJ contributed in the conception and design of the study, helped analyzing and interpreting the data and helped to draft and revise the manuscript. All authors read and approved the final manuscript.

Acknowledgements
This study was supported by grants from the Danish Medical Research Council for Health and Disease, the Novo-Nordisk Foundation, the Lundbeck Foundation and the Danish Heart Association.

Author details
[1]Department of Biomedical Sciences, Faculty of Health and Medical Sciences, The Panum institute, University of Copenhagen, Blegdamsvej 3, DK-2200 Copenhagen N, Denmark. [2]Department of Cardiology, Gentofte Hospital, Copenhagen, Denmark. [3]Department of Veterinary Clinical and Animal Sciences, Faculty of Health and Medical Sciences, University of Copenhagen, Copenhagen, Denmark.

References
1. Segal SS: Regulation of blood flow in the microcirculation. *Microcirculat* 2005, **12**:33–45.
2. Duling BR, Berne RM: Longitudinal gradients in periarteriolar oxygen tension. A possible mechanism for the participation of oxygen in local regulation of blood flow. *Circ Res* 1970, **27**:669–678.
3. Dart C, Standen NB: Activation of ATP-dependent K + channels by hypoxia in smooth muscle cells isolated from the pig coronary artery. *J Physiol* 1995, **483**(Pt 1):29–39.
4. Daut J, Maier-Rudolph W, von Beckerath N, Mehrke G, Gunther K, Goedel-Meinen L: Hypoxic dilation of coronary arteries is mediated by ATP-sensitive potassium channels. *Science* 1990, **247**:1341–1344.
5. Liu Q, Flavahan NA: Hypoxic dilatation of porcine small coronary arteries: role of endothelium and KATP-channels. *Br J Pharmacol* 1997, **120**:728–734.
6. Ngo AT, Jensen LJ, Riemann M, Holstein-Rathlou NH, Torp-Pedersen C: Oxygen sensing and conducted vasomotor responses in mouse cremaster arterioles *in situ*. *Pflug Arch* 2010, **460**:41–53.
7. Archer SL, Rusch NJ: Potassium channels in cardiovascular biology. ; 2001:505–522.
8. Gauthier KM: Hypoxia-induced vascular smooth muscle relaxation: increased ATP-sensitive K + efflux or decreased voltage-sensitive Ca2+ influx? *Am J Physiol Heart Circ Physiol* 2006, **291**:H24–H25.
9. Jackson WF: Hypoxia does not activate ATP-sensitive K + channels in arteriolar muscle cells. *Microcirculation* 2000, **7**:137–145.
10. Franco-Obregon A, Urena J, Lopez-Barneo J: Oxygen-sensitive calcium channels in vascular smooth muscle and their possible role in hypoxic arterial relaxation. *Proc Natl Acad Sci U S A* 1995, **92**:4715–4719.
11. Harder DR, Gebremedhin D, Narayanan J, Jefcoat C, Falck JR, Campbell WB, Roman R: Formation and action of a P-450 4A metabolite of arachidonic acid in cat cerebral microvessels. *Am J Physiol* 1994, **266**:H2098–H2107.
12. Harder DR, Narayanan J, Birks EK, Liard JF, Imig JD, Lombard JH, Roman RJ: Identification of a putative microvascular oxygen sensor. *Circ Res* 1996, **79**:54–61.
13. Kunert MP, Roman RJ, Onso-Galicia M, Falck JR, Lombard JH: Cytochrome P-450 omega-hydroxylase: a potential O(2) sensor in rat arterioles and skeletal muscle cells. *Am J Physiol Heart Circ Physiol* 2001, **280**:H1840–H1845.
14. Wang J, Schmidt JR, Roman RJ, Anjaiah S, Falck JR, Lombard JH: Modulation of vascular O2 responses by cytochrome 450-4A omega-hydroxylase metabolites in Dahl salt-sensitive rats. *Microcirculat* 2009, **16**:345–354.
15. Jarnberg PO, Santesson J, Eklund J: Renal function during neurolept anaesthesia. *Acta Anaesthesiol Scand* 1978, **22**:167–172.
16. Hammer LW, Ligon AL, Hester RL: Differential inhibition of functional dilation of small arterioles by indomethacin and glibenclamide. *Hypertension* 2001, **37**:599–603.
17. Saito Y, Eraslan A, Hester RL: Role of endothelium-derived relaxing factors in arteriolar dilation during muscle contraction elicited by electrical field stimulation. *Microcirculation* 1994, **1**:195–201.
18. Rodrigo GC, Standen NB: ATP-sensitive potassium channels. *Curr Pharm Des* 2005, **11**:1915–1940.
19. Seino S, Miki T: Physiological and pathophysiological roles of ATP-sensitive K + channels. *Prog Biophys Mol Biol* 2003, **81**:133–176.
20. Balwierczak JL, Krulan CM, Kim HS, DelGrande D, Weiss GB, Hu S: Evidence that BKCa channel activation contributes to K + channel opener induced relaxation of the porcine coronary artery. *Naunyn Schmiedebergs Arch Pharmacol* 1995, **352**:213–221.
21. Gardiner SM, Kemp PA, March JE, Fallgren B, Bennett T: Effects of glibenclamide on the regional haemodynamic actions of alpha-trinositol and its influence on responses to vasodilators in conscious rats. *Br J Pharmacol* 1996, **117**:507–515.
22. Meisheri KD, Khan SA, Martin JL: Vascular pharmacology of ATP-sensitive K + channels: interactions between glyburide and K + channel openers. *J Vasc Res* 1993, **30**:2–12.
23. Boegehold MA, Johnson PC: Periarteriolar and tissue PO2 during sympathetic escape in skeletal muscle. *Am J Physiol* 1988, **254**:H929–H936.
24. Johnson PC, Vandegriff K, Tsai AG, Intaglietta M: Effect of acute hypoxia on microcirculatory and tissue oxygen levels in rat cremaster muscle. *J Appl Physiol* 2005, **98**:1177–1184.
25. Lash JM, Bohlen HG: Perivascular and tissue PO2 in contracting rat spinotrapezius muscle. *Am J Physiol* 1987, **252**:H1192–H1202.
26. Raffai G, Wang J, Roman RJ, Anjaiah S, Weinberg J, Falck JR, Lombard JH: Modulation by cytochrome P450-4A omega-hydroxylase enzymes of adrenergic vasoconstriction and response to reduced PO(2) in mesenteric resistance arteries of Dahl salt-sensitive rats. *Microcirculat* 2010, **17**:525–535.
27. Basora N, Boulay G, Bilodeau L, Rousseau E, Payet MD: 20-hydroxyeicosatetraenoic acid (20-HETE) activates mouse TRPC6 channels expressed in HEK293 cells. *J Biol Chem* 2003, **278**:31709–31716.
28. Inoue R, Jensen LJ, Jian Z, Shi J, Hai L, Lurie AI, Henriksen FH, Salomonsson M, Morita H, Kawarabayashi Y, Mori M, Mori Y, Ito Y: Synergistic activation of vascular TRPC6 channel by receptor and mechanical stimulation via phospholipase C/diacylglycerol and phospholipase A2/omega-hydroxylase/20-HETE pathways. *Circ Res* 2009, **104**:1399–1409.
29. Duffy SJ, Castle SF, Harper RW, Meredith IT: Contribution of vasodilator prostanoids and nitric oxide to resting flow, metabolic vasodilation, and flow-mediated dilation in human coronary circulation. *Circulation* 1999, **100**:1951–1957.
30. Huang A, Sun D, Koller A: Shear stress-induced release of prostaglandin H (2) in arterioles of hypertensive rats. *Hypertension* 2000, **35**:925–930.
31. Koller A, Huang A: Development of nitric oxide and prostaglandin mediation of shear stress-induced arteriolar dilation with aging and hypertension. *Hypertension* 1999, **34**:1073–1079.
32. Koller A, Huang A: Impaired nitric oxide-mediated flow-induced dilation in arterioles of spontaneously hypertensive rats. *Circ Res* 1994, **74**:416–421.

Significance of KATP channels, L-type Ca2+ channels and CYP450-4A enzymes in oxygen sensing...

195

33. Nicholson WT, Vaa B, Hesse C, Eisenach JH, Joyner MJ: **Aging is associated with reduced prostacyclin-mediated dilation in the human forearm.** *Hypertension* 2009, **53**:973–978.

34. Edmunds NJ, Marshall JM: **Oxygen delivery and oxygen consumption in rat hindlimb during systemic hypoxia: role of adenosine.** *J Physiol* 2001, **536**:927–935.

35. Edmunds NJ, Moncada S, Marshall JM: **Does nitric oxide allow endothelial cells to sense hypoxia and mediate hypoxic vasodilatation?** *In vivo* and *in vitro* studies. *J Physiol* 2003, **546**:521–527.

36. Edmunds NJ, Marshall JM: **The roles of nitric oxide in dilating proximal and terminal arterioles of skeletal muscle during systemic hypoxia.** *J Vasc Res* 2003, **40**:68–76.

37. Goodwill AG, James ME, Frisbee JC: **Increased vascular thromboxane generation impairs dilation of skeletal muscle arterioles of obese Zucker rats with reduced oxygen tension.** *Am J Physiol Heart Circ Physiol* 2008, **295**:H1522–H1528.

38. Messina EJ, Sun D, Koller A, Wolin MS, Kaley G: **Role of endothelium-derived prostaglandins in hypoxia-elicited arteriolar dilation in rat skeletal muscle.** *Circ Res* 1992, **71**:790–796.

39. Riemann M, Rai A, Ngo AT, Dziegiel MH, Holstein-Rathlou NH, Torp-Pedersen C: **Oxygen-dependent vasomotor responses are conducted upstream in the mouse cremaster microcirculation.** *J Vasc Res* 2011, **48**:79–89.

40. Baudry N, Danialou G, Boczkowski J, Vicaut E: *In vivo* **study of the effect of systemic hypoxia on leukocyte-endothelium interactions.** *Am J Respir Crit Care Med* 1998, **158**:477–483.

41. Frisbee JC, Lombard JH: **Elevated oxygen tension inhibits flow-induced dilation of skeletal muscle arterioles.** *Microvasc Res* 1999, **58**:99–107.

42. Frisbee JC: **Regulation of** *in situ* **skeletal muscle arteriolar tone: interactions between two parameters.** *Microcirculat* 2002, **9**:443–462.

43. Klitzman B, Popel AS, Duling BR: **Oxygen transport in resting and contracting hamster cremaster muscles: experimental and theoretical microvascular studies.** *Microvasc Res* 1983, **25**:108–131.

44. Popel AS: **Mathematical-modeling of oxygen-transport near a tissue surface - effect of the surface Po2.** *Mathematical Biosci* 1981, **55**:231–246.

16

High molecular mass proteomics analyses of left ventricle from rats subjected to differential swimming training

Luiz A O Rocha[1,5], Bernardo A Petriz[1], David H Borges[1], Ricardo J Oliveira[2], Rosangela V de Andrade[1], Gilberto B Domont[4], Rinaldo W Pereira[1,2] and Octávio L Franco[1,3,5*]

Abstract

Background: Regular exercises are commonly described as an important factor in health improvement, being directly related to contractile force development in cardiac cells.

In order to evaluate the links between swimming exercise intensity and cardiac adaptation by using high molecular mass proteomics, isogenic Wistar rats were divided into four groups: one control (CG) and three training groups (TG's), with low, moderate and high intensity of exercises.

In order to evaluate the links between swimming exercise intensity and cardiac adaptation by using high molecular mass proteomics, isogenic Wistar rats were divided into four groups: one control (CG) and three training groups (TG's), with low, moderate and high intensity of exercises.

Results: Findings here reported demonstrated clear morphologic alterations, significant cellular injury and increased energy supplies at high exercise intensities. α-MyHC, as well proteins associated with mitochondrial oxidative metabolism were shown to be improved. α-MyHC expression increase 1.2 fold in high intensity training group when compared with control group. α-MyHC was also evaluated by real-time PCR showing a clear expression correlation with protein synthesis data increase in 8.48 fold in high intensity training group. Other myofibrillar protein, troponin , appear only in high intensity group, corroborating the cellular injury data. High molecular masses proteins such as MRS2 and NADH dehydrogenase, involved in metabolic pathways also demonstrate increase expression, respectily 1.5 and 1.3 fold, in response to high intensity exercise.

Conclusions: High intensity exercise demonstrated an increase expression in some high molecular masses myofibrilar proteins, α-MyHC and troponin. Furthermore this intensity also lead a significant increase of other high molecular masses proteins such as MRS2 and NADH dehydrogenase in comparison to low and moderate intensities. However, high intensity exercise also represented a significant degree of cellular injury, when compared with the individuals submitted to low and moderate intensities.

Keywords: Heart tissue, High molecular mass proteomic, Muscle, Myofibrillar proteins, Swimming training

* Correspondence: ocfranco@pos.ucb.br
[1]Centro de Análises Proteômicas e Bioquímicas, Programa de Pós-Graduação em Ciências Genômicas e Biotecnologia, Universidade Católica de Brasília, Brasília-DF, Brazil
[3]Departamento de Biologia, Universidade Federal de Juiz de Fora, Juiz de Fora-MG, Brazil
Full list of author information is available at the end of the article

Background

The adaptation is a dynamic process with involvement of many circumstances and is an important life mechanism. The cardiac cells of mammals are submitted to a growth phase after birth maturation period defied as cardiac hypertrophy which is characterized by n increase in individual size of the cardiomyocyties without cell division. This pattern of hypertrophy development can be initiated in response to some intrinsic and extrinsic stimuli such mechanical stress, neurohumoral factor, cytokines, ischemia and endocrine disorders [1,2].

These stimuli for heart hypertrophy can be divided in "physiological" cardiac hypertrophy, when is result of exercise for example and "pathological" cardiac hypertrophy, which is associated with cardiovascular diseases [1,2]. The physiological hypertrophy has been classified as a positive increase in heart mass, associated with structural remodeling of components of the ventricular walls to support increase in myocyte size, angiogenesis and changes in fibrilar collagen content and organization, whose enhancer the cardiac pump function.

The cellular and molecular bases behind heart adaptations to exercise are not completely understood, but it is believed that a number of cellular adaptations, intrinsic to the cardiomyocyte, are largely responsible for these changes. The mechanism proposed for this structural adaptation is hypertrophy by increase in functional load [3]. This overload is followed by modifications in the gene expression pattern, activation of signaling pathways which included up regulation in the contractile protein synthesis and his organization into sarcomeric units [1-3]. However, it is not clear what role is played by the impact of differing training intensities on the physiological heart muscle's adaptation, in terms of molecular changes.

In summary the literature describes that one of the most important benefits of exercise, associated to cardio-circulatory system consists in the enhancing of heart work efficiency due to contractile capacity increase. Thus, this study aims to verify the rat cardiac muscle adaptation under different intensities of swimming exercise, focusing on high molecular mass proteomics of *R. novergicus*.

Results and discussion

Measured average values showed a lower lactate accumulation, of 4.6 ($\pm$ 0.7 mmol.L^{-1} in TG_3 in comparison to 5.9 $\pm$ 0.4 mmol.L^{-1} in CG). The two other TG's (data not shown) also showed lower value, [4]. Cardiac fibers from left ventricle of rats in the CG showed a normal size and shape (Additional file 1: Figure S1). Similar data were obtained from left ventricle histological sectioning of rats from TG_1 (Additional file 1: Figure S1), demonstrating no structural alteration in the heart tissue, which indicated lower hypertrophy. Exercise training was also able to induce heart morphological alterations not seen in the untrained group. The small nucleus presented a rounded or in some cases slightly oval shape, indicating no clear pathological alteration which lower hypertrophy. A few morphologic alterations, such as a small sclerotic area with infiltration of granule lipofuscin, characterizing particular metabolic alterations, probably associated with overload were seen in TG_2, (Additional file 1: Figure S1) [5,6]. This pigment is closely associated with oxygen-derived free radicals, which are an important component of muscle fatigue [7] indicating that TG_2 are inducing heart tissue modifications to the detriment of improvement in metabolism. On the other hand, microscopic morphology analysis in TG_3 indicated cellular hypertrophy, showing several modifications such as several areas with increased fibrosis (Additional file 1: Figure S1), evidencing a higher adaptation to exercise overload. This increase suggests that this level of physical activity was stressful to the heart [8,9]. The relative exercise overload is directly associated with oxygen consumption ($VO_{2máx}$) [10,11], because mitochondria are strictly involved in the activation of super-oxide synthesis cascade. It is also worth noting that TG_3 showed an extended area with necrosis and the presence of leucocytes, probably supporting hypertrophy by replacing dead cells with satellite cells (Additional file 1: Figure S1) [12,13]. One important route to hypertrophy of the myocardium directly involves fibroblast proliferation, which stimulates collagen synthesis[14-16]. Increased collagen content is commonly observed with overload pressure and, in certain cases, may negatively impact both diastolic and systolic function [17]. One of the most important benefits of exercise in the cardio-circulatory system is associated with an increase in circulation capability. This upgrade is strictly dependent on contraction increase, carried out by the expression of different heart myosin isoforms [18-22], which will be described below.

Differential electrophoretic analyses of sedentary and exercise-trained cardiac muscle

Since exercise-trained groups showed clear heart tissue alterations, SDS-PAGE was conducted in order to evaluate protein expression modification, showing an apparent quantitative increase in α-MyHC (higher band) and β-MyHC (lower band) expression (Additional file 2: Figure S2), in TG_2 and TG_3 compared to CG. Analyzing overlapped images, it was observed that α-MyHC (Figure 1) increased 1 fold in swimming-trained heart. In order to improve these data, increasing accuracy and leading to an overview of physiologic modifications during swimming exercise training, two-dimensional gels were run by using left ventricles from control and training groups (Additional file 3: Figure S3). Bionumerics™ from Applied Maths matched 177 spots in the 2-DE control group.

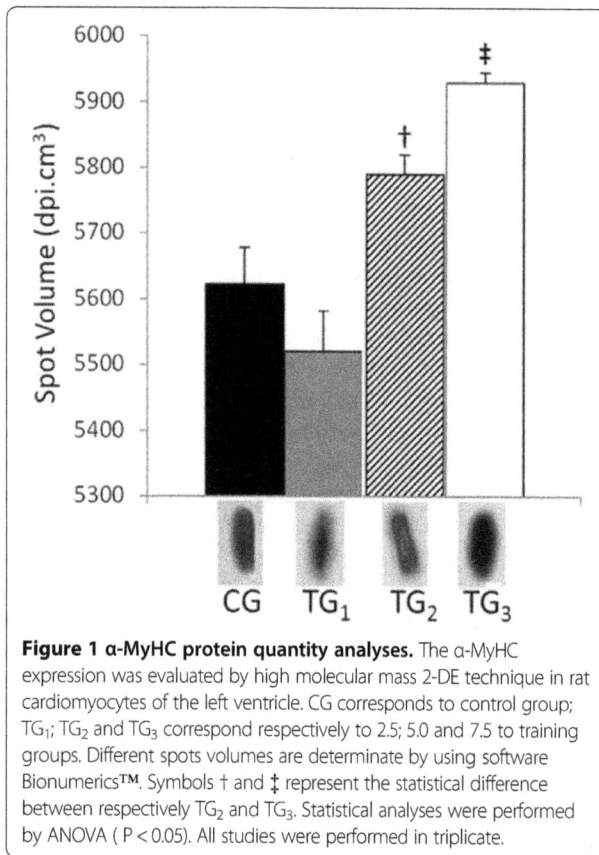

Figure 1 α-MyHC protein quantity analyses. The α-MyHC expression was evaluated by high molecular mass 2-DE technique in rat cardiomyocytes of the left ventricle. CG corresponds to control group; TG_1; TG_2 and TG_3 correspond respectively to 2.5; 5.0 and 7.5 to training groups. Different spots volumes are determinate by using software Bionumerics™. Symbols † and ‡ represent the statistical difference between respectively TG_2 and TG_3. Statistical analyses were performed by ANOVA ($P < 0.05$). All studies were performed in triplicate.

was lower than previously observed in rat heart protein maps (624 spots) submitted to intensity-controlled endurance exercise [11]. This variation could be explained by a different 2-DE technique here utilized, which is focused on evaluation of high molecular mass proteins ranging from 50–220 kDa, while Burninston [11] evaluated most abundant proteins from 14 – 116 kDa. The average coefficient of variation for normalized spot volume gave $R^2 = 0.82$ for biological and 0.94 for technical replicates, showing reliable gel reproducibility. These values are close to the range reported for technical variation for proteomic analyses of muscle homogenate, including skeletal and heart muscle tissues [4,11,26]. Moreover, the average coefficient of variation calculated to compare gels from different groups (CG, TG_1, TG_2 and TG_3) showed a R^2 lower than 0.43, demonstrating the obvious differences in protein maps from rat left ventricles submitted to diverse intensities of training. These proportions were similar to that observed by Burniston [11], evaluating the adaptation of rat cardiac muscle to endurance exercise, despite the different methodologies utilized. While Burniston described the evaluation of proteins from 14 to 116 kDa [27], Our work evaluated proteins varying from 53 to 230 kDa, indicating that protein expression behavior in response of exercise is independent of molecular masses. Moreover, these data are only in agreement with protein maps from rat skeletal muscle [4] and human heart [28]. Furthermore, as previously observed in several reports [4,11], some gene products were identified as multi-spot series exhibiting similar molecular masses but different pI, which may indicate unusual splice variants or states of post-translational modification.

Mass spectrometry protein identification

Of all spots founded seventeen had been considered differentially expressed after swimming training, whereas increase more than one fold and appear in every gel in triplicate. Those were identified by PMF (Table 1) with molecular masses above 56 kDa. These data revealed that the majority (27%) of identified proteins were mitochondrial, one-quarter associated with membrane/

It is known that two MyHC isoforms, α-MyHC and β-MyHC, are expressed in cardiac tissue, and their proportion (normally ~ 70% α-MyHC and 30% β-MyHC) in the rodent myocardium directly influences heart power output [23,24]. Data reported here are consistent with previous results in which MyHC was up regulated in exercise-trained rat hearts [11]. Otherwise, these data contradict those observed during moderate exercise training on skeletal rat muscle suffering chronic heart failure [25]. In this case, MyHC distributions were similar in both groups and training did not alter the MyHC distribution.

We found 162 spots in TG_1, 168 in TG_2 and 186 in TG_3. The number of spots observed in each gel (Table 1),

Table 1 MALDI ToF protein identification

Samples	α-MyHC average C_T	18srRNA average C_T	ΔC_T	$\Delta\Delta C_T$	α-MyHC expression increase in TGs fold related to CG
Control	26.31 ± 0.12	15.21 ± 0.55	11.10 ± 0.32	0.00 ± 0.32	1.00 (0.80-1.25)
TG_1	25.58 ± 0.10	15.16 ± 0.46	10.42 ± 0.27	-0.68 ± 0.27	1.60 (1.33-1.94)
TG_2	25.32 ± 0.06	15.39 ± 0.56	9.92 ± 0.32	-1.18 ± 0.32	2.26 (1.81-2.83)
TG_3	26.28 ± 0.04	18.26 ± 0.63	8.02 ± 0.36	-3.08 ± 0.36	8.48 (6.59-10.91)

Real time PCR evaluating fold change expression of ?-MyHC RNA from training groups (TGs) related to untrained group (CG) calculated by ΔΔCT method. Values were presented as a means ± standard deviation.

extracellular (25%), one-quarter myofibrillar/cytoskeletal (25%) and 23% associated with different functions such as hystocompatibility (Table 1). Besides the evidence, based on protein analysis, of increased expression of α-MyHC in our training groups, we decided to corroborate it using mRNA expression (Table 2). Data here reported showed that training intensity is an important factor for α-MyHC expression. Training groups with overload of 2.5 (TG_1) and 5% (TG_2) showed increased expression of α-MyHC related to untrained group (CG). Respectively, these were increases of 1.60 and 2.26 fold in α-MyHC expression. However, taking in account standard deviation, the increase in TG_1 was 1.33-1.94 and in TG_2 it was 1.81-2.83-fold. The overlap in the upper limit of TG_1 with lower limit in TG_2 shows lower differentiation in these two training groups for α-MyHC expression. The training group with overload of 7.5% (TG_3) showed an 8.48-fold (6.59-10.91) increase.

Aiming to unambiguously differentiate α- and β-MyHC, one ion, which is unique to α-MyHC, of 2036.48 m/z corresponding to residues 1546–1663 (KNAQAHLKDTQL QLDDAVRA) was sequenced from spot 7. Tryptic peptides specifically from β-MyHC were not detected, suggesting that spot 7 is formed by α-MyHC. A similar strategy to elucidate MyHC isoforms has been used before [11]. This result clearly showed a significant increase in α-MyHC expression in proportion to training intensity. A clear cut among TG_3 and the other two training groups was also seen in histopathological analysis and electrophoretic analyses, which showed that TG_3 was clearly able to improve α-MyHC expression (Figure 2). Since α-MyHC up regulation in exercised-trained rat hearts is consistent with previously published data [11,29,30], here we could conclude that intensity, at least in swimming training, is the key to controlling α-MyHC expression and indeed cardiomyocite power output (Figure 1). Other studies using swimming as a training method have suggested that this practice could induce an increase in α-MyHC expression in the rat heart [19]. The same author described little modifications in MyHC isoform content in trained myocardium, despite finding increase in loaded shortening velocity. These results suggest that it is possible to have significant alterations in myocardial contractile function with lower or no change in MyHC isoform expression, as was observed here. However, despite changes in the myosin subunit isoform expression are associated to increase in contractility by an increase in force generation, economy in ATP ratio and increased Ca^{2+} sensitivity, others low molecular weight sarcomeric protein, that they had not been described in this work, like myosin regulatory light chain, troponin-I, troponin-T, alpha-tropomyosin and myosin binding protein-C must be considered for yours relevance for contractile mechanism [31].

Since the 1980s some important studies have reported that an increase in α-MyHC from exercise [32-34] is able to boost cardiomyocyte power output [4,11], especially for myofibrillar proteins [4]. Here, in this report, we used a combination of protein extraction under high salt quantities associated with a long and modified 2D gel run with low acrylamide concentration (8%). These procedures allowed the visualization of high molecular mass protein maps. Otherwise, spot resolution was lower when compared to other muscle tissues' protein maps [4,11]. Similar data were obtained with treadmill-trained rats, in which a 1.9-fold increase of α-MyCH expression was observed [11]. Spot 7 showed 120 kDa of molecular weight, which is approximately half that of the predicted myosin heavy chain complete polypeptide. Furthermore, several MyHC isoforms (17) could share 93% sequence identity [11].

Troponin, which acts as a muscular contraction regulator due to its relationship with calcium molecules, was identified in two different spots (Table 1). It is important to note that, probably, a different troponin species, which showed identical molecular mass (approximately 220 kDa), presented a completely different pI. While one species extracted from spot 14 showed a pI of 4.8, the troponin species from spot 12 had a pI of 9.6 (Table 1). The troponin from spot 12 was only observed in protein maps from rat hearts submitted to intense exercise (TG3), suggesting that only intense exercise is capable of improving its expression at 2-DE detectable levels (data not shown).

Troponin is commonly utilized as a serum muscle injury marker in cardiac insufficiency and, consequently, pathologic hypertrophy [27,35,36]. For Lippi and Banfi, an increase in cTns values might be temporarily responsible for a reversible shed of cardiac blebs. Elevated levels of cTn could be due to ongoing myocardial damage or leakage of myofibrillar components and may reflect the loss of viable cardiac myocytes [37]. Myocyte injury, coronary microvascular dysfunction, and fibroblast and collagen turnover also play an important role in cardiac remodeling; extracellular matrix remodeling takes place in myocardium hypertrophy [38]. Nie et al. [39] suggest a role for exercise-induced increases in ROS in the mediation of cTn. Moreover, oxidative stress in high exercise intensity induced microvascular flow abnormalities, which in turn are associated with an increase in cTn levels observed by microscopic analyses [40]. To support this fact, the presence of an isoform of major histocompatibility complexes, that are strictly associated with immune response in nucleated cells, such as necrosis or hydrolases enzymes, was detected at higher levels in TG_3. This process distinguishes between self-proteins and foreign protein antigens to elicit an effective immune response called antigen-presenting cells [41]. These data, in addition to histological analysis

Table 2 Real time PCR results

Spot	Obs. pI	Exp. pI	Obs. M.M. (kDa)	Exp. M.M. (kDa)	Sequ. Match.	Sequ. not match.	Cover. %	e-value	Swissprot code	Protein	Protein funtion	CG Regul. factor	TG1 Regul. factor	TG1 p-value	TG2 Regul. factor	TG2 p-value	TG3 Regul. factor	TG3 p-value
1	9.0	9.4	≈ 120	122	25	84	23.3	0.4	Q8K4V5	High-affinity immunoglobulin gamma Fc receptor I.	Phagocytes process	1.00	absent	-	absent	-	1.01	0.05
2	8.1	9.2	248	34.4	70	239	22.7	0.3	Q3KRD5	Mitochondrial import receptor subunit TOM34.	Translocase of outer membrane 34 kDa subunit associated to energy synthesis.	1.00	absent	-	absent	-	1.32	0.05
3	6.9	5.9	175	105	33	55	37.	0.1	Q60I07	MHC class I-like located near the LRC, 1.	Immunological leukocyte response.	1.00	absent	-	absent	-	1.00	0.01
4	4.3	9.7	≈ 250	227	65	135	32.5	1.0	AAH83554	Magnesium transporter MRS2.	Mg^{2+} mitochondria's transporter	1.00	1.12	0.05	1.27	0.05	1.53	0.01
5	5.9	5.2	≈ 230	364	63	276	18.6	0.1	Q924V0	Cadherin class 1 receptor.	Immune system.	1.00	absent	-	absent	-	absent	-
6	5.2	5.7	≈ 100	314	72	213	25.3	0.6	BAA18993	N,N,N-dimethylarginine dimethylamino hydrolase.	NO synthetases inhibitor.	1.00	absent	-	1.00	0.05	1.01	0.05
7	6.4	9.1	120	127	630	477	56.9	0.08	Q63356.1	α-Myosin heavy chain.	Primary motor of muscle contraction on cardiac cells.	1.00	1.04	0.05	0.93	0.01	1.24	0.05
8	5.5	9.2	193.9	34.4	54	185	22.6	0.4	Q3KRD5	Mitochondrial import receptor subunit TOM34.	Translocase of outer membrane 34 kDa subunit associated to energy synthesis.	1.00	absent	-	1.47	0.05	1.36	0.05
9	6.9	5.2	192.6	107	698	277	71.6	0.04	AAF37622	Glutamyl aminopeptidase.	Rennin-angiotensin catabolism pathway.	1.00	1.30	0.05	1.10	0.05	1.32	0.05
10	7.3	9.8	213.0	82	48	270	15.1	0.09	CAA40164	NADH dehydrogenase, mitochondrial subunit 1.	Catalyzes the first dehydrogenase reaction in the TCA cycle	1.00	1.07	0.05	1.18	0.05	1.50	0.05
11	5.8	9.4	223.1	46	52	36	59.1	0.1	Q60I18	Major histocompatibility complex class 1.	Immunological leukocyte response.	1.00	absent	-	absent	-	1.12	0.05
12	8.3	9.6	224.9	215	76	135	36.0	1.0	P23693	Troponin I, cardiac muscle.	Muscular contraction regulator by its relation with calcium molecules.	1.00	1.19	0.01	1.05	0.05	1.26	0.001

Table 2 Real time PCR results (Continued)

										Name	Function							
13	5.6	9.2	240.0	34.4	58	185	23.9	1.0	Q3KRD5	Mitochondrial import receptor subunit TOM34.	Associated to energy production.	1.00	absent	-	absent	-	1.42	0.08
14	4.8	9.6	232.2	21	44	167	20.9	2.2	P23693	Troponin I, cardiac muscle.	Muscular contraction regulator by its relation with calcium molecules.	1.00	1.00	0.05	1.00	0.05	1.1	0.05
15	5.5	6.1	249.9	42	26	62	29.5	1.0	Q861Q1	Major histocompatibility complex class 1	Involved in the immunological leukocyte response.	1.00	1.00	0.05	1.02	0.05	1.31	0.05
16	8.6	9.2	261	34.4	73	236	23.6	0.8	Q3KRD5	Mitochondrial import receptor subunit TOM34.	Energy synthesis	1.00	absent	-	absent	-	1.0	0.05
17	4.7	5.2	225	107	66	909	6.8	0.04	AAF37622	Glutamyl aminopeptidase.	Rennin-angiotensin catabolism pathway	1.00	absent	-	1.03	0.05	1.13	0.05

Differential proteins identified by MALDI ToF peptide mass fingerprinting of multiple proteins from rat left ventricles. As a standard, false Discovery rate was calculated as lower than 15%.

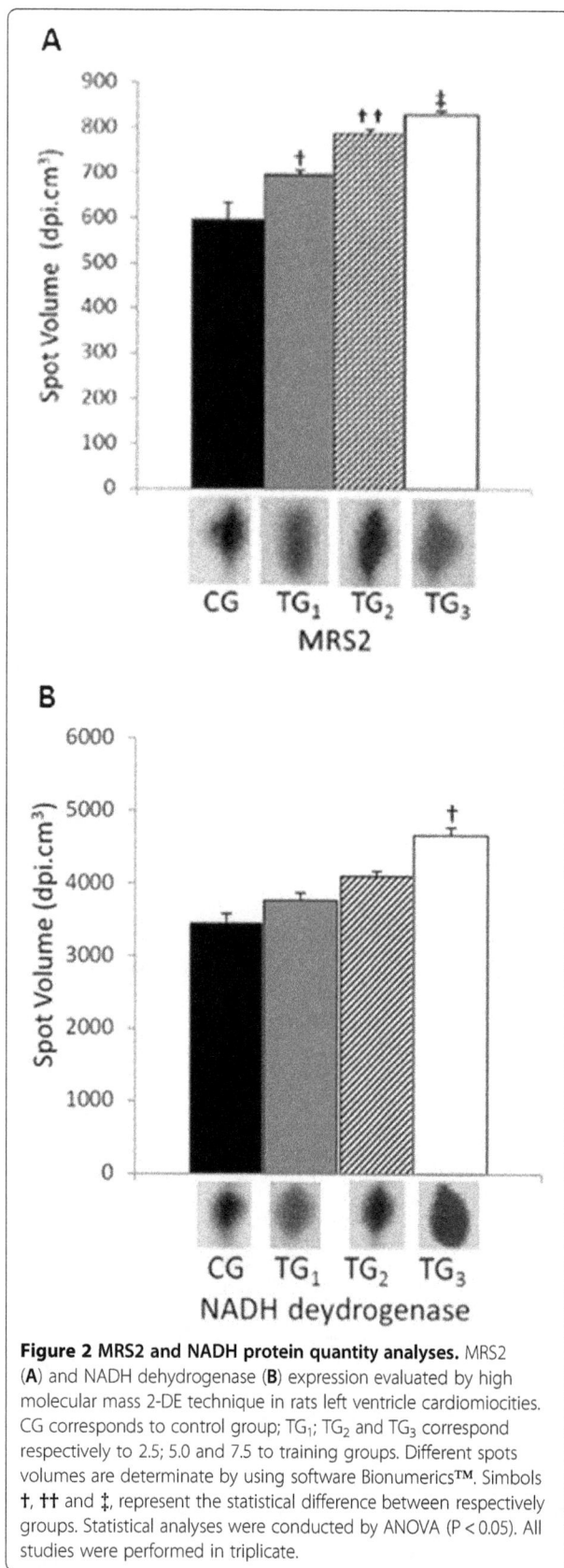

Figure 2 MRS2 and NADH protein quantity analyses. MRS2 (**A**) and NADH dehydrogenase (**B**) expression evaluated by high molecular mass 2-DE technique in rats left ventricle cardiomiocities. CG corresponds to control group; TG_1; TG_2 and TG_3 correspond respectively to 2.5; 5.0 and 7.5 to training groups. Different spots volumes are determinate by using software Bionumerics™. Simbols †, †† and ‡, represent the statistical difference between respectively groups. Statistical analyses were conducted by ANOVA (P < 0.05). All studies were performed in triplicate.

previously described, which show a large necrosis area as well as leucocytes presence, suggested cardiac muscle injury caused by intense exercise (TG_3), leading us to believe that 7.5% overload exercise for 8 weeks brings real benefits to the animal but also causes clear injuries and further decreases in animal health.

Exercise-induced changes in the expression of gene products involved in energy metabolism

An important signal for exercise adaptation consists of greater expression of proteins associated with the oxidative metabolism, such as oxidoreductases, mitochondrial membrane transporters [42]. The mitochondrial internal membrane exerts a fundamental role in oxidative phosphorylation and also in electron transport. Moreover, the translocases move through the mitochondrial membrane and have a logical consequence for an important physiological process known as ATP synthesis [43,44]. In eukaryotic cells, the final stage of nutrients oxidation occurs in mitochondria, with fast oxidation of NADH and $FADH_2$ produced in glycolysis, tricarboxilic cycle, ß-oxidation of fatty acids and amino acid oxidation.

In this study we found the presence of a NADH-dehydrogenase in all training groups and in the control (Table 1; Figure 2), which developed a key role in electron transfer in the respiratory chain to Q coenzyme [45]. The expression of that isoform of NADH dehydrogenase was clearly improved from control groups to more intensely trained rats (Figure 2), leading to 1.30 fold at TG_3. It's important to cite that NADH dehydrogenase here analyses, maybe an isoform and that this up regulation could not be related to all protein class here evaluated. Additionally, it was only in rat hearts from TG_3 group that the synthesis of membranes translocases was observed at detectable levels by the techniques applied here. These translocases are commonly associated with ATP's and H^+ transport to cytosol (Table 1).

Howlett and Willis (cited by [46]) observed that the isocitrate dehydrogenase (IDH) activity is higher in mitochondria from striated muscle, suggesting that it may rely on this enzyme as a regulatory site. This enzyme catalyzes the first dehydrogenase reaction in the TCA cycle and produces $NADH + H^+$, which is the substrate of NADH dehydrogenase. This may explain an over expression of NADH dehydrogenase, as observed in TG_3 in the present study (Figure 2). Although mitochondria exert the essential role of ATP production, they are also the primary source of cellular reactive oxygen species [47,48]. In a recent review Powers and Jackson [49] suggested that common metabolic changes and ROS generation may predominantly occur by contracting skeletal and heart muscle during different exercise protocols. An exception to this rule is an experiment whereby muscle damage occurs, and in this situation, inflammatory processes may play an important role in radical production. It is well accepted that exercise provides intrinsic protection to the heart [50]. Recent reports have associated ROS production with apoptosis after physical effort, a situation in which the apoptotic mitochondrial pathways may play a major role by releasing cytochrome c and activating initiators such as caspases [46]. An increase in mitochondrial oxidant production is generally accepted as a cause of myocardial cell loss via apoptosis and necrosis [50]. These data corroborates with myocite modifications observed in TG_3 by microscopy (Additional file 1: Figure S1), explaining the reduction in exercise benefits during the exercise training stage.

During exercise, H^+ concentration is enhanced, being this process is commonly associated with force generation decline in muscles, also causing a reduction in cross bridge activation by competitively inhibiting Ca^{2+} binding to troponin C. Moreover, proton concentration reduces Ca^{2+} - ATPase re-uptake in sarcoplasm and inhibits myofibrillar ATPase [40]. Mitochondrial ROS generation can lead to a calcium overload, consequently decreased ATP production, and may cause the mitochondrial permeability transition pore (PTP) to open, further decreasing ATP production and releasing cytochrome c. However, the increase of translocases can increase the transport of H^+ reducing the competition with calcium during the exercise, which would make the most of the positive effect of the exercise.

Finally, another important gene product here detected and probably involved in the increase of ATP synthesis consists in an isoform of magnesium homeostasis factor. homolog, MRS2, 1.5 fold (Figure 2, Table 1), a major Mg^{2+} mitochondria's transporter being their function extremely important for respiratory complex I and cell viability maintenance [51]. This protein family is characterized for a conserved GMN C-terminus (Gly-Met-Asn) in the transmembrane domains. Furthermore, this is the region responsible for Mg^{2+} selective filter [52] This divalent ion is abundant inside the cell and plays a fundamental role in many biochemical and regulatory functions being his concentration maintained by an transmembrane electrochemical potential [51]. In cardiac muscle Mg^{2+} may be involved in the ATPase phosphate-release step causing inhibition of myofibril sarcoplasmic reticulum Ca^{2+}-transporting ATPases under anoxia. This last condition could be improved by high intensity contraction in maximal exercise, when the ATP-PCr system can occur to maintain a relatively constant energy supply [53]. This finding in the present study is in accordance with the increase of aerobic capacity by mitochondrial biogenesis and/or workload improvement as a consequence of swimming training but, one more time, it's important to cite that maybe an isoform and that this up- or down regulation could not be related to all protein class here evaluated.

Conclusions

In summary, our study evidenced left ventricular hypertrophy and these data seems to be correlated at molecular levels with proteins of high molecular masses. This increase suggests a clear correlation with the level of intensity which the individuals underwent. It demonstrates that interval training with high intensity compared with low and moderate intensity training led to a remarkable increase in α-MyHC and troponin expressions in the left ventricle of cardiac myocyte of R. norvegicus. Another important data is the significant degree of cellular injury in left ventricle in individual submitted to high intensity, when compared with the individuals submitted to low and moderate intensities. Thus, we conclude that 7.5% overload exercise for 8 weeks may possibly improve contractile function for the animal, but may also cause injuries and consequently, reduce the animal's health. These modifications seem to be related to modifications in contractile and metabolic proteins, previously elucidated by proteomics and molecular analyses. Data here reported add more knowledge to molecular exercise studies.

Methods

Animal group design

All procedures are in accordance with the ethics guidelines for research at the University of Brasília and were approved by the ethics committee (UnbDOC n.48695/ 2010). Twenty isogenic male Wistar adult rats (Rattus novergicus), with age varying from 80–90 days, were equally randomized into four groups, one being the sedentary negative control group (CG) and three the swimming-trained groups (TG's). The control group was maintained in isolated cages receiving water and food ad libitum.

Exercise training protocol

The animals were adapted to the water environment for three weeks, in the same place as the training sessions, in a cylindrical training tank with a smooth surface, measuring 60 cm in diameter by 120 cm in depth, kept at a constant temperature (32 ± 0.5°C). The training period was corporate to 5 consecutive days of 30 min of swimming sessions for 8 weeks . Training groups were characterized by the overloaded applied, respectively 2.5% (TG_1), 5.0% (TG_2) and 7.5% (TG_3) (Figure 3). The overload was determined weekly by individual animal body weight and attached to the animal's chest. Aiming to minimize the animal's stress without promoting physiological adaptations derived from physical exercise, training group animals were submitted to the water environment before the swimming exercise protocol started. At the end of training period, all animals

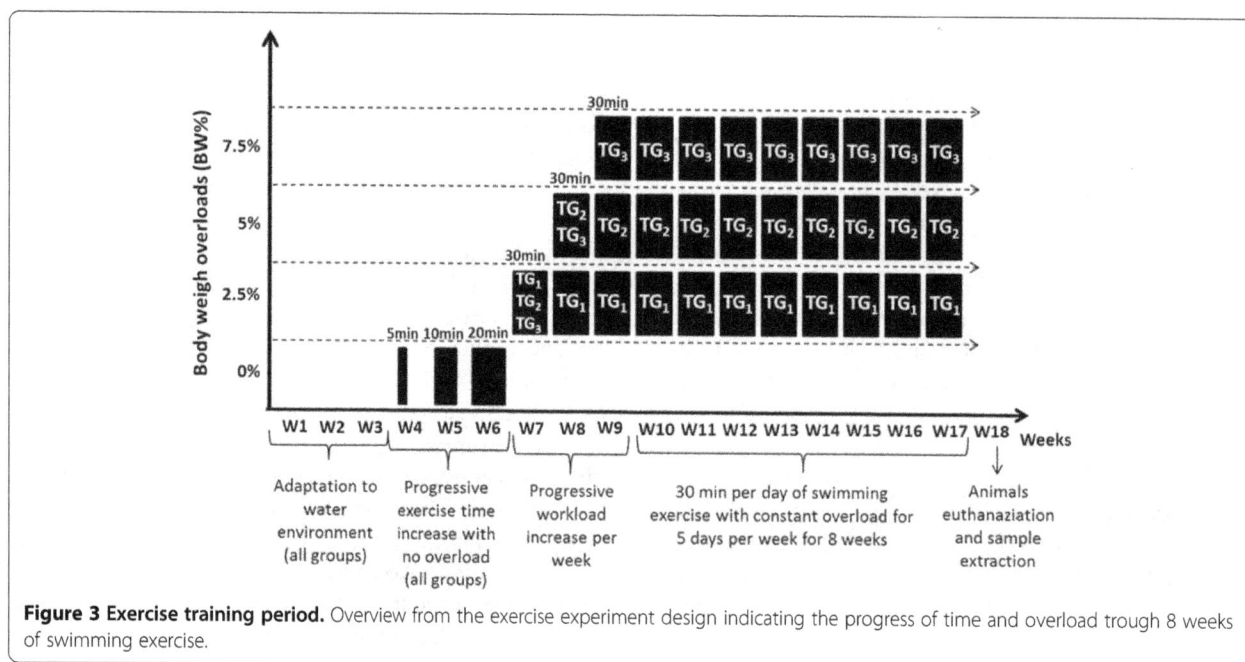

Figure 3 Exercise training period. Overview from the exercise experiment design indicating the progress of time and overload trough 8 weeks of swimming exercise.

immediately underwent euthanasia after the last training session by decapitation after being anaesthetized with 90 mg.Kg^{-1} of ketamin and 10 mg.Kg^{-1} of xilasin provided by muscle injection.

Measuring the animals' training adaptation

In order to verify the animals' training status, lactate was evaluated and used as parameter for rat adaptation to aerobic performance. At the beginning, (in the first week) and at the end (in the last week) of the training process, maximal lactate steady state (MLSS) was measured by an incremental load swimming test with overload increased by 1% of body weight each 3 min, with 90 s of interval until weariness [54]. Moreover, 25 μL of blood samples were collected from a tail tip cut during the exercise tests and deposited in tubes containing 50 μL of 1% sodium fluoride. MLSS was measured in a lactometer model YSI 2700 S™ (Yellow Springs Inc. – USA). The variable maximum lactate used for MLSS identification was 0.07 mM.min^{-1}.

Heart preparation

Complete heart of each animal was removed and placed in an RNAse free sterile apparatus. The left ventricle was separated in three parts. Two were frozen in liquid nitrogen and stored at –80°C until protein and RNA extractions. The third section was stored in 10% formol for 48 h.

Histological sample preparation

After formol (10%) fixation, samples were paraffin embedded and sliced in 3 to 4 μM thickness. After the histological sectioning, tissues were stained with hematoxylin and eosin and further analyzed in an Eclipse E200 POL™ optical microscope (Melville, NY).

Protein extraction

Muscle proteins were extracted from rat heart left ventricles. An amount of 150 mg from each sample was homogenized in 10 mM Tris-EDTA buffer pH 7.4 containing 25 mM sucrose, 2 mM EDTA, and further centrifuged at 1,000 g at 22 to 25°C, as previously described by Short et al. [55]. The pellet, containing the myofibrillar fraction, was re-homogenized in 10 mM Tris–HCl buffer pH 7.2 containing 176 mM KCl and 2 mM EDTA. Bradford's method [56], was used for protein quantification. After that, an aliquot was adjusted to a concentration of 3 mg.ml^{-1} and then dissolved fourfold in sample loading buffer (66 mM Tris–HCl pH 6.7 containing 19 mM EDTA, 1.0% v/v SDS, 0.008% v/v bromophenol blue, 810 mM β-mercaptoethanol and 40% v/v glycerol).

Electrophoretical analyses

SDS-PAGE 12% was performed according to Laemmli [57]. The muscle sample was then loaded on 0.75 mm-thick polyacrylamide gels for protein separation. The discontinuous gel recipe was used, consisting of an 8% separation gel, a 4% stacker gel, and 30% glycerol in the gel matrix. Samples were run in triplicate with CG and TG's samples in adjacent lanes. Gels were run for 20 h at 275 V. Gels were fixed overnight in 50% vol/vol methanol and 10% vol/vol acetic acid. Gels were silver stained using a protocol suggesting by Blum et al. [58] and repeated in triplicate.

Isoelectric focusing and molecular mass separation for 2-DE were conducted according to Gorg et al. [59], with minor modifications obtained from Short et al. [55] using 13 cm immobilized pH gradient (IPG) strips with a 3–11 pH range and a Multiphor II™ electrophoresis system (GE HealthCare). A total of 500 µg of each extract was precipitated using a 2D Clean-Up Kit (GE HealthCare™) and re-suspended in 250 µl solution of 2% CHAPS, 8 M urea, 7 mg.ml^{-1} dithiothreitol (DTT) and 2% IPG Buffer. Strips were hydrated in this solution for 16 hours. Isoelectric focusing was carried out in a gradient mode for 30 min at 500 V, 90 min at 1000 V, 90 min at 3500 V and 6 hours at 3500 V at 2 mA and 5 W. After the first dimension, strips were equilibrated in a solution of 6 M urea, 1% DTT and 2% SDS for 15 min and then applied to gels. A second dimension for high molecular mass proteins was performed in $18 \times 16 \times 0.2$ cm SDS-PAGE 8% gels [55]. Electrophoresis was conducted in a Hoefer system (GE HealthCare™) at 250 V, 40 mA and 10 W for 8 h. The broad range of isoelectric point marker (GE HealthCare™) was also used for subsequent pI identification on gels.

In silico gel analysis

All gels were screened on an HP scanner, model Scanjet 8290 and afterwards analyzed by BioNumerics™ v. 4.5 (Applied Maths™) software. To analyze all the gel images, they were all converted to TIFF files. A calibration curve was applied to convert all colors into gray tones (16-bit, 600 dpi) and convert them into pixel values. All technical replicates were aligned and screened by the software in order to identify the same vectors. Every artifacts and unreliable spots were eliminated by manual inspection. An unreliable spot was defined as not appearing on each of the gel images of the same sample. The spots were located and analyzed by their molecular mass and isoelectric point, concentration and matched by their similarity and spot area and densitometry (volume: pixels per inch) were also counted. In order to define the spot's differential expression a linear regression was performed by the software and a correlation cut off was applied and gels with R^2 lower than 0.8 were discarded. Mean value of spot volume (dpi) from all three replicate were using to describe the spot density and for further comparison of protein expression, taking into account spots with relative volume equal to or bigger than 0.1 dpi. The spots had to present at least a one fold change were select to comparison with the CG 2D gel with the higher R^2. Student's t-test was applied and differences of $p < 0.05$ were considered significant.

Protein identification by MALDI-TOF

All spots defined by technical reproducibility described above and increase or decrease at least one fold when compared to the same spots in control group ($p \leq 0,005$) were excised from gels using a scalpel and each one placed in a 1.5 µl micro tube. Protein in-gel digestion was carried out with Gold sequencing grade trypsin (Promega™) according to Shevchenko et al. [60]. 300 µl of 100% acetonitrile was added to tubes for 5 min. Supernatant was removed and spots were dried in a SpeedVac for 5 min. Samples were incubated for 60 min at 56°C in a solution containing 50 µl of 10 mM DTT and 100 mM NH_4HCO_3. The solution was replaced with 50 µl of 55 mM iodoacetamide and 100 mM NH_4HCO_3 and incubated in darkness for 45 min. Spots were rinsed twice with MilliQ™ water (Millipore™) for 10 min, and exposed to 100 µl of 100% acetonitrile for 5 min. Excess acetonitrile was removed and again spots were dried in a SpeedVac for 5 min. Protein digestion was carried out using 650 ng trypsin diluted in 50 µl of 50 mM NH_4HCO_3 and 6 mM $CaCl_2$, with overnight incubation at 37°C. The peptides derived from tryptic digestion were analyzed as described by Henzel et al. [61] using an UltraFlex II™ MALDI-TOF (Matrix-Assisted Laser Desorption Ionization Time-of-Flight, Bruker Daltonics™, Billerica, MA). A sample of 2 µl was mixed in 6 µl of 0.1% α-cyano-4-hydroxycinnamic acid, 0.1% trifluoroacetic acid dissolved in acetonitrile (1:1). A volume of 0.5 µl was applied to a MALDI plate and dried at room temperature. Spectrometry was operated in a linear mode for MS acquisition and reflected mode for MS/MS acquisitions using modulated power with 200 random shoots. Data were saved in standard Bruker software format. Spots were identified using Peptide Mass Fingerprinting (PMF). Peptide mass lists were produced automated analysis tools of mass spectrometer previously described [62]. Data were smoothed (Gaussian, 2 chan peak width), baseline subtracted (100 chan peak width) and an adaptive ($\times$ 8.0) threshold applied as described by Holloway et al. [63]. Monoisotopic peak (25% centroid) selection was restricted to 15 peptides over 600–40000 m/z, and the peak list searched against the Swiss-Prot database restricted to *Rattus novergicus* databank using a locally implemented MASCOT (www.matrixscience.com) server. The enzyme specificity was trypsin, allowing one missed cleavage, carbamidomethyl modification of cysteine (fixed), oxidation of methionine (variable). Protein identification was accepted based on a significant Mowse score

Quantification of MyHC mRNA by real time qPCR

Total RNA was extracted with the Trizol™ reagent (Invitrogen™, USA) from 25 mg of each animal's ventricle using standard protocol. Total RNA from individual animals from different training groups was pooled together. This provided RNA samples from the untrained group and from the other groups: 2.5% (TG$_1$), 5.0% (TG$_2$) and

7.5% (TG_3). The cDNA was generated using a High Capacity cDNA Archive Kit (Applied Biosystems™) following the manufacturer's instructions. A TaqMan Gene expression assay for myosin, heavy polypeptide 6, cardiac muscle, alpha (*Myh6*, Rn00568304_m1) was bought from Applied Biosystems™ (Foster City, CA). Equal amounts of RNA (0.5 µg) were reverse transcribed using High Capacity cDNA Archive (Applied Biosystems™) and submitted to qPCR. TaqMan assays were carried out with a StepOnePlus instrument (Applied Biosystems™, Foster City, CA) in 20 µl reactions containing 0.5 µl of TaqMan Gene expression Assays (20 ×), 12,5 µl of TaqMan Universal PCR Master Mix (2 ×) and 2 µl of template cDNA (100 ng). After initial denaturation at 95°C for 10 min, amplifications were carried out in 40 cycles at 95°C/15 s and 60°C/1 min. Comparative CT (crossing threshold) method was used to establish differential expression among training groups and control. The constitutive *rRNA18S* gene expression was used for data normalization. Relative quantitation was carried out using $\Delta\Delta C_T$ method based on three technical replicates.

Abbreviations

α-MyHC: α -myosin heavy chain; β- MyHC: β-myosin heavy chain; 2-DE: two-dimensional electrophoresis; ATP: adenosine triphosphate; cDNA: complementary deoxyribonucleic acid; CG: control groups; CHAPS: 3-[(3-cholamidopropyl)dimethylammonio]-1-propanesulfonate; cTn: cardiac troponin; DTT: dithiothreitol; EDTA: ethylenediaminetetraacetic acid; $FADH_2$: flavin adenine dinucleotide, hydroquinone form; IEF: isoelectric focusing; IPG: immobilized pH gradient; MALDI-ToF: matrix-assisted laser desorption ionization time-of-flight; MLC: myosin light chain; MLSS: maximal lactate steady state; Mn-SOD: manganese-superoxide dismutase; mRNA: messenger ribonucleic acid; MS: mass spectrometry; MS/MS: tandem mass spectrometry; MyHC: myosin heavy chain; NADH: nicotinamide adenine dinucleotide at reduced form; NCBI: National Center for Biotechnology Information; PMF: peptide mass fingerprinting; qPCR: real-time polymerase chain reaction; R^2: coefficient of linear regression determination; RNA: ribonucleic acid; SDS-PAGE: sodium dodecyl sulphate polyacrilamide gel electrophoresis; TCA cycle: tricarboxylic acid cycle; TG_1: TG_2 and TG_3, training groups with overload of 2.5%, 5.0% and 7.5% respectively; Tris-EDTA: hydroxymethyl aminomethane-ethylenediaminetetraacetic acid; Tris-HCl: ethylenediaminetetraacetic acid - Hydrochloric acid.

Competing interests

Authors declare there are absolute not political, personal, religious, ideological, academic, intellectual, commercial conflict of interests in this work.

Authors' contributions

LAOR it conceived and participates of design of the study, exercise training, electrophoretical and *in silico* gel analysis and drafted the manuscript. BP participates of exercise training and electrophoretical analyses. DHB does the Histological sample preparation and analyses. RVO helped to draft the manuscript. RV participates of molecular studies (real time qPCR). GD carried out the protein identification by MALDI-TOF. RWP participates of molecular studies (real time qPCR) and helped to draft the manuscript. OLF participates conception and design and coordination of the study and helped to draft the manuscript. All authors read and approved the final manuscript.

Acknowledgments

This work was supported by CNPq, CAPES, FAPDF and UCB.

Author details

[1]Centro de Análises Proteômicas e Bioquímicas, Programa de Pós-Graduação em Ciências Genômicas e Biotecnologia, Universidade Católica de Brasília, Brasília-DF, Brazil. [2]Programa de Pós-Graduação em Educação Física, da Universidade de Brasília. [3]Departamento de Biologia, Universidade Federal de Juiz de Fora, Juiz de Fora-MG, Brazil. [4]Universidade Federal do Rio de Janeiro, Protemics Unit, Rio de Janeiro, Brazil. [5]Pos-graduação em patologia molecular, Universidade de Brasilia, Brasilia, DF, Brazil.

References

1. Iemitsu M, *et al*: Physiological and pathological cardiac hypertrophy induce different molecular phenotypes in the rat. *Am J Physiol Regul Integr Comp Physiol* 2001, **281**(6):R2029–R2036.
2. Vivanco F, *et al*: Proteomics and cardiovascular disease. *Rev Esp Cardiol* 2003, **56**(3):289–302.
3. Bernardo BC, Weeks KL, Pretorius L, McMullen JR: Molecular distinction between physiological and pathological cardiac hypertrophy: experimental findings and therapeutic strategies. *Pharmacol Ther* 2010, **128**(1):191–227.
4. Burniston JG: Changes in the rat skeletal muscle proteome induced by moderate-intensity endurance exercise. *Biochim Biophys Acta* 2008, **1784** (7–8):1077–1086.
5. Bishop JE, Lindahl G: Regulation of cardiovascular collagen synthesis by mechanical load. *Cardiovasc Res* 1999, **42**(1):27–44.
6. Gonzalez A, Lopez B, Diezl J: Myocardial fibrosis in arterial hypertension. *Eur Heart J Suppl* 2002, **4**(suppl_D):D18–D22.
7. Verzola RM, *et al*: Early remodeling of rat cardiac muscle induced by swimming training. *Braz J Med Biol Res* 2006, **39**(5):621–627.
8. Anand IS, Florea VG, Fisher L: Surrogate end points in heart failure. *J Am Coll Cardiol* 2002, **39**(9):1414–1421.
9. Demirel HA, *et al*: Exercise-induced alterations in skeletal muscle myosin heavy chain phenotype: dose–response relationship. *J Appl Physiol* 1999, **86**(3):1002–1008.
10. Joumaa WH, Leoty C: A comparative analysis of the effects of exercise training on contractile responses in fast- and slow-twitch rat skeletal muscles. *J Comp Physiol B* 2002, **172**(4):329–338.
11. Burniston JG: Adaptation of the rat cardiac proteome in response to intensity-controlled endurance exercise. *Proteomics* 2009, **9**(1):106–115.
12. Diffee GM, Chung E: Altered single cell force-velocity and power properties in exercise-trained rat myocardium. *J Appl Physiol* 2003, **94**(5):1941–1948.
13. Scheinowitz M, *et al*: Short- and long-term swimming exercise training increases myocardial insulin-like growth factor-I gene expression. *Growth Horm IGF Res* 2003, **13**(1):19–25.
14. Hashimoto T, *et al*: Expression of MHC-beta and MCT1 in cardiac muscle after exercise training in myocardial-infarcted rats. *J Appl Physiol* 2004, **97**(3):843–851.
15. Herron TJ, Korte FS, McDonald KS: Loaded shortening and power output in cardiac myocytes are dependent on myosin heavy chain isoform expression. *Am J Physiol Heart Circ Physiol* 2001, **281**(3):H1217–H1222.
16. Hinken AC, Korte FS, McDonald KS: Porcine cardiac myocyte power output is increased after chronic exercise training. *J Appl Physiol* 2006, **101**(1):40–46.
17. Guelfi KJ, *et al*: A proteomic analysis of the acute effects of high-intensity exercise on skeletal muscle proteins in fasted rats. *Clin Exp Pharmacol Physiol* 2006, **33**(10):952–957.
18. Gelfi C, *et al*: The human muscle proteome in aging. *J Proteome Res* 2006, **5**(6):1344–1353.
19. Diffee GM: Adaptation of cardiac myocyte contractile properties to exercise training. *Exerc Sport Sci Rev* 2004, **32**(3):112–119.
20. Diffee GM, *et al*: Microarray expression analysis of effects of exercise training: increase in atrial MLC-1 in rat ventricles. *Am J Physiol Heart Circ Physiol* 2003, **284**(3):H830–H837.
21. Lindsey ML, *et al*: A multidimensional proteomic approach to identify hypertrophy-associated proteins. *Proteomics* 2006, **6**(7):2225–2235.

22. White MY, et al: Proteomics of ischemia/reperfusion injury in rabbit myocardium reveals alterations to proteins of essential functional systems. Proteomics 2005, 5(5):1395–1410.

23. Korte FS, et al: Power output is linearly related to MyHC content in rat skinned myocytes and isolated working hearts. Am J Physiol Heart Circ Physiol 2005, 289(2):H801–H812.

24. Herron TJ, McDonald KS: Small amounts of alpha-myosin heavy chain isoform expression significantly increase power output of rat cardiac myocyte fragments. Circ Res 2002, 90(11):1150–1152.

25. Harjola VP, Kiilavuori K, Virkamaki A: The effect of moderate exercise training on skeletal muscle myosin heavy chain distribution in chronic heart failure. Int J Cardiol 2006, 109(3):335–338.

26. Molloy MP, et al: Overcoming technical variation and biological variation in quantitative proteomics. Proteomics 2003, 3(10):1912–1919.

27. Adams JE 3rd, et al: Cardiac troponin I. A marker with high specificity for cardiac injury. Circulation 1993, 88(1):101–106.

28. Westbrook JA, et al: The human heart proteome: Two-dimensional maps using narrow-range immobilised pH gradients. Electrophoresis 2006, 27(8):1547–1555.

29. Rafalski K, Abdourahman A, Edwards JG: Early adaptations to training: upregulation of alpha-myosin heavy chain gene expression. Med Sci Sports Exerc 2007, 39(1):75–82.

30. Jin H, et al: Effects of exercise training on cardiac function, gene expression, and apoptosis in rats. Am J Physiol Heart Circ Physiol 2000, 279(6):H2994–H3002.

31. Schaub MC, et al: Modulation of contractility in human cardiac hypertrophy by myosin essential light chain isoforms. Cardiovasc Res 1998, 37(2):381–404.

32. Malhotra A, et al: Correlation of myosin isoenzyme alterations with myocardial function in physiologic and pathologic hypertrophy. Eur Heart J 1984, 5(Suppl F):61–67.

33. Rupp H: Differential effect of physical exercise routines on ventricular myosin and peripheral catecholamine stores in normotensive and spontaneously hypertensive rats. Circ Res 1989, 65(2):370–377.

34. Rappaport L, et al: Isomyosins, microtubules and desmin during the onset of cardiac hypertrophy in the rat. Eur Heart J 1984, 5(Suppl F):243–250.

35. Agianian B, et al: A troponin switch that regulates muscle contraction by stretch instead of calcium. EMBO J 2004, 23(4):772–779.

36. Liu X, Pollack GH: Stepwise sliding of single actin and Myosin filaments. Biophys J 2004, 86(1 Pt 1):353–358.

37. Lippi G, Banfi G: Exercise-related increase of cardiac troponin release in sports: An apparent paradox finally elucidated? Clin Chim Acta 2010, 411(7–8):610–611.

38. Moreno V, et al: Serum levels of high-sensitivity troponin T: a novel marker for cardiac remodeling in hypertrophic cardiomyopathy. J Card Fail 2010, 16(12):950–956.

39. Nie J, Close G, George KP, Tong TK, Shi Q: emporal association of elevations in serum cardiac troponin T and myocardial oxidative stress after prolonged exercise in rats. Eur J Appl Physiol 2010, 110(6):1299–303.

40. Goette A, et al: Acute atrial tachyarrhythmia induces angiotensin II type 1 receptor-mediated oxidative stress and microvascular flow abnormalities in the ventricles. Eur Heart J 2009, 30(11):1411–20.

41. Smith SC, Allen PM: Expression of myosin-class II major histocompatibility complexes in the normal myocardium occurs before induction of autoimmune myocarditis. Proc Natl Acad Sci USA 1992, 89(19):9131–5.

42. Bye A, et al: Aerobic capacity-dependent differences in cardiac gene expression. Physiol Genomics 2008, 33(1):100–9.

43. Ravi Kiran T, Subramanyam MV, Asha Devi S: Swim exercise training and adaptations in the antioxidant defense system of myocardium of old rats: relationship to swim intensity and duration. Comp Biochem Physiol B Biochem Mol Biol 2004, 137(2):187–96.

44. Vander Heiden MG, et al: Outer mitochondrial membrane permeability can regulate coupled respiration and cell survival. Proc Natl Acad Sci USA 2000, 97(9):4666–71.

45. Vinogradov AD: NADH/NAD + interaction with NADH: ubiquinone oxidoreductase (complex I). Biochim Biophys Acta 2008, 1777(7–8):729–34.

46. Molnar AMA, Pereira-da-Silva L, Macedo DV, Dabbeni-Sala F: Evaluation by blue native polyacrylamide electrophoresis colorimetric staining of the effects of physical exercise on the activities of mitochondrial complexes in rat muscle. Brazilian Journal of sMedical and Biological Researsh 2004, 37(7):939–947.

47. D'Agostino B, et al: Exercise capacity and cytochrome oxidase activity in muscle mitochondria of COPD patients. Respir Med 2010, 104(1):83–90.

48. Raffaello A, Rizzuto R: Mitochondrial longevity pathways. Biochim Biophys Acta 2011, 1813(1):260–8.

49. Powers SK, Jackson MJ: Exercise-Induced Oxidative Stress: Cellular Mechanisms and Impact on Muscle Force Production. Physiol Rev 2008, 88(4):1243–1276.

50. Starnes JWB, Brian D, Olsen, Marissa E: Exercise training decreases rat heart mitochondria free radical generation but does not prevent Ca 2 + –induced dysfunction. Appl Physiol 2007, 102.

51. Starnes JWB, Brian D, Olsen ME: Exercise training decreases rat heart mitochondria free radical generation but does not prevent Ca^{2+}-induced dysfunction. J Appl Physiol 2007, 102(5):1793–1798.

52. Knoop V, et al: Transport of magnesium and other divalent cations: evolution of the 2-TM-GxN proteins in the MIT superfamily. Mol Genet Genomics 2005, 274(3):205–16.

53. Smith GA, et al: The effect of Mg2+ on cardiac muscle function: Is CaATP the substrate for priming myofibril cross-bridge formation and Ca2+ reuptake by the sarcoplasmic reticulum? Biochem J 2001, 354(Pt 3):539–51.

54. Gobatto CA, et al: Maximal lactate steady state in rats submitted to swimming exercise. Comp Biochem Physiol A Mol Integr Physiol 2001, 130(1):21–7.

55. Short KR, et al: Changes in myosin heavy chain mRNA and protein expression in human skeletal muscle with age and endurance exercise training. J Appl Physiol 2005, 99(1):95–102.

56. Bradford MM: A rapid and sensitive method for the quantitation of microgram quantities of protein utilizing the principle of protein-dye binding. Anal Biochem 1976, 72:248–54.

57. Laemmli UK: Cleavage of structural proteins during the assembly of the head of bacteriophage T4. Nature 1970, 227(5259):680–5.

58. Blum H, Beier H, Gross HJ: Improved silver staining of plant proteins, RNA and DNA in polyacrylamide gels. Electrophoresis 1986, 8:93–99.

59. Gorg A, Postel W, Gunther S: The current state of two-dimensional electrophoresis with immobilized pH gradients. Electrophoresis 1988, 9(9):531–46.

60. Shevchenko A, et al: In-gel digestion for mass spectrometric characterization of proteins and proteomes. Nat Protoc 2006, 1(6):2856–60.

61. Henzel WJ, et al: Identifying proteins from two-dimensional gels by molecular mass searching of peptide fragments in protein sequence databases. Proc Natl Acad Sci USA 1993, 90(11):5011–5.

62. Gay S, et al: Peptide mass fingerprinting peak intensity prediction: extracting knowledge from spectra. Proteomics 2002, 2(10):1374–91.

63. Holloway KV, et al: Proteomic investigation of changes in human vastus lateralis muscle in response to interval-exercise training. Proteomics 2009, 9(22):5155–74.

17

Acetate transiently inhibits myocardial contraction by increasing mitochondrial calcium uptake

James F Schooley[1], Aryan M A Namboodiri[1], Rachel T Cox[2], Rolf Bünger[1] and Thomas P Flagg[1*]

Abstract

Background: There is a close relationship between cardiovascular disease and cardiac energy metabolism, and we have previously demonstrated that palmitate inhibits myocyte contraction by increasing K_v channel activity and decreasing the action potential duration. Glucose and long chain fatty acids are the major fuel sources supporting cardiac function; however, cardiac myocytes can utilize a variety of substrates for energy generation, and previous studies demonstrate the acetate is rapidly taken up and oxidized by the heart. In this study, we tested the effects of acetate on contractile function of isolated mouse ventricular myocytes.

Results: Acute exposure of myocytes to 10 mM sodium acetate caused a marked, but transient, decrease in systolic sarcomere shortening ($1.49 \pm 0.20\%$ vs. $5.58 \pm 0.49\%$ in control), accompanied by a significant increase in diastolic sarcomere length (1.81 ± 0.01 μm vs. 1.77 ± 0.01 μm in control), with a near linear dose response in the 1–10 mM range. Unlike palmitate, acetate caused no change in action potential duration; however, acetate markedly increased mitochondrial Ca^{2+} uptake. Moreover, pretreatment of cells with the mitochondrial Ca^{2+} uptake blocker, Ru-360 (10 μM), markedly suppressed the effect of acetate on contraction.

Conclusions: Lehninger and others have previously demonstrated that the anions of weak aliphatic acids such as acetate stimulate Ca^{2+} uptake in isolated mitochondria. Here we show that this effect of acetate appears to extend to isolated cardiac myocytes where it transiently modulates cell contraction.

Background

It is well established that the cardiac myocardium is capable of oxidizing a variety of carbon sources to supply the energy required for continuous contraction. Lipids, carbohydrates, ketone bodies, and amino acids can all support some degree of ATP synthesis in the heart. The loss of metabolic flexibility in the diseased heart may lead to abnormal contractile function. For example, we recently demonstrated that mice overexpressing fatty acid transport protein (FATP4) in the heart have impaired diastolic function [1]. Similarly, acute exposure to long chain fatty acids has been shown to cause a decrease in cardiomyocyte contractility through effects on increases in voltage gated K^+ currents thus causing shortening of the action potential [2].

In a continued effort to understand the relationship of cardiac metabolism and cell function, we set out to test the effects of acetate on contraction. Several studies have examined the effect of acetate on cardiac contraction with equivocal results. In isolated cells, acetate tends to increase cell shortening after 10 minutes of exposure [3]. In isolated papillary muscle and in vivo, sodium acetate has been shown to reduce contractility [4,5], whereas other studies suggest that acetate causes an increase in contractility [6]. The effects of acetate on cardiovascular function in vivo are complicated by the concomitant vasodilatory effects that also must be considered [6]. These mixed results are consistent with the idea that acetate can affect cardiac contractility, but the cellular mechanisms remain poorly understood.

Although it is typically found in low concentrations (~0.2 mM) in non-ruminant mammals [7], acetate oxidation can account for ~10% of the total CO_2 output in humans [8]. Acetate can be converted to acetyl CoA by acetyl CoA sythetase (AceCS2) in the mitochondrial matrix [9] and the resultant acetyl CoA can then enter

* Correspondence: Thomas.Flagg@usuhs.edu
[1]Department of Anatomy, Physiology, and Genetics, Uniformed Services University for the Health Sciences, 4301 Jones Bridge Road, Rm. C-2114, Bethesda 20814, MD, USA
Full list of author information is available at the end of the article

the tricarboxylic acid (TCA) cycle. The heart is unique in that the expression of the mitochondrial AceCS2 is higher than in any other tissue, so the heart is ideally suited to use acetate as a fuel source [9]. Metabolic studies by Randle demonstrate that acetate is rapidly oxidized in the myocardium [10]. In some isolated heart studies, acetate combustion can account for ~90% of total respiration to the exclusion of glucose oxidation [11], although others suggest that at physiological workloads both acetate and glucose are effectively utilized [12]. Acetate can also affect isolated mitochondria independent of its oxidation, where Lehninger and others have demonstrated that exposure to acetate causes a rapid increase in mitochondrial matrix Ca^{2+} and osmotic swelling [13-15].

In this context, we investigated the effects of acetate on cardiac contractility in isolated cardiac myocytes. We tested the effects of acetate throughout a 10 minute exposure. The results demonstrate that acetate inhibits systolic function and increases cell relaxation within 2 minutes of exposure. The decrease in systolic function is transient, however, and contraction amplitude is restored within 10 minutes. These effects are independent of changes in action potential duration; however, the effects of acetate were inhibited by blockade of mitochondrial Ca^{2+} uptake with Ru-360, indicating that acetate causes effects on cardiac contraction by increasing Ca^{2+} uptake into the mitochondria.

Methods
Animal subjects
All animals used in this study were male, aged 2–4 months, C57Bl6/J. All procedures complied with the standards for the care and use of animal subjects as stated in the *Guide for the Care and Use of Laboratory Animals* (NIH publication No. 85–23, revised 1996). Protocols were approved by the USUHS Institutional Animal Care and Use Committee.

Solutions (concentrations in mM)
Normal Tyrode Soution (NT): NaCl, 137; KCl, 5.4; NaH_2PO_4, 0.16; glucose, 10; $MgCl_2$, 0.5; $CaCl_2$, 1.8; HEPES, 5.0; $NaHCO_3$, 3.0; pH 7.35 - 7.4.

Wittenberg Isolation Medium (WIM): NaCl, 116; KCl, 5.3; NaH_2PO_4, 1.2; glucose, 11.6; $MgCl_2$, 3.7; HEPES, 20; L-glutamine, 2.0; $NaHCO_3$, 4.4; KH_2PO_4, 1.5; 1X essential vitamins; 1X amino acids; pH 7.3-7.4.

Myocyte isolation
Isolation of ventricular myocytes was performed as described previously [1,2,16]. Briefly, mice were anesthetized by intra-peritoneal injection with 2,2,2 tribromoethanol (250 mg/kg). Following cervical dislocation, the heart was rapidly excised and the aorta cannulated. The heart was retrogradely perfused with Ca^{2+}-free WIM solution for 5 minutes followed by perfusion with a digestion solution containing 100 µM $CaCl_2$ and 1 mg/mL collagenase (Type 2, Worthington Biochemical). Left ventricular cells were gently dispersed by manual trituration using a pasteur pipette in WIM solution supplemented with bovine serum albumin (1 mg/mL) and 500 µM $CaCl_2$. Cells were washed twice with WIM solution and twice with HEPES-buffered M199 solution and stored at room temperature. Cells were used for experiments within 12 hours of isolation in all cases.

Myocyte contraction measurements
Unloaded sarcomere shortening was measured in freshly isolated ventricular myocytes, as described previously [1,2]. Briefly, isolated myocytes were transferred into a recording chamber mounted on an Olympus X51 inverted microscope and superfused with normal Tyrode solution saturated with room air. Additions to the Tyrode solution are described in the text. The mitochondrial calcium uptake inhibitor, Ru-360, was obtained from EMD Biosciences; all other chemicals were purchased from Sigma. Typically, cells were field stimulated to contract at 1 Hz. When thapsigargin was applied to cells, the stimulation frequency was reduced to 0.5 Hz. Video images were acquired using a Myocam camera and IonWizard software (IonOptix, Inc.). All experiments were performed at room temperature.

Mitochondrial Ca^{2+} measurements
Freshly isolated ventricular myocytes were plated on laminin-coated (100 µg/mL) Mat-Tek dishes for fluorescence imaging. Cells were loaded with Rhod-2-AM (5 µM) for 30 minutes in normal Tyrode solution containing probenecid (500 µM) to inhibit dye export and 200 µM $MnCl_2$ to quench cytoplasmic fluorescence as has been previously reported [17,18]. After loading, cells were washed twice with normal Tyrode solution supplemented with probenecid and 200 µM $MnCl_2$ and transferred to the microscope stage. Cell images were obtained every 10 seconds for 10 minutes. Data were plotted as background-subtracted Rhod-2-AM fluorescence normalized to mean signal during the first 6 images recorded prior to addition of acetate.

Action potential measurements
Action potentials were measured in freshly isolated ventricular myocytes using whole cell current clamp. Briefly, following acquisition of the whole cell mode, cell holding potential was adjusted to –70 mV using current injection. Action potentials were evoked by suprathreshold stimuli (2 nA, 3 msec) delivered at 1 Hz. Action potentials were recorded continuously during 5 minute exposure to acetate followed by 5 minutes washout. Average traces constructed from 25 consecutive action potentials during control, acetate exposure (2 minutes) and washout (5 minutes) were

analyzed. Action potential duration (APD$_{90}$) was determined at 90% repolarization and referenced to the peak of the action potential.

Data analysis

All data were analyzed using ClampFit, IonWizard, ImageJ and Microsoft Excel software and (except where noted) results are presented as mean ± SEM (standard error of the mean). Statistical analysis was performed with built-in functions of Excel or with the Sigma XL software add-in. Statistical tests and p-values are denoted in the figure legend and text where appropriate.

Results

Acute exposure to acetate transiently impairs cardiac contraction and increases diastolic sarcomere length

To test whether the short chain fatty acid, acetate, exerts negative inotropic effects, we continuously monitored average sarcomere length in isolated mouse cardiomyocytes acutely exposed to Tyrode solution containing 10 mM sodium acetate. Three major consequences of acetate exposure were observed. Figure 1 shows that acetate caused a transient decrease in active sarcomere shortening. At two minutes following acetate application, fractional shortening was markedly decreased from 5.6 ± 0.5 to 1.5 ± 0.2 (n = 12, p < 0.001, paired t-test). In the continued presence of acetate, contraction amplitude gradually recovered and returned to baseline after approximately 10 minutes. We also noted a marked increase in fractional sarcomere shortening when acetate was removed from the bath solution.

In addition, exposure to acetate significantly increased the diastolic sarcomere length. We next examined the concentration dependence of the decrease in contraction observed at two minutes and diastolic sarcomere length following the exposure to acetate. Figure 2 shows that the negative inotropic effect of acetate is concentration dependent. Data were fit with a modified Hill equation with an IC$_{50}$ = 5.6 mM and Hill coefficient of 1.4. There was no apparent concentration dependence for the effect on diastolic sarcomere length.

Acetate exposure does not affect the action potential duration

We previously demonstrated that acute exposure to long chain fatty acids shortens the action potential duration principally by increasing outward voltage-dependent K$^+$ currents encoded by K$_v$2.1 and K$_v$1.5, with no effect on IK$_1$ [2]. Considering that short-chain fatty acids might have similar effects on cell excitability, we examined the effect of acetate on the action potential duration (APD$_{90}$) (Figure 3). In contrast to results with palmitate, APD$_{90}$ (24.5 ± 3.2 msec in control) was unaffected by acetate (25.0 ± 3.5 msec, p >0.05, paired t-test), suggesting that a different molecular mechanism underlies the inotropic effects of acetate.

Acetate exposure stimulates mitochondrial Ca^{2+} uptake

It has been shown previously that acetate increases Ca^{2+} uptake in isolated liver and heart mitochondria [13-15]. In this light, we hypothesized that the acute application

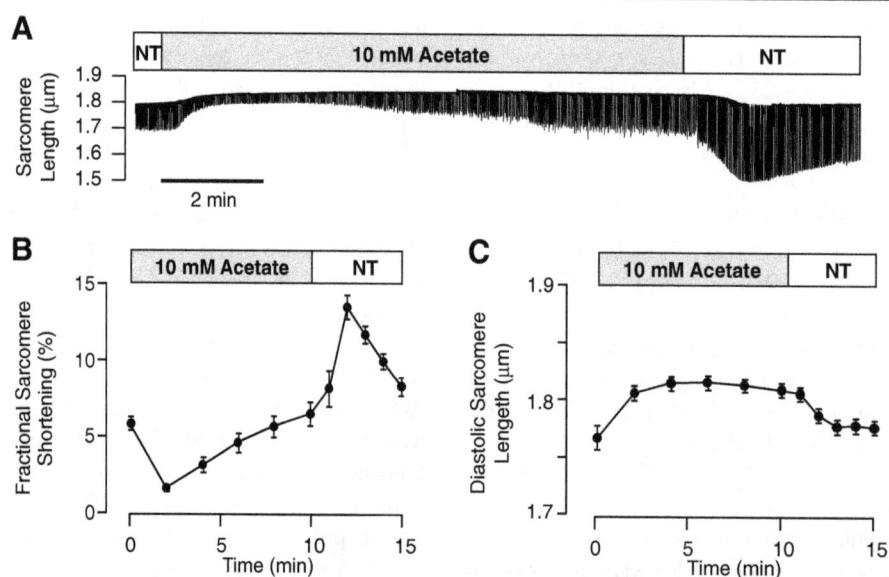

Figure 1 Acetate causes a transient decrease of fractional sarcomere shortening and an increase in diastolic sarcomere length in isolated mouse cardiac myocytes. (A) Representative recording of average sarcomere length assessed continuously throughout application and removal of normal Tyrode solution (NT) supplemented with 10 mM sodium acetate. Summary data from experiments as in **A** (n = 15), illustrating the effects of acetate on **(B)** fractional sarcomere shortening and **(C)** diastolic sarcomere length.

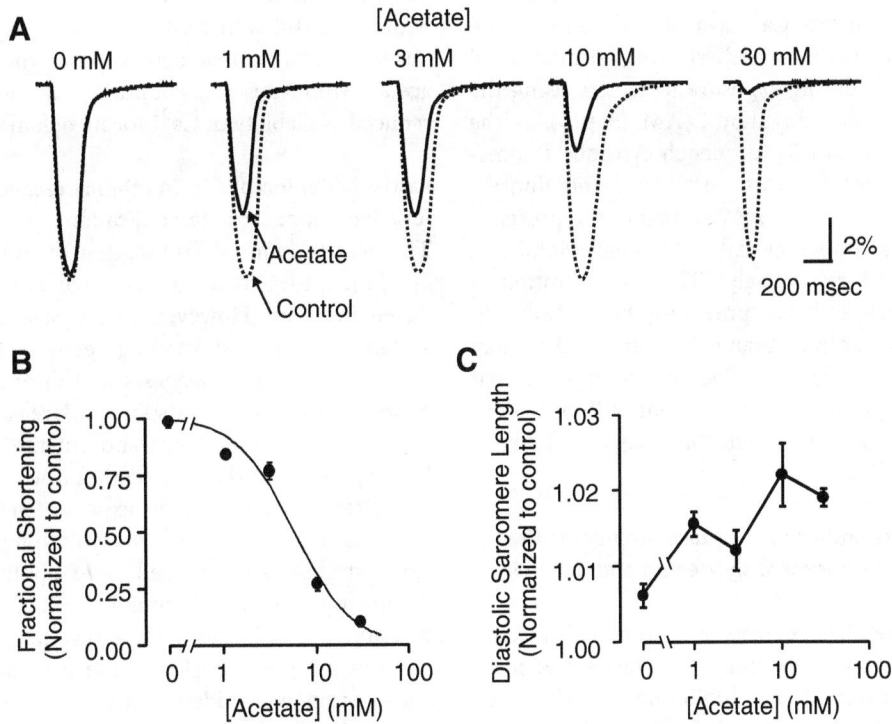

Figure 2 Concentration-dependence of acetate effect on fractional shortening and diastolic sarcomere length. (A) Single averaged contractions acquired in experiments as described in Figure 1 at different concentrations of sodium acetate. Contractions in normal Tyrode (Control, *dotted line*) and at 2 minutes following exposure to acetate solution (Acetate, *solid line*) are shown. 10 mM NaCl, instead of sodium acetate, was added to normal Tyrode to collect the zero acetate data. **(B)** Acetate concentration response curve for maximum contraction inhibition. Data were fit with a modified Hill equation (*solid line*): $FS/FS_0 = 1/(1 + ([Acetate]/IC_{50})^h)$, where IC_{50} is the half-maximal inhibitory concentration of acetate ($IC_{50} = 5.6$ mM) and h is the Hill coefficient (h = 1.3). **(C)** There was no apparent acetate concentration dependence on diastolic sarcomere length.

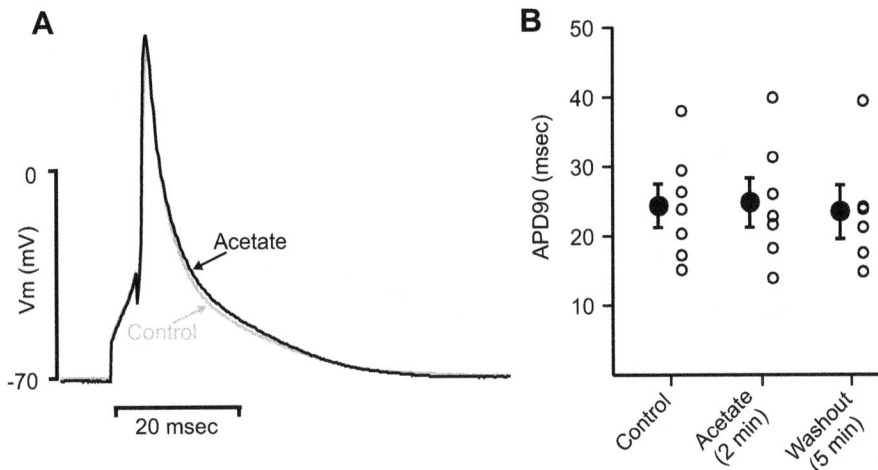

Figure 3 Acetate does not affect the action potential duration (APD$_{90}$). (A) Representative action potentials recorded before (Control, *gray line*) and 2 minutes following acetate exposure (Acetate, *black line*). Action potentials were recorded in whole cell current clamp mode and were evoked suprathreshold current injections. Records are averaged traces from 25 consecutive action potentials. **(B)** Summary APD$_{90}$ data from all (n = 7) experiments as in **A**. Acetate exposure did not affect the APD$_{90}$ (24.5 ± 3.2 msec in acetate vs. 25.0 ± 3.5 msec in control).

of acetate might lead to an increase in mitochondrial Ca^{2+} uptake, leaving less Ca^{2+} available to activate the myofilaments. To test this hypothesis, we first monitored mitochondrial Ca^{2+} during exposure to acetate using the fluorescent Ca^{2+} indicator, Rhod-2 AM (5 µM) in the presence of 200 µM $MnCl_2$ to quench cytosolic fluorescence [17,18]. Figure 4 shows normalized cell fluorescence during exposure to 10 mM acetate in the presence or absence of the mitochondrial Ca^{2+} uptake inhibitor, Ru-360 (n = 9 and 8 respectively). This concentration of Ru-360 was chosen as it has previously been shown to have no effect on transmembrane Ca^{2+} fluxes other than mitochondrial uptake [19,20]. The results indicate that acetate causes a specific increase in Rhod-2 fluorescence consistent with the conclusion that acetate increases mitochondrial Ca^{2+} uptake.

Inhibition of mitochondrial Ca^{2+} uptake attenuates the effects of acetate on fractional shortening and diastolic sarcomere length

If the acetate-dependent increase in mitochondrial Ca^{2+} is responsible for the reduction of myocyte fractional shortening, we reasoned that inhibiting mitochondrial Ca^{2+} uptake would reduce or abolish the effect of acetate on myocyte contraction. To test this hypothesis, we incubated cells for 30 minutes with 10 µM Ru-360, and then measured the effects of acetate on sarcomere shortening. Figure 5 shows that Ru-360 treatment significantly attenuated the effect of acetate on both diastolic sarcomere length and fractional sarcomere shortening. Interestingly, pretreatment with Ru-360 alone also had a marked effect on contractile function prior to acetate exposure. As shown in Figure 5B (inset), fractional sarcomere shortening immediately prior to acetate exposure (time zero) was

13.03 ± 1.17% in cells pretreated with Ru-360 compared with 5.83 ± 0.43% in control cells not exposed to Ru-360. Taken together, these data support the conclusion that acetate stimulates mitochondrial Ca^{2+} uptake, leading to reduced availability of Ca^{2+} for myofilament activation.

Partial inhibition of SERCA inhibits recovery of systolic function during acetate application

The acetate-induced stimulation of mitochondrial Ca^{2+} uptake appears to be the seminal event leading to reduced inotropy. However, in the sustained presence of acetate, fractional shortening recovers to control levels by 10 minutes. This suggests that during the early phase of acetate exposure, cytosolic Ca^{2+} released from the SR bypasses the myofilaments and enters the mitochondria. We hypothesized that the recovery of contraction during the latter phase of acetate exposure reflects refilling of the SR to replace the Ca^{2+} lost to the mitochondria. Previous studies have utilized brief application of 1 µM thapsigargin to partially inhibit SERCA activity [21]. We therefore treated cells with 1 µM thapsigargin for 2–5 minutes prior to transfer to the bath for recording. No thapsigargin was added to the recording solutions. As expected, cell relaxation was markedly slowed by SERCA inhibition and therefore cells were stimulated at 0.5 Hz (instead of 1 Hz) for these experiments (Figure 6). Thapsigargin pretreatment markedly inhibited fractional shortening as expected (Figure 6B, inset), but exposure to acetate still resulted in a decrease in contraction amplitude and increase in diastolic sarcomere length similar to control, untreated cells. It should be noted, however, that the recovery of contraction typically observed during the latter phase of acetate application as well as the transient increase in contraction at washout were

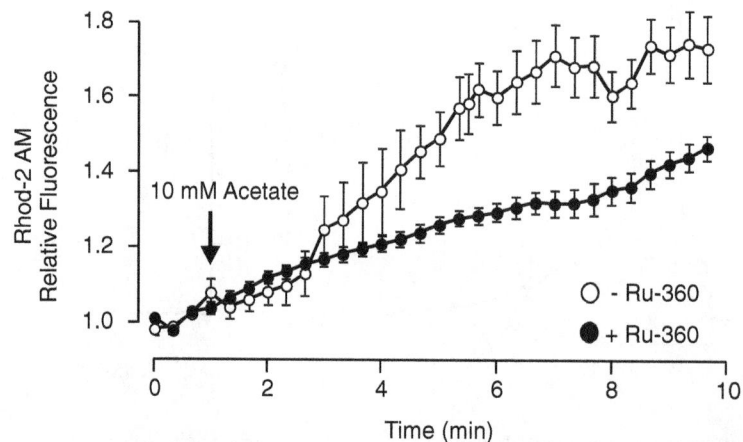

Figure 4 Acetate stimulates mitochondrial Ca^{2+} uptake. Summary of rhod-2-AM fluorescence recorded during exposure to 10 mM sodium acetate in the presence (n = 8) or absence (n = 10) of Ru-360 (10 µM). Background-subtracted fluorescence was normalized to mean fluorescence during the period prior to addition of 10 mM acetate (n =10) or control (no acetate, n = 9). Acetate solution was added at the arrow.

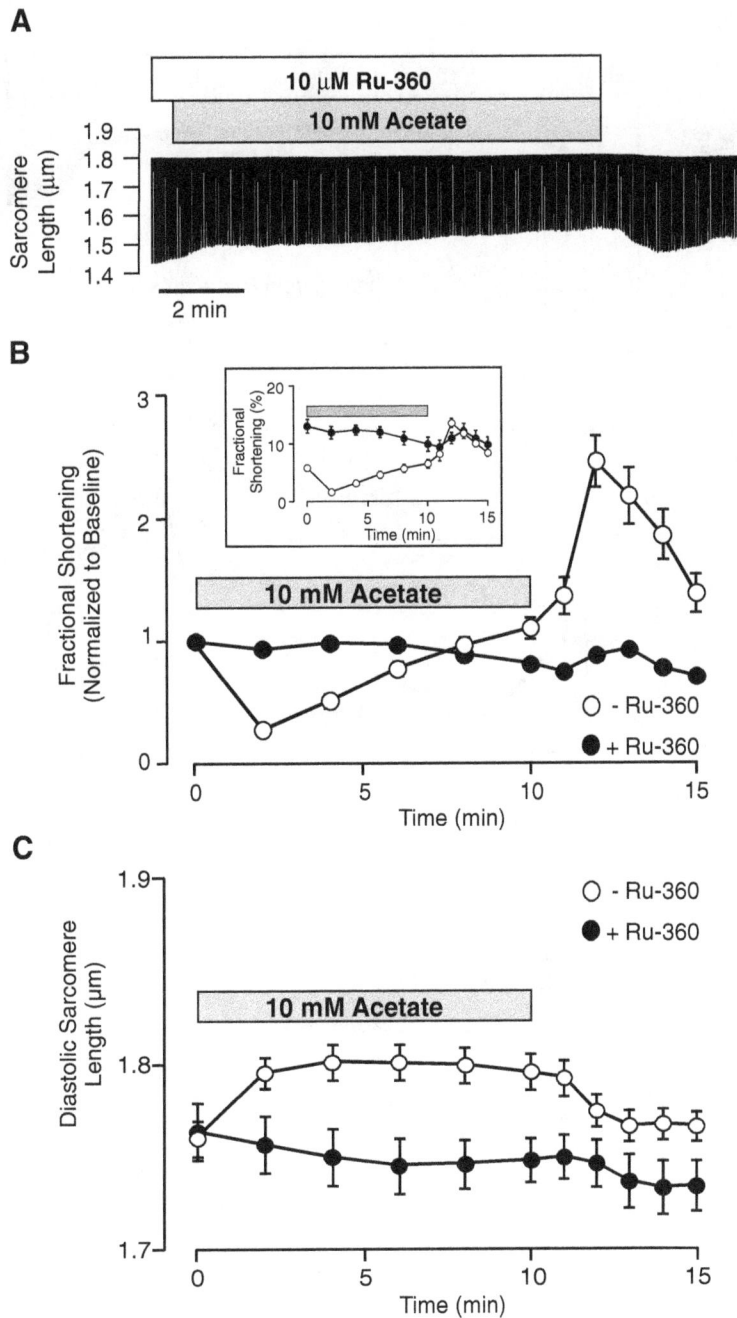

Figure 5 Inhibition of mitochondrial Ca^{2+} uptake with Ru-360 inhibits the effects of acetate on cell contraction. (A) Representative recording of average sarcomere length assessed continuously throughout application and removal of normal Tyrode solution (NT) supplemented with 10 μM sodium acetate in cells pretreated with 10 μM Ru-360 for 30–60 minutes and maintained in Ru-360 throughout the acetate exposure. Summary data from experiments as in **A** (n = 11) illustrate that pretreatment with Ru-360 markedly suppresses the effect of acetate on both (**B**) fractional shortening and (**C**) diastolic sarcomere length.

not observed in experiments where myocytes were briefly exposed to thapsigargin prior to acetate. This finding suggests that the recovery of contraction during acetate treatment reflects refilling of the sarcomplasmic reticulum with Ca^{2+}.

Discussion

Acetate and cardiac function

There have been previous studies that have examined the effects of acetate on cardiovascular function and energetics in different contexts. Consistent with the results

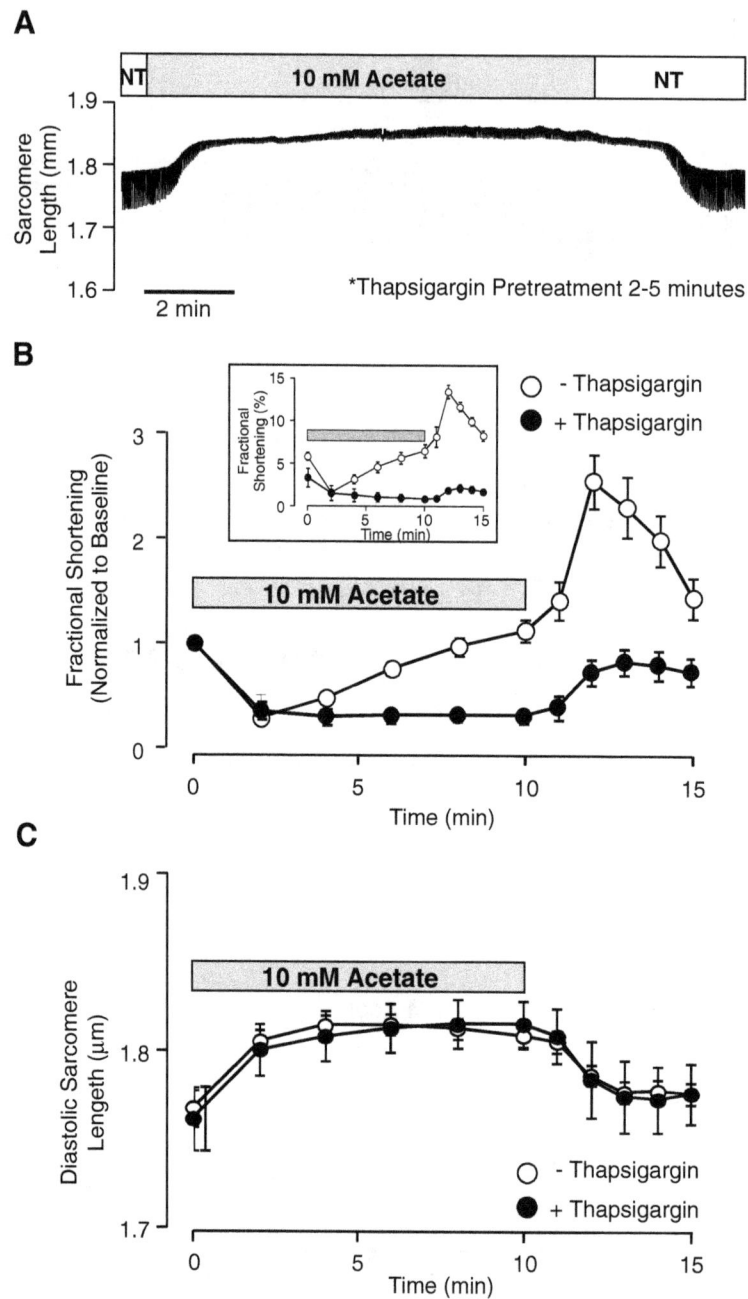

Figure 6 Thapsigargin pretreatment specifically impairs the recovery of contraction during acetate exposure. (A) Representative recording of average sarcomere length assessed continuously throughout application and removal of normal Tyrode solution (NT) supplemented with 10 mM sodium acetate in cells pretreated with thapsigargin (1 μM) for 2–5 minutes. As expected, cell relaxation was markedly slowed so contractions were evoked at 0.5 Hz. **(B & C)** Summary data from experiments as in **A** (n = 9). Thapsigargin pretreatment had no effect on the acetate induced decrease in fractional shortening or increase in diastolic sarcomere length, but markedly blunted the recovery of contraction typically observed from 2–10 minutes during acetate application.

of the present study, acetate is reported to exhibit negative inotropic effects which appear to be transient [4,5]. It should also be noted that acetate infusion can also cause an acute reduction of the blood pressure that is most likely dependent on the increase in AMP associated with the conversion of acetate to acetyl CoA and local release of the vasodilator adenosine [6], complicating the interpretation of experiments in vivo. Nevertheless, the data in the present study indicate that acetate exerts effects on cardiac contraction by directly modulating myocyte function, at least partially independent of energy metabolism.

A possible role for mitochondrial Ca²⁺ uptake in regulating contractile function

The present data provide evidence for a calcium-dependent mechanism linking acetate exposure with contractile function. Unlike the long chain fatty acid palmitate [2], the short chain fatty acid acetate caused no marked change in APD. Instead, we provide evidence that acetate caused a marked increased in mitochondrial Ca^{2+} accumulation. Moreover, the effect of acetate was markedly attenuated by pretreatment of myocytes with Ru-360, an inhibitor of mitochondrial Ca^{2+} uptake. Ru-360 is commonly used to inhibit mitochondrial Ca^{2+} uptake in a number of studies due to its ability to permeate cell membranes and it has been previously shown to have little if any effect on other transmembrane Ca^{2+} transport processes, including SR Ca^{2+} uptake and release, L-type Ca^{2+} channel and sodium calcium exchange function [19]. Our data is consistent with the conclusion that acetate uptake is coupled with an increase in mitochondrial Ca^{2+} and that this decreases, at least transiently, the amount of Ca^{2+} available for contraction of unloaded cardiomyocytes.

Interestingly, the effects of acetate on cell contraction were transient, with complete recovery of fractional shortening within 10 minutes of continuous exposure. This result could imply that as Ca^{2+} is sequestered in the mitochondria in the presence of acetate, additional Ca^{2+} enters the cell and refills the SR Ca^{2+} stores. We found that the acute decrease in contraction amplitude and increase in diastolic sarcomere length were unaffected by pretreatment with thapsigargin to attenuate SERCA activity. Interestingly, however, the *recovery* of depressed myocyte contractility during sustained acetate exposure and the abrupt increase in contraction amplitude due to acetate removal were no longer observed when cells were pretreated with thapsigargin. One possible explanation of this phenomenon is that inhibition of SR Ca^{2+} store replenishment prevents the restoration of fractional shortening.

Acetate effects on mitochondria

Mitochondrial uptake of acetate has been shown to be coupled with increases in Ca^{2+} uptake and swelling [13]. It was proposed that direct transport of phosphate or anions of weak acids like acetate can permeate the mitochondrial membrane generatings a driving force for Ca^{2+} uptake into the mitochondrial matrix. Similar observations demonstrate that acetate or phosphate increase the rate of mitochondrial Ca^{2+} uptake in a concentration dependent manner [14] and that acetate increases mitochondrial Ca^{2+} uptake in heart mitochondria [15]. The data in the present study do not delineate the molecular transporters mediating Ca^{2+} entry into the mitochondria. In addition to the mitochondrial Ca^{2+} uniporter [22], the mitochondrial ryanodine receptor (mRyr) [23], or $Ca^{2+}/H+$ exchanger (Letm1) [24] could play a role in the acetate-induced

increase in mitochondrial Ca^{2+}. Nevertheless, here we present pharmacological evidence showing that acetate is apparently coupled with an increase in mitochondrial Ca^{2+} in isolated cardiac myocytes and it is plausible to assume that this decreases the amount of Ca^{2+} available for contraction.

In isolated mitochondria, acetate also caused osmotic swelling [13]. Given the tight interfibrillar packing of mitochondria in the heart [25,26], acetate associated mitochondrial swelling might also be linked to the observed increase in diastolic sarcomere length. Interestingly, the effect of acetate on diastolic sarcomere length, unlike the effect on contraction, is sustained throughout acetate exposure and shows little concentration dependence. This observation is consistent with the conclusion that acetate causes the mitochondria to swell increasing the sarcomere spacing. While active cell shortening recovers as the SR refills with Ca^{2+}, the mitochondria remain swollen and the increased diastolic sarcomere length is maintained. Given the structural constraints, it seems possible that swelling is physically limited possibly explaining the absence of a clear concentration dependence.

The observed delay from acetate application to initial effects on contraction is similar to the time course for conversion of acetate to acetyl CoA observed by Randle [10]. Acetate has been shown to decrease the phosphorylation potential [27] resulting in decreased free energy from ATP hydrolysis; since the demand likely remains constant, the cell must increase the rate of respiration to cover the difference. This might suggest that acetate oxidation increases mitochondrial respiration with concomitant increases in mitochondrial Ca^{2+}. However, this is very unlikely since substrate availability governs only the pathways used to generate ATP, while workload or demand is the principal determinant of respiration [12,28]. In unloaded myocytes paced at a constant frequency, it is expected that the workload is constant; therefore, it is unlikely that acetate-induced changes in respiration underlie the increase in mitochondrial Ca^{2+} uptake. Rather, we consider the possibility that mitochondrial uptake of the acetate anion is electrically balanced by the uptake of Ca^{2+} in line with the conclusion of others based on experiments with isolated mitochondria [13-15].

Short chain fatty acids like acetate and butyrate may also cause changes in intracellular pH with effects on contraction and SR Ca^{2+} content [29,30]. The current data do not preclude a role for cytoplasm acidification in the effect of acetate on myocyte contraction. However, the observations that acetate increases mitochondrial Ca^{2+} and that pretreatment of cells with Ru-360 markedly attenuates the effects of acetate argues that an acute change in mitochondrial Ca^{2+} uptake, rather than cytoplasmic acidification, is the predominant mechanism underlying the effects of acetate on contraction. Moreover, it is tempting to predict that other anions of weak organic acids (e.g. lactate, butyrate, or pyruvate) may cause similar changes.

Mitochondrial Ca^{2+} uptake and cardiovascular disease

In the heart, mitochondrial Ca^{2+} uptake has been proposed as an important player in regulating cardiac energetics, reactive oxygen species generation and supply–demand matching [31,32]; however, mitochondrial Ca^{2+} overload is also associated with the activation of cell death pathways [33]. Thus a balance in mitochondrial Ca^{2+} loading is required in order to achieve proper regulation of metabolism, but avoid overloading and cell death. In ischemia-reperfusion experiments, excessive Ca^{2+} uptake is associated with a poor outcome, and treatment with Ru-360 to inhibit mitochondrial Ca^{2+} uptake is beneficial [34]. Acetate in this setting would be predicted to have no effect or be detrimental, and this has been shown to be the case [3,35-37]. Conversely, the failing heart has been shown to have reduced mitochondrial Ca^{2+} resulting from increases in cytosolic Na^+ concentrations and increased mitochondrial sodium-calcium exchange activity and blocking mitochondrial Ca^{2+} export (i.e. enhancing mitochondrial Ca^{2+}) is beneficial [38]. The data in the present study suggest that elevating circulating acetate might be an alternative strategy to accomplish this goal, although it should be noted that the study presented here was focused on the transient and not steady state consequences of acetate.

Conclusions

In summary, we have shown that acetate causes an acute but transient reduction in contractile function in isolated cardiac myocytes. Mechanistically, the transient negative inotropic effect appears to result from an acetate-dependent increase in mitochondrial Ca^{2+} uptake. This finding is consistent with the results of Lehninger and others using isolated liver and heart mitochondria, where it has been shown that acetate causes an increase in mitochondrial Ca^{2+} uptake and osmotic swelling [13-15]. Here we show that this effect appears to extend into intact, hydraulically unloaded cardiomyocytes, possibly suggesting a novel way to modulate mitochondrial Ca^{2+} homeostasis in the intact heart in vivo.

Competing interests

The authors declare that they have no competing interests.

Authors' contributions

JS performed the cell shortening experiments and analyzed data. AN participated in the design of the study and manuscript revision. RC performed mitochondrial Ca^{2+} uptake measurements and analyzed data. RB participated in the design of the study, data interpretation, and manuscript revision. TF performed electrophysiology experiments, cell shortening experiments, analyzed data, and drafted the manuscript. All authors read and approved the final manuscript.

Acknowledgements

This work was supported by funding from the Henry M. Jackson Foundation (to TPF) and the Department of Defense (R0702O to TPF).

Disclaimer

The views expressed are those of the authors and do not reflect the official policy or position of the Uniformed Services University of the Health Sciences, the Department of the Defense, or the United States governmen.

Author details

[1]Department of Anatomy, Physiology, and Genetics, Uniformed Services University for the Health Sciences, 4301 Jones Bridge Road, Rm. C-2114, Bethesda 20814, MD, USA. [2]Department of Biochemistry and Molecular Biology, Uniformed Services University for the Health Sciences, Bethesda 20814, MD, USA.

References

1. Flagg TP, Cazorla O, Remedi MS, Haim TE, Tones MA, Bahinski A, Numann RE, Kovacs A, Schaffer JE, Nichols CG, Nerbonne JM: Ca2 + –independent alterations in diastolic sarcomere length and relaxation kinetics in a mouse model of lipotoxic diabetic cardiomyopathy. *Circ Res* 2009, 104(1):95–103.
2. Haim TE, Wang W, Flagg TP, Tones MA, Bahinski A, Numann RE, Nichols CG, Nerbonne JM: Palmitate attenuates myocardial contractility through augmentation of repolarizing Kv currents. *J Mol Cell Cardiol* 2010, 48(2):395–405.
3. Martin BJ, Valdivia HH, Bunger R, Lasley RD, Mentzer RM Jr: Pyruvate augments calcium transients and cell shortening in rat ventricular myocytes. *Am J Physiol* 1998, 274(1 Pt 2):H8–H17.
4. Kirkendol PL, Pearson JE, Bower JD, Holbert RD: Myocardial depressant effects of sodium acetate. *Cardiovasc Res* 1978, 12(2):127–136.
5. Jacob AD, Elkins N, Reiss OK, Chan L, Shapiro JI: Effects of acetate on energy metabolism and function in the isolated perfused rat heart. *Kidney Int* 1997, 52(3):755–760.
6. Liang CS, Lowenstein JM: Metabolic control of the circulation. Effects of acetate and pyruvate. *J Clin Invest* 1978, 62(5):1029–1038.
7. Ballard FJ: Supply and utilization of acetate in mammals. *Am J Clin Nutr* 1972, 25(8):773–779.
8. Skutches CL, Holroyde CP, Myers RN, Paul P, Reichard GA: Plasma acetate turnover and oxidation. *J Clin Invest* 1979, 64(3):708–713.
9. Fujino T, Kondo J, Ishikawa M, Morikawa K, Yamamoto TT: Acetyl-CoA synthetase 2, a mitochondrial matrix enzyme involved in the oxidation of acetate. *J Biol Chem* 2001, 276(14):11420–11426.
10. Randle PJ, England PJ, Denton RM: Control of the tricarboxylate cycle and its interactions with glycolysis during acetate utilization in rat heart. *Biochem J* 1970, 117(4):677–695.
11. Williamson JR: Effects of insulin and starvation on the metabolism of acetate and pyruvate by the perfused rat heart. *Biochem J* 1964, 93(1):97–106.
12. Taegtmeyer H, Hems R, Krebs HA: Utilization of energy-providing substrates in the isolated working rat heart. *Biochem J* 1980, 186(3):701–711.
13. Lehninger AL: Role of phosphate and other proton-donating anions in respiration-coupled transport of Ca2+ by mitochondria. *Proc Natl Acad Sci U S A* 1974, 71(4):1520–1524.
14. Reed KC, Bygrave FL: A kinetic study of mitochondrial calcium transport. *Eur J Biochem* 1975, 55(3):497–504.
15. Harris EJ: Anion/calcium ion ratios and proton production in some mitochondrial calcium ion uptakes. *Biochem J* 1978, 176(3):983–991.
16. Flagg TP, Charpentier F, Manning-Fox J, Remedi MS, Enkvetchakul D, Lopatin A, Koster J, Nichols C: Remodeling of excitation-contraction coupling in transgenic mice expressing ATP-insensitive sarcolemmal K-ATP channels. *Am J Physiol Heart Circ Physiol* 2004, 286(4):H1361–H1369.
17. Pan X, Liu J, Nguyen T, Liu C, Sun J, Teng Y, Fergusson MM, Rovira II, Allen M, Springer DA, Aponte AM, Gucek M, Balaban RS, Murphy E, Finkel T: The physiological role of mitochondrial calcium revealed by mice lacking the mitochondrial calcium uniporter. *Nat Cell Biol* 2013, 15(12):1464–1472.

18. Miyata H, Silverman HS, Sollott SJ, Lakatta EG, Stern MD, Hansford RG: **Measurement of mitochondrial free Ca2+ concentration in living single rat cardiac myocytes.** *Am J Physiol* 1991, **261**(4 Pt 2):H1123–H1134.

19. Matlib MA, Zhou Z, Knight S, Ahmed S, Choi KM, Krause-Bauer J, Phillips R, Altschuld R, Katsube Y, Sperelakis N, Bers DM: **Oxygen-bridged dinuclear ruthenium amine complex specifically inhibits Ca2+ uptake into mitochondria in vitroand in situ in single cardiac myocytes.** *J Biol Chem* 1998, **273**(17):10223–10231.

20. Zhou Z, Bers D: **Time course of action of antagonists of mitochondrial Ca uptake in intact ventricular myocytes.** *Pflugers Arch* 2002, **445**(1):132–138.

21. Bode EF, Briston SJ, Overend CL, O'Neill SC, Trafford AW, Eisner DA: **Changes of SERCA activity have only modest effects on sarcoplasmic reticulum Ca2+ content in rat ventricular myocytes.** *J Physiol* 2011, **589**(19):4723–4729.

22. Marchi S, Pinton P: **The mitochondrial calcium uniporter complex: molecular components, structure and physiopathological implications.** *J Physiol* 2014, **592**(Pt 5):829–839.

23. Beutner G, Sharma VK, Giovannucci DR, Yule DI, Sheu SS: **Identification of a ryanodine receptor in rat heart mitochondria.** *J Biol Chem* 2001, **276**(24):21482–21488.

24. Jiang D, Zhao L, Clapham DE: **Genome-Wide RNAi Screen Identifies Letm1 as a Mitochondrial Ca2+/H+ Antiporter.** *Science* 2009, **326**(5949):144–147.

25. Lukyanenko V, Chikando A, Lederer WJ: **Mitochondria in cardiomyocyte Ca2+ signaling.** *Int J Biochem Cell Biol* 2009, **41**(10):1957–1971.

26. Ong S-B, Hausenloy DJ: **Mitochondrial morphology and cardiovascular disease.** *Cardiovasc Res* 2010, **88**(1):16–29.

27. Kang YH, Mallet RT, Bunger R: **Coronary autoregulation and purine release in normoxic heart at various cytoplasmic phosphorylation potentials: disparate effects of adenosine.** *Pflugers Arch* 1992, **421**(2–3):188–199.

28. Neely JR, Denton RM, England PJ, Randle PJ: **The effects of increased heart work on the tricarboxylate cycle and its interactions with glycolysis in the perfused rat heart.** *Biochem J* 1972, **128**(1):147–159.

29. Bountra C, Vaughan-Jones RD: **Effect of intracellular and extracellular pH on contraction in isolated, mammalian cardiac muscle.** *J Physiol* 1989, **418**:163–187.

30. O'Neill SC, Eisner DA: **pH-dependent and -independent effects inhibit Ca2 + –induced Ca2+ release during metabolic blockade in rat ventricular myocytes.** *J Physiol* 2003, **550**(2):413–418.

31. Balaban RS: **Cardiac energy metabolism homeostasis: role of cytosolic calcium.** *J Mol Cell Cardiol* 2002, **34**(10):1259–1271.

32. Liu T, O'Rourke B: **Regulation of mitochondrial Ca2+ and its effects on energetics and redox balance in normal and failing heart.** *J Bioenerg Biomembr* 2009, **41**(2):127–132.

33. Garcia-Dorado D, Ruiz-Meana M, Inserte J, Rodriguez-Sinovas A, Piper HM: **Calcium-mediated cell death during myocardial reperfusion.** *Cardiovasc Res* 2012, **94**(2):168–180.

34. Garcia-Rivas Gde J, Carvajal K, Correa F, Zazueta C: **Ru360, a specific mitochondrial calcium uptake inhibitor, improves cardiac post-ischaemic functional recovery in rats in vivo.** *Br J Pharmacol* 2006, **149**(7):829–837.

35. Mallet RT, Sun J, Knott EM, Sharma AB, Olivencia-Yurvati AH: **Metabolic cardioprotection by pyruvate: recent progress.** *Exp Biol Med (Maywood)* 2005, **230**(7):435–443.

36. Bunger R, Mallet RT: **Mitochondrial pyruvate transport in working guinea-pig heart. Work-related vs carrier-mediated control of pyruvate oxidation.** *Biochim Biophys Acta* 1993, **1151**(2):223–236.

37. Bunger R, Mallet RT, Hartman DA: **Pyruvate-enhanced phosphorylation potential and inotropism in normoxic and postischemic isolated working heart. Near-complete prevention of reperfusion contractile failure.** *Eur J Biochem* 1989, **180**(1):221–233.

38. Liu T, O'Rourke B: **Enhancing mitochondrial Ca2+ uptake in myocytes from failing hearts restores energy supply and demand matching.** *Circ Res* 2008, **103**(3):279–288.

18

Regulation of Locomotor activity in fed, fasted, and food-restricted mice lacking tissue-type plasminogen activator

Jessica A. Krizo[1], Linley E. Moreland[1], Ashutosh Rastogi[1], Xiang Mou[2], Rebecca A. Prosser[3] and Eric M. Mintz[1*]

Abstract

Background: Circadian rhythms of physiology and behavior are driven by a circadian clock located in the suprachiasmatic nucleus of the hypothalamus. This clock is synchronized to environmental day/night cycles by photic input, which is dependent on the presence of mature brain-derived neurotrophic factor (BDNF) in the SCN. Mature BDNF is produced by the enzyme plasmin, which is converted from plasminogen by the enzyme tissue-type plasminogen activator (tPA). In this study, we evaluate circadian function in mice lacking functional tPA.

Results: tPA$^{-/-}$ mice have normal circadian periods, but show decreased nocturnal wheel-running activity. This difference is eliminated or reversed on the second day of a 48-h fast. Similarly, when placed on daily cycles of restricted food availability the genotypic difference in total wheel-running activity disappears, and tPA$^{-/-}$ mice show equivalent amounts of food anticipatory activity to wild type mice.

Conclusions: These data suggest that tPA regulates nocturnal wheel-running activity, and that tPA differentially affects SCN-driven nocturnal activity rhythms and activity driven by fasting or temporal food restriction.

Keywords: Circadian, Food anticipatory activity, Wheel-running

Background

Circadian rhythms of physiology and behavior are driven by a circadian clock located in the suprachiasmatic nucleus of the hypothalamus (SCN) [1, 2]. The SCN is directly innervated by retinal ganglion cells, which provide the entrainment signals that synchronize SCN rhythms with the environmental light-dark (LD) cycle [3–5]. The signal transduction pathway that conveys photic information to the SCN is dependent on the activation of the trkB receptor by brain-derived neurotrophic factor (BDNF) [6]. The production of the mature form of BDNF in the brain is at least partly dependent on the extracellular activity of tissue-type plasminogen activator (tPA), which converts plasminogen to plasmin, which in turn catalyzes the conversion of proBDNF to mBDNF [7]. Both BDNF and trkB are found in the SCN [6, 8, 9].

BDNF signaling deficits lead to a decrease in light induced phase shifts [10], and trkB antagonists in the SCN block light induced phase shifts of the circadian clock in vivo [11] and glutamate-induced phase shifts in vitro [9]. Further, tPA inhibition in vitro decreases glutamate-induced phase shifts [9]. These findings suggest that tPA activity is important for regulating glutamate induced phase shifts. Surprisingly, mice that lack tPA have normal free-running periods and normal phase-shifting responses to light pulses, though they do show slower entrainment to a large shift of the light-dark cycle [12]. This suggests that any deficiency in entrainment in these mice is modest. However, in the course of screening tPA knockout mice (tPA$^{-/-}$) for their circadian phenotype, we noted that overall wheel-running activity appeared to be reduced compared to wild type mice. Mice that lack BDNF in adulthood are hyperactive [13], suggesting the possibility that depressed activity in tPA$^{-/-}$ mice occurs via a BDNF-independent mechanism.

BDNF also has been implicated in regulating the brain's adaptations to energetic challenges [14]. When food availability is restricted to a narrow window of time

* Correspondence: emintz@kent.edu

[1]Department of Biological Sciences, Kent State University, Kent, OH 44242, USA

Full list of author information is available at the end of the article

per day, rodents exhibit a behavior known as food antici-patory activity [15], which occurs for a 2-3 h period prior to food availability. This activity appears to be driven by a food-entrainable circadian oscillator, and persists in the absence of a functional SCN [16, 17] or critical components of the molecular circadian clock mechanism [18, 19]. A number of neuroendocrine regu-latory factors contribute to the appearance of food anticipatory activity (for a review, see [20]), however, the underlying mechanisms are still poorly understood. Because the loss of tPA reduces neuronal plasticity, and due to its known, but limited effects on SCN entrain-ment pathways, we hypothesized that mice lacking tPA would have difficulty adapting to timed restricted feed-ing regimes.

Methods

Animals

Animals used in this study were age-matched across each experimental group in each study. Two to four-month old male C57BL/6 J wildtype mice (tPA$^{+/+}$) and tPA knockout mice (tPA$^{-/-}$) (bred from stock purchased from Jackson Laboratory (Bar Harbor, ME), backcrossed to C57BL/6 J) were used in all experiments. Variation in age is based on the length of study and animal availabil-ity, however, in all studies genotypes were age matched. No animals were used in more than one experiment. Animals were individually housed in Plexiglas cages equipped with a running wheel. Animals were housed at a temperature of 20 °C and had access to water ad libitum. Food was also available ad libitum except as indicated below. All animal use protocols in this study were approved by the Kent State Institutional Animal Care and Use Committee and were performed in accord-ance with the recommendations in the Guide for the Care and Use of Laboratory Animals of the National Institutes of Health.

Assessment of mature BDNF in the SCN

To assess in vivo protein expression, SCN tissue was dissected from mouse brains at zeitgeber time (ZT) 4 (4 h after lights on) and ZT 12 and immediately frozen for later Western blot assay as described before [9]. Harvested tissue was homogenized in ice-chilled HEPES-based extraction buffer containing a protease inhibitor cocktail (1 mM phenylmethylsulfonyl fluoride, 10 mg/mL aprotinin, 15 mg/mL leupeptin, 10 mg/mL pepstatin). For BDNF immunoblots, tissue was prepared in Tris-based denaturing extraction buffer [4 M urea, 0.02 M dithiothreitol, 0.05 M Tris, pH 7.4, 2% sodium dodecyl sulfate (SDS)]. The tissue extract sample was separated into aliquots and stored at − 80 °C. Protein content of the extract was determined by the bicinchoni-nic acid method (BCA; Pierce). Tissue samples were

mixed with loading buffer (pH 6.8 Tris, SDS, bromophe-nol blue, glycerol), and subjected to SDS–polyacrylamide gel electrophoresis. Proteins were electrotransferred onto nitrocellulose membranes, which were then incu-bated with blocking buffer [10% solution of non-fat dry milk in phosphate-buffered saline with Tween-20 (PBST, 8 mM Na$_2$HPO$_4$, 150 mM NaCl, 2 mM KH$_2$PO$_4$, 3 mM KCl, 0.05% Tween-20, pH 7.4)]. The membranes were probed with primary antibodies diluted in a 2.0% solution of non-fat dry milk in PBST, followed by goat anti-rabbit horseradish peroxidase-conjugated secondary antibody at appropriate dilutions in the same buffer. Signals were revealed by enzyme-catalyzed chemilumin-escence (Pierce, IL, USA). The amount of protein loaded in each lane was assessed by probing for α-tubulin, so all protein expression was calculated as levels relative to α-tubulin. Control experiments included running paral-lel lanes loaded with the corresponding native proteins (positive controls), and probing membranes with primary antibodies pre-incubated with the native protein to test for cross-reactivity and to establish the specificity of the antibody samples. Rabbit anti-α-tubulin antibodies were obtained from Santa Cruz Biochemicals (Santa Cruz, CA, USA). Rabbit anti-proBDNF antibody was ob-tained from Millipore (MA, USA) and rabbit anti-BDNF antibody was from Alomone Labs (Jerusalem, Israel). We differentiated between pro- and mBDNF proteins by using respectively specific antibodies as well as by their distinct sizes. proBDNF was identified as ~37kD bands, while mBDNF ~15kD bands.

Restricted feeding

Following a two-week baseline activity recording period, mice were deprived of food for 48 h. Mice were then given four days of free food access before food removal at lights off (ZT 12). Subsequently, food was presented to mice at ZT 6 and removed at ZT 10. This was contin-ued for eight to ten days at which point experimental protocol varied as detailed below. Body weight was mea-sured during baseline activity, following fast, following free feeding period and after restricted feeding.

Activity measurement

All cages were equipped with either traditional stainless steel 6 in. diameter running wheels or 6.10 in. running wheel discs. Traditional running wheel data was collected as revolutions per minute with ClockLab (Actimetrics, Wilmette, IL) and running disc data was collected with Med Associates (St. Albans, VT); data was qualified and quantified using ClockLab. Experiments in regular LD cycles were performed using the running wheels and the skeleton photoperiod data in the supple-mentary data file used the running discs. Due to differ-ences in data collection between wheels, comparisons between studies using different wheels were not made. The use of two different wheel systems was necessary in order to complete the studies in a timely manner. Activity profiles were calculated as an average activity per animal and per genotype as follows: baseline, averaged 4 day baseline and restricted feeding averaged over days three through eight. Activity profiles were created using total revolutions per hour as a percentage of total 24 h baseline activity. Food anticipatory activity (FAA) was defined as activity measured during the 3 h (ZT 3-6) prior to food presentation. This 3 h period was chosen based on a review of the FAA literature and to provide for a consistent measurement interval.

Assessment of baseline activity profiles in a 12:12 LD cycle

Mice were housed in a 12:12 LD cycle and activity profiles were assessed, both in absolute terms and as a percentage of the 24-h mean for each animal.

Food anticipatory activity in tPA$^{-/-}$ mice under light-dark conditions

Male tPA$^{+/+}$ and tPA$^{-/-}$ mice were maintained in a standard 12:12 light-dark cycle and underwent the food restriction protocol described above.

Assessment of circadian phase during food restriction

Male tPA$^{+/+}$ and tPA$^{-/-}$ mice were placed in a skeleton photoperiod after being entrained to a 12:12 light-cycle. Mice were divided into four groups, tPA$^{+/+}$ RF and tPA$^{-/-}$ RF were food restricted and tPA$^{+/+}$ and tPA$^{-/-}$ ad/ libitum feeding groups (AL) had continuous access to food. After ten days of restricted feeding, mice were released into constant dark conditions with continuous access to food. Mice were allowed to free run for two weeks before phase was measured.

Food intake changes during restricted feeding

Male age matched tPA$^{+/+}$ and tPA$^{-/-}$ mice were individually housed in small Plexiglas cages with metal grated cage liners and a PVC pipe for comfort. Weight and food intake was measured daily to generate a baseline. Mice then were food restricted and weight and food intake was measured daily. Body composition analysis was completed with the use of an EchoMRI (Echo Medical Systems, Houston, TX) for baseline, after fast, and before and after restricted feeding. EchoMRI measured fat mass and lean mass, with lean mass being calculated as total body mass minus fat mass.

Statistical analysis

Analyses were performed using NCSS 10 software (Kaysville, UT). Comparisons between groups were performed using one-way and two-way ANOVA with repeated measures where appropriate. Planned comparisons between genotypes throughout the 24-h cycle were assessed using Fisher's LSD test if the ANOVA showed a statistically significant interaction between genotype and clock time. Fisher's LSD is used because the time-series data being analyzed have a strong serial correlation and this results in most other tests being overly conservative. Significance was ascribed if $p < 0.05$.

Results

Assessment of mBDNF/proBDNF ratio in the SCN

First, we established whether there was a reduction in mBDNF levels in the SCN of tPA$^{-/-}$ mice. For these experiments, SCN tissue was isolated from tPA$^{+/+}$ and tPA$^{-/-}$ mice at ZT 4 and ZT 12 and immediately transferred into extraction buffer for protein analysis. SCN content of pro- and mBDNF from tPA$^{-/-}$ and tPA$^{+/+}$ mice was quantified and normalized to α-tubulin. Then an mBDNF to proBDNF ratio was computed as the index for relative mBDNF quantity. There was a significant main effect of genotype ($F_{1,8} = 7.88$, $p = 0.023$) (Fig. 1), but not ZT ($F_{1,8} = 1.29$, $p = 0.29$) or an interaction ($F_{1,8} = 0.42$, $p = 0.53$), indicating reduced conversion of proBDNF to mBDNF in tPA$^{-/-}$ mice.

Reeintrainment to an advance of the LD cycle

We previously reported that tPA$^{-/-}$ mice took longer to adjust to a 12-h shift of the LD cycle than did tPA$^{+/+}$ mice [12]. However, these shifts represent only the phase delaying effects of light. To measure the impact of the loss of tPA on phase advances, we measured the time to adjust to a 6-h advance of the LD cycle (Fig. 2). tPA$^{-/-}$ mice took significantly longer (8.1 ± 0.7 days) than tPA$^{+/+}$ (5.9 ± 0.5 days) to reentrain to the shifted LD cycle ($t_{17} = 2.57$, $p = 0.02$). We also exposed the animals to a 6-h phase delay, but due to suppression of activity by

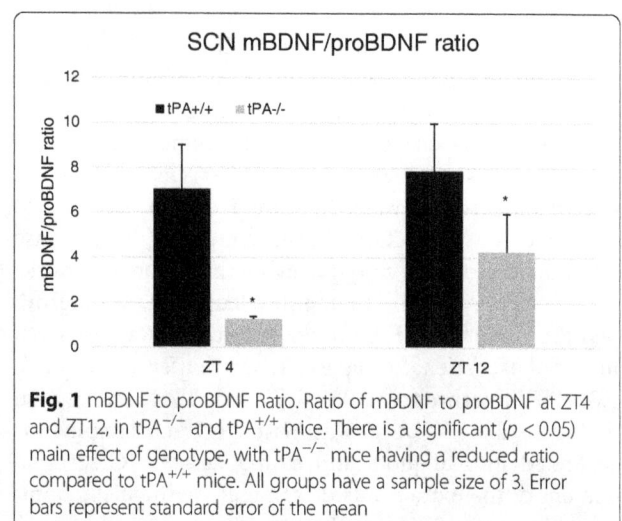

Fig. 1 mBDNF to proBDNF Ratio. Ratio of mBDNF to proBDNF at ZT4 and ZT12, in tPA$^{-/-}$ and tPA$^{+/+}$ mice. There is a significant ($p < 0.05$) main effect of genotype, with tPA$^{-/-}$ mice having a reduced ratio compared to tPA$^{+/+}$ mice. All groups have a sample size of 3. Error bars represent standard error of the mean

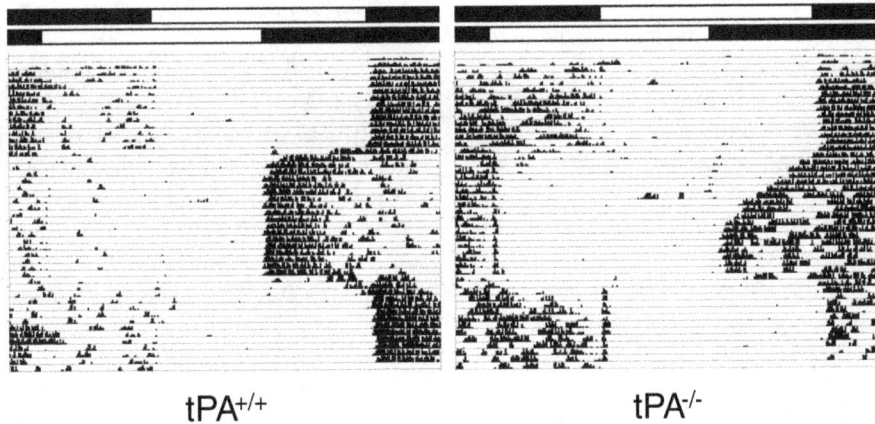

Fig. 2 Simulated Jet Lag. Representative actograms showing a 6 h advance and a 6 h delay of the light-dark cycle in both genotypes

light (masking) an accurate assessment of reentrainment time could not be performed.

Locomotor activity during timed restricted feeding

During baseline measurements both tPA$^{+/+}$ and tPA$^{-/-}$ mice exhibit typical patterns of nocturnal locomotor activity. Nocturnal activity was divided into two discrete bouts of locomotor activity, a high level of activity in early to mid-night ending in a drop of locomotor activity followed by a brief increase in activity ending gradually at ZT 24. However, the level of activity was reduced in tPA$^{-/-}$ mice during the first part of the dark phase in LD (Fig. 3a and b) from ZT12-17 ($F_{23,575} = 2.63$, $p < 0.001$). Food availability had an effect on both the pattern and

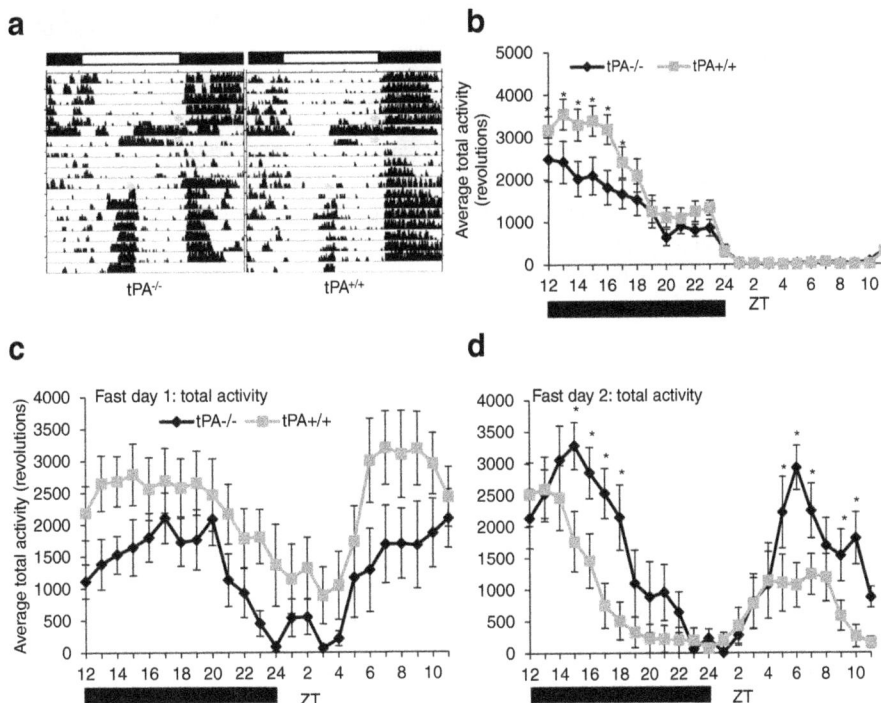

Fig. 3 Activity During LD – Baseline and Fasting. Representative actograms (**a**) of food restriction protocol in tPA$^{-/-}$ and tPA$^{+/+}$ mice in LD. Arrows indicate onset and offset of fast and beginning of restricted feeding. Fast includes food removal at ZT 12 and return 48 h later at ZT 12. Average 24 h activity profile (**b**), bar indicates dark phase; locomotor activity is higher in tPA$^{+/+}$ ($n = 13$) than tPA$^{-/-}$ ($n = 14$) at ZT 12-17 ($p < 0.05$). During fast day 1 total locomotor activity (**c**) is higher in tPA$^{+/+}$ ($n = 8$) than tPA$^{-/-}$ ($n = 7$) ($p < 0.05$) with no effect of time of day. During fast day 2 (**d**) total locomotor activity is significantly higher in tPA$^{-/-}$ ($n = 8$) than tPA$^{+/+}$ ($n = 8$) during both the night (ZT15-18) and the day (ZT 5-7, 9-10) ($p < 0.001$). Error bars represent standard error of the mean

level of locomotor activity in tPA$^{+/+}$ and tPA$^{-/-}$ mice. Food deprivation led to increased diurnal activity across genotypes on both days. When food was removed at ZT 12 locomotor activity was suppressed compared to baseline activity during the first portion of the dark phase. tPA$^{-/-}$ mice had decreased activity compared to tPA$^{+/+}$ mice on LD fast day one ($F_{1,22} = 4.57$, $p = 0.044$)(Fig. 3c). During fast day two locomotor activity increased significantly over tPA$^{+/+}$ (Fig. 3d) during both night (ZT 15-18) and day (ZT 5-7, 9, 10) ($F_{23,529} = 2.23$, $p < 0.001$). There was no difference in weight loss between genotypes (Fig. 4a) (tPA$^{-/-}$: $- 20.6\% \pm .008$ and tPA$^{+/+}$: $- 21.7\% \pm .009$, $t_{29} = 0.937$, $p = 0.399$). During restricted feeding the baseline differences in raw locomotor activity between genotypes disappeared (Fig. 5) and there was no difference in nocturnal or food anticipatory activity levels ($F_{23,547} = 1.18$, $p = 0.253$). Following restricted feeding tPA$^{-/-}$ mice gained less weight than tPA$^{+/+}$ mice, but this difference was not statistically significant (Fig. 4b)(tPA$^{-/-}$: $-.9\% \pm .01$ and tPA$^{+/+}$: $2.91\% \pm .02$, $t_{28} = - 1.65$, $p = 0.109$).

This experiment was repeated, except that the light cycle utilized was a skeleton photoperiod, which is 15 min of light only at the beginning and end of a 12 h "day". This design examines whether activity during the day is being suppressed, or "masked", by the presence of light. The results from this experiment did not substantially differ from those obtained in standard light/dark conditions (Additional file 1).

Assessment of circadian phase during food restriction

The effect of timed restricted feeding on the SCN can be masked by light. When released to constant darkness following restricted or ad libitum feeding there was no genotypic effect on free-running period ($F_{1,23} = 0.60$, $p = 0.447$) (Fig. 6a and b). However, RF treatment had an aftereffect

on free-running period, shortening the free-running period of RF groups (tPA$^{-/-}$ RF: 23.77 ± 0.036, tPA$^{+/+}$ RF: 23.75 ± 0.019) compared to AL groups (tPA$^{-/-}$ AL: 23.84 ± 0.073, tPA$^{+/+}$ AL: 23.91 ± 0.026) ($F_{1,23} = 8.49$, $p = 0.008$). Activity data were also analyzed to determine if the underlying nocturnal activity rhythm was advanced in food restricted mice, which would not be observable in LD due to the masking effect of light on activity but which could subsequently be predicted by the onsets of activity upon release into DD. There was no evidence of an underlying shift in the phase angle of entrainment toward food presentation in LD$_{sk}$ across genotypes ($F_{1,23} = 2.24$, $p = 0.148$) or treatment ($F_{1,23} = 0.024$, $p = 0.631$) (tPA$^{-/-}$ RF: $-.33 \pm 0.339$, tPA$^{+/+}$ RF: $.24 \pm 0.194$, tPA$^{-/-}$ AL: $-.40 \pm 0.188$, tPA$^{+/+}$ AL: $-.01 \pm 0.203$) (Fig. 6c). Additionally, no difference in phase angle of entrainment was seen between genotypes following release from RF in LD to constant conditions (tPA$^{-/-}$ RF $= - 0.24 \pm 0.154$, tPA$^{+/+}$ RF $= 0.15 \pm 0.262$)($t_{14} = 1.383$, $p = 0.1882$) (Fig. 6d).

Food intake analysis

Since differences in FAA might reflect differences in the motivation for feeding, we compared food intake in tPA$^{-/-}$ and tPA$^{+/+}$ mice. There was no difference in food intake (tPA$^{-/-}$: 4.65 g $\pm$ .09 g tPA$^{+/+}$: 4.79 g $\pm$ .07 g) during standard LD conditions with food available ad libitum ($t_{18} = 0.045$, $p = 0.964$). During ad libitum feeding following food deprivation there was no difference in food intake (tPA$^{-/-}$: 5.76 g $\pm$ .19 g tPA$^{+/+}$: 5.70 g $\pm$ .15 g) ($t_{18} = 0.21$, $p = 0.83$). During restricted feeding food intake in tPA$^{-/-}$ mice was reduced compared to tPA$^{+/+}$ (tPA$^{-/-}$: 2.14 g $\pm$ .06 g, tPA$^{+/+}$ 2.73 g $\pm$ .11 g) ($t_{18} = 4.656$, $p < 0.001$) (Fig. 7a). There are no significant genotypic differences in weight at baseline (tPA$^{-/-}$ $= 29.21$ g $\pm$ .58 g, tPA$^{+/+}$ $= 28.43$ g $\pm$ .44 g) ($t_{18} = 1.073$, $p = 0.297$ or following RF (tPA$^{-/-}$ $= 26.27$ g $\pm$ .41 g, tPA$^{+/+}$ $= 26.91$ g $\pm$ .47 g) ($t_{18} = 1.031$, $p = 0.316$) (Fig. 7b).

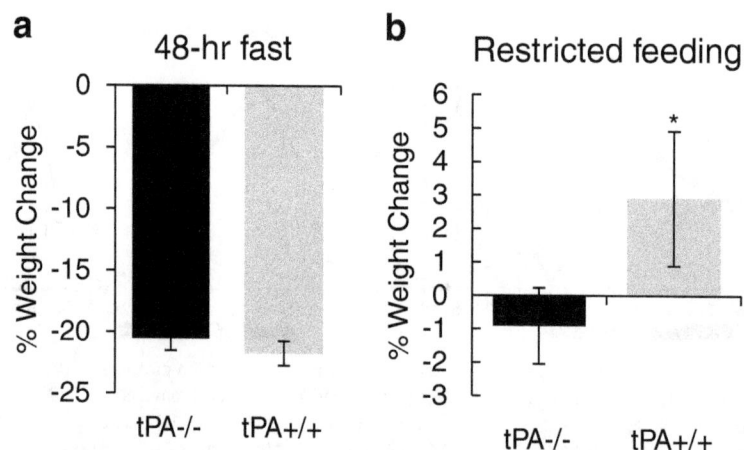

Fig. 4 Body Weight Comparison. Weight changes between genotypes are consistent following a 48-h fast (**a**); following restricted feeding (**b**) tPA$^{+/+}$ increased in weight more than tPA$^{-/-}$ ($p < 0.05$). Sample sizes are 15-16 per group. Error bars represent standard error of the mean

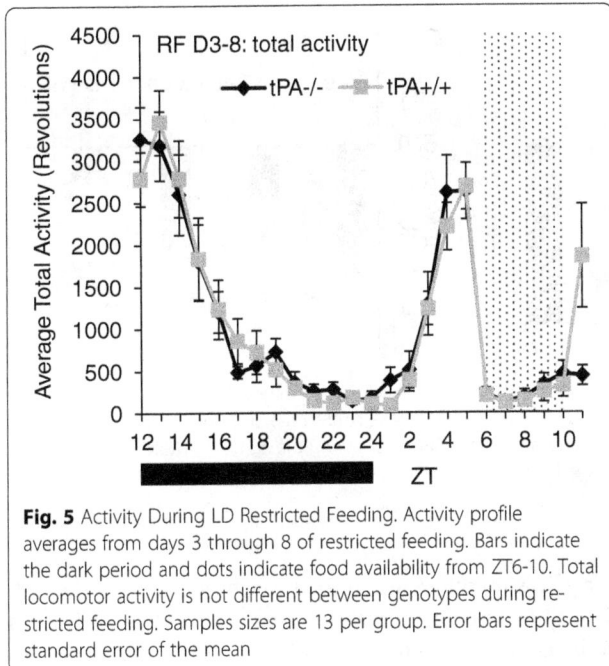

Fig. 5 Activity During LD Restricted Feeding. Activity profile averages from days 3 through 8 of restricted feeding. Bars indicate the dark period and dots indicate food availability from ZT6-10. Total locomotor activity is not different between genotypes during restricted feeding. Samples sizes are 13 per group. Error bars represent standard error of the mean

While $tPA^{-/-}$ mice weighed slightly more than $tPA^{+/+}$ after 48 h of food deprivation, the difference was not statistically significant ($tPA^{-/-} = 23.62 \pm .51$, $tPA^{+/+} = 22.22 \pm .44$) ($t_{18} = 2.081$, $p = 0.0519$). Changes in weight following food deprivation were due to changes in lean mass regardless of genotype. $tPA^{-/-}$ mouse lean mass change was less than $tPA^{+/+}$ ($tPA^{-/-} = -3.265$ g $\pm .23$ g, $tPA^{+/+} = -3.7076$ g $\pm .27$ g) ($t_{18} = 3.919$, $p = 0.001$). There was no difference in the loss of fat mass between genotypes ($tPA^{-/-} = 1.243$ g $\pm .11$ g, $tPA^{+/+} = -1.1872$ g $\pm .20$ g) ($t_{18} = -0.453$, $p = 0.657$). Following RF there was no genotypic difference in lean mass change ($tPA^{-/-} = -2.753$ g $\pm .10$ g, $tPA^{+/+} = -2.714$ g $\pm .45$ g)($t_{18} = 0.223$, $p = 0.823$) but fat mass change differed between genotypes ($tPA^{-/-} = -.78$ g $\pm .26$ g, $tPA^{+/+} = .3533$ g $\pm .10$ g) ($t_{18} = 4.097$, $p < 0.001$) (Fig. 7c).

Discussion

This research was initiated with the goal of examining the role of tPA in regulating circadian rhythms of activity, particularly with regard to circadian clock-driven responses to restricted feeding. The results, however, suggest a more subtle role for tPA in modulating the circadian rhythm of

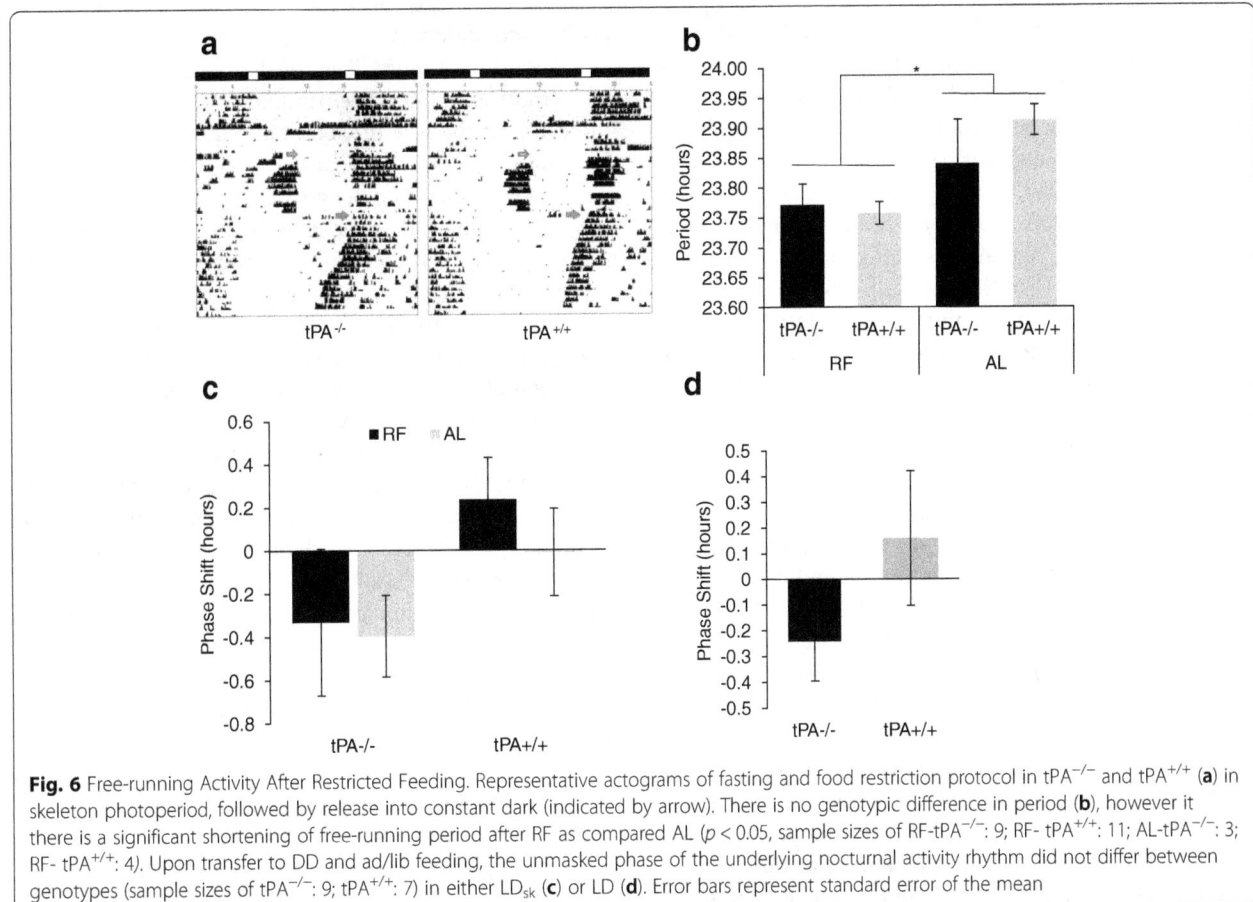

Fig. 6 Free-running Activity After Restricted Feeding. Representative actograms of fasting and food restriction protocol in $tPA^{-/-}$ and $tPA^{+/+}$ (**a**) in skeleton photoperiod, followed by release into constant dark (indicated by arrow). There is no genotypic difference in period (**b**), however it there is a significant shortening of free-running period after RF as compared AL ($p < 0.05$, sample sizes of RF-$tPA^{-/-}$: 9; RF- $tPA^{+/+}$: 11; AL-$tPA^{-/-}$: 3; RF- $tPA^{+/+}$: 4). Upon transfer to DD and ad/lib feeding, the unmasked phase of the underlying nocturnal activity rhythm did not differ between genotypes (sample sizes of $tPA^{-/-}$: 9; $tPA^{+/+}$: 7) in either LD_{sk} (**c**) or LD (**d**). Error bars represent standard error of the mean

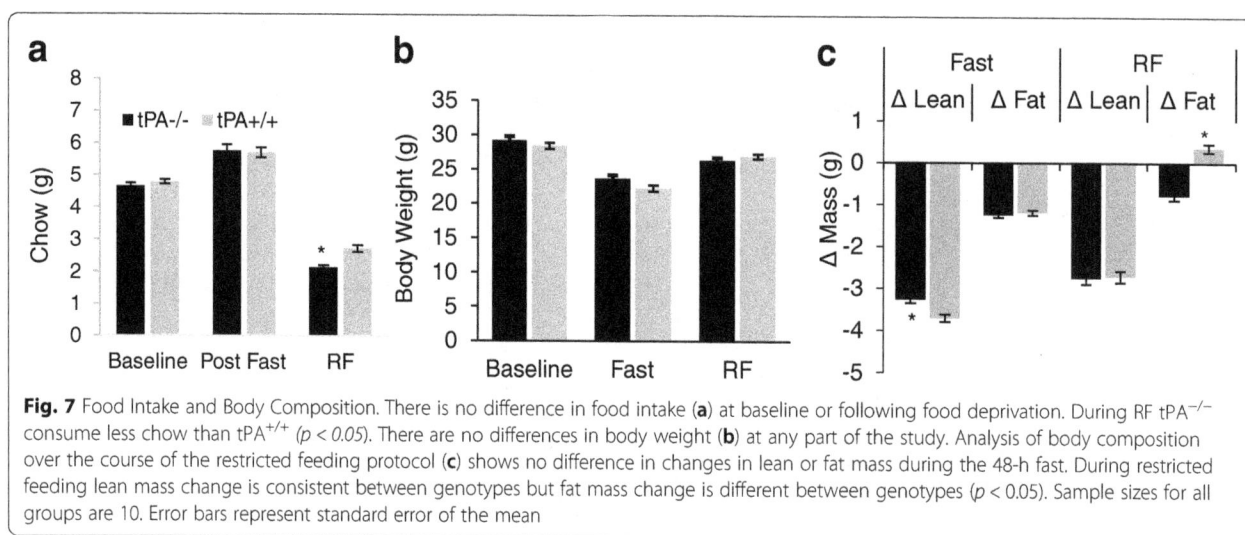

Fig. 7 Food Intake and Body Composition. There is no difference in food intake (**a**) at baseline or following food deprivation. During RF tPA$^{-/-}$ consume less chow than tPA$^{+/+}$ (p < 0.05). There are no differences in body weight (**b**) at any part of the study. Analysis of body composition over the course of the restricted feeding protocol (**c**) shows no difference in changes in lean or fat mass during the 48-h fast. During restricted feeding lean mass change is consistent between genotypes but fat mass change is different between genotypes (p < 0.05). Sample sizes for all groups are 10. Error bars represent standard error of the mean

locomotor activity output. The loss of tPA should have a significant impact on the ability of animals to entrain to light cycles, through reduced BDNF levels [6, 9]. However, recent data suggests that urokinase-type plasminogen activity may substitute for tPA in the tPA$^{-/-}$ mice [12]. Our initial finding was that tPA$^{-/-}$ mice had reduced nocturnal wheel-running under a standard 12:12 LD cycle. It is likely that this results from the deficiency in mature BDNF in these mice. The positive link between BDNF and locomotor activity has been examined largely in the context of animal models of depression [21, 22], but not explicitly for the motivated behavior of voluntary wheel-running. However, we might have expected tPA$^{-/-}$ mice to show deficits in circadian entrainment, given the reduction in mBDNF and the importance of mBDNF to the circadian clock's photic signaling system [6, 10]. We interpret this to mean that the residual mBDNF remaining is sufficient to allow for normal entrainment of the circadian clock by light. This residual BDNF is produced by the activation of plasmin by enzymes other than tPA, such as urokinase-type plasminogen activator [12] or other enzymes that perform this function such as kallikreins [23].

Interestingly, reduced wheel-running in the tPA$^{-/-}$ mice was reversed on day two of a 48-h fast. During fasting, both tPA$^{+/+}$ and tPA$^{-/-}$ mice show a second daily peak of activity during the light phase of the light-dark cycle. On day one of the fast, activity is elevated during the light phase in both genotypes, but is still reduced in tPA$^{-/-}$ mice. On day two, however, nocturnal wheel-running in tPA$^{+/+}$ mice is reduced while it is increased in tPA$^{-/-}$ mice, suggesting an increased activity in response to the energetic deficit. The timing of the behavior also seems to be somewhat altered on day two, with the peak in dark-phase locomotor activity delayed slightly in tPA$^{-/-}$ mice. Despite the difference in locomotor activity, however,

there was no difference in total weight loss during the fast. The phenomenon of fast-induced increases in activity in rodents is well documented [24], however, our data suggests a role for tPA in the neural processes that regulate this behavior, in a manner distinct from circadian clock-mediated locomotor activity. Furthermore, the increase in wheel-running in tPA$^{-/-}$ mice on day 2 of the fast provides evidence that the decrease in wheel-running under baseline conditions is not due to any kind of physical deficiency, but is more likely related to processes relating to the motivation for wheel-running.

Because of the role tPA plays in regulating plasticity in the brain [25], we had anticipated that tPA$^{-/-}$ mice might have some difficulty adapting to a timed restricted feeding schedule, however, this turned out not to be an issue. Timed restricted feeding totally eliminated the difference in wheel-running activity between tPA$^{-/-}$ and tPA$^{+/+}$ mice. A strong bout of activity in the 3 h prior to food presentation was observed in both genotypes, with a compensatory decrease in activity during the latter half of the dark phase. There was a small but statistically significant difference in the change in body weight during the restricted feeding regime, with weight increasing slightly in tPA$^{+/+}$ mice but not in tPA$^{-/-}$ mice. It could be that increases in locomotor activity in tPA$^{-/-}$ mice compared to baseline resulted in increased energy expenditure, however, given the short-term nature (~ 10 days) of the restricted feeding period we are reluctant to attribute much functional importance to this finding. It is also worth noting that the food anticipatory activity bout that appears during restricted feeding represents a consolidation of the increased daytime activity seen during fasting into a temporally coherent bout.

After a period of restricted feeding, we released mice into ad/lib feeding and constant darkness to assess the phase of the underlying nocturnal activity rhythm. We found no genotypic differences in free-running period, or phase at the time of the photoperiod transition, suggesting that SCN function was largely unaffected by restricted feeding. However, we did note that restricted feeding had an aftereffect on free-running period in the subsequent constant dark period, irrespective of genotype, in the form of a shortening of the period of the wheel-running rhythm. Since this rhythm is driven by the SCN, it suggests periods of restricted feeding may have a more subtle, long-lasting effect on the SCN.

As a result of seeing small differences in the change in body weight between genotypes during restricted feeding, we conducted a separate study on food intake. The protocol for this experiment differed from the locomotor activity studies in that the mice were housed in cages without running wheels, but which were designed for more accurate assessment of food intake. We found no genotypic differences in food intake during baseline conditions or during refeeding after a 48 h fast. However, total food intake was significantly reduced in restricted feeding as compared to ad/lib, and was reduced in tPA$^{-/-}$ mice compared to tPA$^{+/+}$. This manifested as a small decrease in fat mass in tPA$^{-/-}$ mice that was not present in tPA$^{+/+}$. These data do suggest that from an energetic standpoint the tPA$^{-/-}$ mice have a slightly decreased ability to adapt to restricted feeding, but the lack of a difference in the fasted animals suggests that the difference is not metabolic but is more likely behavioral.

Conclusions

Overall, the data presented here suggests that the effects of tPA on locomotor activity are primarily mediated by actions in the brain. The most likely route for these effects is through tPA's regulation of mature BDNF production, and that tPA's actions are stimulatory for wheel-running locomotor activity. Locomotor activity increases production of BDNF [26, 27]. From our studies, it is not possible to identify where in the brain tPA might be acting to influence these patterns of locomotor activity. The current literature regarding tPA's functions in modulating hypothalamic-driven behaviors is sparse; further investigations into the location of tPA's action in the brain may reveal important pathways that show divergence between locomotor activity driven by circadian rhythms and those driven by energetic demands.

Abbreviations
BDNF: Brain-derived neurotrophic factor; FAA: food anticipatory activity; LD: light-dark; SCN: suprachiasmatic nucleus; tPA: tissue-type plasminogen activator; TrkB: Tropomyosin receptor kinase B; ZT: zeitgeber time

Acknowledgements
The authors would like to thank Will Huffman for his assistance with this work.

Funding
Support was provided National Science Foundation grant IOS-1021957 to EMM and the Donald Akers Fellowship to RAP.

Authors' contributions
JAK collected, analyzed, and interpreted the data on locomotor activity, and was a major contributor in writing the manuscript. LEM collected and analyzed locomotor activity data. AR performed the simulated jet lag experiment and assisted in editing the manuscript. XM performed the assay for mBDNF in the SCN and assisted in editing the manuscript. RAP analyzed BDNF data and assisted in interpretation of data and editing the manuscript. EMM supervised the overall project, analyzed and interpreted the data, and was a major contributor in writing the manuscript. All authors read and approved the final manuscript.

Competing interests
The authors declare that they have no competing interests.

Author details
[1]Department of Biological Sciences, Kent State University, Kent, OH 44242, USA. [2]Department of Molecular and Cellular Biology, Baylor College of Medicine, Houston, TX 77030, USA. [3]Department of Biochemistry and Cellular and Molecular Biology, University of Tennessee, Knoxville, TN 37996, USA.

References
1. Stephan FK, Zucker I. Circadian rhythms in drinking behavior and locomotor activity of rats are eliminated by hypothalamic lesions. Proc Natl Acad Sci U S A. 1972;69(6):1583–6.
2. Moore RY, Eichler VB. Loss of a circadian adrenal corticosterone rhythm following suprachiasmatic lesions in the rat. Brain Res. 1972;42(1):201–6.
3. Stephan F, Nunez AA. Role of retino-hypothalamic pathways in the entrainment of drinking rhythms. Brain Res Bull. 1976;1(5):495–7.
4. Pickard GE. The afferent connections of the suprachiasmatic nucleus of the golden hamster with emphasis on the retinohypothalamic projection. J Comp Neurol. 1982;211(1):65–83.
5. Morin LP, Allen CN. The circadian visual system, 2005. Brain Res Rev. 2006; 51(1):1–60.
6. Liang FQ, Allen G, Earnest D. Role of brain-derived neurotrophic factor in the circadian regulation of the suprachiasmatic pacemaker by light. J Neurosci. 2000;20(8):2978–87.
7. Pang PT, Teng HK, Zaitsev E, Woo NT, Sakata K, Zhen SH, Teng KK, Yung WH, Hempstead BL, Lu B. Cleavage of proBDNF by tPA/plasmin is essential for long-term hippocampal plasticity. Science. 2004;306(5695):487–91.
8. Liang FQ, Walline R, Earnest DJ. Circadian rhythm of brain-derived neurotrophic factor in the rat suprachiasmatic nucleus. Neurosci Lett. 1998; 242(2):89–92.
9. Mou X, Peterson CB, Prosser RA. Tissue-type plasminogen activator-plasmin-BDNF modulate glutamate-induced phase-shifts of the mouse suprachiasmatic circadian clock in vitro. Eur J Neurosci. 2009;30(8):1451–60.
10. Allen GC, Qu XY, Earnest DJ. TrkB-deficient mice show diminished phase shifts of the circadian activity rhythm in response to light. Neurosci Lett. 2005;378(3):150–5.
11. Michel S, Clark JP, Ding JM, Colwell CS. Brain-derived neurotrophic factor and neurotrophin receptors modulate glutamate-induced phase shifts of the suprachiasmatic nucleus. Eur J Neurosci. 2006;24(4):1109–16.
12. Cooper JM, Rastogi A, Krizo JA, Mintz EM, Prosser RA. Urokinase-type plasminogen activator modulates mammalian circadian clock phase regulation in tissue-type plasminogen activator knockout mice. Eur J Neurosci. 2017;45(6): 805–15.
13. Chan JP, Unger TJ, Byrnes J, Rios M. Examination of behavioral deficits triggered by targeting Bdnf in fetal or postnatal brains of mice. Neuroscience. 2006;142(1):49–58.
14. Marosi K, Mattson MP. BDNF mediates adaptive brain and body responses to energetic challenges. Trends Endocrinol Metab. 2014;25(2):89–98.
15. Bolles RC, Stokes LW. Rat's anticipation of diurnal and a-diurnal feeding. J Comp Physiol Psychol. 1965;60(2):290–4.
16. Marchant EG, Mistlberger RE. Anticipation and entrainment to feeding time in intact and SCN-ablated C57BL/6j mice. Brain Res. 1997;765(2):273–82.

17. Stephan FK, Swann JM, Sisk CL. Anticipation of 24-hr feeding schedules in rats with lesions of the Suprachiasmatic nucleus. Behav Neural Biol. 1979;25(3):346–63.

18. Storch KF, Weitz CJ. Daily rhythms of food-anticipatory behavioral activity do not require the known circadian clock. Proc Natl Acad Sci U S A. 2009; 106(16):6808–13.

19. Pendergast JS, Nakamura W, Friday RC, Hatanaka F, Takumi T, Yamazaki S. Robust food anticipatory activity in BMAL1-deficient mice. PLoS One. 2009;4(3)

20. Patton DF, Mistlberger RE. Circadian adaptations to meal timing: neuroendocrine mechanisms. Front Neurosci. 2013;7:185.

21. Siuciak JA, Lewis DR, Wiegand SJ, Lindsay RM. Antidepressant-like effect of brain-derived neurotrophic factor (BDNF). Pharmacol Biochem Behav. 1997; 56(1):131–7.

22. Shirayama Y, ACH C, Nakagawa S, Russell DS, Duman RS. Brain-derived neurotrophic factor produces antidepressant effects in behavioral models of depression. J Neurosci. 2002;22(8):3251–61.

23. de Souza LR, M Melo P, Paschoalin T, Carmona AK, Kondo M, Hirata IY, Blaber M, Tersariol I, Takatsuka J, Juliano MA, et al. Human tissue kallikreins 3 and 5 can act as plasminogen activator releasing active plasmin. Biochem Biophys Res Commun. 2013;433(3):333–7.

24. Richter CP. A behavioristic study of the activity of the rat. Williams & Wilkins Company: Baltimore; 1922.

25. Salazar IL, Caldeira MV, Curcio M, Duarte CB. The role of proteases in Hippocampal synaptic plasticity: putting together small pieces of a complex puzzle. Neurochem Res. 2016;41(1-2):156–82.

26. Ieraci A, Mallei A, Musazzi L, Popoli M. Physical exercise and acute restraint stress differentially modulate hippocampal brain-derived neurotrophic factor transcripts and epigenetic mechanisms in mice. Hippocampus. 2015;25(11): 1380–92.

27. Wrann CD, White JP, Salogiannnis J, Laznik-Bogoslavski D, Wu J, Ma D, Lin JD, Greenberg ME, Spiegelman BM. Exercise induces hippocampal BDNF through a PGC-1alpha/FNDC5 pathway. Cell Metab. 2013;18(5):649–59.

Ryanodine-induced vasoconstriction of the gerbil spiral modiolar artery depends on the Ca^{2+} sensitivity but not on Ca^{2+} sparks or BK channels

Gayathri Krishnamoorthy[1], Katrin Reimann[1,2] and Philine Wangemann[1*]

Abstract

Background: In many vascular smooth muscle cells (SMCs), ryanodine receptor-mediated Ca^{2+} sparks activate large-conductance Ca^{2+}-activated K^+ (BK) channels leading to lowered SMC $[Ca^{2+}]_i$ and vasodilation. Here we investigated whether Ca^{2+} sparks regulate SMC global $[Ca^{2+}]_i$ and diameter in the spiral modiolar artery (SMA) by activating BK channels.

Methods: SMAs were isolated from adult female gerbils, loaded with the Ca^{2+}-sensitive flourescent dye fluo-4 and pressurized using a concentric double-pipette system. Ca^{2+} signals and vascular diameter changes were recorded using a laser-scanning confocal imaging system. Effects of various pharmacological agents on Ca^{2+} signals and vascular diameter were analyzed.

Results: Ca^{2+} sparks and waves were observed in pressurized SMAs. Inhibition of Ca^{2+} sparks with ryanodine increased global Ca^{2+} and constricted SMA at 40 cmH_2O but inhibition of Ca^{2+} sparks with tetracaine or inhibition of BK channels with iberiotoxin at 40 cmH_2O did not produce a similar effect. The ryanodine-induced vasoconstriction observed at 40 cmH_2O was abolished at 60 cmH_2O, consistent with a greater Ca^{2+}-sensitivity of constriction at 40 cmH_2O than at 60 cmH_2O. When the Ca^{2+}-sensitivity of the SMA was increased by prior application of 1 nM endothelin-1, ryanodine induced a robust vasoconstriction at 60 cmH_2O.

Conclusions: The results suggest that Ca^{2+} sparks, while present, do not regulate vascular diameter in the SMA by activating BK channels and that the regulation of vascular diameter in the SMA is determined by the Ca^{2+}-sensitivity of constriction.

Keywords: Ca^{2+} spark, Ca^{2+} sensitivity, Spiral modiolar artery, Ryanodine, Vascular diameter, BK channels, Tetracaine

Background

Cochlear function is sensitive to dynamic changes in cochlear blood flow that is responsible for the delivery of oxygen and glucose and the removal of CO_2 [1, 2]. Regulation of cochlear blood flow is essential for hearing and is important as a treatment strategy for the restoration of hearing loss in humans [3–8]. Homeostatic regulation of blood flow in the cochlear capillary beds is achieved by the dynamic adjustment of the vascular diameter or "tone" of pre-capillary arteries and arterioles against systemic changes of pressure, nerve and metabolic activity [9–14]. The mechanisms involved in such regulation of the spiral modiolar artery, the principal artery of the cochlear blood supply, remain to be elucidated.

Smooth muscle cells of most arteries exhibit "Ca^{2+} sparks", which are transient local elevations of Ca^{2+} caused by the opening of ryanodine receptors (RyRs) in the sarcoplasmic reticulum (SR) [15, 16]. In most smooth muscle cells, Ca^{2+} sparks activate BK channels, leading to membrane hyperpolarization, reduced activity of L-type voltage-dependent Ca^{2+} channels (VDCCs),

---

* Correspondence: wange@vet.ksu.edu
[1]Anatomy & Physiology Department, Cell Physiology Laboratory, Kansas State University, 228 Coles Hall, Manhattan, Kansas 66506-5802, USA
Full list of author information is available at the end of the article

decrease in $[Ca^{2+}]_i$ and smooth muscle relaxation [15, 17–19]. Thus, the triad of Ca^{2+} sparks, VDCCs and BK channels effectively regulates intracellular Ca^{2+} to oppose vasoconstriction and maintain blood flow to the underlying tissue. Activation of BK channels by Ca^{2+} sparks is a potent vasodilatory mechanism to regulate SMC global $[Ca^{2+}]_i$ and vascular diameter and a prominent feature in blood vessels of the cerebral, kidney, mesenteric and cardiac microcirculation [17–21].

We have recently demonstrated Ca^{2+} sparks in smooth muscle cells of the intact SMA [22]. In this study, we investigate whether Ca^{2+} sparks regulate the global Ca^{2+} and vascular diameter in the SMA. Our results demonstrate that Ca^{2+} sparks are also present in the pressurized SMA but do not regulate vasodilation of the SMA by activating BK channels. Instead, the effects produced by ryanodine, which eliminates Ca^{2+} sparks, are dictated by the pressure-dependent changes in the Ca^{2+} sensitivity of contraction.

Methods

Ethics statement

All procedures involving animals were approved by the Institutional Animal Care and Use Committee at Kansas State University (IACUC#: 2961 and 3245).

Isolation of the spiral modiolar artery (SMA)

Female gerbils between the ages of 4 to 12 weeks (Charles River, Wilmington, MA) were anesthetized with tri-bromo-ethanol (560 mg/kg i.p.) and sacrificed by decapitation. Auditory bullae were harvested and the spiral modiolar arteries (SMAs) separated from the cochlea by microdissection in HEPES-buffered physiological saline solution (PSS) at 4 C°.

Pressurization and superfusion

Segments of the SMA were pressurized and perfused in a custom-built bath chamber using a variable hydrostatic pressure column connected to a motorized set of concentric glass pipettes (Wangemann Instruments, Kansas State University, KS) mounted on an inverted microscope (Axiovert 200, Carl Zeiss, Göttingen, Germany) [12]. Briefly, arteries were held by a holding pipette and luminally perfused with a perfusion pipette at one end while the other end was occluded using a blunt glass pipette. All pipettes were prepared using a custom-built micro-forge. The pressurized vessel was superfused in the bath with either HEPES-buffered PSS at a rate of 1.6 ml/min, permitting one complete exchange of the bath volume (~70 μl) within ~3 s. Experiments were conducted at 37 °C. Bath temperature was maintained by a triple heating system consisting of regulating the temperatures of the superfusate (8-line heater, CL-100, Warner Instruments, Hamden, CT, USA), the bath

chamber (TC 324B, Warner Instruments) and the microscope objective (TC 324B, Warner Instruments).

Measurements of cytosolic Ca^{2+} signals

Cytosolic Ca^{2+} signals in SMCs were monitored as spatial and temporal changes in the fluorescence intensity of the indicator dye fluo4. For loading the dye, pressurized vessel segments were incubated in 2.5 μM fluo4-AM (Invitrogen, Carlsbad, CA, USA) for 15 min at 37 ° C, followed by wash and superfusion with HEPES-buffered PSS. The dye loaded virtually exclusively into SMCs. Fluo4 was excited by a 488 nm argon laser. Fluorescence emissions were filtered by a 488 notch and two long-pass filters (490 nm and 505 nm) and recorded by a photomultiplier through an open pinhole (LSM 510 Meta, Carl Zeiss).

Ca^{2+} sparks

Ca^{2+} sparks in SMCs of pressurized SMA were detected in frame scans and line scans. For frame scans, tangential images of the vascular wall (32.14 μm × 10.04 μm) were recorded using an oil-immersion objective (Plan-Neofluar 40× 1.3 N.A., Carl Zeiss) at a temporal resolution of ~61 images/s (16.3 ms/frame) and a spatial resolution of 0.25 μm × 0.25 μm per pixel. Spark sites were identified using custom-designed software, SparkAn, developed by Dr. Adrian D. Bonev (University of Vermont, VT, USA) in IDL 5.0.2 (Research Systems, Boulder, CO) and kindly provided for use by Dr. Adrian D. Bonev and Dr. Mark T. Nelson (University of Vermont). Ca^{2+} sparks were detected by dividing an area spanning 2.01 μm (8 pixels) × 2.01 μm (8 pixels) in each frame by a baseline (F_0) that was obtained by averaging 10 frames without Ca^{2+} spark activity. Spark traces and 2-dimensional pseudo-color images were obtained as F/F_0. 3-dimensional ratio images were generated by SparkAn.

Line-scan recordings of 5 s duration each were performed at a Ca^{2+} spark site to determine the temporal parameters of Ca^{2+} sparks in SMCs. Lines (0.15 μm × 12.4 μm) were recorded using an oil-immersion objective (Plan-Neofluar 40× 1.3 N.A.) at a temporal resolution of ~521 lines per second (0.82 ms per line). For spark measurements at different pressures, three 5 s line-scans were performed first at 60 cmH$_2$O, followed by three line-scans at 40 cmH$_2$O, followed by three line scans at 60 cmH$_2$O. Time intervals between consecutive line-scans were 15 s to allow for recovery. Time intervals between pressure-changes were 45 s. For experiments in ryanodine and tetracaine, 10 μM ryanodine or 100 μM tetracaine was introduced after the third line-scan in PSS and scans were resumed after 2 min. Recordings were analyzed as described earlier [11]. For presentation, a single 5 s line-scan image was contrast-enhanced to highlight the occurrence of Ca^{2+} spark events.

Determination of length and height of smooth muscle cells

To calculate Ca^{2+} spark density, cell length and cell height of single SMCs were estimated from scanned images of pressurized SMA loaded with BCECF (Sigma-Aldrich). SMC length and height were determined to be 132 ± 17 µm and 3.2 ± 0.1 µm based on images of 9 vessels that each covered 20 – 30 cells. These values correspond to a cell volume of ~1 pl, which is consistent with SMCs from other vessels [15].

Simultaneous measurements of vascular diameter and global cytosolic Ca^{2+}

Pressurized vessels (40 or 60 cmH$_2$O), loaded with the indicator dye fluo4 as described above, were superfused with HEPES-buffered PSS. To record the inner diameter of pressurized vessels simultaneously with changes in the global cytosolic Ca^{2+} in SMCs, images (225 µm × 225 µm) were recorded using an oil-immersion objective (Plan-Neofluar 40× 1.3 N.A.) with a temporal resolution of 1 image/s (983 ms/frame) and a spatial resolution of 0.44 µm × 0.44 µm per pixel. In addition to filtering and recording fluorescence emissions as described above, the transmitted light from the argon laser was detected by a second photomultiplier. Inner diameter was measured by automatic edge detection by a method developed and described in Reimann et al. 2011 [12]. Inner diameter (ID) was detected from acquired real time transmitted light images, using a custom written data acquisition program (Dr. W. Gil Wier, University of Maryland). Edge detection data were analyzed using a custom written analysis program in Origin 6.0 (Dr. P. Wangemann, Kansas State University). Inner diameter changes were normalized against the average of 30 data points obtained in PSS at the beginning of the experiment (basal vascular tone). Fluorescence intensity values from 5–10 SMCs per pressurized vessel were averaged and normalized between the fluorescence values in Ca^{2+} free solution and the fluorescence value in PSS before the addition of drugs according to the formula Norm $Ca^{2+} = (([Ca^{2+}]_i - [Ca^{2+}]_0)/([Ca^{2+}]_{PSS} - [Ca^{2+}]_0)) + 1$, where $[Ca^{2+}]_0$ is marked b and $[Ca^{2+}]_{PSS}$ is marked in Figs. 2b, 3b, 3e, 4b, 5b, and 7b. a

Ca^{2+} sensitivity

Simultaneous measurements of diameter and global cytosolic Ca^{2+} were performed to determine the Ca^{2+}-sensitivity of constrictions. In these experiments, following equilibration in HEPES-buffered PSS for 15 min, arteries were superfused with saline solutions containing 0, 1, 3 and 10 mM Ca^{2+} in 2 min steps, first at 60 cmH$_2$O followed by the same protocol at 40 cmH$_2$O. Data points for concentration curves were obtained by averaging diameter and fluorescence intensity

measurements over the last 30s of each Ca^{2+} step and normalizing against the average value obtained in PSS at 60 cmH$_2$O. Data points from individual vessels were fitted to a modified Hill equation:

$$Dia = Base + \frac{(Max\text{–}Base) \times [Ca^{2+}]^h}{\left([FC_{50}]^h + [Ca^{2+}]^h\right)}$$

where Dia is the normalized diameter, Max is the diameter at 60 cmH$_2$O in PSS containing 1 mM Ca^{2+}, $Base$ is the maximum achievable constriction with respect to Max for the female gerbil SMA estimated from previous observations [23], $[Ca^{2+}]$ is the normalized cytosolic $Ca^2$$^+$ concentration, h is the slope coefficient, and FC_{50} is the fold-change in the global cytosolic Ca^{2+} concentration that is necessary for a half-maximal constriction. The slope coefficient h was set to -5.2 and Max was clamped to 100%. Two FC_{50} values, one each for 60 cmH$_2$O and 40 cmH$_2$O, were obtained for each experiment. For presentation, normalized Ca^{2+} and diameter data were averaged and fitted with the equation above using average FC_{50} values.

Solutions and drugs

HEPES-buffered PSS contained (in mM): 150 NaCl, 5 HEPES, 3.6 KCl, 1 MgCl$_2$, 1 CaCl$_2$ and 5 glucose, pH adjusted to 7.4 at 37 °C. Ca^{2+}-free solutions were devoid of CaCl$_2$ and contained 1 mM EGTA. 100 µM papaverine hydrochloride (Pap) was added to the Ca^{2+} free solution wherever indicated. Stock solutions of ryanodine (Ryn, 20 mM, Enzo Life Sciences, NY or Santa Cruz Biotechnologies, Santa Cruz, CA), tetracaine (Tet, 100 mM, Sigma- Aldrich), paxilline (Pax, 10 mM, Sigma-Aldrich) and papaverine (Pap, 250 mM, Sigma-Aldrich) were prepared in DMSO and stored at -20 °C and freshly diluted to target concentration in solution when required taking care that the final DMSO concentration in solution did not exceed 0.1%. Endothelin-1 (ET-1, 1 µM, Sigma-Aldrich) and iberiotoxin (IbTx, 2 µM, Alomone Labs, Jerusalem, Israel) were always freshly prepared in PSS for immediate use.

Results

Ca^{2+} sparks in the pressurized spiral modiolar artery

Ca^{2+} sparks and waves were recently reported in the intact unpressurized gerbil SMA [22]. We now report $Ca^2$$^+$ sparks and Ca^{2+} waves in SMCs of the pressurized gerbil SMA (Fig. 1). Ca^{2+} spark sites were consistently observed in frame scans (Fig. 1a), with super Ca^{2+} sparks, of larger cross-sectional area and longer duration of elevated Ca^{2+} observed occasionally, which may reflect the combined synchronized activity of two or more closely spaced Ca^{2+} sparks sites. The average spatial area of

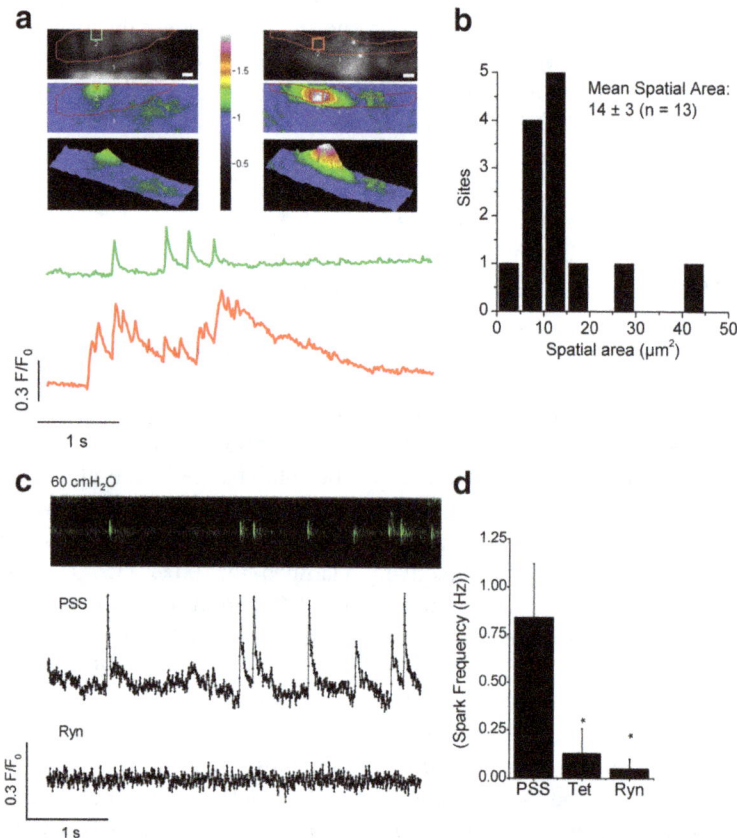

Fig. 1 Ca²⁺ sparks in smooth muscle cells of the pressurized spiral modiolar artery. **a** Ca²⁺ spark site captured during a 5 s frame scan of SMCs in a pressurized (60 cmH₂O) SMA. Grey panel (*top panels*) depicts the average of 10 frames that do not contain a Ca²⁺ spark. Outline (*in red*) depicts the visible portion of the cell. Scale bar = 2 μm. Pseudo-color image depicts an average (*left middle panel*) and a large (*right middle panel*) Ca²⁺ spark at its peak. Regions of interest (ROIs) are 2 μm × 2 μm. (*Bottom panels*) show a 3D rendering of the 2D images. Traces (*green and red*) represent the fluorescence intensity changes occurring at the corresponding ROIs shown in the panels above. **b** Histogram showing the distribution of the calculated spatial area of Ca²⁺ spark sites. **c** Contrast-adjusted 5 s line-scan recording of a Ca²⁺ spark site in a SMC of a pressurized (60 cmH₂O) SMA and the corresponding fluorescence intensity traces recorded in PSS and in the presence of 10 μM ryanodine (Ryn). **d** Spark frequency in PSS (*n* = 9), 100 μM tetracaine (Tet, *n* = 3) and 10 μM ryanodine (Ryn, *n* = 4)

spark sites was 14 ± 3 μm², corresponding to a spatial width of ~4 μm. Two out of 13 recorded Ca²⁺ spark sites had larger spatial areas between 25 – 50 μm² (Fig. 1b). An average of 1.3 ± 0.2 Ca²⁺ spark sites were present in 200 ± 10 μm² of recorded area ($n = 10$), corresponding to ~47% of one cell, giving a spark density of 2.8 ± 0.3 spark sites/cell. The frequency of Ca²⁺ spark occurrence per site and other temporal parameters were measured in pressurized SMA using line-scans (Fig. 1c). Spark frequency per site increased from 0.6 Hz to 0.9 Hz, as pressure increased from 40 cmH₂O to 60 cmH₂O (Table 1). However, increasing pressure from 40 to 60 cmH₂O did not alter the spark amplitude, the rise-

time or the half-time of decay (Table 1). Ca²⁺ sparks were completely eliminated in the presence of 10 μM ryanodine (Fig. 1c) and significantly decreased in frequency in the presence of 100 μM tetracaine (Fig. 1d). Ca²⁺ oscillations exhibiting wave-like phenomena were also observed in SMCs and were likewise abolished by application of 10 μM ryanodine (Fig. 2a).

Effects of inhibitors of Ca²⁺ sparks and BK channels on global Ca²⁺ and vascular diameter of the SMA

In most arteries, inhibition of Ca²⁺ sparks and/or BK channels has been shown to increase SMC global Ca²⁺ to cause a robust vasoconstriction in a non-additive

Table 1 Parameters of Ca²⁺ sparks

Pressure (cmH₂O)	Frequency per site (Hz)	Amplitude (F/F₀)	Rise-Time (ms)	Half-decay-time (ms)
40	0.6 ± 0.1 (*n* = 17)	1.53 ± 0.03 (*n* = 65)	18.3 ± 0.7 (*n* = 65)	19.8 ± 1.2 (*n* = 64)
60	[a] 0.9 ± 0.1 (*n* = 17)	1.49 ± 0.03 (*n* = 110)	16.9 ± 0.3 (*n* = 110)	17.8 ± 0.8 (*n* = 110)

[a] indicates significance between parameter values measured at 40 and 60 cmH₂O

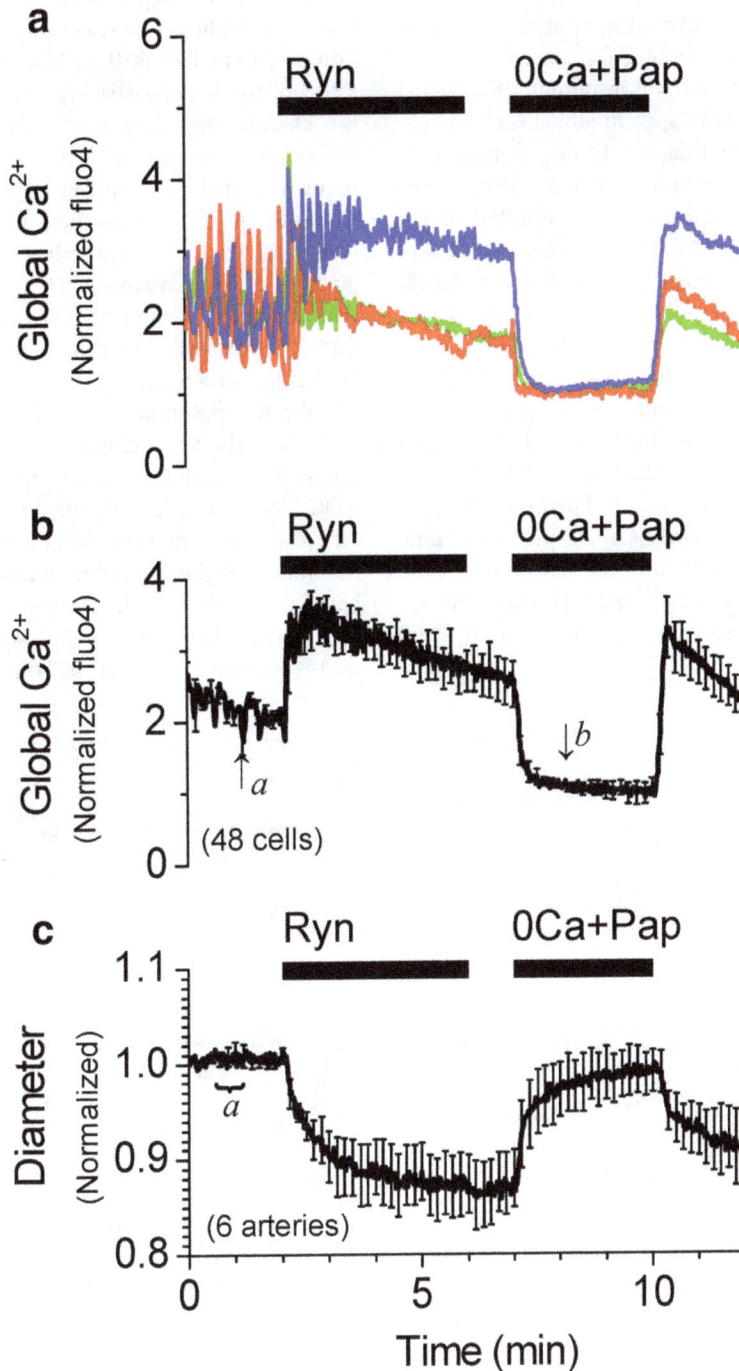

Fig. 2 Inhibition of Ca^{2+} sparks with ryanodine increases the global $[Ca^{2+}]_i$ and constricts the SMA. **a** Representative recordings of $[Ca^{2+}]_i$ changes from single smooth muscle cells from a pressurized (40 cmH$_2$O) SMA in response to 10 µM ryanodine (Ryn). **b** Average of normalized traces of $[Ca^{2+}]_i$ changes at 40 cmH$_2$O (48 cells). Traces in **a** and **b** were normalized as described in Methods. **c** Average trace of corresponding changes in vascular diameter (6 arteries). Diameter changes were normalized to the average of values recorded between 30–60 s (average value indicated by 'a' was set to 1). $[Ca^{2+}]_i$ and diameter data were simultaneously acquired at 1 s intervals, however, for clarity, error bars (sem) are plotted only every 10 s

fashion, reflecting that Ca^{2+} sparks and BK channels are part of the same mechanism to hyperpolarize the membrane and limit Ca^{2+} influx, leading to vasorelaxation

[17, 18, 20]. In the pressurized (40 cmH$_2$O) SMA, application of 10 µM ryanodine inhibited Ca^{2+} sparks and appeared to similarly increase the average global cytosolic

Ca^{2+} followed by a robust vasoconstriction (Fig. 2). However, application of 100 μM tetracaine, another known inhibitor of ryanodine receptors and Ca^{2+} sparks [24], or application of 100 nM iberiotoxin, a potent BK channel inhibitor, did not cause any change in global Ca^{2+} or vascular diameter similar to that produced by ryanodine (Fig. 3). Activation of BK channels is dependent on the local $[Ca^{2+}]_i$ as well as the membrane potential of the smooth muscle membrane [25]. It is possible that lack of an effect of iberiotoxin is a consequence of unopened BK channels caused by a hyperpolarized resting membrane potential in the smooth muscle cells of the SMA. To account for such a possibility, the pressurized SMA was superfused with PSS solution containing 30 mM K^+. High K^+ induced a transient increase in the global $[Ca^{2+}]_i$ and vasoconstriction. Under these conditions, 100 nM iberiotoxin remained without effect (Fig. 4). Furthermore, contrary to the effect at 40 cmH_2O, 10 μM ryanodine increased global Ca^{2+} modestly and did not constrict the SMA pressurized at 60 cmH_2O (Fig. 5), even though spark frequency is increased significantly from 40 to 60 cmH_2O (Table 1).

These effects suggest that, unlike cerebral arteries, the ryanodine-induced increase in global Ca^{2+} and constriction at 40 cmH_2O in the SMA may not be attributed to a loss of the hyperpolarizing influence of the Ca^{2+} spark-BK channel signaling mechanism. Under these conditions, ryanodine-sensitive Ca^{2+} sparks do not appear to regulate global Ca^{2+} and vascular tone via BK channels in the SMA. This raises the question as to the mechanism involved in the ryanodine-induced increase in the global Ca^{2+} and vasoconstriction. It is to be expected that at least a portion of the global Ca^{2+} is the result of Ca^{2+} influx via voltage-dependent Ca^{2+} channels (VDCCs), which are open at the physiological resting membrane potential in SMCs. Evidence for active VDCCs in the SMA comes from the observation of a decrease in global Ca^{2+} upon application of a reversible VDCC inhibitor, 2 μM nifedipine, in the presence of 100 μM tetracaine (Fig. 3d and e). It is possible that the remainder of the ryanodine-induced increase in the global Ca^{2+} is the result of ryanodine receptor-mediated Ca^{2+} release from the sarcoplasmic reticulum (SR). It is well-established that at a concentration of 10 μM,

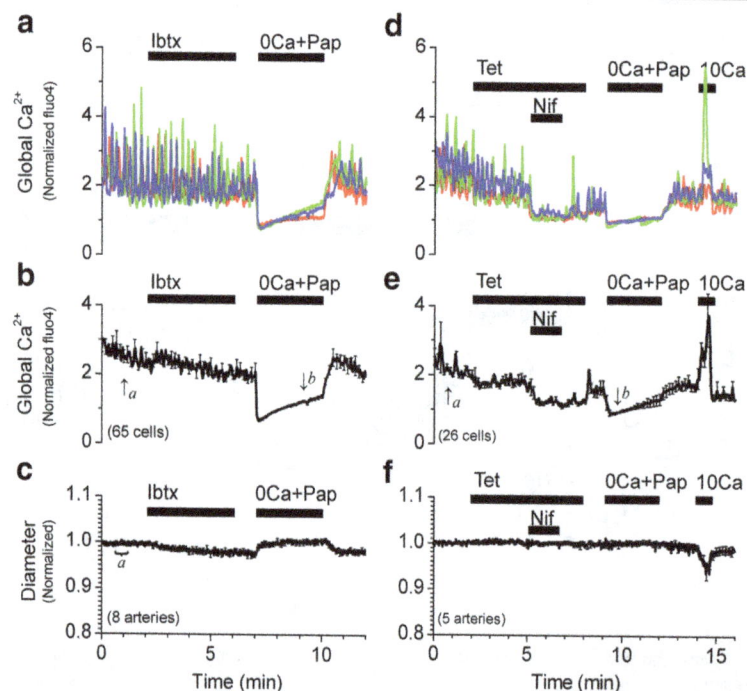

Fig. 3 Inhibition of BK channels with iberiotoxin or inhibition of Ca^{2+} sparks with tetracaine does not increase the global $[Ca^{2+}]_i$ or constrict the SMA at 40 cmH_2O. **a** Representative recordings of $[Ca^{2+}]_i$ changes from single smooth muscle cells from a pressurized (40 cmH_2O) SMA in response to 100 nM Ibtx. **b** Average of normalized traces of $[Ca^{2+}]_i$ changes in the presence of Ibtx (65 cells). Traces in **a** and **b** were normalized as described in Methods. **c** Average trace of corresponding changes in vascular diameter in the presence of Ibtx (8 arteries). **d** Representative recordings of $[Ca^{2+}]_i$ changes from single smooth muscle cells from a pressurized (40 cmH_2O) SMA in response to 100 μM Tet and 1 μM nifedipine (Nif). **e** Average of normalized traces of $[Ca^{2+}]_i$ changes at 40 cmH_2O (26 cells). Traces in **d** and **e** were normalized as described in Methods. **f** Average trace of corresponding changes in vascular diameter (5 arteries) in the presence of Tet and Nif. Diameter changes were normalized to the average of values recorded between 30–60s (value indicated by 'a' was set to 1). $[Ca^{2+}]_i$ and diameter data were simultaneously acquired at 1 s intervals, however, for clarity, error bars (sem) are plotted only every 10s

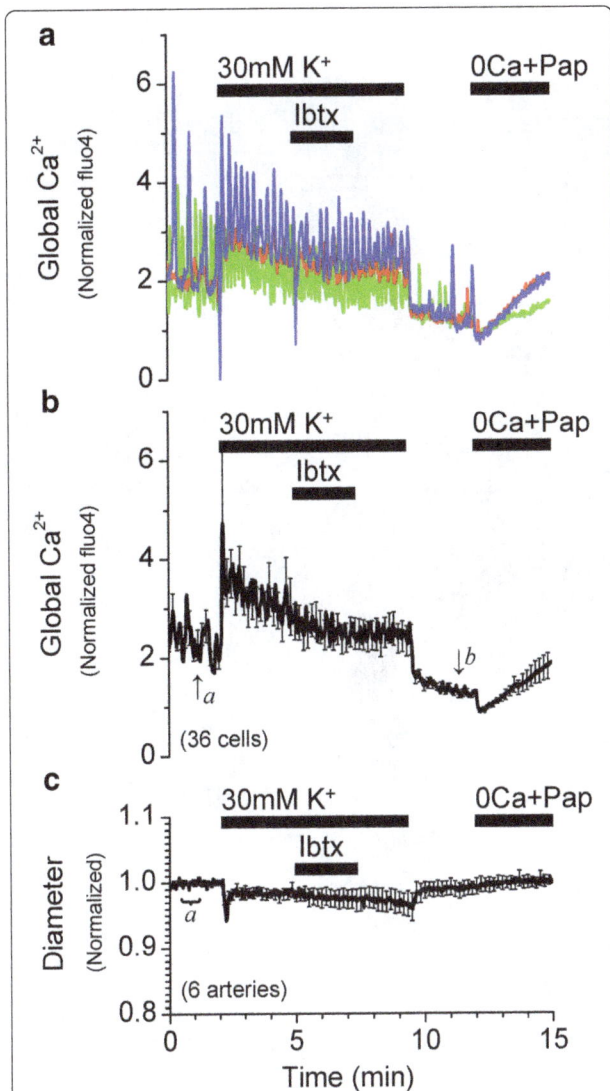

Fig. 4 Inhibition of BK channels in the presence of high K+ does not increase the global [Ca^{2+}]$_i$ or constrict the SMA. **a** Representative recordings of [Ca^{2+}]$_i$ changes from single smooth muscle cells from a pressurized (40 cmH$_2$O) SMA in the presence of PSS containing 30 mM K+ and 100 nM Ibtx. **b** Average of normalized traces of [Ca^{2+}]$_i$ changes in the presence of PSS containing 30 mM K+ and Ibtx (36 cells). Traces in **a** and **b** were normalized as described in Methods. **c** Average trace of corresponding changes in vascular diameter (6 arteries). Diameter changes were normalized to the average of values recorded between 30 – 60 s (value indicated by 'a' was set to 1). [Ca^{2+}]$_i$ and diameter data were simultaneously acquired at 1 s intervals, however, for clarity, error bars (sem) are plotted only every 10 s

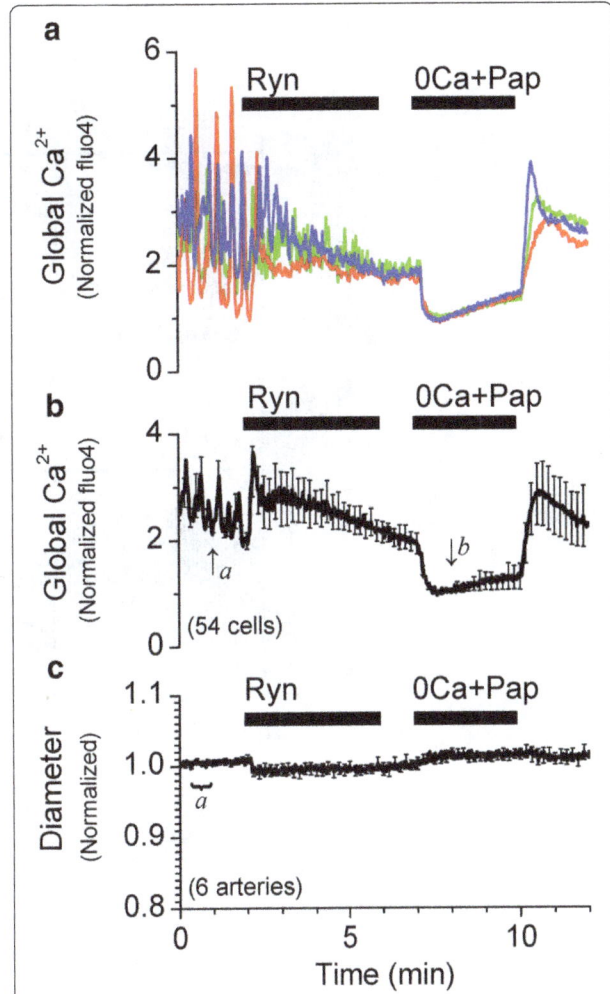

Fig. 5 Inhibition of Ca^{2+} sparks with ryanodine results in a modest increase in global [Ca^{2+}]$_i$ but does not constrict the SMA at 60 cmH$_2$O. **a** Representative recordings of [Ca^{2+}]$_i$ changes from single smooth muscle cells from a pressurized (60 cmH$_2$O) SMA superfused with HEPES-buffered PSS in response to 10 μM Ryn. **b** Average of normalized traces of [Ca^{2+}]$_i$ changes at 60 cmH$_2$O (54 cells). Traces in **a** and **b** were normalized as described in Methods. **c** Average trace of corresponding changes in vascular diameter (6 arteries). Diameter changes were normalized to the average of values recorded between 30 – 60 s (average value indicated by 'a' was set to 1). [Ca^{2+}]$_i$ and diameter data were simultaneously acquired at 1 s intervals, however, for clarity, error bars (sem) are plotted only every 10 s

ryanodine binds to open ryanodine receptors and modifies the channel to lock them in an irreversible sub-conductance state of 234 pS [16, 26] that inhibits Ca^{2+} release and instead "leaks" SR Ca^{2+} into the cytosol. This is reflected in the transient increase in global Ca^{2+} immediately upon application of 10 μM ryanodine, followed by a slowly decaying plateau

phase devoid of Ca^{2+} oscillations, indicating the relatively slow emptying of the SR through the partially open ryanodine receptors (Fig. 2a and b).

It is to be noted that the ryanodine-induced vasoconstriction continues to increase as the corresponding average global Ca^{2+} plateaus and then decreases (Fig. 2b and c). Indeed, the maximum vasoconstriction corresponds to the least increase in global Ca^{2+} induced by ryanodine, suggesting an increase in the Ca^{2+} sensitivity

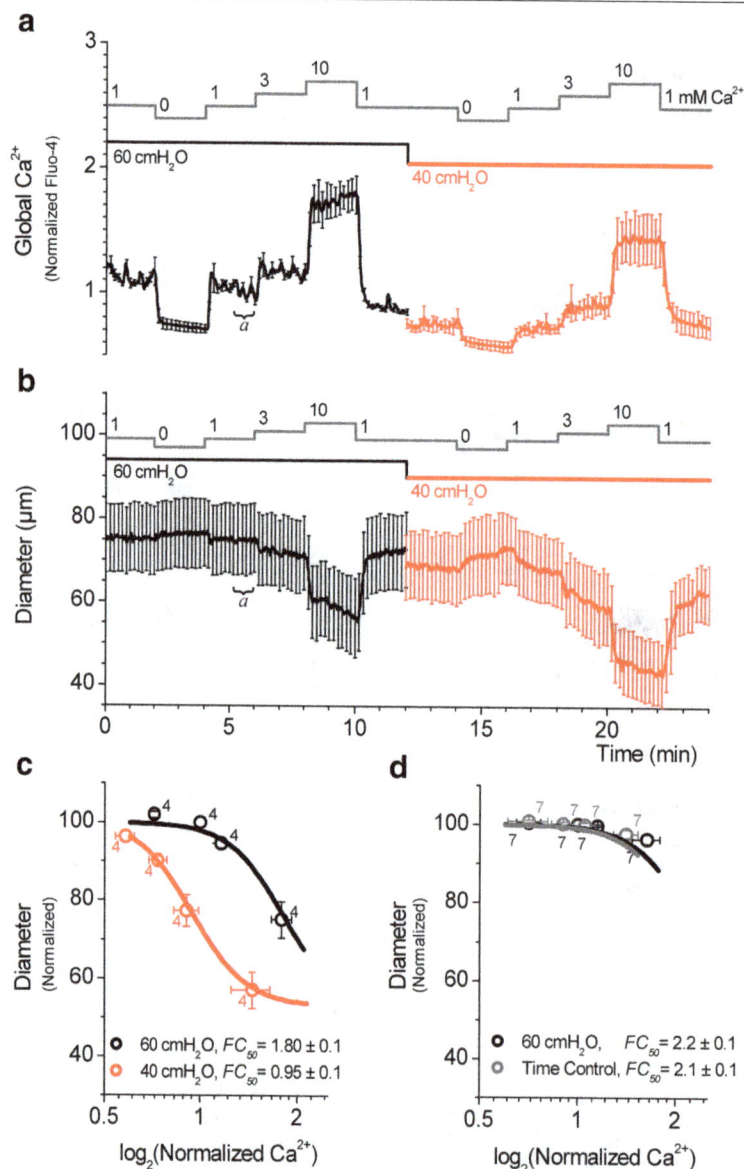

Fig. 6 Ca^{2+} sensitivity of the SMA decreases with increase in pressure. **a, b** Vascular diameter and $[Ca^{2+}]_i$ changes in the presence of 0, 1, 3 and 10 mM Ca^{2+} were simultaneously measured from vessel segments pressurized at 60 cmH_2O (black trace) followed by 40 cmH_2O (*red trace*), as indicated. **a** Summary of changes in $[Ca^{2+}]_i$ measured as changes in fluorescence intensity. **b** Summary of corresponding diameter measurements first at 60 cmH_2O and then at 40 cmH_2O (4 arteries). Data were acquired at 1 s intervals, however, for clarity, error bars (sem) are plotted only every 10s. **c** Ca^{2+} sensitivity of SMA at 60 cmH_2O (*black trace*) and 40 cmH_2O (*red trace*). **d** Ca^{2+} sensitivity of SMA at 60 cmH_2O (*black trace*) and time control at 60 cmH_2O (*grey trace*). Numbers next to symbols represent the number of arteries. For **c** and **d**, average FC_{50} values are given as mean ± sem. Data points for normalized $[Ca^{2+}]_i$ and diameter were obtained by averaging diameter and fluorescence intensity measurements over the last 30 s of each Ca^{2+} step and normalizing these values against the average value obtained in PSS containing 1 mM Ca^{2+} at 60 cmH_2O (denoted as 'a')

of constriction following the initial increase in the global Ca^{2+}. In other words, the constriction induced by ryanodine at 40 cmH_2O may be attributed to enhanced Ca^{2+} sensitivity of the SMA that is able to respond to the ryanodine-induced increase in intracellular Ca^{2+} with vasoconstriction. The observation that the ryanodine-induced constriction at 40 cmH_2O is enhanced (Fig. 2c) compared to that at 60 cmH_2O (Fig. 5c) suggests that

the Ca^{2+} sensitivity at 40 cmH_2O may be greater than at 60 cmH_2O.

Ca^{2+} sensitivity of the SMA decreases with increasing pressure

The Ca^{2+} sensitivity at 40 and 60 cmH_2O was determined from simultaneous measurements of the cytosolic Ca^{2+} and the vascular diameter. The cytosolic Ca^{2+}

concentration was manipulated by altering the Ca^{2+} concentration in the superfusate (Fig. 6a and b). Normalized cytosolic Ca^{2+} and corresponding vascular diameter measurements were plotted against each other and fitted to the Hill equation. A decrease in the pressure from 60 to 40 cmH_2O shifted the Ca^{2+}-diameter relationship to the left on the Ca^{2+} axis, indicating a dramatic increase in the Ca^{2+} sensitivity, with nearly 2-fold decrease in the Ca^{2+} required for a half-maximal constriction at 40 cmH_2O compared to that at 60 cmH_2O (Fig. 6c), whereas a time control repeated at 60 cmH_2O did not (Fig. 6d). Thus, the modest increase in global Ca^{2+} caused by ryanodine at 60 cmH_2O was insufficient to constrict the SMA at this pressure, whereas the enhanced Ca^{2+} sensitivity at 40 cmH_2O allowed for a robust constriction for an increase in global Ca^{2+}.

Endothelin enhances the ryanodine-induced vasoconstriction

The result above implies that conditions that increase the Ca^{2+} sensitivity at 60 cmH_2O would increase the ryanodine-induced vasoconstriction. Consequently, the SMA pressurized at 60 cmH_2O was first exposed to 1 nM endothelin-1 (ET-1) for 1 min. It has been previously shown that endothelin-1 acts via ET_A receptors to increase the Ca^{2+} sensitivity of the SMA in a rho-kinase dependent manner [27]. ET-1 caused a transient increase in the cytosolic Ca^{2+} concentration and a persistent vasoconstriction, consistent with an increase in the Ca^{2+} sensitivity (Fig. 7). Under these conditions, 10 μM ryanodine caused a vasoconstriction that was enhanced compared to that observed in the absence of ET-1 (Fig. 5). These results support the concept that ryanodine increases global Ca^{2+} and constricts the SMA when the Ca^{2+} sensitivity is high. Ca^{2+} sensitivity of SMC contraction is hence a critical factor in the regulation of the vascular diameter of the SMA in response to changes in pressure and cytosolic global Ca^{2+}.

Discussion

Salient findings of the present study are 1) Ca^{2+} spark frequency in the pressurized SMA increases with pressure; 2) Inhibition of Ca^{2+} sparks with ryanodine increases global Ca^{2+} and causes a robust vasoconstriction, however, ryanodine-induced effects on global Ca^{2+} and vascular diameter are not reproduced by other inhibitors of Ca^{2+} sparks or by inhibitors of BK channels as would be expected if Ca^{2+} sparks activated BK channels to regulate membrane potential, global Ca^{2+} and vascular diameter. 3) The ryanodine-induced vasoconstrictions depends on the Ca^{2+} sensitivity, which is higher at 40 cmH_2O compared to that at 60 cmH_2O and can be enhanced with endothelin-1.

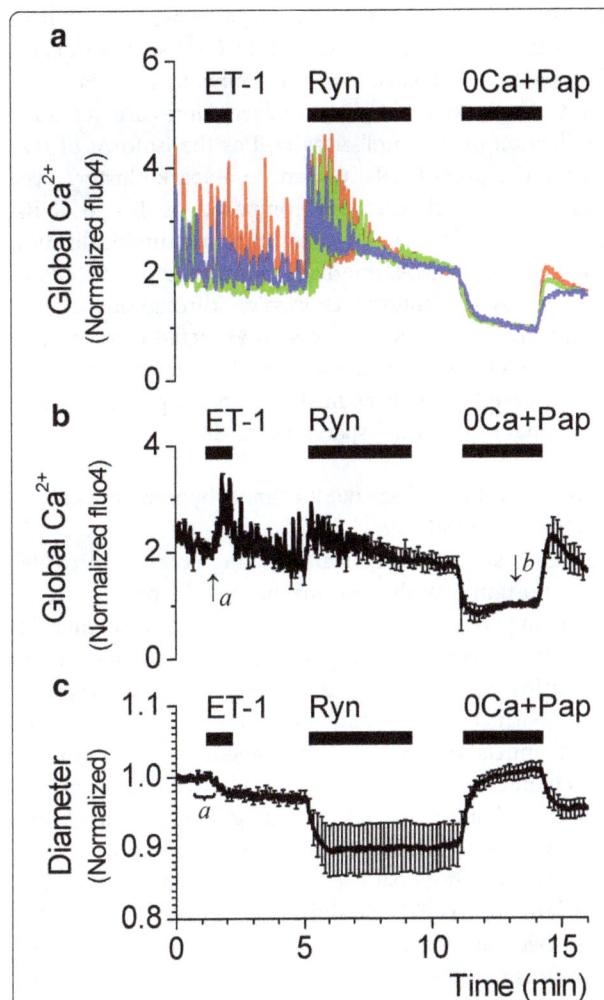

Fig. 7 Inhibition of Ca^{2+} sparks with ryanodine increases global Ca^{2+} and constricts SMA at 60 cmH_2O following an increase in Ca^{2+} sensitivity by endothelin-1. **a** Representative recordings of cytosolic Ca^{2+} changes from single smooth muscle cells from a SMA loaded with fluorescent dye fluo4 and pressurized to 60 $cmH2O$ in response to 10 μM ryanodine after treatment with 1 nM endothelin-1 (ET-1). **b** Average of normalized traces of cytosolic Ca^{2+} changes at 60 cmH_2O (64 cells from 7 arteries). Traces in **a** and **b** were normalized as described in Methods. **c** Average trace of corresponding changes in vascular diameter of SMA pressurized at 60 cmH_2O (15 arteries). Diameter changes were normalized to the average of values recorded between 30–60 s (value indicated by 'a' was set to 1). Ca^{2+} and diameter data were simultaneously acquired at 1 s intervals, however, for clarity, error bars (sem) are plotted only every 10 s

Ca^{2+} sparks

Ca^{2+} sparks in the pressurized SMA occurred with a lower frequency than in unpressurized SMA [22], but with a similar frequency, spatial width and spark site density as observed in smooth muscle cells of cerebral pial arteries [15, 19, 28] and pressurized mesenteric arteries [21, 29]. The increase in Ca^{2+} spark frequency in response to a 20 cmH_2O (~ 14 mmHg) increase in pressure, is also consistent with observations made in cerebral arteries [28]. However, as in unpressurized SMA, the time of half decay of Ca^{2+} sparks was far shorter (~17–19 ms) than that observed for Ca^{2+} sparks in cerebral arteries, but closer to that found in rat heart [16, 30]. Ca^{2+} spark amplitudes and decay times are generally a reflection of the number as well as the isoform of ryanodine receptors (RyRs) present in a spark cluster. Typically, Ca^{2+} spark sites are composed of 4 – 6 RyRs, giving a punctate staining pattern in immunolocalization studies. In the SMA, the distribution pattern of RyRs in SMCs shows a uniform expression throughout the SR rather than a punctate expression expected of ryanodine receptors clustered in spark sites [22] and may underlie the observed differences in the temporal properties and functional role of Ca^{2+} sparks in the SMA.

Absence of the Ca^{2+} spark/BK channel hyperpolarizing mechanism in the SMA

The Ca^{2+} spark/BK channel signaling complex provides an important vasodilatory mechanism in preventing or mitigating pressure- or agonist-induced vasoconstrictions in arteries. This negative feedback mechanism in regulating vascular tone is evident from observations that pharmacological inhibition of Ca^{2+} sparks and/or BK channels or SMC-specific genetic manipulation of BK channel or RyR expression leads to the loss of this hyperpolarizing signal leading to membrane depolarization, increased VDCC activation, increase in Ca^{2+} influx and global Ca^{2+} and enhanced vasoconstriction [18, 20, 31–33]. However, Ca^{2+} sparks have not always been linked to a hyperpolarizing or vasodilatory mechanism. Other studies have observed excitatory roles for Ca^{2+} sparks and RyR-mediated Ca^{2+} release in small diameter arterioles. Kur et al. [24] reported that, contrary to the conventional hyperpolarizing mechanism, Ca^{2+} sparks in retinal arterioles combined to form Ca^{2+} waves and enhanced the myogenic tone. Westcott et al. [34] reported SMCs of murine cremaster muscle feed arterioles to express diffused staining of RyRs without manifesting Ca^{2+} sparks and no coupling with BK channels, while SMCs of upstream feed arteries exhibited clustered staining of RyRs, robust Ca^{2+} sparks and spatial and functional coupling to BK channels, indicating heterogeneity of RyR function within the same vascular tree. In the SMA, the effects of ryanodine on global Ca^{2+} and vascular diameter at 40 cmH_2O seemed to suggest, at first, a vasodilatory mechanism for Ca^{2+} sparks acting via BK channels. However, the failure of tetracaine, an RyR inhibitor, which inhibits Ca^{2+} sparks without depleting the SR, and iberiotoxin, a BK channel inhibitor, to produce similar effects on global Ca^{2+} and diameter as ryanodine (Figs. 2 and 3) combined with the non-effect of BK channel inhibition following membrane depolarization by external application of high K^+ (Fig. 4) or increase in pressure (Fig. 5) disproves the regulation of vascular tone of the SMA by the Ca^{2+} spark/BK channel mechanism.

Regulation of vascular tone by Ca^{2+} sensitivity

Changes in SMC global Ca^{2+} have generally been accepted as the central mechanism regulating SMC contractility in the development of pressure-dependent myogenic tone [35]. More recently, the contribution of Ca^{2+}-independent processes that regulate the Ca^{2+} sensitivity of the myofilament in the development of myogenic tone have been better described [36]. In cerebral and skeletal resistance arteries, increases in intravascular pressure are associated with increases in the Ca^{2+} sensitivity achieved by balancing the relative activities of myosin light chain kinase and myosin light chain phosphatase in a PKC and rho-kinase-dependent manner. Such changes in Ca^{2+} sensitivity further augment the Ca^{2+}-dependent myogenic vasoconstrictions [36–40]. We have previously shown that myogenic tone in the male, but not female, gerbil SMA is regulated not by changes in the SMC global Ca^{2+} but by rho-kinase-mediated changes in the Ca^{2+} sensitivity of contraction, which was revealed under inhibition of NO-mediated signaling [23]. The present study shows that the regulation of vascular tone in the female gerbil SMA is also determined by the Ca^{2+} sensitivity of the myofilament, with the crucial difference that increase in intravascular pressure significantly lowered the Ca^{2+} sensitivity (Fig. 7). This finding is consistent with the development of small myogenic tones with increasing intravascular pressures in the SMA [12]. Rho-kinase-dependent regulation of Ca^{2+} sensitivity also plays a significant role in mediating the vascular effects of endogenous vasoconstrictors and agonists [41–43]. Further studies are required to elucidate the mechanisms underlying the relationship between pressure and Ca^{2+} sensitivity in the SMA.

Conclusions

In conclusion, in this study, we have shown in the gerbil spiral modiolar artery that Ca^{2+} sparks, while present, do not regulate vascular tone and global Ca^{2+} by activating BK channels. Instead, ryanodine-receptor mediated increases in global Ca^{2+} and vasoconstriction depend on the Ca^{2+} sensitivity of SMC contraction, which is enhanced at lower pressures or by regulating rho-kinase activity.

It remains to be seen whether such mechanisms of vascular tone regulation as described in this study are applicable to spiral modiolar arteries in general or particularly unique to the gerbil spiral modiolar artery. Gerbils are commonly favored over other rodents such as mice and rats as hearing models for investigations into the causes for age-related hearing loss involving pathological changes in both peripheral and central auditory

Ryanodine-induced vasoconstriction of the gerbil spiral modiolar artery depends on the Ca2+ sensitivity...

237

system components. Gerbils are uniquely suited for such investigations as they exhibit sensitive hearing in the low frequency ranges (below 4 kHz) that are relevant for human auditory perception, compared to the much higher thresholds in mice and rats for the same frequency range [44]. Thus, the differences observed in the regulation of the gerbil SMA by Ca^{2+} sparks and BK channels compared to the observations made in arteries from other extensively studied rodent species become relevant in the choice of appropriate models for future interpretation of hearing studies and pharmacological interventions.

Funding
This study was supported by NIH-R01-DC04280 to PW and by Fortüne 2339-0-0 (University of Tuebingen, Tuebingen, Germany) to KR. The Confocal Microscopy Core facility was supported by the College of Veterinary Medicine at Kansas State University and by NIH-P20-RR017686.

Authors' contributions
GK and PW conceived and designed the study. GK collected and analyzed the data. KR collected and analyzed the data for Ca^{2+} sparks in ryanodine and Ca^{2+} sensitivity at different pressures. PW wrote the software code for data analysis. GK, KR and PW wrote the manuscript. All authors have read and agreed to the final version of the manuscript.

Competing interests
The authors declare that they have no competing interests.

Author details
[1]Anatomy & Physiology Department, Cell Physiology Laboratory, Kansas State University, 228 Coles Hall, Manhattan, Kansas 66506-5802, USA. [2]Department of Otolaryngology–Head and Neck Surgery, Tübingen Hearing Research Centre, and Molecular Physiology of Hearing, University of Tübingen, Tübingen, Germany.

References
1. Wangemann P. Supporting sensory transduction: cochlear fluid homeostasis and the endocochlear potential. J Physiol. 2006;576(Pt 1):11–21.
2. Wing KG, Harris JD, Stover A, Brouillette JH. Effects of changes in arterial oxygen and carbon dioxide upon cochlear microphonics. J Comp Physiol Psychol. 1953;46(5):352–7.
3. Heigl F, Hettich R, Suckfuell M, Luebbers CW, Osterkorn D, Osterkorn K, Canis M. Fibrinogen/LDL apheresis as successful second-line treatment of sudden hearing loss: a retrospective study on 217 patients. Atheroscler Suppl. 2009;10(5):95–101.
4. Nakashima T, Naganawa S, Sone M, Tominaga M, Hayashi H, Yamamoto H, Liu X, Nuttall AL. Disorders of cochlear blood flow. Brain Res Brain Res Rev. 2003;43(1):17–28.
5. Nishimura T, Nario K, Hosoi H. Effects of intravenous administration of prostaglandin E_1 and lipo-prostaglandin E_1 on cochlear blood flow in guinea pigs. Eur Arch Otorhinolaryngol. 2002;259(5):253–6.
6. Scherer EQ, Yang J, Canis M, Reimann K, Ivanov K, Diehl CD, Backx PH, Wier WG, Strieth S, Wangemann P, Voigtlaender-Bolz J, Lidington D, Bolz SS. Tumor necrosis factor-alpha enhances microvascular tone and reduces blood flow in the cochlea via enhanced sphingosine-1-phosphate signaling. Stroke. 2010;41(11):2618–24.
7. Arpornchayanon W, Canis M, Ihler F, Settevendemie C, Strieth S. TNF-alpha inhibition using etanercept prevents noise-induced hearing loss by improvement of cochlear blood flow in vivo. Int J Audiol. 2013;52(8):545–52.
8. Ihler F, Bertlich M, Sharaf K, Strieth S, Strupp M, Canis M. Betahistine exerts a dose-dependent effect on cochlear stria vascularis blood flow in guinea pigs in vivo. PLoS One. 2012;7(6):e39086.
9. Gruber DD, Dang H, Shimozono M, Scofield MA, Wangemann P. Alpha1A-adrenergic receptors mediate vasoconstriction of the isolated spiral modiolar artery in vitro. Hear Res. 1998;119(1–2):113–24.
10. Wangemann P, Gruber DD. The isolated in vitro perfused spiral modiolar artery: pressure dependence of vasoconstriction. Hear Res. 1998;115(1–2):113–8.
11. Wangemann P, Cohn ES, Gruber DD, Gratton MA. Ca^{2+}-dependence and nifedipine-sensitivity of vascular tone and contractility in the isolated superfused spiral modiolar artery in vitro. Hear Res. 1998;118(1-2):90–100.
12. Reimann K, Krishnamoorthy G, Wier WG, Wangemann P. Gender differences in myogenic regulation along the vascular tree of the gerbil cochlea. PLoS One. 2011;6(9):e25659.
13. Wu T, Dai M, Shi XR, Jiang ZG, Nuttall AL. Functional expression of P2X4 receptor in capillary endothelial cells of the cochlear spiral ligament and its role in regulating the capillary diameter. Am J Physiol Heart Circ Physiol. 2011;301(1):H69–78.
14. Dai M, Yang Y, Shi X. Lactate dilates cochlear capillaries via type V fibrocyte-vessel coupling signaled by nNOS. Am J Physiol Heart Circ Physiol. 2011; 301(4):H1248–54.
15. Nelson MT, Cheng H, Rubart M, Santana LF, Bonev AD, Knot HJ, Lederer WJ. Relaxation of arterial smooth muscle by calcium sparks. Science. 1995; 270(5236):633–7.
16. Cheng H, Lederer WJ. Calcium sparks. Physiol Rev. 2008;88(4):1491–545.
17. Jaggar JH, Wellman GC, Heppner TJ, Porter VA, Perez GJ, Gollasch M, Kleppisch T, Rubart M, Stevenson AS, Lederer WJ, et al. Ca^{2+} channels, ryanodine receptors and Ca^{2+}-activated K^+ channels: a functional unit for regulating arterial tone. Acta Physiol Scand. 1998;164(4):577–87.
18. Knot HJ, Standen NB, Nelson MT. Ryanodine receptors regulate arterial diameter and wall $[Ca^{2+}]$ in cerebral arteries of rat via Ca^{2+}-dependent K^+ channels. J Physiol. 1998;508(Pt 1):211–21.
19. Perez GJ, Bonev AD, Patlak JB, Nelson MT. Functional coupling of ryanodine receptors to KCa channels in smooth muscle cells from rat cerebral arteries. J Gen Physiol. 1999;113(2):229–38.
20. Nelson MT, Quayle JM. Physiological roles and properties of potassium channels in arterial smooth muscle. Am J Physiol. 1995;268(4 Pt 1):C799–822.
21. Krishnamoorthy G, Sonkusare SK, Heppner TJ, Nelson MT. Opposing roles of smooth muscle BK channels and ryanodine receptors in the regulation of nerve-evoked constriction of mesenteric resistance arteries. Am J Physiol Heart Circ Physiol. 2014;306(7):H981–8.
22. Krishnamoorthy G, Regehr K, Berge S, Scherer EQ, Wangemann P. Calcium sparks in the intact gerbil spiral modiolar artery. BMC Physiol. 2011;11:15.
23. Reimann K, Krishnamoorthy G, Wangemann P. NOS inhibition enhances myogenic tone by increasing rho-kinase mediated Ca^{2+} sensitivity in the male but not the female gerbil spiral modiolar artery. PLoS One. 2013;8(1): e53655.
24. Kur J, Bankhead P, Scholfield CN, Curtis TM, McGeown JG. Ca^{2+} sparks promote myogenic tone in retinal arterioles. Br J Pharmacol. 2013;168(7): 1675–86.
25. Cui J, Yang H, Lee US. Molecular mechanisms of BK channel activation. Cell Mol Life Sci. 2009;66(5):852–75.
26. Buck E, Zimanyi I, Abramson JJ, Pessah IN. Ryanodine stabilizes multiple conformational states of the skeletal muscle calcium release channel. J Biol Chem. 1992;267(33):23560–7.
27. Scherer EQ, Wangemann P. ET_A receptors in the gerbil spiral modiolar artery. Adv Otorhinolaryngol. 2002;59:58–65.
28. Jaggar JH. Intravascular pressure regulates local and global Ca^{2+} signaling in cerebral artery smooth muscle cells. Am J Physiol Cell Physiol. 2001;281(2): C439–48.
29. Miriel VA, Mauban JR, Blaustein MP, Wier WG. Local and cellular Ca^{2+} transients in smooth muscle of pressurized rat resistance arteries during myogenic and agonist stimulation. J Physiol. 1999;518(Pt 3):815–24.
30. Lukyanenko V, Gyorke S. Ca^{2+} sparks and Ca^{2+} waves in saponin-permeabilized rat ventricular myocytes. J Physiol. 1999;521(Pt 3):575–85.

31. Brenner R, Perez GJ, Bonev AD, Eckman DM, Kosek JC, Wiler SW, Patterson AJ, Nelson MT, Aldrich RW. Vasoregulation by the beta1 subunit of the calcium-activated potassium channel. Nature. 2000;407(6806):870–6.

32. Evanson KW, Bannister JP, Leo MD, Jaggar JH. LRRC26 is a functional BK channel auxiliary gamma subunit in arterial smooth muscle cells. Circ Res. 2014;115(4):423–31.

33. Lohn M, Jessner W, Furstenau M, Wellner M, Sorrentino V, Haller H, Luft FC, Gollasch M. Regulation of calcium sparks and spontaneous transient outward currents by RyR3 in arterial vascular smooth muscle cells. Circ Res. 2001;89(11):1051–7.

34. Westcott EB, Goodwin EL, Segal SS, Jackson WF. Function and expression of ryanodine receptors and inositol 1,4,5-trisphosphate receptors in smooth muscle cells of murine feed arteries and arterioles. J Physiol. 2012;590(8): 1849–69.

35. Davis MJ, Hill MA. Signaling mechanisms underlying the vascular myogenic response. Physiol Rev. 1999;79(2):387–423.

36. Schubert R, Lidington D, Bolz SS. The emerging role of Ca^{2+} sensitivity regulation in promoting myogenic vasoconstriction. Cardiovasc Res. 2008; 77(1):8–18.

37. Johnson RP, El-Yazbi AF, Takeya K, Walsh EJ, Walsh MP, Cole WC. Ca^{2+} sensitization via phosphorylation of myosin phosphatase targeting subunit at threonine-855 by Rho kinase contributes to the arterial myogenic response. J Physiol. 2009;587(Pt 11):2537–53.

38. Moreno-Dominguez A, Colinas O, El-Yazbi A, Walsh EJ, Hill MA, Walsh MP, Cole WC. Ca^{2+} sensitization due to myosin light chain phosphatase inhibition and cytoskeletal reorganization in the myogenic response of skeletal muscle resistance arteries. J Physiol. 2013;591(5):1235–50.

39. Sward K, Mita M, Wilson DP, Deng JT, Susnjar M, Walsh MP. The role of RhoA and Rho-associated kinase in vascular smooth muscle contraction. Curr Hypertens Rep. 2003;5(1):66–72.

40. Lagaud G, Gaudreault N, Moore ED, Van Breemen C, Laher I. Pressure-dependent myogenic constriction of cerebral arteries occurs independently of voltage-dependent activation. Am J Physiol Heart Circ Physiol. 2002; 283(6):H2187–95.

41. Ito K, Shimomura E, Iwanaga T, Shiraishi M, Shindo K, Nakamura J, Nagumo H, Seto M, Sasaki Y, Takuwa Y. Essential role of rho kinase in the Ca^{2+} sensitization of prostaglandin $F_{2\alpha}$-induced contraction of rabbit aortae. J Physiol. 2003;546(Pt 3):823–36.

42. Baek I, Jeon SB, Kim J, Seok YM, Song MJ, Chae SC, Jun JE, Park WH, Kim IK. A role for Rho-kinase in Ca-independent contractions induced by phorbol-12,13-dibutyrate. Clin Exp Pharmacol Physiol. 2009;36(3):256–61.

43. El-Yazbi AF, Johnson RP, Walsh EJ, Takeya K, Walsh MP, Cole WC. Pressure-dependent contribution of Rho kinase-mediated calcium sensitization in serotonin-evoked vasoconstriction of rat cerebral arteries. J Physiol. 2010; 588(Pt 10):1747–62.

44. Gleich O, Strutz J. The Mongolian gerbil as a model for the analysis of peripheral and central age-dependent hearing loss. In: Naz S, editor. Hearing loss. Rijeka, Croatia: InTech. 2012. doi:10.5772/33569.

Permissions

The contributors of this book come from diverse backgrounds, making this book a truly international effort. This book will bring forth new frontiers with its revolutionizing research information and detailed analysis of the nascent developments around the world.

We would like to thank all the contributing authors for lending their expertise to make the book truly unique. They have played a crucial role in the development of this book. Without their invaluable contributions this book wouldn't have been possible. They have made vital efforts to compile up to date information on the varied aspects of this subject to make this book a valuable addition to the collection of many professionals and students.

This book was conceptualized with the vision of imparting up-to-date information and advanced data in this field. To ensure the same, a matchless editorial board was set up. Every individual on the board went through rigorous rounds of assessment to prove their worth. After which they invested a large part of their time researching and compiling the most relevant data for our readers.

The editorial board has been involved in producing this book since its inception. They have spent rigorous hours researching and exploring the diverse topics which have resulted in the successful publishing of this book. They have passed on their knowledge of decades through this book. To expedite this challenging task, the publisher supported the team at every step. A small team of assistant editors was also appointed to further simplify the editing procedure and attain best results for the readers.

Apart from the editorial board, the designing team has also invested a significant amount of their time in understanding the subject and creating the most relevant covers. They scrutinized every image to scout for the most suitable representation of the subject and create an appropriate cover for the book.

The publishing team has been an ardent support to the editorial, designing and production team. Their endless efforts to recruit the best for this project, has resulted in the accomplishment of this book. They are a veteran in the field of academics and their pool of knowledge is as vast as their experience in printing. Their expertise and guidance has proved useful at every step. Their uncompromising quality standards have made this book an exceptional effort. Their encouragement from time to time has been an inspiration for everyone.

The publisher and the editorial board hope that this book will prove to be a valuable piece of knowledge for researchers, students, practitioners and scholars across the globe.

Contributors

Jennifer A Sanders
Department of Pediatrics, Rhode Island Hospital and Brown University, Providence, RI 02903, USA

Philip A Gruppuso
Department of Pediatrics, Rhode Island Hospital and Brown University, Providence, RI 02903, USA
Department of Molecular Biology, Cell Biology and Biochemistry, Brown University, Providence, RI 02912, USA

Christoph Schorl and John M Sedivy
Department of Molecular Biology, Cell Biology and Biochemistry, Brown University, Providence, RI 02912, USA
Center for Genomics and Proteomics, Brown University, Providence, RI 02912, USA

Ajay Patel
Department of Pathology, MacNeal Hospital, Berwyn, IL, USA

Sebastian Benkhoff and Ralf P Brandes
Institute for Cardiovascular Physiology, Vascular Research Centre, Fachbereich Medizin, Goethe University, Frankfurt (Main), Germany

Rainer U Pliquett
Institute for Cardiovascular Physiology, Vascular Research Centre, Fachbereich Medizin, Goethe University, Frankfurt (Main), Germany
Department of Nephrology, Clinic of Internal Medicine 2, University Clinic Halle, Martin Luther University Halle-Wittenberg, Ernst-Grube-Str. 40, Halle (Saale) 06120, Germany

Oliver Jung
Institute for Cardiovascular Physiology, Vascular Research Centre, Fachbereich Medizin, Goethe University, Frankfurt (Main), Germany
Department of Nephrology, Goethe University, Frankfurt (Main), Germany

Lisa M Schwiebert
Departments of Cell Developmental and Integrative Biology, University of Alabama at Birmingham, 1918 University Blvd, Birmingham, AL 35294-0005, USA
Gregory Fleming James Cystic Fibrosis (CF) Research Center, University of Alabama at Birmingham, 1918 University Blvd, Birmingham 35294-0005AL, USA

Akos Zsembery
Departments of Cell Developmental and Integrative Biology, University of Alabama at Birmingham, 1918 University Blvd, Birmingham, AL 35294-0005, USA
Gregory Fleming James Cystic Fibrosis (CF) Research Center, University of Alabama at Birmingham, 1918 University Blvd, Birmingham 35294-0005AL, USA
Department of Experimental Human Physiology, Semmelweis University, Budapest, Hungary

Torry A Tucker
Departments of Cell Developmental and Integrative Biology, University of Alabama at Birmingham, 1918 University Blvd, Birmingham, AL 35294-0005, USA
Gregory Fleming James Cystic Fibrosis (CF) Research Center, University of Alabama at Birmingham, 1918 University Blvd, Birmingham 35294-0005AL, USA
Department of Biochemistry, University of Texas Health Sciences Center at Tyler, Tyler, TX, USA

Erik M Schwiebert
Departments of Cell Developmental and Integrative Biology, University of Alabama at Birmingham, 1918 University Blvd, Birmingham, AL 35294-0005, USA
Gregory Fleming James Cystic Fibrosis (CF) Research Center, University of Alabama at Birmingham, 1918 University Blvd, Birmingham 35294-0005AL, USA
DiscoveryBioMed, Inc, Birmingham, AL, USA

James A Fortenberry
Gregory Fleming James Cystic Fibrosis (CF) Research Center, University of Alabama at Birmingham, 1918 University Blvd, Birmingham 35294-0005AL, USA

Philippe Cettour-Rose, Carole Bezençon, Christian Darimont and Sami Damak
Nestlé Research Center, Verschez-les-Blanc, Lausanne 1000, Switzerland

Johannes le Coutre
Nestlé Research Center, Verschez-les-Blanc, Lausanne 1000, Switzerland
Organization for Interdisciplinary Research Projects, The University of Tokyo, Tokyo, Japan

Sven Martin Jørgensen, Aleksei Krasnov, Jacob Torgersen and Gerrit Timmerhaus
Nofima AS, N-1431 Ås, Norway

Harald Takle
Nofima AS, N-1431 Ås, Norway
AVS Chile S.A., Casilla 300, Puerto Varas, Chile

Vicente Castro
AVS Chile S.A., Casilla 300, Puerto Varas, Chile

Ernst Morten Hevrøy
National Institute of Nutrition and Seafood Research (NIFES), N-5817 Bergen, Nordnes, Norway

Tom Johnny Hansen
Institute of Marine Research, Matre Research Station, N-5984 Matredal, Norway

Sissel Susort
Skretting Norway AS, Sentrum N-4002 Stavanger, Norway

Olav Breck
Marine Harvest Norway AS, Sandviksbodene 78, N-5035 Bergen, Norway

Kristin J Speaker and Monika Fleshner
Department of Integrative Physiology, University of Colorado at Boulder, 1725 Pleasant Street, Boulder Colorado 80309, USA

Wouter Eilers
Institute for Biomedical Research into Human Movement and Health, Manchester Metropolitan University, John Dalton Building, Oxford Road, M1 5GD Manchester, United Kingdom

Arnold de Haan
Institute for Biomedical Research into Human Movement and Health, Manchester Metropolitan University, John Dalton Building, Oxford Road, M1 5GD Manchester, United Kingdom
Laboratory for Myology, MOVE Research Institute Amsterdam, Faculty of Human Movement Sciences, VU University Amsterdam, Van der Boechorststraat 7, 1081 BT Amsterdam, The Netherlands

Martin Flck
Institute for Biomedical Research into Human Movement and Health, Manchester Metropolitan University, John Dalton Building, Oxford Road, M1 5GD Manchester, United Kingdom
Laboratory for Muscle Plasticity, Department of Orthopaedics, University of Zurich, Balgrist University Hospital, Forchstrasse 340, 8008 Zurich, Switzerland

Richard T Jaspers
Laboratory for Myology, MOVE Research Institute Amsterdam, Faculty of Human Movement Sciences, VU University Amsterdam, Van der Boechorststraat 7, 1081 BT Amsterdam, The Netherlands

Cline Ferri and Paola Valdivieso
Laboratory for Muscle Plasticity, Department of Orthopaedics, University of Zurich, Balgrist University Hospital, Forchstrasse 340, 8008 Zurich, Switzerland

Britt-Marie Iresjö and Kent Lundholm
Department of Surgery Sahlgrenska University Hospital Kir., Metabol lab Bruna Stråket 20-413 45, Gothenburg, Sweden

Johan Svensson and Claes Ohlsson
Department of InternalMedicine, Sahlgrenska Academy, University of Gothenburg, Gothenburg, Sweden

Barbara Serrano-Flores, Edith Garay, Francisco G Vázquez-Cuevas and Rogelio O Arellano
Departamento de Neurobiología Celular y Molecular, Instituto de Neurobiología, Universidad Nacional Autónoma de México, Boulevard Juriquilla 3001, Juriquilla Querétaro, Querétaro, C.P. 76230, Mexico

Richard Head
CSIRO Preventative Health Flagship, CSIRO, North Ryde, NSW 2113, Australia

Janet M Shaw, and Trevor Lockett
CSIRO Preventative Health Flagship, CSIRO, North Ryde, NSW 2113, Australia
CSIRO, Food and Nutritional Sciences, North Ryde, NSW 2113, Australia

Caroline A Kerr
CSIRO Preventative Health Flagship, CSIRO, North Ryde, NSW 2113, Australia
CSIRO, Food and Nutritional Sciences, North Ryde, NSW 2113, Australia

Graduate School of Medicine, University of Wollongong, Wollongong, NSW, Australia

Barney M Hines
CSIRO Preventative Health Flagship, CSIRO, North Ryde, NSW 2113, Australia
CSIRO Division of Livestock Industries, Queensland Biosciences Precinct, St Lucia, Queensland 4067, Australia

Robert Dunne and Lauren M Bragg
CSIRO Preventative Health Flagship, CSIRO, North Ryde, NSW 2113, Australia
CSIRO, Mathematical and Information Sciences, North Ryde, New South Wales 1670, Australia

Julie Clarke
CSIRO Preventative Health Flagship, CSIRO, North Ryde, NSW 2113, Australia
CSIRO Food and Nutritional Sciences, Adelaide 5000, South Australia

Konstantinos Petsanis, Athanasios Chatzisotiriou, Dorothea Kapoukranidou and Maria Albani
Department of Physiology, Faculty of Medicine, Aristotle University of Thessaloniki, Thessaloniki, Greece

Constantina Simeonidou
Department of Experimental Physiology, Faculty of Medicine, Aristotle University of Thessaloniki, Thessaloniki, Greece

Dimitrios Kouvelas
nd Department of Pharmacology, Faculty of Medicine, Aristotle University of Thessaloniki, Thessaloniki, Greece

Michelle L Verant and Jeffrey M Lorch
Department of Pathobiological Sciences, School of Veterinary Medicine, University of Wisconsin-Madison, 2015 Linden Dr., Madison, Wisconsin, USA

David S Blehert
US Geological Survey National Wildlife Health Center, 6006 Schroeder Rd., Madison, Wisconsin, USA

Carol U Meteyer
US Geological Survey National Wildlife Health Center, 6006 Schroeder Rd., Madison, Wisconsin, USA
US Geological Survey National Center, Environmental Health, 12201Sunrise Valley Dr., Reston, Virginia, USA

John R Speakman
Institute of Biological and Environmental Sciences, University of Aberdeen, Aberdeen, Scotland, UK

Paul M Cryan
US Geological Survey Fort Collins Science Center, 2150 Centre Ave. Building C, Fort Collins, Colorado, USA

Tohru Saeki, Kosuke Sato, Shiho Ito and Keisuke Ikeda
Laboratory of Molecular Nutrition, Kyoto Prefectural University, Nakaragi, Shimogamo, Sakyo-ku, Kyoto 606-8522, Japan

Ryuhei Kanamoto
Laboratory of Molecular Nutrition, Kyoto Prefectural University, Nakaragi, Shimogamo, Sakyo-ku, Kyoto 606-8522, Japan
Laboratory of Physiological Function of Food, Division of Food Science and Biotechnology, Graduate School of Agriculture, Kyoto University, Gokasho, Uji city, Kyoto Prefecture 611-0011, Japan

Paul Fransen, Dorien M Schrijvers, Wim Martinet and Guido R Y De Meyer
Laboratory of Physiopharmacology, University of Antwerp, Universiteitsplein 1 Building T, 2.18, Wilrijk B-2610, Belgium

Cor E Van Hove, Johanna van Langen and Hidde Bult
Laboratories of Pharmacology, University of Antwerp, Antwerp, Belgium

Anh Thuc Ngo, Mads Riemann and Niels-Henrik Holstein-Rathlou
Department of Biomedical Sciences, Faculty of Health and Medical Sciences,The Panum institute, University of Copenhagen, Blegdamsvej 3, DK-2200 Copenhagen N, Denmark

Christian Torp-Pedersen
Department of Cardiology, Gentofte Hospital, Copenhagen, Denmark

Lars Jørn Jensen
Department of Veterinary Clinical and Animal Sciences, Faculty of Health and Medical Sciences, University of Copenhagen, Copenhagen, Denmark

Bernardo A Petriz, David H Borges and Rosangela V de Andrade
Centro de Análises Proteômicas e Bioquímicas, Programa de Pós-Graduação em Ciências Genômicas e Biotecnologia, Universidade Católica de Brasília, Brasília-DF, Brazil

Rinaldo W Pereira
Centro de Análises Proteômicas e Bioquímicas, Programa de Pós-Graduação em Ciências Genômicas e Biotecnologia, Universidade Católica de Brasília, Brasília-DF, Brazil
Programa de Pós-Graduação em Educação Física, da Universidade de Brasília

Octávio L Franco
Centro de Análises Proteômicas e Bioquímicas, Programa de Pós-Graduação em Ciências Genômicas e Biotecnologia, Universidade Católica de Brasília, Brasília-DF, Brazil
Departamento de Biologia, Universidade Federal de Juiz de Fora, Juiz de Fora-MG, Brazil
Pos-graduação em patologia molecular, Universidade de Brasilia, Brasilia, DF, Brazil

Luiz A O Rocha
Centro de Análises Proteômicas e Bioquímicas, Programa de Pós-Graduação em Ciências Genômicas e Biotecnologia, Universidade Católica de Brasília, Brasília-DF, Brazil
Pos-graduação em patologia molecular, Universidade de Brasilia, Brasilia, DF, Brazil

Ricardo J Oliveira
Programa de Pós-Graduação em Educação Física, da Universidade de Brasília

Gilberto B Domont
Universidade Federal do Rio de Janeiro, Protemics Unit, Rio de Janeiro, Brazil

James F Schooley, Aryan M A Namboodiri, Rolf Bünger and Thomas P Flagg
Department of Anatomy, Physiology, and Genetics, Uniformed Services University for the Health Sciences, 4301 Jones Bridge Road, Rm. C-2114, Bethesda 20814, MD, USA

Rachel T Cox
Department of Biochemistry and Molecular Biology, Uniformed Services University for the Health Sciences, Bethesda 20814, MD, USA

Jessica A. Krizo, Linley E. Moreland, Ashutosh Rastogi and Eric M. Mintz
Department of Biological Sciences, Kent State University, Kent, OH 44242, USA

Xiang Mou
Department of Molecular and Cellular Biology, Baylor College of Medicine, Houston, TX 77030, USA

Rebecca A. Prosser
Department of Biochemistry and Cellular and Molecular Biology, University of Tennessee, Knoxville, TN 37996, USA

Gayathri Krishnamoorthy and Philine Wangemann
Anatomy and Physiology Department, Cell Physiology Laboratory, Kansas State University, 228 Coles Hall, Manhattan, Kansas 66506-5802, USA

Katrin Reimann
Anatomy and Physiology Department, Cell Physiology Laboratory, Kansas State University, 228 Coles Hall, Manhattan, Kansas 66506-5802, USA
Department of Otolaryngology–Head and Neck Surgery, Tübingen Hearing Research Centre, and Molecular Physiology of Hearing, University of Tübingen, Tübingen, Germany

Index